AMERICAN PSYCHIATRIC ASSOCIATION
Practice Guidelines for the Treatment of Psychiatric Disorders

COMPENDIUM
2000

D0939405

AMERICAN PSYCHIATRIC ASSOCIATION

Practice Guidelines for the Treatment of Psychiatric Disorders

COMPENDIUM
2000

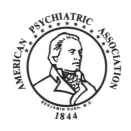

Published by the
American Psychiatric Association
Washington, D.C.

Manufactured in the United States of America on acid-free paper

04 03 02 01   5 4 3 2

American Psychiatric Association
1400 K Street, N.W.
Washington, DC 20005
www.psych.org

Library of Congress Cataloging-in-Publication Data
American Psychiatric Association.
     American Psychiatric Association practice guidelines for the treatment of psychiatric disorders : compendium 2000. — 1st ed.
          p. ; cm.
     Includes bibliographical references and index.
     ISBN 0-89042-312-1 (casebound : alk. paper) — ISBN 0-89042-315-6 (softbound : alk. paper)
     1. Mental illness—Diagnosis. 2. Mental illness—Diagnosis—Decision making. I. Title: Practice guidelines for the treatment of psychiatric disorders. II. Title.
     [DNLM: 1. Mental Disorders—therapy. 2. Mental Disorders—diagnosis. WM 400 A5131a 2000]
     RC469.A52 2000
     616.89—dc21

                                                                                    00-024850

British Library Cataloguing in Publication Data
A CIP record is available from the British Library.

Hardback ISBN 0-89042-312-1
Paperback ISBN 0-89042-315-6

AMERICAN PSYCHIATRIC ASSOCIATION
STEERING COMMITTEE ON PRACTICE GUIDELINES

JOHN S. MCINTYRE, M.D.
Chair

SARA C. CHARLES, M.D.
Vice-Chair

DEBORAH A. ZARIN, M.D.
Director, Office of Quality Improvement and Psychiatric Services

Kenneth Altshuler, M.D.
Ian Cook, M.D.
C. Deborah Cross, M.D.
Helen Egger, M.D.
Louis Alan Moench, M.D.
Allan Tasman, M.D.
Stuart Twemlow, M.D.
Sherwyn Woods, M.D.
Joel Yager, M.D.

CONSULTANTS AND LIAISONS

Thomas Bittker, M.D. (Liaison)
Paula Clayton, M.D. (Consultant)
Amarendra Das, M.D., Ph.D. (Liaison)
Laurie Flynn (Consultant)
Marcia Goin, M.D. (Liaison)
Marion Goldstein, M.D. (Consultant)
Sheila Hafter Gray, M.D. (Consultant)
Herbert Meltzer, M.D. (Consultant)
Grayson Norquist, M.D. (Consultant)

Roger Peele, M.D. (Consultant)
Susan Stabinsky, M.D. (Consultant)
Robert Johnston, M.D. (Area I)
James Nininger, M.D. (Area II)
John Urbaitis, M.D. (Area III)
Anthony D'Agostino, M.D. (Area IV)
Jennifer Berg, M.D. (Area V)
Lawrence Lurie, M.D. (Area VI)
R. Dale Walker, M.D. (Area VII)

STAFF

Rebecca M. Thaler, M.P.H., C.H.E.S.
Project Manager

Leslie Seigle Davis
Project Manager

Petrina B. Marcus
Project Coordinator

The Steering Committee on Practice Guidelines
expresses its appreciation to
Deborah A. Zarin, M.D.,
whose knowledge, talents, dedication, and constant attention
have been central to the development of the
practice guidelines included in this volume.
Dr. Zarin was director of the Practice Guideline Project
from 1992 to 1999.

▶ NOTE TO THE READER

Each practice guideline included in this book contains several sections. In addition to sections containing diagnostic, epidemiologic, and other background information, the guidelines each include two categories of sections that are likely to be of particular interest to most readers: detailed reviews of the safety and efficacy of available treatments, and sections that contain treatment recommendations for the "typical" patient as well as for patients with special clinical circumstances. The organization of these guidelines has evolved over time. To help the reader find the sections of particular interest, a "Note to the Reader" that outlines how that particular guideline is organized is included opposite the table of contents for each guideline.

CONTENTS

STATEMENT OF INTENT

The APA Practice Guidelines are not intended to be construed or to serve as a standard of medical care. Standards of medical care are determined on the basis of all clinical data available for an individual case and are subject to change as scientific knowledge and technology advance and patterns evolve. These parameters of practice should be considered guidelines only. Adherence to them will not ensure a successful outcome in every case, nor should they be construed as including all proper methods of care or excluding other acceptable methods of care aimed at the same results. The ultimate judgment regarding a particular clinical procedure or treatment plan must be made by the psychiatrist in light of the clinical data presented by the patient and the diagnostic and treatment options available.

These practice guidelines have been developed by psychiatrists who are in active clinical practice. In addition, some contributors are primarily involved in research or other academic endeavors. It is possible that through such activities some contributors have received income related to treatments discussed in this guideline. A number of mechanisms are in place to minimize the potential for producing biased recommendations due to conflicts of interest. The guideline has been extensively reviewed by members of APA as well as by representatives from related fields. Contributors and reviewers have all been asked to base their recommendations on an objective evaluation of the available evidence. Any contributor or reviewer who has a potential conflict of interest that may bias (or appear to bias) his or her work has been asked to notify the APA Office of Quality Improvement and Psychiatric Services. This potential bias is then discussed with the work group chair and the chair of the Steering Committee on Practice Guidelines. Further action depends on the assessment of the potential bias.

INTRODUCTION

John S. McIntyre, M.D.
Deborah A. Zarin, M.D.
Sara C. Charles, M.D.

This volume contains 10 practice guidelines developed by the American Psychiatric Association (APA). Each of these practice guidelines has been published in *The American Journal of Psychiatry* and also as an individual monograph. Two of the guidelines included (for major depressive disorder and eating disorders) are revisions of previously published APA practice guidelines. Following the practice guideline on evaluation of adults, the other practice guidelines are presented in the order in which the categories of disorder appear in DSM-IV.

The term *practice guideline* refers to a set of patient care strategies developed to assist physicians in clinical decision making. The APA is continually developing new and revised guidelines, which will be published as they are completed. Currently in development are practice guidelines for borderline personality disorder, HIV/AIDS, and geriatric issues.

Readers should note that these parameters of care are indeed "guidelines" and are not intended to be "standards of care." These guidelines do not necessarily include all proper methods of care for a particular disorder. The ultimate judgment concerning the selection and implementation of a specific plan of treatment must be made by the psychiatrist in light of the clinical data presented by the patient and the diagnostic and treatment options available. Further description of the intended role of the practice guidelines can be found in the Statement of Intent (p. xi).

Although the APA has published specific recommendations about the practice of psychiatry since 1851, the commitment of resources to the practice guideline development process over the past decade represents a qualitative change in the APA's role in establishing guidelines. Such a change raises many questions.

Why Is the APA Developing Practice Guidelines?

For nearly 150 years, the APA's fundamental aim in developing practice guidelines has been to assist psychiatrists in their clinical decision making, with the ultimate goal of improving the care of patients. The explosion of knowledge in our field over the last several decades amplifies the value of these guidelines. Furthermore, the current health care climate is characterized by concerns about quality of care, access to care, and cost. Efforts to respond to these problems by exerting external control over the types and amount of care that can be provided have led to new concerns about the quality of the data on which such efforts are based and the process by which the data are used to determine "appropriate" or "reimbursable" care. The realization that both treatment and reimbursement decisions are occurring without systematic scientific and clinical input has led the APA, along with many other medical specialty societies, to accelerate the process of documenting clearly and concisely what is known and what is not known about the treatment of patients. Although there are a number of other groups, including the federal and state governments, managed care organizations, and care delivery systems, that are also developing practice guidelines, the APA has decided that the psychiatric profession should take the lead in describing the best treatments and the range of appropriate treatments available to patients with mental illnesses.

How Are Practice Guidelines Developed?

The APA practice guidelines are developed under the direction of the Steering Committee on Practice Guidelines. The process is designed to ensure the development of reliable and valid guidelines and is consistent with the recommendations of the American Medical Association and the Institute of Medicine. It is characterized by rigorous scientific review of the available literature, widespread review of iterative drafts, and ultimate approval by the APA Assembly and Board of Trustees. The APA is committed to revising the guidelines at 5- to 10-year intervals. A revision may be accelerated if there is substantial new evidence suggesting a change in preferred treatment approaches. The development process is fully described in the Appendix (p. 699).

What Are the Potential Benefits of This Project?

Ultimately, the aim of practice guidelines is to improve patient care. Although some have argued that no guidelines should be promulgated until "all the data are in," this is not possible given the pressure of clinical and administrative decisions. Guidelines should help practicing psychiatrists determine what is known today about how best to help their patients. In addition, psychiatrists and those charged with the allocation of health care resources must try to make the best possible decisions on the basis of currently available data. Well-developed guidelines can help in these efforts.

Toward the end of helping patients, guidelines can have other beneficial effects. They are a vehicle for educating psychiatrists, other medical and mental health professionals, and the general public about appropriate and inappropriate treatments. By demonstrating that the quality of evidence for psychiatric treatments is on par with (and in many cases exceeds) that for other medical care, guidelines contribute to the credibility of the field. Guidelines identify those areas in which critical information is lacking and in which research could be expected to improve clinical decisions. Finally, guidelines can help those charged with overseeing the utilization and reimbursement of psychiatric services to develop more scientifically based and clinically sensitive criteria.

What Are the Possible Risks?

The APA reasons that the risks of this project are small and are considerably outweighed by the benefits. One risk is that the guidelines can be misinterpreted and misused by third parties in a way that will ultimately harm patients. Although this risk rightfully concerns many psychiatrists, it is the judgment of the Steering Committee, the Assembly, and the Board of Trustees that the existence of guidelines helps to clarify the sources of disagreement between treating psychiatrists and reviewers and their use can be a great improvement over the use of "secret" criteria or criteria developed through less objective procedures. In addition, many have expressed the concern that guidelines can "homogenize" the care of patients and detract from psychiatrists' freedom to shape treatment in ways that they feel best suit their individual patients. Inevitably, there is a tension in writing guidelines between the desire for specificity and the desire to allow for the consideration of individual clinical circumstances. These concerns must be balanced in such a way that allows psychiatrists to make appropriate clinical decisions. This very important issue is addressed in the Statement of Intent that begins each individually published guideline. Finally, there are concerns that the APA-approved guidelines may lead to an increase in malpractice claims. At this time, legal experts have mixed opinions about the impact of guidelines on the volume and severity of malpractice suits. However, in fact, some medical specialties that have been developing guidelines over the past two decades report that guidelines seem to have had the positive effect of fewer claims and, for at least one specialty, lower malpractice insurance premiums. Since the publication of APA's first practice guideline in 1993, the Steering Committee has been monitoring the potential impact of the guidelines on malpractice actions and has not noted any trends suggesting an increase in the number or severity of malpractice claims that might be attributed to the existence of APA-approved guidelines.

How Can We Improve the Current Process?

Since the inception of the APA project in 1989, the practice guideline development process has evolved significantly. Specifically, the activities of the work groups developing the guidelines have been made more explicit, and the nature of the reviewers' input has been standardized. Also, the format of each guideline has evolved over the past several years. In the two most recently developed guidelines (the revisions of the eating disorders and the major depressive disorder practice guidelines), the recommendations covering treatment, including the formulation of a treatment plan, are now presented before background information and the evidence that supports these recommendations. This change in format was based on input from psychiatrists and is designed to make the guidelines more "user-friendly."

However, certain principles remain crucial to further improvement. Clearly, practice guidelines should be based on objective data whenever possible. Such data are of two types: well-designed research studies and systematically identified clinical wisdom. Systematic reviews of the literature are an essential part of this work. However, efforts to synthesize studies in any given area are hampered by the uneven quantity and quality of research, by problems in generalizing from a literature largely derived from tertiary care research settings to more typical clinical practice, by the inherent difficulty in conducting controlled studies of some treatments for some populations, and by the difficulty in characterizing "clinical consensus." These issues are being partially addressed through the use of the APA's Practice Research Network (PRN). The PRN involves a panel of more than 800 psychiatrists in the full range of practice settings who cooperate to gather data and conduct clinical research. Practice research networks are also being used in other areas of medicine (e.g., family practice and pediatrics) to gather data from practice settings of relevance to the development of guidelines. For example, data about prevailing practice patterns and patient outcomes can be systematically gathered and incorporated into the guidelines. In addition, the impact of guidelines on psychiatric practice and patient outcomes can be assessed; ultimately, it should be possible to determine whether guidelines improve patient care. Currently, a major thrust of the APA project is to explore, devise, and test educational and dissemination strategies that will increase psychiatrists' use of the guidelines in daily practice.

Quick Reference Guides and Patient/Family Guides

In further attempts to increase the use and usefulness of the practice guidelines, the APA now publishes with each guideline a quick reference guide and a patient/family guide.

The quick reference guide is a summary and synopsis of the guideline's major recommendations and is presented in an algorithmic format. The quick reference guide is designed to assist psychiatrists in using the material presented in the full-text guideline.

The patient/family guide closely follows the information contained in the APA guideline and is designed to help patients and their families learn more about their illness and thus become more active and productive partners in their treatment.

Conclusions

The practice guidelines included in this volume represent an important step in the development of an "evidence-based psychiatry." The development of better research tools, the accumulation of new research data, the systematic identification of best clinical practice, and the iterative improvement of the process for developing practice guidelines will contribute to the continual development of better practice guidelines to aid psychiatrists in their clinical decision making.

PRACTICE GUIDELINE FOR THE
Psychiatric Evaluation of Adults

WORK GROUP ON PSYCHIATRIC EVALUATION OF ADULTS

Barry S. Fogel, M.D., Co-Chair
Ronald Shellow, M.D., Co-Chair

Renee Binder, M.D.
Jack Bonner III, M.D.
Leah Dickstein, M.D.
Gerald Flamm, M.D.
Marc Galanter, M.D.
Anthony Lehman, M.D.
Francis Lu, M.D.
Michael Popkin, M.D.
George Wilson, M.D.

▶ NOTE TO THE READER

This practice guideline is organized into five main sections: Purpose of Evaluation, Site of the Clinical Evaluation, Domains of the Clinical Evaluation, Evaluation Process, and Special Considerations that arise when conducting a psychiatric evaluation.

This practice guideline was approved in July 1995 and was published in *The American Journal of Psychiatry* in November 1995.

CONTENTS

SUMMARY

The following summary is intended to provide an overview of the organization and scope of recommendations in this practice guideline. The psychiatric evaluation of patients requires the consideration of many factors and cannot adequately be reviewed in a brief summary. The reader is encouraged to consult the relevant portions of the guideline when specific recommendations are sought. This summary is not intended to stand by itself.

This guideline focuses on the purpose, site, domains, and process of clinical psychiatric evaluations. General psychiatric evaluations, emergency evaluations, and clinical consultations, conducted in inpatient, outpatient, and other settings, are discussed. The domains of these evaluations include the reason for the evaluation, history of the present illness, past psychiatric history, general medical history, psychosocial/developmental history (personal history), social history, occupational history, family history, review of systems, physical examination, mental status examination, functional assessment, diagnostic tests, and information derived from the interview process.

Processes by which information is obtained and integrated to address the aims of the evaluation are described. Methods of obtaining information discussed include the patient interview; use of collateral sources; use of structured interviews, questionnaires, and rating scales; use of diagnostic, including psychological and neuropsychological, tests; use of the multidisciplinary team; examination under medication and/or restraint; and the physical examination. The process of assessment includes diagnosis and case formulation, formulation of the initial treatment plan, decisions regarding treatment-related legal and administrative issues, addressing of systems issues, and consideration for sociocultural diversity.

Other special considerations discussed include interactions with third-party payers, privacy and confidentiality, legal and administrative issues in institutions, and evaluation of elderly persons.

INTRODUCTION

Psychiatric evaluations vary according to their purpose. This guideline is intended primarily for general, emergency, and consultation evaluations for clinical purposes. It is applicable to evaluations conducted by a psychiatrist with adult patients, age 18 or older, although sections may be applicable to younger patients. Other psychiatric evaluations (including forensic, child custody, and disability evaluations) are not the focus of this guideline.

The guideline presumes familiarity with basic principles of psychiatric diagnosis and treatment planning as outlined in standard, contemporary psychiatric textbooks and taught in psychiatry residency training programs. It was developed following a review of contemporary references and emphasizes areas of consensus in the field.

While there is broad agreement that each element of the extensive general evaluation described in the guideline may be relevant or even crucial in a particular case, the specific emphasis of a given evaluation will vary according to its purpose and the problem presented by the patient. Consideration of the domains outlined in this guideline is part of a general psychiatric evaluation, but the content, process, and documentation must be determined by applying the professional skill and judgment of the psychiatrist. The performance of a particular set of clinical procedures does not assure the adequacy of a psychiatric evaluation, nor does their omission imply that the evaluation is deficient. The particular emphasis or modifications applied by the psychiatrist to the generic evaluation offered in this guideline should be consonant with the aims of the evaluation, the setting of practice, the patient's presenting problem, and the ever-evolving knowledge base concerning clinical assessment and clinical inference. It is important to emphasize that the scope and detail of clinically appropriate documentation also will vary with the patient, setting, clinical situation, and confidentiality issues. Because of the great variation in these factors, this guideline does not include recommendations regarding the content or frequency of documentation. These determinations must be based on the specific circumstances of the evaluation.

I. PURPOSE OF EVALUATION

The purpose and conduct of a psychiatric evaluation depend on who requests the evaluation, why it is requested, and the expected future role of the psychiatrist in the patient's care. Three types of clinical psychiatric evaluations are discussed: 1) general psychiatric evaluation, 2) emergency evaluation, and 3) clinical consultation. In addition, general principles to guide the conduct of evaluations for administrative or legal purposes are reviewed. At times there may be a conflict between the need to establish an effective working relationship with the patient and the need to efficiently obtain comprehensive information. To the extent that the psychiatrist expects to directly provide care to the patient, the establishment of an effective working relationship with the patient may take precedence over the comprehensiveness of the initial interview or interviews. In these instances, emphasis is placed on obtaining information needed for immediate clinical recommendations and decisions (1).

A. GENERAL PSYCHIATRIC EVALUATION

A general psychiatric evaluation has as its central component a face-to-face interview with the patient. The interview-based data are integrated with data that may be obtained through other components of the evaluation, such as a review of medical records, a physical examination, diagnostic tests, and history from collateral sources. A general evaluation usually takes more than 1 hour to complete, depending on the complexity of the problem and the patient's ability and willingness to work cooperatively with the psychiatrist. Several meetings with the patient may be necessary. Evaluations of lesser scope may be appropriate when the psychiatrist is called on to address a specific, limited diagnostic or therapeutic issue.

The aims of a general psychiatric evaluation are 1) to establish a psychiatric diagnosis, 2) to collect data sufficient to permit a case formulation, and 3) to develop an initial treatment plan, with particular consideration of any immediate interventions that may be needed to ensure the patient's safety, or, if the evaluation is a reassessment of a patient in long-term treatment, to revise the plan of treatment in accord with new perspectives gained from the evaluation.

B. EMERGENCY EVALUATION

The emergency psychiatric evaluation occurs in response to the occurrence of thoughts or feelings that are intolerable to the patient, or behavior that prompts urgent action by others, such as violent or self-injurious behavior, threats of harm to self or others, failure to care for oneself, deterioration of mental status, bizarre or confused behavior, or intense expressions of distress (2). The aims of the emergency evaluation include the following:

1. To establish a provisional diagnosis of the mental disorder most likely to be responsible for the current emergency, and to identify other diagnostic possibilities requiring further evaluation in the near term, including general medical conditions to be further assessed as potential causes of or contributors to the patient's mental condition.

2. To identify social, environmental, and cultural factors relevant to immediate treatment decisions.
3. To determine the patient's ability and willingness to cooperate with further assessment and treatment, what precautions are needed if there is a substantial risk of harm to self or others, and whether involuntary treatment is necessary.
4. To develop a plan for immediate treatment and disposition, with determination of whether the patient requires treatment in a hospital or other supervised setting and what follow-up will be required if the patient is not hospitalized.

The emergency evaluation varies greatly in length and may on occasion exceed several hours. Patients who will be discharged to the community after emergency evaluation may require more extensive evaluation in the emergency setting than those who will be hospitalized.

Patients presenting for emergency psychiatric evaluation have a high prevalence of combined general medical and psychiatric illness, recent trauma, substance use and substance-related conditions, and cognitive impairment disorders. These diagnostic possibilities deserve careful consideration. General medical and psychiatric evaluations should be coordinated so that additional medical evaluation can be requested or initiated by the psychiatrist on the basis of diagnostic or therapeutic considerations arising from the psychiatric history and interview. In many emergency settings, patients initially are examined by a nonpsychiatric physician to exclude acute general medical problems. Such examinations usually are limited in scope and rarely are definitive. Therefore, the psychiatrist may need to request or initiate further general medical evaluation to address diagnostic concerns that emerge from the psychiatric evaluation (3, 4).

▶ C. CLINICAL CONSULTATION

Clinical consultations are evaluations requested by other physicians or health care professionals, patients, families, or others for the purpose of assisting in the diagnosis, treatment, or management of a patient with a suspected mental disorder or behavioral problem. These evaluations may be comprehensive or may be focused on a relatively narrow question, such as the preferred medication for treatment of a known mental disorder in a patient with a particular general medical condition. Psychiatric evaluations for consultative purposes use the same data sources as general evaluations. Consideration is given to information from the referring source on the specific problem leading to the consultation, the referring source's aims for the consultation, information that the psychiatrist may be able to obtain regarding the patient's relationship with the primary clinician, and the resources and constraints of those currently treating the patient. Also, in the case of a consultation regarding a mental or behavioral problem in a patient with a general medical illness, information about that illness, its treatment, and its prognosis is relevant. The patient should be informed that the purpose of the consultation is to advise the party who requested it.

The aim of the consultative psychiatric evaluation is to provide clear and specific answers to the questions posed by the party requesting the consultation (5, 6). These include 1) a psychiatric diagnosis when relevant to the question posed to the consultant; 2) treatment advice, when requested, at a level of specificity appropriate to the needs of the treating clinician; and 3) recommendation for a change in treatment (e.g., in site of treatment) when the consultant finds a major diagnostic or therapeutic issue not raised by the requester but of concern to the patient or of likely relevance to treatment outcome.

The evaluation should respect the patient's relationship with the primary clinician and should encourage positive resolution of conflicts between the patient and the primary clinician if these emerge as an issue.

▶ D. OTHER CONSULTATIONS

Other psychiatric consultations are directed toward the resolution of specific legal, administrative, or other nonclinical questions. While the details of these evaluations, such as forensic evaluations, child custody evaluations, and disability evaluations, are beyond the scope of this guideline, several general principles apply. First, the evaluee usually is not the psychiatrist's patient and there are limits to confidentiality implicit in the aims of the evaluation; accordingly, the aims of the evaluation and the scope of disclosure should be addressed with the evaluee at the start of the interview (7, 8). Second, questions about the evaluee's legal status and legal representation should be resolved before the assessment begins, if possible. Third, many such consultations rely heavily, or even entirely, on documentary evidence or data from collateral sources. The quality and potential biases of such data should be taken into account.

The aims of these psychiatric consultations are 1) to answer the requester's question to the extent possible with the data obtainable and 2) to make a psychiatric diagnosis if it is relevant to the question.

II. SITE OF THE CLINICAL EVALUATION

▶ A. INPATIENT SETTINGS

The scope, pace, and depth of inpatient evaluation depend on the patient population served by the inpatient service, the goals of the hospitalization, and the role of the inpatient unit within the overall system of mental health services available to the patient (9). For example, a general hospital psychiatric unit specializing in patients with combined medical and psychiatric illness will necessarily do a relatively rapid general medical evaluation of all admitted patients (10). The evaluation of stable chronic general medical conditions in a long-stay setting for the chronically mentally ill might proceed at a slower pace than in a psychiatric-medical specialty unit in a general hospital.

When a patient is admitted by someone other than the treating psychiatrist, the reason for continued hospitalization should be promptly reviewed. The necessity for hospitalization should be carefully assessed, and alternative treatment settings should be considered.

From the outset, inpatient evaluations should include consideration of discharge planning (9). If the posthospitalization disposition is not apparent, the evaluation should identify both patient factors and community resources that would be relevant to a viable dispositional plan and should identify the problems that could impede a suitable disposition. If the patient was referred to the hospital by another clinician, the inpatient evaluation should be viewed in part as a consultation to the referring source (9). Special attention is given to unresolved diagnostic issues requiring data collection in an inpatient setting.

B. OUTPATIENT SETTINGS

Evaluation in the outpatient setting usually differs in intensity from inpatient evaluation, because of less frequent interviews, less involvement of other professionals, and less immediate availability of laboratory services and consultants from other medical specialties. Also, the psychiatrist in the outpatient setting has substantially less opportunity to directly observe the patient's behavior and to implement protective interventions when necessary. For this reason, during the period of evaluation the outpatient evaluator should continually reassess whether the patient requires hospitalization and whether unresolved questions about the patient's general medical status require more rapid assessment. A decision to change the setting for continued evaluation should be based on the patient's current mental status and behavior.

Advantages of the outpatient setting include economy, greater patient autonomy, and the potential for a longer longitudinal perspective on the patient's symptoms. However, the lack of continuous direct observation of behavior limits the obtainable data on how the patient's behavior appears to others. The involvement of family or significant others as collateral sources in the evaluation process deserves consideration. When substance use is suspected, data from collateral observers, drug screens, and/or determination of blood alcohol levels may be especially important.

C. GENERAL MEDICAL SETTINGS

Evaluations on general medical (i.e., nonpsychiatric) inpatient units allow for some direct behavioral observation by staff and for some safeguards against self-injurious or other violent behavior by patients. However, the level of behavioral observation and potential intervention against risky behavior tends to be less than on psychiatric inpatient units.

Psychiatric interviews on general medical-surgical units often are compromised by interruptions and lack of privacy. These problems sometimes can be mitigated by careful scheduling of interviews and using a space on the unit where the patient and the psychiatrist can meet privately.

Documentation of psychiatric evaluations in general medical charts should be sensitive to the standards of confidentiality of the nonpsychiatric medical sector and the possibility that charts may be read by persons who are not well informed about psychiatric issues. Information written in general medical charts should be confined to that necessary for the general medical team and should be expressed with a minimum of technical terms.

D. OTHER SETTINGS

Evaluations conducted in other settings, such as partial hospital settings, residential treatment facilities, home care services, nursing homes, long-term care facilities, schools, and prisons, are affected by a number of factors: 1) the level of behavioral observations available and the quality of those observations, 2) the availability of privacy for conducting interviews, 3) the availability of general medical evaluations and diagnostic tests, 4) the capacity to conduct the evaluation safely, and 5) the likelihood that information written in facility records will be understood and kept confidential.

In light of these factors, it is necessary to consider whether a particular setting permits an evaluation of adequate speed, safety, accuracy, and confidentiality to meet the needs of the patient.

III. DOMAINS OF THE CLINICAL EVALUATION

General psychiatric evaluations involve a systematic consideration of the broad domains described in this guideline, and they vary in scope and intensity. The intensity with which each domain is assessed depends on the purpose of the evaluation and the clinical situation. An evaluation of lesser scope may be appropriate when its purpose is to answer a circumscribed question. Such an evaluation may involve a particularly intense assessment of one or more domains especially relevant to the reason for the evaluation.

▶ A. REASON FOR THE EVALUATION

The purpose of the evaluation influences the focus of the examination and the form of documentation. The reason for the evaluation usually includes (but may not be limited to) the chief complaint of the patient, elicited in sufficient detail to permit an understanding of the patient's specific goals for the evaluation. If the symptoms are of long standing, the reason for seeking treatment at this specific time is relevant; if the evaluation was occasioned by a hospitalization, the reason for the hospitalization is also relevant.

▶ B. HISTORY OF THE PRESENT ILLNESS

The history of the present illness is a chronologically organized history of current symptoms or syndromes, recent exacerbations or remissions, available details of previous treatments, and the patient's response to those treatments. In consideration of the information obtained, the patient's current mental state may be relevant. If the patient was or is in treatment with another clinician, the effects of that relationship on the current illness, including transference and countertransference issues, are considered. Factors that the patient believes to be precipitating, aggravating, or otherwise modifying the illness are also pertinent.

▶ C. PAST PSYCHIATRIC HISTORY

The past psychiatric history includes a chronological summary of all past episodes of mental illness and treatment, including psychiatric syndromes not formally diagnosed at the time, previously established diagnoses, treatments offered, and responses to treatment. The dose, duration of treatment, efficacy, side effects, and patient's adherence to previously prescribed medications are part of the past psychiatric history. Past medical records frequently contain relevant data.

The chronological summary also includes episodes when the patient was functionally impaired or seriously distressed by mental or behavioral symptoms, even if no formal treatment occurred. Such episodes frequently can be identified by asking the patient about the past use of psychotropic drugs prescribed by a nonpsychiatric physician, prior suicide attempts or other self-destructive behavior, and otherwise unexplained episodes of social or occupational disability.

▶ D. GENERAL MEDICAL HISTORY

The general medical history includes available information on known general medical illnesses (e.g., hospitalizations, procedures, treatments, and medications) and undiagnosed health problems that have caused the patient major distress or functional impairment. This includes history of any episodes of important physical injury or trauma; sexual and reproductive history; and any history of neurologic disorders, allergies, drug sensitivities, and conditions causing pain and discomfort. Of particular importance is a specific history regarding diseases, and symptoms of diseases, that have a high prevalence among individuals with the patient's demographic characteristics and background, e.g., infectious diseases in users of intravenous drugs or pulmonary and cardiovascular disease in people who smoke. Information regarding all current and recent medications is part of the general medical history.

E. HISTORY OF SUBSTANCE USE

The psychoactive substance use history includes past and present use of both licit and illicit psychoactive substances, including but not limited to alcohol, caffeine, nicotine, marijuana, cocaine, opiates, sedative-hypnotic agents, stimulants, solvents, and hallucinogens. Relevant information includes the quantity and frequency of use and route of administration; the pattern of use (e.g., episodic versus continual; solitary versus social); functional, interpersonal, or legal consequences of use; tolerance and withdrawal phenomena; any temporal association between substance use and present psychiatric illness; and any self-perceived benefits of use. Obtaining an accurate substance use history often involves a gradual, nonconfrontational approach to inquiry with multiple questions seeking the same information in different ways and/or the use of slang terms for drugs, patterns of use, and drug effects.

F. PSYCHOSOCIAL/DEVELOPMENTAL HISTORY (PERSONAL HISTORY)

The personal history reviews the stages of the patient's life, with special attention to developmental milestones and to patterns of response to normative life transitions and major life events. The patient's history of formal education and history of important cultural and religious influences on the patient's life are obtained. Any involvement with the juvenile or criminal justice system is noted. A sexual history is obtained, as well as any history of physical, emotional, sexual, or other abuse or trauma (11–13). Any experiences related to political repression, war, or a natural disaster are also relevant.

An assessment of the patient's past and present levels of functioning in family and social roles (e.g., marriage, parenting, work, school) (14–16) includes the following information: number and ages of any children; capacity to meet the needs of dependent children in general and during psychiatric crises, if these are likely to occur; and the overall health, including mental health, of the children, especially when the patient's psychiatric condition is likely to affect the children through genetic or psychosocial mechanisms or to impede the patient's ability to recognize and attend to the needs of a child.

G. SOCIAL HISTORY

The social history includes the patient's living arrangements and currently important relationships. Emphasis is given to relationships, both familial and nonfamilial, that are relevant to the present illness, act as stressors, or have the potential to serve as resources for the patient. Also included is a history of any formal involvement with social agencies or the courts, as well as details of any current litigation or criminal proceedings.

H. OCCUPATIONAL HISTORY

The occupational history describes the sequence of jobs held by the patient, reasons for job changes, and the patient's current or most recent employment, including whether current or recent jobs have involved unusual physical or psychological stress, toxic materials, a noxious environment, or shift work. Relevant data about military experience would include volunteer versus draftee status, whether the patient experienced combat, discharge status, awards, disciplinary actions, and whether the patient suffered injury or trauma while in service.

I. FAMILY HISTORY

The family history includes available information about general medical and psychiatric illness in close relatives, including disorders that may be familial or may strongly affect the family environment. This information includes any history of mood disorder, psychosis, suicide, and substance use disorders, as well as any treatment received and response to treatment. Items of current family health status that are of emotional importance to the patient are identified.

J. REVIEW OF SYSTEMS

The review of systems includes current symptoms not already identified in the history of the present illness. Also relevant are sleep, appetite, vegetative symptoms of mood disorder, pain and discomfort, systemic symptoms such as fever and fatigue, and neurologic symptoms, if any of these have not already been covered in the history of the present illness. In addition, common symptoms of diseases for which the patient is known to be at particular risk because of historical, genetic, environmental, or demographic factors are a relevant part of the review of systems.

K. PHYSICAL EXAMINATION

A physical examination is needed to evaluate the patient's general medical (including neurological) status. The scope and intensity necessary will vary according to clinical circumstances. An understanding of the patient's general medical condition is important in order to 1) properly assess the patient's psychiatric symptoms and their potential cause, 2) determine the patient's need for general medical care, and 3) choose among psychiatric treatments that can be affected by the patient's general medical status (4, 17). The physical examination includes sections concerning the following:

1. General appearance and nutritional status.
2. Vital signs.
3. Head and neck, heart, lungs, abdomen, and extremities.
4. Neurological status, including cranial nerves, motor and sensory function, gait, coordination, muscle tone, reflexes, and involuntary movements.
5. Skin, with special attention to any stigmata of trauma, self-injury, or drug use.

6. Any body area or organ system that is specifically mentioned in the history of the present illness or review of systems or that is relevant to determining the current status of problems mentioned in the past medical history.

Additional items may be added to the examination to address specific diagnostic concerns or to screen a member of a clinical population at risk for a specific disease. For example, a mentally retarded adult might be assessed for recognizable patterns of malformation.

L. MENTAL STATUS EXAMINATION

The mental status examination is a systematic collection of data based on observation of the patient's behavior during the interview and before and after the interview while the patient is in the psychiatrist's view. Responses to specific questions are an important part of the mental status examination, particularly in the assessment of cognition (18).

The purpose of the mental status examination is to obtain evidence of current symptoms and signs of mental disorders from which the patient might be suffering. Further, evidence is obtained regarding the patient's insight, judgment, and capacity for abstract reasoning, to inform decisions about treatment strategy and the choice of an appropriate treatment setting. The mental status examination contains the following core elements:

1. The patient's appearance and general behavior.
2. The patient's expressions of mood and affect.
3. Characteristics of the patient's speech and language (e.g., rate, rhythm, structure, flow of ideas, and pathologic features such as tangentiality, vagueness, incoherence, or neologisms).
4. The patient's rate of movement and the presence of any purposeless, repetitive, or unusual movements or postures.
5. The patient's current thoughts and perceptions, including the following:

   a. Spontaneously expressed worries, concerns, thoughts, impulses, and perceptual experiences.
   b. Cognitive and perceptual symptoms of specific mental disorders, usually elicited by specific questioning and including hallucinations, delusions, ideas of reference, obsessions, and compulsions.
   c. Suicidal, homicidal, violent, or self-injurious thoughts, feelings, or impulses. If present, details are elicited regarding their intensity and specificity, when they occur, and what prevents the patient from acting them out (19).

6. Features of the patient's associations, such as loose or idiosyncratic associations and self-contradictory statements.
7. The patient's understanding of his or her current situation.
8. Elements of the patient's cognitive status, including the following:

   a. Level of consciousness.
   b. Orientation.
   c. Attention and concentration.
   d. Language functions (naming, fluency, comprehension, repetition, reading, writing).

e. Memory.
f. Fund of knowledge (appropriate to sociocultural and educational background).
g. Calculation (appropriate to educational attainment).
h. Drawing (e.g., copying a figure or drawing a clock face).
i. Abstract reasoning (e.g., explaining similarities or interpreting proverbs).
j. Executive (frontal system) functions (e.g., list making, inhibiting impulsive answers, resisting distraction, recognizing contradictions).
k. Quality of judgment.

While systematic assessment of cognitive functions is an essential part of the general psychiatric evaluation, the level of detail necessary and the appropriateness of particular formal tests depend on the purpose of the evaluation and the psychiatrist's clinical judgment.

▶ M. FUNCTIONAL ASSESSMENT

For persons with chronic diseases, and particularly those with multiple comorbid conditions, structured assessment of physical and instrumental function may be useful in assessing disease severity and treatment outcome (20). Functional assessments include assessment of physical activities of daily living (e.g., eating, using the toilet, transferring, bathing, and dressing) and instrumental activities of daily living (e.g., driving or using public transportation, taking medication as prescribed, shopping, managing one's own money, keeping house, communicating by mail or telephone, and caring for a child or other dependent) (21, 22). Impairments in these activities can be due to physical or cognitive impairment or to the disruption of purposeful activity by the symptoms of mental illness.

Formal functional assessments facilitate the delineation of the combined effects of multiple illnesses and chronic conditions on patient's lives, and such assessments provide a severity measure that is congruent with patients' and families' experience of disability. In addition, functional assessment facilitates the monitoring of treatment by assessing important beneficial and adverse effects of treatment.

Formal functional assessment may be appropriate for patients who are evidently disabled by old age or by chronic physical or mental illness.

▶ N. DIAGNOSTIC TESTS

Laboratory tests are included in a psychiatric evaluation when they are necessary to establish or exclude a diagnosis, to aid in the choice of treatment, or to monitor treatment effects or side effects (23, 24). Relevant test results are documented in the evaluation, and their importance for diagnosis and treatment is indicated in the case formulation or treatment plan (see section IV.A.4).

▶ O. INFORMATION DERIVED FROM THE INTERVIEW PROCESS

The face-to-face interview provides the psychiatrist with a sample of the patient's interpersonal behavior and emotional processes that can either support or qualify diagnostic inferences from the history and examination and can also aid in prognosis and treatment planning. Important information can be derived by observing the ways in which the patient minimizes or exaggerates certain aspects of his or her history, whether particular questions appear to evoke hesitation or signs of discomfort, and the patient's general style of relating. Further observations concern the patient's ability to communicate about emotional issues, the defense mechanisms the patient uses when discussing emotionally important topics, and the patient's responses to the psychiatrist's comments and to other behavior, such as the psychiatrist's handling of interruptions or time limits.

IV. EVALUATION PROCESS

▷ **A. METHODS OF OBTAINING INFORMATION**

1. Patient interview

The psychiatrist's primary assessment tool is the direct face-to-face interview of the patient: evaluations based solely on review of records and interviews of persons close to the patient are inherently limited. The interview should be done in a manner that optimizes the ability to support the patient's attempts to tell his or her story, while simultaneously obtaining the necessary information. Empirical studies of the interview process suggest that the most comprehensive and accurate information emerges from a combination of a) open-ended questioning with empathic listening and b) structured inquiry about specific events and symptoms (25–28). When the purpose is a general evaluation, beginning with open-ended, empathic inquiry about the patient's concerns usually is best. Patient satisfaction with open-ended inquiry is greatest when the psychiatrist provides feedback to the patient at one or more points during the interview. Structured, systematic questioning has been shown to be especially helpful in eliciting information about substance use and about traumatic life events and in ascertaining the presence or absence of specific symptoms and signs of particular mental disorders (29–32).

The psychiatrist should discuss with the patient the purpose of the evaluation. The psychiatrist should also consider whether the time planned for the interview is adequate for the aims of the evaluation and should prioritize the aims or extend the time accordingly. A high priority should be given to the assessment of the patient's safety and the identification of any general medical or mental disorders requiring urgent treatment; the patient's most pressing concerns should also receive a high priority whenever possible. The specific method and sequence of the interview is left to the psychiatrist's clinical judgment. Since the aim of evaluative interviews often is to develop an alliance with the patient, certain inquiries might be limited initially in the service of that alliance.

The evaluation ought to be performed in a manner that is sensitive to the patient's individuality, identifying issues of development, culture, ethnicity, gender, sexual orientation, familial/genetic patterns, religious/spiritual beliefs, social class, and physical and social environment influencing the patient's symptoms and behavior (also refer to section IV.B.5). Interpreters other than family members should be used if possible when the psychiatrist and the patient do not share a common language (including sign language in persons with impaired hearing). Interpreters with mental health experience and awareness of the patient's culture can provide the best information (33). The interpreter should be instructed to translate the patient's own words and to avoid paraphrasing except as needed to translate the correct meaning of idioms and other culture-specific expressions.

2. Use of collateral sources

The psychiatrist should always consider using collateral sources of information. Collateral information is particularly important for patients with impaired insight, including those with substance use disorders or cognitive impairment, and is essential for treatment planning for patients requiring a high level of assistance or supervision because of impaired function or unstable behavior. Nonetheless, the confidentiality of the patient should be respected, except when immediate safety concerns are paramount. Family members, other important people in the patient's life, and records of prior medical and/or psychiatric treatment are frequently useful sources of information. The extent of the collateral interviews and the extent of prior record review should be commensurate with the purpose of the evaluation, the ambitiousness of the diagnostic and therapeutic goals, and the difficulty of the case.

3. Use of structured interviews, questionnaires, and rating scales

Structured interviews, standardized data forms, questionnaires, and rating scales can be useful tools for diagnostic assessment and evaluation of treatment outcome. Structured interviews increase the reliability of determining that diagnostic criteria for a particular mental disorder are present; rating scales permit quantification of symptom severity. Potential cultural, ethnic, gender, social, and age biases are relevant to the selection of standardized interviews and rating scales and the interpretation of their results (34–37).

However, these tools are not a substitute for the clinician's narrative or judgment (38, 39). In particular, diagnostic and treatment decisions for patients whose conditions approach but do not reach diagnostic criteria for major psychiatric syndromes rely heavily on clinical judgment. Clinical impressions of treatment response should consider the relative importance of specific symptoms to the patient's function and well-being and the relative impact of specific symptoms on the patient's social environment.

4. Use of diagnostic tests, including psychological and neuropsychological tests

Diagnostic tests used during a psychiatric evaluation include those that do the following:

a. Detect or rule out the presence of a disorder or condition that has treatment consequences. Examples include urine screens for substance use disorders, neuropsychological tests to ascertain the presence of a learning disability, and brain imaging tests to ascertain the presence of a structural neurological abnormality.

b. Determine the relative safety and/or appropriate dose of potential alternative treatments. For example, tests of hematologic, thyroid, renal, and cardiac function in a patient with bipolar disorder may be needed to help the clinician choose among available mood-stabilizing medications.

c. Provide a baseline that will be useful in monitoring treatment response. For example, a baseline ECG may be required to facilitate the detection of tricyclic antidepressant effects on cardiac conduction.

In each of these cases, the potential utility of a test is determined by the following:

a. The probability that the disorder or condition under question is currently present or the probability that a condition may occur at a later date and require a baseline measure for detection. This may be thought of as the prevalence of the condition in a population of similar patients.
b. The probability that the test will correctly detect the condition if it is present.
c. The probability that the test will incorrectly identify a condition that is not present.
d. The treatment implications of the potential correct and incorrect test results. The treatment implications may be nil if the test detects a condition that is already known to be present on the basis of clinical examination or history or if it detects a condition that has no impact on treatment.

Given the wide range of clinical situations that are evaluated by psychiatrists, there are no general guidelines about which tests should be "routinely" done. Rather, the principles already discussed, as well as patient preferences, should be applied. Although each patient should be considered individually, it is sometimes possible to apply "clinical rules." For example, in some cases tests may be ordered on the basis of the setting (e.g., patients seen in emergency rooms of large city hospitals may be at high risk for certain conditions that warrant diagnostic tests), the clinical presentation (e.g., certain tests are warranted for patients with new onset of delirium), or the potential treatments (e.g., patients may need certain tests before initiation of lithium therapy).

5. Working with multidisciplinary teams

Multidisciplinary teams participate in general evaluations in most institutional settings and in many outpatient clinics. When working with a multidisciplinary team, the attending psychiatrist integrates both primary data and evaluative impressions of team members in arriving at a diagnosis and case formulation. It is crucial that the psychiatrist's diagnosis and case formulation rely on data recorded in the medical record and not rest primarily on undocumented impressions of other members of the team.

Systematic observations of patients' behavior by staff are a diagnostic asset of controlled settings, such as hospitals, partial hospital settings, residential treatment facilities, and other institutions. In these settings the psychiatrist may suggest to other team members specific observations that may be particularly relevant to the diagnosis or treatment plan. Several types of observations may be recorded, according to the patient's specific situation.

a) General observations

These are relevant to all patients in all settings and include notes on patients' behavior, complaints and statements, cooperativeness with or resistance to staff, sleep/wake patterns, and self-care.

b) Diagnosis-specific observations

These are observations relevant to confirming a diagnosis or assessing the severity, complications, or subtype of a disorder. Examples include recording of signs of withdrawal in an alcohol-dependent patient and observations during meals for patients with eating disorders.

c) Patient-specific observations

These are observations aimed at assessing a clinical hypothesis. An example is observation of behavior following a family meeting, for a patient in whom family conflicts are suspected of having contributed to a psychotic relapse.

d) Observations of response to treatment interventions

Examples include systematic recording of a target behavior in a trial of behavior therapy, observations of the effects of newly prescribed medications, and nurse-completed rating scales to measure changes after behavioral or psychotherapeutic interventions.

6. Examination under medication and/or restraint

The initial evaluation of a severely ill patient sometimes requires the use of psychotropic medication, seclusion, and/or physical restraint in order to provide for the safety of the patient and/or others, to allow collection of diagnostic information, and to enable the conduct of a physical examination and diagnostic testing. Resort to such measures should be justified by the urgency of obtaining the information and should be in compliance with applicable laws. The psychiatrist should consider how any special circumstances of the interview or examination may influence clinical findings; parts of the examination that cannot be completed or that are grossly influenced by the use of medication, seclusion, and/or restraint should be repeated if possible when the patient is able to cooperate.

7. Physical examination

The physical examination may be performed by the psychiatrist or another physician. Moreover, the psychiatrist may supplement an examination by another physician (e.g., perform a focused neurological examination). The psychiatrist should be informed about the scope and pertinent findings of examinations performed by other physicians. Considerations influencing the decision of whether the psychiatrist will personally perform the physical examination include potential effects on the psychiatrist-patient relationship, the purposes of the evaluation, and the psychiatrist's proficiency in performing physical examinations.

The psychiatrist's close involvement in the patient's general medical evaluation and ongoing care can improve the patient's care by promoting cooperation, facilitating follow-up, and permitting prompt reexamination of symptomatic areas when symptoms change.

In most cases, the physical examination by a psychiatrist should be chaperoned. Particular caution is warranted in the physical examination of persons with histories of physical or sexual abuse or with other features that could increase the possibility of the patient's being distressed as a result of the examination (e.g., a patient with an erotic or paranoid transference to the psychiatrist). All but limited examinations of such patients should be chaperoned.

▶ B. THE PROCESS OF ASSESSMENT

The actual assessment process during a psychiatric evaluation usually involves the development of initial impressions and hypotheses during the interview and their continual testing and refinement on the basis of information obtained throughout the interview and from mental status examination, diagnostic testing, and other sources (40).

1. Diagnosis and case formulation

On the basis of information obtained in the evaluation, a differential diagnosis is developed. The differential diagnosis comprises conditions (including personality disorders or personality traits) described in the current edition of the *Diagnostic and*

Statistical Manual of Mental Disorders (DSM) of the American Psychiatric Association. The DSM classification and the specific diagnostic criteria are meant to serve as guidelines to be informed by clinical judgment in the categorization of the patient's condition(s) and are not meant to be applied in a cookbook fashion. (Other issues in the use of DSM and its application in developing a psychiatric diagnosis are discussed in DSM-IV, pp. xv–xxv and 1–13 [41].) General medical conditions are established through history, examination, medical records, conferences with or referrals to other physicians, diagnostic tests, and independent examinations performed by the psychiatrist. A multiaxial system of diagnosis provides a convenient format for organizing and communicating the patient's current clinical status, other factors affecting the clinical situation, the patient's highest level of past functioning, and the patient's quality of life (41, pp. 25–31).

Information is obtained and compiled to permit an assessment of the patient's adaptive strengths, stressors implicated in the present illness, and support available in the patient's environment. The method of deriving this information should be sensitive to the patient's individuality, identifying issues of development, culture, ethnicity, gender, sexual orientation, familial/genetic patterns, religious/spiritual beliefs, social class, and physical and social environment influencing the patient's symptoms and behavior.

The case formulation includes information specific to the individual patient that goes beyond what is conveyed by the diagnosis. The scope and depth of the formulation vary with the purpose of the evaluation. Elements commonly include psychosocial and developmental factors that may have contributed to the present illness; the patient's particular strengths and weaknesses; social resources and the ability to form and maintain relationships; issues related to culture, ethnicity, gender, sexual orientation, and religious/spiritual beliefs; likely precipitating or aggravating factors in the illness; and preferences, opinions, and biases of the patient relevant to the choice of a treatment (33, 42–53). Additional elements may be based on a specific model of psychopathology and treatment, e.g., psychodynamic or behavioral. The diagnosis and case formulation together facilitate the development of a treatment plan.

2. Initial treatment plan

A psychiatrist conducting an evaluation to guide treatment should include an initial treatment plan that includes answers to the questions that were posed and/or a plan for obtaining additional necessary information.

The initial treatment plan begins with an explicit statement of the diagnostic, therapeutic, and rehabilitative goals for treatment. In the case of patients who initially will be treated in an inpatient or partial hospital setting, this implies apportioning the therapeutic task between a hospital phase and a posthospital phase. On the basis of the goals, the plan specifies further diagnostic tests and procedures, further systematic observations to be made, and specific therapeutic modalities to be applied.

All potentially effective treatments should be considered. More detailed consideration of the risks and benefits of treatment options may be needed in the following circumstances: when a relatively risky, costly, or unusual treatment is under consideration; when involved parties disagree about the optimal course of treatment; when the patient's motivation or capacity to benefit from potential treatment alternatives is in question; when the treatment would be involuntary or when other legal or administrative issues are involved; or when external constraints limit available treatment options.

3. Decisions regarding treatment-related legal and administrative issues

Within the scope of general evaluation, certain areas might require special emphasis if there is an outstanding legal or administrative issue. Assessment should be undertaken with these issues in mind. Discussions of informed consent, if carried out during the evaluation for the purpose of treatment planning, require documentation. Thus, when a patient's competence to consent to treatment is in question, questioning to determine mental status should be extended to include items that test the patient's decision-making capacity.

On the basis of the history, examination, symptoms, diagnosis, and case formulation, the psychiatrist makes and justifies decisions regarding voluntary versus involuntary status; the patient's capacity to make treatment-related decisions; the appropriateness and/or necessity of the site, intensity, and duration of the treatment chosen; and the level of supervision necessary for safety.

4. Addressing systems issues

In addition to generating goals for the patient's diagnosis and individual treatment, the evaluation may lead to the development of goals for intervention with the family, other important people in the patient's life, other professionals (e.g., therapists), general medical providers, and governmental or social agencies (e.g., community mental health centers or family service agencies). Goals are developed in response to data from the initial evaluation indicating that various aspects of the care system have an important role in the patient's illness and treatment. Plans may be needed for addressing problems in the care system that are seen as important to the patient's illness, symptoms, function, or well-being and that appear amenable to modification. These plans should consider feasibility, the patient's wishes, and the willingness of other people to be involved.

5. Consideration for sociocultural diversity

The process of psychiatric evaluation must take into consideration and respect the diversity of American subcultures and must be sensitive to the patient's ethnicity and place of birth, gender, social class, sexual orientation, and religious/spiritual beliefs (54). Respectful evaluation involves an empathic, nonjudgmental attitude toward the patient's explanation of illness, concerns, and background. An awareness of one's possible biases or prejudices about patients from different subcultures and an understanding of the limitations of one's knowledge and skills in working with such patients may lead to the identification of situations calling for consultation with a clinician who has expertise concerning a particular subculture (41, pp. 843–849; 55–57). Further, the potential effect of the psychiatrist's sociocultural identity on the attitude and behavior of the patient should be taken into account in the formulation of a diagnostic opinion.

V. SPECIAL CONSIDERATIONS

▶ ## A. INTERACTIONS WITH THIRD-PARTY PAYERS AND THEIR AGENTS

Third-party payers and their agents frequently request data from psychiatric evaluations to make determinations about whether a hospital admission or a specific treatment modality will be covered by a particular insurance plan. Despite the blanket consents to release information to payers that most patients must sign to obtain insurance benefits, the psychiatrist should, whenever feasible, inform the patient what specific information has been requested and obtain specific consent to the release of that information. With valid consent, the psychiatrist may release information to a third-party reviewer, supplying the third-party reviewer with sufficient information to understand the rationale for the treatment and why it was selected over potential alternatives. The psychiatrist may withhold information about the patient not directly relevant to the utilization review or preauthorization decision.

B. PRIVACY AND CONFIDENTIALITY

Psychiatrists should follow APA standards for confidentiality in dealing with the results of psychiatric evaluations. Evaluations should be conducted in the most private setting compatible with the safety of the patient and others. The identity and presence of persons other than the psychiatrist at a diagnostic interview should be explained to the patient, and the presence of these persons should be acceptable to the patient unless compelling clinical or safety reasons justify overriding the patient's objection. Psychiatrists should not make audiotape or videotape recordings of patient interviews without the knowledge and consent of the patient or the patient's legal guardian (58).

C. LEGAL AND ADMINISTRATIVE ISSUES IN INSTITUTIONS

When a patient is admitted to a hospital or other residential setting, the patient's legal status should be promptly clarified. It should be established whether the admission is voluntary or involuntary, whether the patient gives or withholds consent to evaluation and recommended treatment, and whether the patient appears able to make treatment-related decisions. If there is a potential legal impediment to necessary treatment, action should be taken to resolve the issue.

In every institution, whether public or private, fiscal and administrative considerations limit treatment options. Usually there are constraints on length of stay and on the intensity of services available. Further constraints can arise from the absence or inadequate funding of aftercare services or of a full continuum of care. The initial assessment of treatment needs should not be confounded unduly with concerns about financing or availability of services, although the actual treatment may represent a compromise between optimal treatment and external constraints. When this results in a major negative effect on patient care, efforts should be made to find alternatives and the patient, family, and/or third-party payer should be informed of the limitations of the current treatment setting and/or resources. A common example is the situation in which a patient's safety requires a level of supervision not available in a given facility. Another example is when a patient requires a general medical workup that cannot be carried out in a freestanding psychiatric facility and requires the patient's transfer to a general hospital.

D. EVALUATION OF ELDERLY PERSONS

While advanced chronological age alone does not necessitate a change in the approach to the psychiatric evaluation, the strong association of old age with chronic disease and related impairments may increase the need for emphasis on certain aspects of the evaluation. The general medical history and evaluation, cognitive mental status examination, and functional assessment may need to be especially detailed because of the high prevalence of disease-related disability, use of multiple medications, cognitive impairment, and functional impairment in older people. The psychiatrist should attempt to identify all of the general medical and personal care providers involved with the patient and to obtain relevant information from them if the patient consents. The personal and social history includes coverage of common late-life issues, including the loss of a spouse or partner, the loss of friends or close relatives, residential moves, the new onset of disabilities, financial concerns related to illness or disability, and intergenerational issues, such as informal caregiving or financial transfers between members of different generations.

The psychiatrist may need to accommodate the evaluation to patients who cannot hear adequately. Amplification, a quieter interview room, and enabling lip reading are possible means to do this. When elderly patients are brought for psychiatric evaluation by a family member, special effort may be necessary to ensure them of the opportunity to talk to the psychiatrist alone.

VI. DEVELOPMENT PROCESS

The development process is detailed in the Appendix to this volume. Key features of the process included the following:

- a literature review (see the following description);
- initial drafting by a work group that included psychiatrists with clinical and research expertise in psychiatric evaluation;
- the production of multiple drafts with widespread review, in which 32 organizations and over 106 individuals submitted comments (see section VII);
- approval by the APA Assembly and Board of Trustees; and
- planned revisions at 3- to 5-year intervals.

Two types of literature were reviewed. Major texts published since 1983 on general psychiatry or psychiatric evaluation were identified by using the card catalogue at a medical school library. Primary sources and major review articles were identified by using MEDLINE (1973–1993) and PsycLIT (1987–1993) and using references given in the texts. Key words for computer searches included the following:

Diagnostic Interview Schedule
   and evaluation
Interview-Psychological (including Psychiatric)
   and family history
   and adult
   and forensic
   and methods
   and initial
Mental-Disorders-Diagnosis
   and interview
   and physical examination
   and outcome
   and tests

Mental Status Examination
Psychiatric-status-rating scales
Psychiatric
   and validity
   and admission
Psychological
   and discharge
   and evaluation
   and emergency
   and interview

The literature search was augmented by numerous references suggested by reviewers. It showed a predominance of expert opinion and psychometric studies of specific tests, with a small number of studies linking the evaluation process to clinical outcome.

VII. INDIVIDUALS AND ORGANIZATIONS THAT SUBMITTED COMMENTS

Paul Stuart Appelbaum, M.D.
Bernard S. Arons, M.D.
Boris M. Astrachan, M.D.
Joseph Autry, M.D.
F.M. Baker, M.D., M.P.H.
Richard Balon, M.D.
Ruth T. Barnhouse, M.D.
Cole Barton, Ph.D.
Jerome S. Beigler, M.D.
Jules R. Bemporad, M.D.
Charles H. Blackinton, M.D.
Mary C. Blehar, Ph.D.
Linda Bond, M.D.
Barbara A. Bonorden, M.S.
William H. Bristow, Jr., M.D.
John W. Buckley, M.D.
Robert Paul Cabaj, M.D.
Claudio Cepeda, M.D.
Daniel S. Chaffin, M.D.
Gordon H. Clark, Jr., M.D.
Norman Clemens, M.D.
Jacquelyn T. Coleman
John D. Cone, M.D.
Namir Damluji, M.D.
Carol Dashoff
Dave M. Davis, M.D.
Barbara G. Deutsch, M.D.

Park Dietz, M.D., Ph.D.
Richard S. Epstein, M.D.
Lois T. Flaherty, M.D.
Jean-Guy Fontaine, M.D.
Robert Fusco, M.D.
Glen Owens Gabbard, M.D.
Donald Gallant, M.D.
Elizabeth Galton, M.D.
Elena Garralda, Ph.D.
Jerry H. Gelbart, M.D.
Earl L. Giller, M.D., Ph.D.
Katharine Gillis, M.D.
Linda G. Gochfeld, M.D.
Stephen M. Goldfinger, M.D.
Larry S. Goldman, M.D.
Melvin G. Goldzband, M.D.
James Goodman, M.D.
Tracy R. Gordy, M.D.
Sheila Hafter Gray, M.D.
David Arlen Gross, M.D.
J.D. Hamilton, M.D.
Edward Hanin, M.D.
Steven C. Hayes, Ph.D.
Michel Hersen, M.D.
Steven K. Hoge, M.D.
Jeffrey S. Janofsky, M.D.
Mary A. Jansen, Ph.D.

Brad Johnson, M.D.
Robert A. Kimmich, M.D.
Donald F. Klein, M.D.
Thomas M. Kozak, Ph.D.
Kachigere Krishnappa, M.D.
Jeremy Lazarus, M.D.
Robert L. Leon, M.D.
William L. Licamele, M.D.
Elliot D. Luby, M.D.
Velandy Manohar, M.D.
John C. Markowitz, M.D.
Ronald L. Martin, M.D.
Jerome A. Motto, M.D.
Charles B. Mutter, M.D.
Carol Nadelson, M.D.
Henry Nasrallah, M.D.
James E. Nininger, M.D.
George W. Paulson, M.D.
Herbert S. Peyser, M.D.
Katharine Phillips, M.D.
Edward Pinney, M.D.
Ghulam Qadir, M.D.
Jonas R. Rappeport, M.D.
Victor I. Reus, M.D.
Richard E. Rhoden, M.D.
Michelle Riba, M.D.
Barbara R. Rosenfeld, M.D.

Pedro Ruiz, M.D.
James Ray Rundell, M.D.
Jo-Ellyn M. Ryall, M.D.
Joseph D. Sapira, M.D.
Jerome M. Schnitt, M.D.
Marc A. Schuckit, M.D.
Paul M. Schyve, M.D.
Stephen Shanfield, M.D.
Sheldon N. Siegel, M.D.
Edward Silberman, M.D.
Andrew Edward Skodol II, M.D.
Stanley L. Slater, M.D.
Terry Stein, M.D.
Nada L. Stotland, M.D.
Paul Summergrad, M.D.
Margery Sved, M.D.
Kenneth J. Tardiff, M.D.
William R. Tatomer, M.D., M.P.H.
Clark Terrell, M.D.
Ole Johannes Thienhaus, M.D., M.B.A.
Josef H. Weissberg, M.D.
Joseph J. Westermeyer, M.D., Ph.D.
Robert M. Wettstein, M.D.
Rhonda Whitson, R.R.A.
Howard V. Zonana, M.D.

American Academy of Child and Adolescent Psychiatry
American Academy of Neurology
American Academy of Psychiatrists in Alcoholism and Addiction
American Academy of Psychiatry and the Law
American Academy of Psychoanalysis
American Association of Community Psychiatrists
American Association of Psychiatric Administrators
American Association of Psychiatrists From India
American Association of Suicidology
American College of Emergency Physicians
American Medical Association
American Nurses Association
American Psychoanalytic Association
American Psychological Association
American Psychosomatic Society
American Sleep Disorders Association
American Society for Adolescent Psychiatry
American Society of Addiction Medicine
American Society of Clinical Hypnosis
Association for Academic Psychiatry
Association for Child Psychoanalysis
Association for the Advancement of Behavior Therapy
Association of Gay and Lesbian Psychiatrists

Center for Substance Abuse Prevention
Department of Veterans Affairs
Joint Commission on Accreditation of Healthcare Organizations
National Association of Veterans Affairs Chiefs of Psychiatry
National Institute of Mental Health
Pakistan Psychiatric Society of North America
Royal College of Psychiatrists
Society of Biological Psychiatry
Substance Abuse and Mental Health Services Administration

VIII. REFERENCES

The following coding system is used to indicate the nature of the supporting evidence in the summary recommendations and references:

[A]   *Randomized clinical trial.* A study of an intervention in which subjects are prospectively followed over time; there are treatment and control groups; subjects are randomly assigned to the two groups; both the subjects and the investigators are blind to the assignments.

[B]   *Clinical trial.* A prospective study in which an intervention is made and the results of that intervention are tracked longitudinally; study does not meet standards for a randomized clinical trial.

[C]   *Cohort or longitudinal study.* A study in which subjects are prospectively followed over time without any specific intervention.

[D]   *Case-control study.* A study in which a group of patients is identified in the present and information about them is pursued retrospectively or backward in time.

[E]   *Review with secondary data analysis.* A structured analytic review of existing data, e.g., a meta-analysis or a decision analysis.

[F]   *Review.* A qualitative review and discussion of previously published literature without a quantitative synthesis of the data.

[G]   *Other.* Textbooks, expert opinion, case reports, and other reports not included above.

1. Margulies A, Havens LL: The initial encounter: what to do first? Am J Psychiatry 1981; 138:421–428 [F]

2. Bassuk EL: The diagnosis and treatment of psychiatric emergencies. Compr Ther 1985; 11(7):6–12 [F]

3. Hall RC, Gardner ER, Popkin MK, Lecann AF, Stickney SK: Unrecognized physical illness prompting psychiatric admission: a prospective study. Am J Psychiatry 1981; 138:629–635 [C]

4. Anfinson TJ, Kathol RG: Laboratory and neuroendocrine assessment in medical-psychiatric patients, in Psychiatric Care of the Medical Patient. Edited by Stoudemire A, Fogel BS. New York, Oxford University Press, 1993 [F]

5. Garrick TR, Stotland NL: How to write a psychiatric consultation. Am J Psychiatry 1982; 139:849–855 [G]

6. Karasu TB, Plutchik R, Conte H, Siegel B, Steinmuller R, Rosenbaum M: What do physicians want from a psychiatric consultation service? Compr Psychiatry 1977; 18:73–81 [C]

7. Appelbaum PS, Gutheil TG: Clinical Handbook of Psychiatry and the Law. Baltimore, Williams & Wilkins, 1991 [F]

8. Group for the Advancement of Psychiatry: The Mental Health Professional and the Legal System: Report 131. Washington, DC, Group for the Advancement of Psychiatry, 1991 [F]

9. Sederer LI: Brief hospitalization, in American Psychiatric Press Review of Psychiatry, vol 11. Edited by Tasman A, Riba MB. Washington, DC, American Psychiatric Press, 1992 [F]

10. Fogel BS, Summergrad P: Evolution of the medical-psychiatric unit in the general hospital, in Handbook of Studies on General Hospital Psychiatry. Edited by Judd FK, Burrows GD, Lipsitt DR. New York, Elsevier, 1991 [G]

11. Lowenstein RJ: An office mental status examination for complex chronic dissociative symptoms and multiple personality disorder. Psychiatr Clin North Am 1991; 14:567–604 [G]

12. Herman JL: Trauma and Recovery. New York, Basic Books, 1992, pp 115–129 [G]

13. March JS: What constitutes a stressor: the "Criterion A" issue, in Posttraumatic Stress Disorder: DSM-IV and Beyond. Edited by Davison JRT, Foa EB. Washington, DC, American Psychiatric Press, 1993 [F]

14. Rey JM, Stewart GW, Plapp JM, Bashir MR, Richards IN: Validity of Axis V of DSM-III and other measures of adaptive function. Acta Psychiatr Scand 1988; 77:535–542 [C]

15. Sohlberg S: There's more in a number than you think: new validity data for the Global Assessment Scale. Psychol Rep 1989; 64:455–461 [F]

16. Harder DW, Strauss JS, Greenwald DF, Kokes RF, Ritzler BA, Gift TE: Predictors of outcome among adult psychiatric first admissions. J Clin Psychol 1992; 46:119–128 [C]

17. Schiffer RB, Klein RF, Sider RC: The Medical Evaluation of Psychiatric Patients. New York, Plenum, 1988, pp 3–33 [G]

18. Trzepacz PJ, Baker RW: The Psychiatric Mental Status Examination. New York, Oxford University Press, 1993, pp 3–12 [G]

19. Tardiff K: The current state of psychiatry in the treatment of violent patients. Arch Gen Psychiatry 1992; 49:493–499 [G]

20. Applegate WB, Blass JP, Williams TF: Instruments for the functional assessment of older patients. N Engl J Med 1990; 322:1207–1214 [F]

21. Katz S: Assessing self-maintenance: activities of daily living, mobility, and instrumental activities of daily living. J Am Geriatr Soc 1983; 31:721–727 [F]

22. American Psychiatric Association: Position statement on the role of psychiatrists in assessing driving ability (official actions). Am J Psychiatry 1995; 152:819 [G]

23. Anfinson TJ, Kathol RG: Screening laboratory evaluation in psychiatric patients: a review. Gen Hosp Psychiatry 1992; 14:248–257 [F]

24. White AJ, Barraclough B: Benefits and problems of routine laboratory investigations in adult psychiatric admissions. Br J Psychiatry 1989; 155:65–72 [F]

25. Cox A, Hopkinson K, Rutter M: Psychiatric interviewing techniques, II—naturalistic study: eliciting factual information. Br J Psychiatry 1981; 138:283–291 [C]

26. Hopkinson K, Cox A, Rutter M: Psychiatric interviewing techniques, III—naturalistic study: eliciting feelings. Br J Psychiatry 1981; 138:406–415 [C]

27. Cox A, Rutter M, Holbrook D: Psychiatric interviewing techniques, V—experimental study: eliciting factual information. Br J Psychiatry 1981; 139:29–31 [B]

28. Cox A, Holbrook D, Rutter M: Psychiatric interviewing techniques, VI—experimental study: eliciting feelings. Br J Psychiatry 1981; 139:144–152 [B]

29. Maier W, Philipp M, Buller R: The value of structured clinical interviews. Arch Gen Psychiatry 1988; 45:963–964 [C]

30. Robins L: Diagnostic grammar and assessment: translating criteria into questions. Psychol Med 1989; 19:57–68 [F]

31. Watson CG, Juba MP, Manifold V, Kucala T, Anderson PE: The PTSD interview: rationale, description, reliability, and concurrent validity of a DSM-III-based technique. J Clin Psychol 1991; 47:179–188 [C]

32. Skre I, Onstad S, Torgersen S, Kringlen E: High interrater reliability for the Structured Clinical Interview for DSM-III-R axis I (SCID I). Acta Psychiatr Scand 1991; 84:167–173 [C]

33. Westermeyer JJ: Cross-cultural psychiatric assessment, in Culture, Ethnicity, and Mental Illness. Edited by Gaw AC. Washington, DC, American Psychiatric Press, 1993 [F]

34. Escobar JI, Burnam A, Karno M, Forsythe A, Landsverk J, Golding JM: Use of the Mini-Mental State Examination (MMSE) in a community population of mixed ethnicity: cultural and linguistic artifacts. J Nerv Ment Dis 1986; 174:607–614 [C]

35. Lopez S, Nunez JA: Cultural factors considered in selected diagnostic criteria and interview schedules. J Abnorm Psychol 1987; 96:270–272 [F]

36. Flaherty JA, Gaviria FM, Pathak D, Mitchell T, Wintrob R, Richman JA, Birz S: Developing instruments for cross-cultural psychiatric research. J Nerv Ment Dis 1988; 176:257–263 [F]

37. Roberts RE, Rhoades HM, Vernon SW: Using the CES-D Scale to screen for depression and anxiety: effects of language and ethnic status. Psychiatry Res 1990; 31:69–83 [C]

38. Kovess V, Sylla O, Fournier L, Flavigny V: Why discrepancies exist between diagnostic interviews and clinicians' diagnoses. Soc Psychiatry Psychiatr Epidemiol 1992; 27:185–191 [C]

39. Harrington R, Hill J, Rutter M, John K, Fudge H, Zoccolillo M, Weissman M: The assessment of lifetime psychopathology: a comparison of two interviewing styles. Psychol Med 1988; 18:487–493 [C]

40. Nurcombe B, Fitzhenry-Coor I: How do psychiatrists think? clinical reasoning in the psychiatric interview: a research and education project. Aust NZ J Psychiatry 1982; 16:13–24 [F]

41. American Psychiatric Association: Diagnostic and Statistical Manual of Mental Disorders, 4th ed (DSM-IV). Washington, DC, APA, 1994 [G]

42. Perry S, Cooper AM, Michels R: The psychodynamic formulation: its purpose, structure, and clinical application. Am J Psychiatry 1987; 144:543–550 [F]

43. Barrett DH, Abel GG, Rouleau JL, Coyne BJ: Behavioral therapy strategies with medical patients, in Psychiatric Care of the Medical Patient. Edited by Stoudemire A, Fogel BS. New York, Oxford University Press, 1993

44. Miller NE: Behavioral medicine: symbiosis between laboratory and clinic. Annu Rev Psychol 1983; 34:1–31

45. Powell G (ed): The Psychosocial Development of Minority Group Children. New York, Brunner-Mazel, 1983 [F]

46. Dickstein L: New perspectives on human development, in American Psychiatric Press Review of Psychiatry, vol 10. Edited by Tasman A, Goldfinger S. Washington, DC, American Psychiatric Press, 1991 [F]

47. Gaw A (ed): Culture, Ethnicity, and Mental Illness. Washington, DC, American Psychiatric Press, 1993 [G]

48. Notman M, Nadelson C: Women and Men: New Perspectives on Gender Differences. Washington, DC, American Psychiatric Press, 1991 [F]

49. Stein T: Changing perspectives on homosexuality, in American Psychiatric Press Review of Psychiatry, vol 12. Edited by Oldham J, Riba M, Tasman A. Washington, DC, American Psychiatric Press, 1993 [F]

50. McGoldrick M, Pearce J, Giordano J (eds): Ethnicity and Family Therapy. New York, Guilford Press, 1982 [G]

51. Barnhouse R: How to evaluate patients' religious ideation, in Psychiatry and Religion: Overlapping Concerns. Edited by Robinson L. Washington, DC, American Psychiatric Press, 1986 [G]

52. Kroll J, Sheehan W: Religious beliefs and practices among 52 psychiatric inpatients in Minnesota. Am J Psychiatry 1989; 146:67–72 [C]

53. Westermeyer J: Psychiatric Care of Migrants: A Clinical Guide. Washington, DC, American Psychiatric Press, 1989 [G]
54. Gonzalez CA, Griffith EEH, Ruiz P: Cross-cultural issues in psychiatric treatment, in Treatments of Psychiatric Disorders, 2nd ed. Edited by Gabbard GO. Washington, DC, American Psychiatric Press, 1995
55. Pinderhughes E: Understanding Race, Ethnicity and Power. New York, Free Press, 1988 [F]
56. American Psychiatric Association: Guidelines regarding possible conflict between psychiatrists' religious commitments and psychiatric practice (official actions). Am J Psychiatry 1990; 147:542 [G]
57. American Psychiatric Association: Position statement on bias-related incidents (official actions). Am J Psychiatry 1993; 150:686 [G]
58. Macbeth JE, Wheeler AM, Sither JW, Onek JN: Legal and Risk Management Issues in the Practice of Psychiatry. Washington, DC, American Psychiatric Press, 1994 [F]

PRACTICE GUIDELINE FOR THE
Treatment of Patients With Delirium

WORK GROUP ON DELIRIUM

Paula Trzepacz, M.D., Chair

William Breitbart, M.D.
John Franklin, M.D.
James Levenson, M.D.
D. Richard Martini, M.D.
Philip Wang, M.D. (Consultant)

▶ NOTE TO THE READER

In this practice guideline, treatment recommendations are discussed in sections IV and V and are summarized in section I. Data regarding the safety and efficacy of available treatments are reviewed in section III.

This practice guideline was approved in December 1998 and was published in *The American Journal of Psychiatry* in May 1999.

CONTENTS

INTRODUCTION

This practice guideline seeks to summarize data regarding the care of patients with delirium. It begins at the point where the psychiatrist has diagnosed a patient as suffering from delirium according to the DSM-IV criteria for the disorder. The purpose of this guideline is to assist the psychiatrist in caring for a patient with delirium.

Psychiatrists care for patients with delirium in many different settings and serve a variety of functions. In many cases, a psychiatrist will serve as a consultant to the attending physician and will not have primary responsibility for the patient. This guideline reviews the treatment that patients with delirium may need. The psychiatrist should either provide or advocate for the appropriate treatments. In addition, many patients have comorbid conditions that cannot be described completely with one DSM diagnostic category. Therefore, the psychiatrist caring for patients with delirium should consider, but not be limited to, the treatments recommended in this practice guideline.

DEVELOPMENT PROCESS

This practice guideline was developed under the auspices of the Steering Committee on Practice Guidelines. The process is detailed in the Appendix to this volume. Key features of the process include the following:

- a comprehensive literature review (description follows) and development of evidence tables;
- initial drafting by a work group that included psychiatrists with clinical and research expertise in delirium;
- the production of multiple drafts with widespread review, in which 12 organizations and over 83 individuals submitted comments (see section VI);
- approval by the APA Assembly and Board of Trustees; and
- planned revisions at 3- to 5-year intervals.

A computerized search of the relevant literature from MEDLINE, PsycINFO, and EMBASE was conducted.

The first literature search was conducted by searching MEDLINE for the period 1966 to April 1996 and used the key words "organic mental disorders," "psychotic," "delirium," "delusions," "acute organic brain syndrome," "alcohol amnestic disorder," "psychoses," "substance-induced," and "intensive care psychosis" with "haloperidol," "droperidol," "antipsychotic agents," "physostigmine," "tacrine," "cholinergic agents," "benzodiazepines," "thiamine," "folic acid," "vitamin b 12," "vitamins," "morphine," "paralysis," "electroconvulsive therapy," "risperidone," and "neuroleptic malignant syndrome." A total of 954 citations were found.

A second search in MEDLINE was completed for the period 1995 to 1998 and used the key words "delirium," "dementia," "amnestic," "cognitive disorders," and "delusions" with "haloperidol," "droperidol," "antipsychotic agents," "physostigmine," "tacrine," "cholinergic agents," "benzodiazepines," "vitamins," "morphine," "paralysis," "electroconvulsive therapy," "risperidone," and "neuroleptic malignant syndrome." A total of 1,386 citations were found.

The literature search conducted by using PsycINFO covered the period 1967 to November 1998 and used the key words "delirium" and "treatment & prevention" with "psychosocial," "behavioral," "restraint," "seclusion," "isolation," "structure," "support," "sensory deprivation," "orient," "reorient," and "delirium tremens." A total of 337 citations were found.

An additional literature search was conducted by using EMBASE for the period 1985 to November 1998 and used the key word "delirium" with "vitamins," "morphine," "paralysis," "electroconvulsive therapy," and "neuroleptic malignant syndrome." A total of 156 citations were found.

I. SUMMARY OF RECOMMENDATIONS

The following executive summary is intended to provide an overview of the organization and scope of recommendations in this practice guideline. The treatment of patients with delirium requires the consideration of many factors and cannot be adequately reviewed in a brief summary. The reader is encouraged to consult the relevant portions of the guideline when specific treatment recommendations are sought. This summary is not intended to stand on its own.

A. CODING SYSTEM

Each recommendation is identified as falling into one of three categories of endorsement, indicated by a bracketed Roman numeral following the statement. The three categories represent varying levels of clinical confidence regarding the recommendations:

[I]   Recommended with substantial clinical confidence.
[II] Recommended with moderate clinical confidence.
[III] May be recommended on the basis of individual circumstances.

B. GENERAL CONSIDERATIONS

Delirium is primarily a disturbance of consciousness, attention, cognition, and perception but can also affect sleep, psychomotor activity, and emotions. It is a common psychiatric illness among medically compromised patients and may be a harbinger of significant morbidity and mortality. The treatment of patients with delirium begins with an essential array of psychiatric management tasks designed to provide immediate interventions for urgent general medical conditions, identify and treat the etiology of the delirium, ensure safety, and improve the patient's functioning. Environmental and supportive interventions are also generally offered to all patients with delirium and are designed to reduce factors that may exacerbate delirium, to reorient patients, and to provide them with support. Somatic interventions largely consist of pharmacologic treatment with high-potency antipsychotic medications. Other somatic interventions may be of help in particular cases of delirium due to specific etiologies or with particular clinical features.

1. Psychiatric management

Psychiatric management is an essential feature of treatment for delirium and should be implemented for all patients with delirium [I]. The specific tasks that constitute psychiatric management include the following: coordinating the care of the patient with other clinicians; identifying the underlying cause(s) of the delirium; initiating immediate interventions for urgent general medical conditions; providing treatments that address the underlying etiology of the delirium; assessing and ensuring the safety of the patient and others; assessing the patient's psychiatric status and monitoring it on an ongoing basis; assessing individual and family psychological and social characteristics; establishing and maintaining a supportive therapeutic stance with the patient, the family, and other clinicians; educating the patient, family, and other clinicians regarding the illness; and providing postdelirium management to support the patient and family and providing education regarding risk factors for future episodes.

2. Environmental and supportive interventions

These interventions are generally recommended for all patients with delirium [I]. Environmental interventions are designed to reduce or eliminate environmental factors that exacerbate delirium. They include providing an optimal level of environmental stimulation, reducing sensory impairments, making environments more familiar, and providing environmental cues that facilitate orientation. Cognitive-emotional supportive measures include providing patients with reorientation, reassurance, and information concerning delirium that may reduce fear or demoralization. In addition to providing such supportive interventions themselves, it may be helpful for psychiatrists to inform nursing staff, general medical physicians, and family members of their importance.

3. Somatic interventions

The choice of somatic interventions for delirium will depend on the specific features of a patient's clinical condition, the underlying etiology of the delirium, and any associated comorbid conditions [I]. Antipsychotic medications are often the pharmacologic treatment of choice [I]. Haloperidol is most frequently used because it has few anticholinergic side effects, few active metabolites, and a relatively small likelihood of causing sedation and hypotension. Haloperidol may be administered orally, intramuscularly, or intravenously and may cause fewer extrapyramidal symptoms when administered intravenously. Haloperidol can be initiated in the range of 1–2 mg every 2–4 hours as needed (0.25–0.50 mg every 4 hours as needed for elderly patients), with titration to higher doses for patients who continue to be agitated. For patients who require multiple bolus doses of antipsychotic medications, continuous intravenous infusions of antipsychotic medication may be useful (e.g., haloperidol bolus, 10 mg i.v., followed by continuous intravenous infusion of 5–10 mg/hour; lower doses may be required for elderly patients). For patients who require a more rapid onset of action, droperidol, either alone or followed by haloperidol, can be considered. Recently some physicians have used the newer antipsychotic medications (risperidone, olanzapine, and quetiapine) in the treatment of patients with delirium. Patients receiving antipsychotic medications for delirium should have their ECGs monitored [I]. A QT_c interval greater than 450 msec or more than 25% over baseline may warrant a cardiology consultation and reduction or discontinuation of the antipsychotic medication.

Benzodiazepine treatment as a monotherapy is generally reserved for delirium caused by withdrawal of alcohol or sedative-hypnotics [I]. Patients with delirium who can tolerate only lower doses of antipsychotic medications may benefit from the combination of a benzodiazepine and antipsychotic medication [III].

Other somatic interventions may be considered for patients with delirium who have particular clinical conditions or specific underlying etiologies. Cholinergics such as physostigmine may be useful in delirium known to be caused specifically by anticholinergic medications [II]. Paralysis, sedation, and mechanical ventilation may be required for agitated patients with delirium and hypercatabolic conditions [III]. Palliative treatment with opiates may be needed by patients with delirium for whom pain is an aggravating factor [III]. Multivitamin replacement should be given to patients with delirium for whom there is the possibility of B vitamin deficiencies (e.g., those who are alcoholic or malnourished) [II].

II. DISEASE DEFINITION, EPIDEMIOLOGY, AND NATURAL HISTORY

▶ A. DEFINITION AND CLINICAL FEATURES

The essential features of delirium include disturbances of consciousness, attention, cognition, and perception. The disturbance develops over a short period of time (usually hours to days) and tends to fluctuate during the course of the day. Following are the DSM-IV criteria for delirium (1):

A. Disturbance of consciousness (i.e., reduced clarity of awareness of the environment) with reduced ability to focus, sustain, or shift attention.

B. A change in cognition (such as memory deficit, disorientation, language disturbance) or the development of a perceptual disturbance that is not better accounted for by a preexisting, established, or evolving dementia.

C. The disturbance develops over a short period of time (usually hours to days) and tends to fluctuate during the course of the day.

According to DSM-IV, delirium frequently represents a sudden and significant decline from a previous level of functioning and cannot be better accounted for by a preexisting or evolving dementia. There is usually evidence from the history, physical examination, or laboratory tests that the delirium is a direct physiological consequence of a general medical condition, substance intoxication or withdrawal, use of a medication, toxin exposure, or a combination of these factors. The disorders included in the DSM-IV delirium section have a common symptom presentation of a disturbance in consciousness and cognition but are differentiated by etiology:

1. Delirium due to a general medical condition.
2. Substance-induced delirium.
3. Delirium due to multiple etiologies.
4. Delirium not otherwise specified.

The disturbance in consciousness or arousal can be manifested by a reduced clarity or awareness of the environment that does not reach the level of stupor or coma. In addition, the ability to focus, sustain, or shift attention is frequently impaired and may result in the patient's being easily distracted.

There is also an accompanying decline in other areas of cognition. Cognitive deficits can include memory and visuoconstructional impairment, disorientation, or language disturbance. Memory impairment is most commonly evident in recent memory. Disorientation is usually manifested as disorientation to time (e.g., thinking it is morning in the middle of the night) or place (e.g., thinking one is at home rather than in the hospital). Disorientation to other persons occurs commonly, but disorientation to self is rare. It may be difficult for the clinician to fully assess cognitive function because the patient is inattentive and incoherent. Obtaining information from the medical chart, medical staff, and other informants, particularly family members, is often helpful in these circumstances.

Dysarthria is a frequent speech and language disturbance, and dysnomia (i.e., impaired ability to name objects), dysgraphia (i.e., impaired ability to write), or even frank aphasia may be observed.

Perceptual disturbances may include misinterpretations, illusions, or hallucinations. For example, the patient may see the nurse mixing intravenous solutions and conclude the nurse is trying to poison him or her (misinterpretation); the folds of the bedclothes may appear to be animate objects (illusion); or the patient may see a group of people around the bed when no one is actually there (hallucination). Although visual misperceptions and hallucinations are most common in delirium, auditory, tactile, gustatory, and olfactory misperceptions or hallucinations can also occur. Misperceptions range from simple and uniform to highly complex. A patient with delirium may have a delusional conviction of the reality of a hallucination and exhibit emotional and behavioral responses consistent with the hallucination's content.

B. ASSOCIATED FEATURES

Other commonly associated features of delirium include disturbances of sleep, psychomotor activity, and emotion. Disturbances in the sleep-wake cycle observed in delirium include daytime sleepiness, nighttime agitation, and disturbances in sleep continuity. In some cases, complete reversal of the night-day sleep-wake cycle or fragmentation of the circadian sleep-wake pattern can occur.

Delirium is often accompanied by disturbed psychomotor activity. Lipowski (2, 3) clinically described two subtypes of delirium based on psychomotor activity and arousal levels. These delirium subtypes included the "hyperactive" (or agitated, hyperalert) subtype and the "hypoactive" (lethargic, hypoalert) subtype. Others have included a "mixed" delirium subtype with alternating features of both. Ross et al. (4) suggested that the hyperactive form is more often characterized by hallucinations, delusions, agitation, and disorientation, while the hypoactive form is characterized by confusion and sedation and is less often accompanied by hallucinations, delusions, or illusions. Comparable levels of cognitive impairment have been observed with both motoric subtypes.

The delirious individual may also exhibit emotional disturbances, such as anxiety, fear, depression, irritability, anger, euphoria, and apathy. There may be affective lability, with rapid and unpredictable shifts from one emotional state to another.

Depending on the etiology, delirium can be associated with a number of nonspecific neurological abnormalities, such as tremor, myoclonus, asterixis, and reflex or muscle tone changes. For example, nystagmus and ataxia may accompany delirium due to medication intoxications; cerebellar signs, myoclonus, and generalized hyperreflexia may be seen with lithium intoxication; cranial nerve palsies may occur with Wernicke's encephalopathy; and asterixis may be observed with renal or hepatic insufficiency. The background rhythm seen on EEG is typically abnormal, usually showing generalized slowing. However, in alcohol or sedative-hypnotic withdrawal, the EEG usually shows fast activity. In addition, laboratory findings that are characteristic of associated or etiological general medical conditions (or intoxication or withdrawal states) may be seen.

C. DIFFERENTIAL DIAGNOSIS

The differential diagnosis of patients with features of delirium is discussed in the delirium section of DSM-IV. The most common issue in differential diagnosis is whether the patient has dementia rather than delirium, has delirium alone, or has a delirium superimposed on a preexisting dementia. Cognitive disturbances, such as memory impairment, are common to both delirium and dementia; however, the patient with dementia usually is alert and does not have the disturbance of consciousness or arousal that is characteristic of delirium. The temporal onset of cognitive deficit symptoms and the temporal course and reversibility of cognitive impairments are helpful in distinguishing between delirium and dementia. The severity of delirium symptoms characteristically fluctuates during a 24-hour period, while dementia symptoms generally do not. Information from medical records, other caregivers, and family members may be helpful in determining whether a dementia was present before the onset of a delirium.

▶ D. PREVALENCE AND COURSE

The prevalence of delirium in the hospitalized medically ill ranges from 10% to 30%. In the hospitalized elderly, the delirium prevalence ranges from 10% to 40% (2). As many as 25% of hospitalized cancer patients (5) and 30%–40% of hospitalized AIDS patients (6) develop delirium. As many as 51% of postoperative patients develop delirium (7), and up to 80% of patients with terminal illnesses develop delirium near death (8). Patients who have just had surgery, particularly cardiotomy, hip surgery, or a transplant, and patients with burns, dialysis, or central nervous system lesions are at increased risk for delirium.

Some patients manifest subclinical delirium or prodromal symptoms such as restlessness, anxiety, irritability, distractibility, or sleep disturbance in the days before the onset of overt delirium. Prodromal symptoms may progress to full-blown delirium over 1 to 3 days. The duration of symptoms of delirium has been reported to range from less than 1 week to more than 2 months (9–14). Typically the symptoms of delirium resolve within 10–12 days; however, up to 15% of patients with delirium have symptoms that persist for up to 30 days and beyond (10). Elderly patients with delirium may be more likely to have a prolonged course, with symptom durations frequently exceeding 1 month (11, 12).

While the majority of patients recover fully, delirium may progress to stupor, coma, seizures, or death, particularly if untreated. Full recovery is less likely in the elderly, with estimated rates of full recovery by the time of discharge varying from 4% to 40% (9, 15). Persistent cognitive deficits are also quite common in elderly patients recovering from delirium, although such deficits may be due to preexisting dementia that was not fully appreciated (9). Similarly, in a study of delirium in AIDS patients Fernandez et al. (16) found that only 27% had complete recovery of cognitive function, possibly because of underlying AIDS dementia.

Delirium in the medically ill is associated with significant morbidity. Medically ill patients, particularly the elderly, have a significantly increased risk of developing complications, such as pneumonia and decubitus ulcers, resulting in longer hospital stays (17, 18). In postoperative patients, delirium is a harbinger of limited recovery and poor long-term outcome. Patients who develop delirium, particularly after orthopedic surgery, are at increased risk for postoperative complications, longer postoperative recuperation periods, longer hospital stays, and long-term disability (19, 20). Seizures may occur in delirium, particularly among patients with alcohol or sedative-hypnotic withdrawal, cocaine intoxication, head trauma, hypoglycemia, strokes, or extensive burns (21).

Delirium in the medically ill is also associated with an increased mortality rate (22, 23). Elderly patients who develop delirium during a hospitalization have been estimated to have a 22%–76% chance of dying during that hospitalization (22, 24). Patients who develop delirium during a hospitalization also have a very high rate of death during the months following discharge. Several studies suggest that up to 25% of patients with delirium die within 6 months and that their mortality rate in the 3 months after diagnosis is 14 times as high as the mortality rate for patients with affective disorders (25, 26).

E. CAUSES

The disorders included in the delirium section of DSM-IV have a common symptom presentation but are differentiated according to presumed etiology (see table 1 for a list of common etiologies).

1. Due to a general medical condition

In determining that delirium is due to a general medical condition, the clinician must first establish the presence of a general medical condition and then establish that the delirium is etiologically related. A careful and comprehensive assessment is necessary to make this judgment. A temporal association between the onset, exacerbation, or remission of the general medical condition and that of the delirium is a helpful guide. Evidence from the literature that suggests the condition in question can be directly associated with the development of delirium is also useful. Delirium can be associated with many different general medical conditions, each of which has characteristic physical examination and laboratory findings. When these are present they may help confirm the relationship between delirium and the general medical condition. General medical conditions commonly causing delirium are shown in table 1.

TABLE 1. Underlying Conditions Commonly Associated With Delirium

Type	Disorder
Central nervous system disorder	Head trauma Seizures Postictal state Vascular disease (e.g., hypertensive encephalopathy) Degenerative disease
Metabolic disorder	Renal failure (e.g., uremia) Hepatic failure Anemia Hypoxia Hypoglycemia Thiamine deficiency Endocrinopathy Fluid or electrolyte imbalance Acid-base imbalance
Cardiopulmonary disorder	Myocardial infarction Congestive heart failure Cardiac arrhythmia Shock Respiratory failure
Systemic illness	Substance intoxication or withdrawal Infection Neoplasm Severe trauma Sensory deprivation Temperature dysregulation Postoperative state

2. Due to substance use or withdrawal

Delirium is frequently due to substance use or withdrawal (27). Substances with the potential to cause delirium include both agents that are not usually regarded as having psychoactive properties and those with established psychoactive properties. Delirium that occurs during substance intoxication may arise within minutes to hours after ingestion of high doses of drugs such as cocaine or hallucinogens; other drugs, such as alcohol, barbiturates, or meperidine, may cause delirium after intoxication is sustained for several days. During substance intoxication, the potential for additional agents with anticholinergic activity to cause delirium is increased. Usually the delirium resolves as the intoxication ends or within hours to days thereafter. Delirium associated with substance withdrawal develops as fluid and tissue concentrations of the substance decrease after reduction of sustained, high-dose use of certain substances. Substance-withdrawal delirium can also occur after the reduction of lower doses in patients having poor clearance, experiencing drug interactions, or taking combinations of drugs. The duration of the delirium usually varies with the half-life of the substance involved. Longer-acting substances usually are associated with less severe but more protracted withdrawal and may not have an onset of withdrawal symptoms for days or weeks after use of the substance is discontinued. Substance-withdrawal delirium may continue for only a few hours or may persist for as long as 2–4 weeks.

Table 2 lists substances associated with delirium, including substances of abuse, prescription medications, and toxins.

3. Due to multiple etiologies

Delirium, particularly in the critically ill and in elderly hospitalized patients, often has multiple etiologies (25). Francis and Kapoor (28) found that while 56% of elderly patients with delirium had a single definite or probable etiology for delirium, the remaining 44% had an average of 2.8 etiologies per patient.

4. Due to unspecified etiology

Occasionally, no clear etiology is immediately apparent. Often, unrecognized medication use or substance abuse is the cause of an intoxication or withdrawal delirium, and sometimes a rare cause of delirium, such as disseminated intravascular coagulation, is eventually revealed. There has been some controversy as to whether particular settings can themselves cause delirium (e.g., there has been speculation that the intensive care environment can cause "intensive care unit psychosis"). Koponen et al. (11) found a clear organic etiology in 87% of patients with delirium, and they found relatively little evidence that delirium was caused primarily by environmental factors.

F. USE OF FORMAL MEASURES

Although standard psychiatric, general medical, and neurological histories and examinations are usually sufficient to diagnose and evaluate the severity of delirium, they can be supplemented by assessments using formal instruments. A large number of delirium assessment methods have been designed, some intended for clinical evaluations and others for research. Detailed reviews of the psychometric properties of instruments, as well as suggestions for choosing among instruments for particular clinical evaluations or research purposes, are available (29–31). Four types of instruments are briefly mentioned in the following sections: tests that screen for delirium symptoms, delirium diagnostic instruments, delirium symptom severity ratings, and some experimental laboratory tests.

TABLE 2. Substances That Can Cause Delirium Through Intoxication or Withdrawal

Category	Substance
Drugs of abuse	Alcohol
	Amphetamines
	Cannabis
	Cocaine
	Hallucinogens
	Inhalants
	Opioids
	Phencyclidine
	Sedatives
	Hypnotics
	Other
Medications	Anesthetics
	Analgesics
	Antiasthmatic agents
	Anticonvulsants
	Antihistamines
	Antihypertensive and cardiovascular medications
	Antimicrobials
	Antiparkinsonian medications
	Corticosteroids
	Gastrointestinal medications
	Muscle relaxants
	Immunosuppressive agents
	Lithium and psychotropic medications with anticholinergic properties
Toxins	Anticholinesterase
	Organophosphate insecticides
	Carbon monoxide
	Carbon dioxide
	Volatile substances, such as fuel or organic solvents

1. Screening instruments

Several tools have been developed to screen for delirium symptoms among patients, and most have been designed to be administered by nursing staff. These may aid in the recognition of delirium, especially in nursing homes, where physician visits are less frequent. The number of delirium symptoms covered, the specificity of items for delirium, and the complexity of administration all vary. Screening instruments include the Clinical Assessment of Confusion—A (CAC-A) (32), the Confusion Rating Scale (CRS) (33), the MCV Nursing Delirium Rating Scale (MCV-NDRS) (34), and the NEECHAM Confusion Scale (35).

2. Diagnostic instruments

Investigators have designed a variety of instruments to make a formal diagnosis of delirium. These instruments consist of operationalized delirium criteria from a variety of diagnostic systems, often in the form of a checklist incorporating information from patient observation and the medical record (e.g., DSM-III-R, DSM-IV, ICD-9, and ICD-10). The rate of delirium diagnosis obtained by using these diagnostic instruments varies according to both the diagnostic system that was used and the particular way in which the authors chose to operationalize the criteria. One structured diagnostic interview schedule, the Delirium Symptom Interview (DSI), can be administered by lay interviewers and used in epidemiological studies (36). Other delirium diagnostic instruments include the Confusion Assessment Method (CAM) (37), Delirium Scale (Dscale) (38), Global Accessibility Rating Scale (GARS) (39), Organic Brain Syndrome Scale (OBS) (40), and Saskatoon Delirium Checklist (SDC) (41).

3. Delirium symptom severity rating scales

Several instruments have been developed to rate the severity of delirium symptoms. Ratings are generally based both on behavioral symptoms and on confusion and cognitive impairment. Rating the severity of delirium over time may be useful for monitoring the effect of an intervention or plotting the course of a delirium over time. These scales have also been used to make the diagnosis of delirium by considering patients with scores above a specified cutoff to have the diagnosis. Such rating scales include the Delirium Rating Scale (DRS) (42) and the Memorial Delirium Assessment Scale (MDAS) (43).

4. Laboratory tests

Several laboratory evaluations have been investigated for possible use in evaluating delirium. With the exception of the EEG, these tests are experimental and currently appropriate only for research purposes. For several decades, investigators have observed EEG changes in patients with delirium (44). EEG changes consist mainly of generalized slowing, although low-voltage fast activity is seen in some types of delirium, such as delirium tremens (45). The presence of EEG abnormalities has fairly good sensitivity for delirium (in one study, the sensitivity was found to be 75%), but their absence does not rule out the diagnosis; thus, the EEG is no substitute for careful clinical observation. Among the experimental laboratory tests that have been investigated for use in delirium, those that appear to show some promise include brain imaging (46, 47) and measures of serum anticholinergic activity (48).

III. TREATMENT PRINCIPLES AND ALTERNATIVES

Several therapeutic modes are employed in the treatment of delirium and are discussed in this section. First, the cornerstone of treatment, psychiatric management, is defined and its components are described. Treatment of the delirium itself involves a set of environmental and supportive interventions and specific pharmacologic treatments. Environmental manipulations are generally designed to help reorient the patient and modulate the degree of stimulation. Supportive measures are designed to provide patient, family, and friends with both reassurance and education regarding the nature, temporal course, and sequelae of delirium.

▶ ### A. PSYCHIATRIC MANAGEMENT

Psychiatric management involves an array of tasks that the psychiatrist should seek to ensure are performed for all patients with delirium. A psychologically informed understanding of the patient and the family may facilitate these tasks. These tasks are designed to facilitate the identification and treatment of the underlying cause(s) of delirium, improve the patient's level of functioning, and ensure the safety and comfort of patients and others. In many cases, the psychiatrist will be part of, or a consultant to, a multidisciplinary team and should encourage the administration of the full range of needed treatments.

1. Coordinate with other physicians caring for the patient

Delirium frequently heralds a medical emergency, and patients are usually managed in an acute-care hospital setting. For some patients with milder symptoms, once the etiology of delirium has been identified and general medical management has begun, psychiatric and general medical management can take place in an alternative setting (e.g., skilled nursing facility, home, hospice). The psychiatrist is commonly asked to consult when a patient develops delirium on a general medical or surgical unit in the hospital; however, delirium may also present as an emergency in either the psychiatric outpatient or inpatient setting.

The appropriate treatment of delirium involves interventions to search for and correct underlying causes, as well as relieve current symptoms. Joint and coordinated management of the patient with delirium by the psychiatrist and internist, neurologist, or other primary care or specialty physicians will frequently help ensure appropriate comprehensive evaluation and care.

2. Identify the etiology

An essential principle in the psychiatric management of delirium is the identification and correction of the etiologic factors. Careful review of the patient's medical history and interview of family members or others close to the patient may provide some direction. Appropriate laboratory and radiological investigations such as those listed in table 3 may be necessary to determine the underlying cause(s) of delirium. The choice of specific tests to be undertaken will depend on the results of the clinical evaluation.

3. Initiate interventions for acute conditions

A patient with delirium may have life-threatening general medical conditions that demand therapeutic intervention even before a specific or definitive etiology is determined. In addition to ensuring that diagnostic tests essential to identifying the cause of delirium are ordered, when acting as a consultant, the psychiatrist should raise the level of awareness of the general medical staff concerning the potential morbidity and mortality associated with delirium. Increased observation and monitoring of the patient's general medical condition should include frequent monitoring of vital signs, fluid intake and output, and levels of oxygenation. A patient's medications should be carefully reviewed; nonessential medications should be discontinued, and doses of needed medications should be kept as low as possible.

4. Provide other disorder-specific treatment

The goal of diagnosis is to discover reversible causes of delirium and prevent complications through prompt treatment of these specific disorders. One must give a high priority to identifying and treating such disorders as hypoglycemia, hypoxia or anoxia, hyperthermia, hypertension, thiamine deficiency, withdrawal states, and anticholinergic-induced or other substance-induced delirium. Examples of specific reversible causes of delirium and treatments for these disorders appear in table 4.

5. Monitor and ensure safety

Behavioral disturbances, cognitive deficits, and other manifestations of delirium may endanger patients or others. Psychiatrists must assess the suicidality and violence potential of patients and implement or advocate interventions to minimize these risks (e.g., remove dangerous items, increase surveillance and supervision, and institute

TABLE 3. Assessment of the Patient With Delirium[a]

Domain	Measure
Physical status	History Physical and neurological examinations Review of vital signs and anesthesia record if postoperative Review of general medical records Careful review of medications and correlation with behavioral changes
Mental status	Interview Cognitive tests, e.g., clock face, digit span, Trailmaking tests
Basic laboratory tests—consider for all patients with delirium	Blood chemistries: electrolytes, glucose, calcium, albumin, blood urea nitrogen (BUN), creatinine, SGOT, SGPT, bilirubin, alkaline phosphatase, magnesium, PO_4 Complete blood count (CBC) Electrocardiogram Chest X-ray Measurement of arterial blood gases or oxygen saturation Urinalysis
Additional laboratory tests— ordered as indicated by clinical condition	Urine culture and sensitivity (C&S) Urine drug screen Blood tests, e.g., venereal disease research laboratory (VDRL), heavy metal screen, B_{12} and folate levels, lupus erythematosus (LE) prep, antinuclear antibody (ANA), urinary porphyrins, ammonia, human immunodeficiency virus (HIV) Blood cultures Measurement of serum levels of medications, e.g., digoxin, theophylline, phenobarbital, cyclosporine Lumbar puncture Brain computerized tomography (CT) or magnetic resonance imaging (MRI) Electroencephalogram (EEG)

[a]From guidelines by Trzepacz and Wise (49).

pharmacotherapy). Suicidal behaviors are often inadvertent in delirium and occur in the context of cognitive impairment and/or in response to hallucinations or delusions. Additional assessments of a patient's risk for falls, wandering, inadvertent self-harm, etc., should also be made with appropriate measures taken to ensure safety.

Whenever possible, means other than restraints, such as sitters, should be used to prevent the delirious patient from harming himself or herself, others, or the physical environment. Restraints themselves can increase agitation or carry risks for injuries and should be considered only when other means of control are not effective or appropriate (50). A patient who is restrained should be seen as frequently as is necessary to monitor changes in the patient's condition (51). The justification for initiating restraints and continuing use of restraints should be documented in the patient's medical record. Additional rules may apply in some jurisdictions, and the psychiatrist should become familiar with applicable regulations and institutional policies (52).

6. Assess and monitor psychiatric status

The psychiatrist must periodically assess the patient's delirium symptoms, mental status, and other psychiatric symptoms. The symptoms and behavioral manifestations of delirium can fluctuate rapidly, and regular monitoring will allow for the adjustment of treatment strategies.

TABLE 4. Examples of Reversible Causes of Delirium and Their Treatments

Condition	Treatment
Hypoglycemia or delirium of unknown etiology where hypoglycemia is suspected	Tests of blood and urine for diagnosis Thiamine hydrochloride, 100 mg i.v. (before glucose) 50% glucose solution, 50 ml i.v.
Hypoxia or anoxia, e.g., due to pneumonia, obstructive or restrictive pulmonary disease, cardiac disease, hypotension, severe anemia, or carbon monoxide poisoning	Immediate oxygen
Hyperthermia, e.g., temperature above 40.5°C or 105°F	Rapid cooling
Severe hypertension, e.g., blood pressure of 260/150 mm Hg, with papilledema	Prompt antihypertensive treatment
Alcohol or sedative withdrawal	Appropriate pharmacologic intervention Thiamine, intravenous glucose, magnesium, phosphate, and other B vitamins, including folate
Wernicke's encephalopathy	Thiamine hydrochloride, 100 mg i.v., followed by thiamine daily, either intravenously or orally
Anticholinergic delirium	Withdrawal of offending agent In severe cases, physostigmine should be considered unless contraindicated

Important behavioral issues that must be addressed include depression, suicidal ideation or behavior, hallucinations, delusions, aggressive behavior, agitation, anxiety, disinhibition, affective lability, cognitive deficits, and sleep disturbances. It is helpful to record serial assessments of mental status and symptoms over time, as these may indicate the effectiveness of interventions and new or worsening medical conditions. A structured or semistructured instrument, such as those described in section II.F, may aid in the systematic completion of this task.

7. Assess individual and family psychological and social characteristics

Knowledge of the patient's and the family's psychodynamic issues, personality variables, and sociocultural environment may aid in dealing effectively with specific anxieties and reaction patterns on the part of both the patient and the family. This understanding may be based on prior acquaintance with the patient, current interviews or interaction with the patient or family, and/or history from the family.

8. Establish and maintain alliances

It is important for the psychiatrist who is treating the patient with delirium to establish and maintain a supportive therapeutic stance. Understanding the underlying affect, concerns, and premorbid personality of the patient is frequently helpful in maintaining a supportive alliance. A solid alliance with the family is also desirable, as family members are a critical source of potential support for patients and information on patients who may be unable to give reliable histories. Establishing strong alliances with the multiple clinicians and caregivers frequently involved in the care of delirious medically ill patients is also crucial.

9. Educate patient and family regarding the illness

Educating patients and families regarding delirium, its etiology, and its course is an important role for psychiatrists involved in the care of patients with delirium. Patients may vary in their ability to appreciate their condition; however, providing reassurance that delirium is usually temporary and that the symptoms are part of a medical condition may be extremely beneficial to both patients and their families. Specific educational and supportive interventions are discussed in more detail in the following paragraphs.

Nursing staff make frequent observations of patients over time, which places them in an excellent position to detect the onset and monitor the course of delirium. Education of nursing staff on each shift regarding the clinical features and course of delirium can be an important task for psychiatrists.

Because of the behavioral problems accompanying delirium, there may be a tendency for some general medical physicians to overlook underlying general medical problems contributing to a patient's delirium and to consider the problem to be entirely in the realm of the psychiatrist. In such instances, providing education to other physicians regarding the underlying physiological etiologies of delirium may be an important task for the psychiatrist.

10. Provide postdelirium management

Following recovery, patients' memory for the experience and events of the delirium is variable. Some patients gradually or abruptly lose all apparent recall of the delirious experience, while others have vivid, frightening recollections. Explanations regarding delirium, its etiology, and its course should be reiterated. Supportive interventions that are a standard part of psychiatric management following a traumatic experience should be used for those with distressing postdelirium symptoms. Following recovery, all patients who have experienced delirium should be educated about the apparent cause of their delirium (when this could be identified) so that the patient, family, and subsequent physicians can be made aware of risk factors that may lead to delirium in the future. Psychotherapy focused on working through the experience of the delirium may, at times, be necessary to resolve anxiety, guilt, anger, depression, or other emotional states. These states may be compounded by the patient's preexisting psychological, social, or cultural characteristics.

B. ENVIRONMENTAL AND SUPPORTIVE INTERVENTIONS

1. Environmental interventions

Management of delirium includes a specific array of interventions by nursing, psychological, general medical, and psychiatric staff that can be broadly categorized as environmental interventions. The general goals are to reduce environmental factors that exacerbate delirium, confusion, and misperception while providing familiarity and an optimal level of environmental stimulation. While there is no empirical evidence that the environment by itself causes delirium, certain environmental conditions may exacerbate delirium.

"Timelessness" in hospital intensive care units (ICUs), i.e., a similar environment regardless of the time of day, appears to contribute to disorganization of sleep-wake cycles, which in turn aggravates fatigue and confusion. Some ICUs have introduced windows, while others change the lighting to cue night versus day. The ICU can be a very noisy environment, with beeps, alarms, pumps, respirators, overhead paging, resuscitation efforts, etc. The confused patient with delirium may become overstimulated by too much noise, and efforts should be made to reduce this whenever possible. On the other hand, understimulation from the environment may leave the patient with delirium undistracted from his or her own internal disorganized perceptions and thoughts; too quiet an environment may exacerbate delirium. It is important to provide a regular amount of modest stimulation (vocal, visual, tactile) to the patient with delirium.

Delirium can also be aggravated by sensory impairments, including visual impairment (53) and auditory impairment (54). By restoring a patient's glasses or hearing aid, one may substantially reduce the manifestations of delirium. Ensuring that there is an analog clock and a calendar that the patient can see will further facilitate orientation. Steps that render the environment more familiar and less alien, such as bringing in family photographs or favorite objects from home (e.g., stuffed animals) or actually having family members there when possible, are also helpful. Especially in a room that may be dark at night, nightlights can help reduce anxiety.

There is some empirical evidence that these environmental interventions can reduce the severity of delirium and improve outcomes (55–58). While there are no large, rigorous, randomized controlled trials, these environmental interventions are widely endorsed because of clinical experience and the lack of adverse effects. Although the value of environmental interventions is widely recognized, they remain substantially underutilized (59).

2. Structure and support for the patient

Nursing, psychological, general medical, and psychiatric staff and family members can also provide cognitive-emotional support designed to strengthen any retained adaptive cognitive functioning that the patient possesses. The goal of these interventions is to reduce anxiety and the unfamiliar while providing understanding and support.

Central to providing cognitive and emotional support are efforts to deal with disorientation. All who come in contact with the patient should provide reorientation, which entails reminding the patient in an unpressured manner of where he or she is, the date and time, and what is happening to him or her.

The patient's emotional reaction to symptoms of delirium can itself be a significant aggravating factor. The patient should be told that the symptoms are temporary and reversible and do not reflect a persistent psychiatric disorder. Similarly, the perception of cognitive deficits may lead patients to conclude that they have suffered brain damage. Unless the delirium is thought to be due to a major stroke or injury or to another event that may cause permanent brain injury, all who have contact with the patient should reassure her or him that these deficits are common and reversible symptoms associated with the particular illness, surgery, or other treatment.

There have been no large clinical trials examining the efficacy of cognitive and emotional support in delirium. However, as with environmental interventions, increased use of these currently underutilized supportive measures has been encouraged on the basis of clinical experience, common sense, and lack of adverse effects (59).

3. Support and education for the family

Educating patients' friends and family about delirium is extremely helpful since they may have the same worries as the patient (e.g., the patient has a permanent psychiatric illness or is brain damaged) and become frightened and demoralized instead of being hopeful and encouraging the patient (60).

It may be useful to recommend that family and friends spend time in the patient's room and bring familiar objects from home to help orient the patient and help him or her feel secure.

► C. SOMATIC INTERVENTIONS

The primary treatment of the symptoms of delirium is largely pharmacologic. The high-potency antipsychotic medication haloperidol is most frequently employed, although other pharmacologic and somatic interventions have been used in particular instances. Recently, there has been increased use of risperidone (61, 62). The available studies of the efficacy and other outcomes from use of these treatments for patients with delirium are reviewed in this section.

Several important points should be considered when evaluating the evidence for specific somatic interventions. While haloperidol has been the most studied pharmacologic treatment, few studies have used a standardized definition of delirium (e.g., based on DSM-IV criteria). In addition, few investigations have used reliable and valid delirium symptom rating measures to assess symptom severity before and after intervention.

For somatic treatments other than haloperidol, there have been no large, prospective trials or studies including a control group. Information regarding the efficacy of these treatments comes mainly from small case series or case reports; interpretation of the results from many of these case presentations is also made difficult by the use of nonstandardized definitions of delirium or informal measures of delirium symptom severity.

1. Antipsychotics

a) Goals and efficacy

Antipsychotics have been the medication of choice in the treatment of delirium. Evidence for their efficacy has come from numerous case reports and uncontrolled trials (63, 64). A series of controlled trials also showed that antipsychotic medications can be used to treat agitation and psychotic symptoms in medically ill and geriatric patient populations (65–69). However, most of these trials were not conducted with patients who had clearly or consistently defined delirium; in some studies, agitation and disorientation were the sole criteria and symptom assessments ranged from questionnaires to simple identification without symptom descriptions.

A randomized, double-blind, comparison trial by Breitbart et al. (70) identified delirium by using standardized clinical measures, and it demonstrated the clinical superiority of antipsychotic medications over benzodiazepines in delirium treatment. The Delirium Rating Scale, Mini-Mental State examination, and DSM-III-R were used to make the diagnosis in 244 hospitalized AIDS patients. The subjects were randomly assigned to one of three medications: chlorpromazine, haloperidol, and lorazepam. There were statistically significant decreases in scores on the Delirium Rating Scale after 2 days in the haloperidol and chlorpromazine groups but not in the lorazepam group (the mean decreases in scores were 8.0, 8.5, and 1.0, respectively). The improvement in delirium symptoms observed among those treated with antipsychotic medications occurred quickly, usually before the initiation of interventions directed at the medical etiologies of the delirium.

Droperidol, a butyrophenone with a rapid onset of action and relatively short half-life that is more sedating than haloperidol, has also been found to be an effective treatment for hospitalized patients with agitation, although not necessarily delirium (71). Results of two double-blind clinical trials comparing droperidol to haloperidol suggest that a more rapid response may be obtained with droperidol. Resnick and Burton (72) reported that 30 minutes after intramuscular injections, 81% of patients initially treated with 5 mg of haloperidol required a second injection, compared to only 36% of patients initially given 5 mg of droperidol. Thomas and colleagues (69), comparing 5 mg i.m. of droperidol to 5 mg i.m. of haloperidol, found significantly decreased combativeness among the droperidol treatment group after 10, 15, and 30 minutes. There has been very little study of the newer antipsychotic medications (risperidone, olanzapine, and quetiapine) in the treatment of delirium. Although there have been several case reports of use of risperidone for patients with delirium (61, 62, 73, 74), there have been no published clinical trials of any of the new antipsychotic medications for patients with delirium.

b) Side effects

Phenothiazines can be associated with sedation, anticholinergic effects, and α-adrenergic blocking effects that can cause hypotension; each of these side effects may complicate delirium. Butyrophenones, particularly haloperidol and droperidol, are considered the safest and most effective antipsychotics for delirium. Haloperidol, a high-potency dopamine-blocking agent with few or no anticholinergic side effects, minimal cardiovascular side effects, and no active metabolites, has generally been considered the antipsychotic medication of first choice in the treatment of delirium. High-potency antipsychotic medications also cause less sedation than the phenothiazines and therefore are less likely to exacerbate delirium. Although droperidol may have the advantages of a more rapid onset of action and a shorter half-life than haloperidol, droperidol is associated with greater sedation and hypotensive effects (75).

The use of antipsychotic medications can be associated with neurological side effects, including the development of extrapyramidal side effects, tardive dyskinesia, and neuroleptic malignant syndrome. However, there is some evidence to suggest that extrapyramidal side effects may be less severe when antipsychotic medications are administered intravenously (76). One case series involved 10 consecutive general medical inpatients receiving doses of oral or intravenous haloperidol at approximately 10 mg/day. Four patients were given intravenous medication, and six were given oral doses. Although delirium was not identified as the reason for treatment, five patients met diagnostic criteria by description. There was no significant difference in the incidence of akathisia, but the group receiving intravenous medication experienced less severe extrapyramidal symptoms. Neither method of administration resulted in acute dystonic reactions or changes in blood pressure or pulse rate (76).

Haloperidol used in the treatment of delirium has been found in some instances to lengthen the QT interval, which can lead to torsades de pointes, a form of polymorphic ventricular tachycardia that can degenerate to ventricular fibrillation and sudden death. Estimates of the incidence of torsades de pointes among patients with delirium treated with intravenous haloperidol have ranged from four out of 1,100 patients (77) to eight out of 223 patients (78). Although development of this serious event has been associated with higher intravenous doses (>35 mg/day) of haloperidol, it is important to note that torsades de pointes has also been reported with low-dose intravenous haloperidol and oral haloperidol as well (78, 79). Droperidol has also been associated with lengthening of the QT interval, and it may also be associated with torsades de pointes and sudden death.

Other side effects of antipsychotic medication use can rarely include lowering of the seizure threshold, galactorrhea, elevations in liver enzyme levels, inhibition of leukopoiesis, neuroleptic malignant syndrome, and withdrawal movement disorders.

c) Implementation

Although different antipsychotic medications can be given orally, intramuscularly, or intravenously, in emergency situations or when there is lack of oral access, intravenous administration may be most effective. In addition, as described in the preceding section on side effects, there is some evidence that antipsychotic medications may cause less severe extrapyramidal side effects when administered intravenously (76). Intravenous administration of haloperidol has not yet received approval by the Food and Drug Administration (FDA).

There have been few studies to determine the optimal doses of antipsychotic medications in the treatment of delirium. On the basis of doses used in several studies, starting haloperidol in the range of 1–2 mg every 2–4 hours as needed has been suggested (80). Low doses, for example as low as 0.25–0.50 mg of haloperidol every 4 hours as needed, have been suggested for elderly patients (81). On the other hand, severely agitated patients may require titration to higher doses. Bolus intravenous haloperidol doses exceeding 50 mg with total daily doses up to 500 mg have been reported, and they were associated with minimal effects on heart rate, respiratory rate, blood pressure, and pulmonary artery pressure and minimal extrapyramidal side effects (82, 83).

Several studies (75, 84) have examined the use of continuous intravenous infusions of haloperidol or droperidol among agitated medically ill patients who have required multiple bolus intravenous injections of antipsychotic medications. The results indicate that this means of administration can be safe and may help avoid some of the complications associated with repeated bolus dosing (e.g., hypotension). The authors of one study (84) recommended continuous infusion of haloperidol for patients who required more than eight 10-mg haloperidol boluses in 24 hours or more than 10 mg/hour for more than 5 consecutive hours. They suggested initiating haloperidol with a bolus dose of 10 mg followed by continuous infusion at 5–10 mg/hour.

Because antipsychotic medications used in the treatment of delirium have occasionally been found to lengthen the QT interval, possibly leading to torsades de pointes, ventricular fibrillation, and sudden death, recommendations for medication management include a baseline ECG with special attention paid to the length of the QT_c interval. A prolongation of the QT_c interval to greater than 450 msec or to greater than 25% over that in previous ECGs may warrant telemetry, a cardiology consultation, and dose reduction or discontinuation (85, 86). It has also been recommended that serum levels of magnesium and potassium be monitored in critically ill patients, especially those whose baseline QT_c interval is 440 msec or longer, those who are receiving other drugs that increase the QT interval, or those who have electrolyte disturbances (87).

2. Benzodiazepines

a) Goals and efficacy

Few controlled studies have evaluated the efficacy of benzodiazepines as a monotherapy (i.e., not in combination with other pharmacotherapies) for the treatment of delirium. The limited data that are available suggest that benzodiazepine monotherapy may be ineffective as a treatment for general cases of delirium caused by a variety of etiologies. For example, the comparison by Breitbart et al. (70), described in section III.C.1, indicated that lorazepam, given alone, was less effective as a treatment for delirium than either haloperidol or chlorpromazine.

Although there appears to be little evidence to support the use of benzodiazepines alone for general cases of delirium, there may be certain types of delirium for which benzodiazepines have advantages and are preferable. For example, benzodiazepines are the treatment of choice for delirium related to alcohol or benzodiazepine withdrawal. Other specific clinical circumstances in which benzodiazepines may be useful include instances when there is a need for a medication that can raise the seizure threshold (unlike antipsychotics, which lower the seizure threshold) or when anticholinergic side effects or akathisia associated with antipsychotics would seriously exacerbate a patient's condition.

There have been several reports of the combination of antipsychotics and benzodiazepines for the treatment of delirium, and the results indicate that this combination may decrease medication side effects and potentially increase clinical effectiveness in special populations, for example severely ill cancer patients or AIDS patients. Results of several open studies using intravenous haloperidol along with intravenous lorazepam suggest that the combined treatment is more efficacious, with a shorter duration of the delirium and fewer extrapyramidal symptoms, than intravenous haloperidol alone (16, 63, 88). Most of these studies defined delirium according to DSM criteria but did not use standardized assessment tools.

b) Side effects

The adverse effects of benzodiazepines on mental status have received some attention. Marcantonio et al. (89) demonstrated an association between benzodiazepine use and postoperative delirium in a prospective study of psychoactive medications given to patients admitted for elective noncardiac procedures. Long-acting benzodiazepines in particular posed problems. Benzodiazepines have been associated with sedation, behavioral disinhibition, amnesia, ataxia, respiratory depression, physical dependence, rebound insomnia, withdrawal reactions, and delirium. Geriatric populations are at greater risk for the development of these complications; children and adolescents may also be at increased risk for disinhibition reactions, emotional lability, increased anxiety, hallucinations, aggression, insomnia, euphoria, and incoordination (16, 90, 91).

Benzodiazepines are generally contraindicated in delirium from hepatic encephalopathy due to accumulation of glutamine, which is related chemically to γ-aminobutyric acid (GABA). Benzodiazepines should also be avoided, or used with caution, in patients with respiratory insufficiency. For patients who have hepatic insufficiency or are taking other medications metabolized by the cytochrome P450 system, benzodiazepines that are predominantly metabolized by glucuronidation (lorazepam, oxazepam, and temazepam) should be used when a benzodiazepine is required.

c) Implementation

When benzodiazepines are used, relatively short-acting medications with no active metabolites (e.g., lorazepam) should be selected.

Few studies have investigated the optimal dose of benzodiazepines for the treatment of delirium. However, the dose must be carefully considered, given the possibility that benzodiazepines may exacerbate symptoms of delirium. In cases of delirium due specifically to alcohol or sedative-hypnotic withdrawal, higher doses of benzodiazepines and benzodiazepines with longer half-lives may be required.

In a report of a case series of 20 critically ill cancer patients for which benzodiazepines and antipsychotics were administered together, Adams et al. (63) suggested that treatment be started with 3 mg i.v. of haloperidol followed immediately by 0.5–1.0 mg i.v. of lorazepam. Additional doses and the frequency are then titrated to the patient's degree of improvement. For example, Adams et al. stated that if little or no improvement is observed within 20 minutes, an additional dose of 5 mg i.v. of haloperidol and 0.5–2.0 mg i.v. of lorazepam can be given. In some cases of severe agitation, the eventual doses of both medications have been quite large (e.g., daily doses of lorazepam between 20 and 30 mg and of haloperidol between 100 and 150 mg).

3. Cholinergics

a) Goals and efficacy

Anticholinergic mechanisms have been implicated in the pathogenesis of many medication-induced deliriums. In addition, anticholinergic mechanisms may be involved in delirium from hypoxia, hypoglycemia, thiamine deficiency, traumatic brain injury, and stroke (49). However, cholinergic medications have been used in a very limited fashion to treat delirium, almost exclusively in cases of delirium clearly caused by anticholinergic medications. Physostigmine, a centrally active cholinesterase inhibitor, has been used most often, with tacrine and donepezil receiving less attention.

In one prospective study (92), physostigmine reversed delirium among 30 patients in a postanesthesia recovery room, in whom either atropine or scopolamine had caused the delirium. In four single case reports of delirium diagnosed by clinical interviews, physostigmine reversed the delirium resulting from ranitidine (93), homatropine eyedrops (94), benztropine (95), and meperidine (96).

In a single case study (97), tacrine reversed delirium induced by anticholinergic medication. Newer cholinesterase inhibitors with fewer side effects than tacrine have not been studied for treatment of delirium.

b) Side effects

Many side effects of cholinesterase inhibitors are caused by cholinergic excess; such effects include bradycardia, nausea, vomiting, salivation, and increased gastrointestinal acid. Physostigmine can cause seizures, particularly if intravenous administration is too rapid (98). Tacrine has been associated with asymptomatic increases in liver enzyme levels. A threefold increase has been observed in approximately 30% of patients and is generally reversible with discontinuation of treatment; 5%–10% of patients develop more marked (e.g., tenfold) but still generally reversible increases in liver enzyme levels that warrant discontinuation of tacrine treatment (99).

c) Implementation

Physostigmine is usually administered parenterally. Doses that have been used in studies of delirium have included intravenous or intramuscular injections ranging from 0.16 to 2.00 mg and continuous intravenous infusions of 3 mg/hour (92–96).

In the single case study of tacrine used to reverse delirium induced by anticholinergic medication, 30 mg i.v. was used (97).

4. Vitamins

Certain vitamin deficiencies are commonly described as causing delirium. Consequently, one would expect such deliria to reverse at least to some extent with repletion of the deficient vitamin. Although this has not been subjected to rigorous trials, there are some case reports and case series supporting this effect. A malnourished hemodialysis patient with nicotinamide deficiency had a paranoid delirium that responded to parenteral nicotinamide, 500 mg/day (100). Bahr et al. (101) reported that of two chronic alcoholic patients with B vitamin deficiency, malnutrition, and central pontine myelinolysis, one improved quickly with intravenous vitamins. Thiamine deficiency delirium (DSM-III-R) was treated with vitamin B complex in six of 13 elderly medically ill patients, but only one patient had a dramatic response to treatment (102).

In one randomized controlled trial (103), 26 elderly patients undergoing orthopedic surgery received treatment with intravenous vitamins B and C preoperatively and postoperatively and were compared to 32 age-matched surgical control subjects who did not receive vitamins. There was no difference between the intervention and control groups in the incidence of postoperative confusion (39% versus 38%) or in the preoperative thiamine status as determined by serum assays.

In general, any patient with delirium who has a reason to be B vitamin deficient (e.g., alcoholic or malnourished) should be given multivitamin replacement.

5. Morphine and paralysis

Hypoxia, fatigue, and the metabolic consequences of overexertion all exacerbate delirium. Such hypercatabolic conditions are likely to accompany certain causes of agitated delirium (e.g., hyperdynamic heart failure, adult respiratory distress syndrome, hyperthyroid storm). For such patients and for any cases of agitated delirium unresponsive to other pharmacologic interventions, the patient may require a paralytic agent and mechanical ventilation. This improves oxygenation and reduces skeletal muscle exertion. The patient is usually heavily sedated. Morphine (or other opiate) is also an important palliative treatment in cases of delirium where pain is an aggravating factor (104). However, some opiates can exacerbate delirium, particularly through their metabolites, which possess anticholinergic activity (89). Among opiates, meperidine and fentanyl are particularly anticholinergic.

6. ECT

ECT has not been shown to be an effective treatment for general cases of delirium. Earlier case reports and case series had significant limitations: standardized diagnostic criteria and rating scales were not used; patients with schizophrenia, mania, postpartum psychosis, or psychotic depression were included and diagnosed with delirium because they had disorganized thinking and cognition; and few details concerning the manner in which ECT was performed were provided (105–111).

There is limited evidence for ECT as a treatment for particular cases of delirium due to specific etiologies. MEDLINE literature searches identified two case reports of ECT use for the delirium that is a component of neuroleptic malignant syndrome. In one study (112), the delirium symptoms improved in 24 of 29 patients with neuroleptic malignant syndrome who were treated with ECT. In the second study (113), 26 of 31 patients with neuroleptic malignant syndrome who were treated with ECT and hydration were described as having improved delirium symptoms. ECT has been studied in small samples of patients with delirium tremens. In one older study (109), 10 patients receiving ECT and conventional treatment had a shorter duration of delirium symptoms than 10 patients receiving conventional treatment alone (mean, 0.85 versus 2.8 days, respectively). In one case report (106), a patient with delirium tremens who had not responded to high-dose benzodiazepine treatment was described as recovering after ECT. In two case reports (114, 115), patients with protracted courses of delirium after traumatic brain injuries improved after receiving ECT. Because of the lack of compelling evidence, as well as the availability of alternative means of management, ECT is not presently used in the United States for treatment of delirium tremens.

In addition to the very limited evidence that ECT is an effective treatment for delirium, there may be considerable risks with ECT in medically unstable patients. For these reasons, ECT should be considered only rarely for patients with delirium due to specific etiologies such as neuroleptic malignant syndrome and should not be considered initially as a substitute for more conservative and conventional treatments. ECT itself may carry a risk of both postictal delirium (lasting minutes to hours) and interictal delirium (lasting days) after the procedure (116–120). Beyond that time period, ECT can also exacerbate cognitive deficits, such as memory impairment. Certain patient populations at higher risk for these adverse effects from ECT include patients with Parkinson's disease (particularly those taking carbidopa), Huntington's disease, or caudate or other basal ganglia strokes (119, 121–125).

IV. FORMULATION AND IMPLEMENTATION OF A TREATMENT PLAN

After the diagnosis of delirium is made (see section II) a treatment plan is developed. The components of the treatment plan and factors that go into a psychiatrist's choice of treatment recommendations are discussed in this section. Although the treatment of delirium involves multiple modalities, certain components are essential and should be implemented with all patients. Other components of treatment may involve a choice between specific therapies, and this choice should be guided by a careful assessment of the patient's clinical condition, etiology, and comorbid conditions.

A. PSYCHIATRIC MANAGEMENT

Psychiatric management is the cornerstone of successful treatment for delirium and should be implemented for all patients with delirium. The goals of psychiatric management are similar for all patients with delirium and involve facilitating the identification and treatment of underlying etiologies, improving patient functioning and comfort, and ensuring the safety of patients and others. The specific elements (see section III.A) include coordinating care with other clinicians; ensuring that the etiology is identified; ensuring that interventions for acute conditions are initiated; ensuring that disorder-specific treatments are provided; monitoring and ensuring safety; assessing and monitoring psychiatric status; establishing and maintaining supportive therapeutic alliances with patients, families, and other treaters; educating the patient and family regarding the illness; and postdelirium management.

B. CHOICE OF SPECIFIC ENVIRONMENTAL AND SUPPORTIVE INTERVENTIONS

One aspect of the management of delirium involves environmental interventions and cognitive-emotional support provided by nursing, general medical, and psychiatric treaters. The general goals of environmental interventions are to remove factors that exacerbate delirium while providing familiarity and an optimal level of environmental stimulation; the general goals of supportive management include reorientation, reassurance, and education concerning delirium. Specific examples of environmental and supportive interventions are given in section III.B. These interventions are recommended for all patients with delirium, on the basis of some formal evidence but mainly because of the value observed through clinical experience and the absence of adverse effects.

C. CHOICE OF SOMATIC INTERVENTION

The specific features of a patient's clinical condition, the underlying cause(s) of the delirium, and associated conditions may be used by the psychiatrist to determine the choice of specific somatic therapy. Antipsychotic medications are the pharmacologic treatment of choice in most cases of delirium because of their efficacy in the treatment of psychotic symptoms. Haloperidol is most frequently used because of its short half-life, few or no anticholinergic side effects, no active metabolites, and lower likelihood of causing sedation. Haloperidol may be administered orally or intramuscularly, but it appears to cause fewer extrapyramidal side effects when administered intravenously. An optimal dose range for patients with delirium has not been determined. Initial doses of haloperidol in the range of 1–2 mg every 2–4 hours as needed have been used, and even lower starting doses (e.g., 0.25–0.50 mg every 4 hours as needed) are suggested for elderly patients. Titration to higher doses may be required for patients who continue to be agitated. Although total daily intravenous doses in the hundreds of milligrams have been given under closely monitored conditions, much lower doses usually suffice. Continuous intravenous infusions of antipsychotic medications can be used for patients who have required multiple bolus doses of antipsychotic medications. Initiating haloperidol with a bolus dose of 10 mg followed by continuous intravenous infusion of 5–10 mg/hour has been suggested. Droperidol, either alone or followed by haloperidol, can be considered for patients with delirium and acute agitation for whom a more rapid onset of action is required. The ECG should be monitored in patients receiving antipsychotic medications for delirium, and a QT_C interval longer than 450 msec or more than 25% over baseline may warrant a cardiology consultation and consideration of discontinuation of the antipsychotic medication. The availability of new antipsychotic medications (risperidone, olanzapine, and quetiapine) with their different side effect profiles has led some physicians to use these agents for the treatment of delirium.

Benzodiazepines can exacerbate symptoms of delirium and, when used alone for general cases of delirium, have been shown to be ineffective. For these reasons, benzodiazepines as monotherapies are reserved for specific types of patients with delirium for which these medications may have particular advantages. For example, benzodiazepines are used most frequently to treat patients with delirium that has been caused by withdrawal of alcohol or benzodiazepines. When a benzodiazepine is used, medications such as lorazepam, which are relatively short-acting and have no active metabolites, are preferable. Combining a benzodiazepine with an antipsychotic medication can be considered for patients with delirium who can only tolerate lower doses of antipsychotic medications or who have prominent anxiety or agitation. Combined treatment can be started with 3 mg i.v. of haloperidol followed immediately by 0.5–1.0 mg i.v. of lorazepam and then adjusted according to the patient's degree of improvement.

Other somatic interventions have been suggested for patients with delirium who have particular clinical conditions or specific underlying etiologies; however, few data are available regarding the efficacy of these interventions in treating delirium. There is some suggestion that cholinergics such as physostigmine and tacrine may be useful in delirium caused by anticholinergic medications. Agitated patients with delirium with hypercatabolic conditions (e.g., hyperdynamic heart failure, adult respiratory distress syndrome, hyperthyroid storm) may require paralysis and mechanical ventilation. For patients with delirium in whom pain is an aggravating factor, palliative treatment with an opiate such as morphine is recommended. ECT may be a treatment consideration in a few cases of delirium due to a specific etiology such as neuroleptic malignant syndrome; any potential benefit of ECT should be weighed against the risks of ECT for patients who are often medically unstable. Any patient with delirium with a reason to be deficient in B vitamins (e.g., alcoholic or malnourished) should be given multivitamin replacement.

▶ D. ISSUES OF COMPETENCY AND CONSENT

Decisions regarding the care of patients with delirium are often complex because of risks associated with treatments, and these decisions frequently have to be made quickly because of the seriousness of the underlying general medical conditions. Unfortunately, delirium intermittently affects consciousness, attention, and cognition and can impair a patient's decisional capacity (i.e., the ability to make decisions as determined by a clinician's evaluation) or competence (i.e., the ability to make decisions as determined by a court of law) (126, 127).

The presence or diagnosis of delirium does not in itself mean that a patient is incompetent or lacks capacity to give informed consent (128). Instead, a determination of decisional capacity or competence to give informed consent involves formal assessment of a patient's understanding about the proposed intervention (including the intervention's risks, benefits, and alternatives) and the consequences of the decisions to be made.

Decision-making guidelines have been suggested for patients with delirium who lack decisional capacity or competence to give informed consent (129). The urgency with which treatment is needed and the risks and benefits of treatments can be used by the treating physician to choose between several alternative courses of action. In medical emergencies requiring prompt intervention, the first alternative is to treat the patient with delirium without informed consent, under the common law doctrine of implied consent (i.e., that treatment may be provided in medical emergencies without informed consent if it is appropriate treatment that a reasonable person would want). In nonemergency situations, the clinician should obtain input or consent from surrogates. Involving interested family members can be especially helpful for choosing among equally beneficial interventions that involve low or moderate risks. The opinion of a second clinician can be useful for making decisions involving more uncertainty or interventions associated with greater risks. Obtaining the consultation of a hospital's administrator, risk manager, or legal counsel may also provide a means for reassuring family members and the treatment team that reasonable decisions are being made. For decisions that involve significant risks or substantial disagreements involving family members, a court-appointed guardian can be sought if time permits. In more emergent cases, an urgent hearing with a judge may be required. All assessments of a patient's decisional capacity or competence and the reasons for a particular course of action should be documented in the patient's medical record.

V. CLINICAL FEATURES INFLUENCING TREATMENT

▶ A. COMORBID PSYCHIATRIC DISORDERS

Delirium is often misdiagnosed as depression or dementia. These disorders can be diagnosed during a delirium only when the patient's history reveals symptoms that clearly existed before the delirium onset. When delirium is comorbid with other psychiatric disorders, the delirium should be treated first and the treatments for these other disorders, such as antidepressant or anxiolytic medications, should be minimized or not begun until the delirium is resolved. Medications for psychiatric disorders can both be the cause of delirium and exacerbate or contribute to delirium from other causes.

B. COMORBID GENERAL MEDICAL CONDITIONS

1. AIDS/HIV

Approximately 30%–40% of hospitalized AIDS patients develop delirium (6, 16, 70). Early reports concerning the increased sensitivity of AIDS patients to the extrapyramidal side effects of dopamine-blocking antipsychotic drugs have made clinicians cautious in using high doses of antipsychotics, such as haloperidol (130, 131). At lower doses, antipsychotics such as haloperidol and chlorpromazine have been demonstrated to be safe and effective with minimal extrapyramidal side effects (70).

2. Liver disease

The liver is the body's detoxifying organ for drugs and other molecules. Hepatic insufficiency significantly affects the metabolism of many medications. Most psychotropic medications undergo hepatic transformation. In addition, the liver produces albumin and other plasma proteins that transport bound medications in the bloodstream. When these protein levels decrease because of liver dysfunction, unbound medications can enter tissues at an accelerated rate—including crossing the blood-brain barrier—and can also be more available for catabolism or excretion. Thus, the former effect may alter therapeutic effects or cause side effects, while the latter may result in less therapeutic effect than expected at a given dose.

Haloperidol undergoes metabolism by the P450 2D6 enzyme system, which reduces it to reduced haloperidol. The latter is in equilibrium with the parent drug. In addition, glucuronidation is an important route of metabolism of haloperidol (132). This suggests that its pharmacokinetics in patients with liver insufficiency would be similar to those in other patients when used to treat delirium.

On the other hand, many benzodiazepines require oxidation by the liver. The exceptions are lorazepam, temazepam, and oxazepam, which require only glucuronidation. It is therefore preferred that benzodiazepines requiring only glucuronidation be used to treat delirium secondary to sedative-hypnotic or alcohol withdrawal in patients who have liver insufficiency. Of these, lorazepam is usually chosen because it is well absorbed when given orally, intramuscularly, or intravenously.

C. ADVANCED AGE

The elderly are particularly vulnerable to delirium due to changes in brain function, multiple general medical problems, polypharmacy, reduced hepatic metabolism of medications, multisensory declines, and brain disorders such as dementia. Conducting a careful medical evaluation that includes particular attention to a patient's level of oxygenation, possible occult infection (e.g., urinary tract infection), and the possible role of medications is an essential initial approach to the management of delirium in the elderly. Medications with anticholinergic effects are often the culprit; however, even medications not generally recognized as possessing anticholinergic effects (e.g., meperidine, digoxin, and ranitidine) can be responsible (133–135). Nursing home patients are at particular risk of delirium.

Low doses of antipsychotic medication usually suffice in treating delirium in elderly patients, for example, beginning with 0.5 mg haloperidol once or twice a day. The benefits of restraints may be greater for elderly patients than for younger patients because of the greater risk of falls and hip fractures in older populations; hip and other fractures often carry a grim prognosis for elderly patients, who may never return to independent functioning. On the other hand, the risks associated with restraints may be greater among the elderly, and other means to prevent falls should be considered if possible. When extrapyramidal side effects occur early in the treatment of delirium, Lewy body dementia should be considered in the differential diagnosis.

VI. REVIEWERS AND REVIEWING ORGANIZATIONS

Larry Altstiel, M.D.
Varda Peller Backus, M.D.
William T. Beecroft, M.D.
Jeffrey L. Berlant, M.D.
D. Peter Birkett, M.D.
Charles H. Blackinton, M.D.
Mel Blaustein, M.D.
Barton J. Blinder, M.D.
Harold E. Bronheim, M.D.
Thomas Markham Brown, M.D.
Stephanie Cavanaugh, M.D.
Christopher C. Colenda, M.D.
Dave M. Davis, M.D.
Horace A. DeFord, M.D.
Prakash Desai, M.D.
Joel E. Dimsdale, M.D.
Ann Maxwell Eward, Ph.D.
Laura J. Fochtmann, M.D.
David G. Folks, M.D.
Gilles L. Fraser, Pharm.D.
Richard K. Fuller, M.D.
Dolores Gallagher-Thompson
Larry Goldman, M.D.
Sheila Hafter Gray, M.D.
Robert M. Greenberg, M.D.
Jon E. Gudeman, M.D.
Edward Hanin, M.D.
Carla T. Herrerias, M.P.H.
Daniel W. Hicks, M.D.
John Hughes, M.D.
Keith Isenberg, M.D.
Sue C. Jacobs, Ph.D.
Sandra Jacobson, M.D.

Leslie Dotson Jaggers, Pharm.D.
Charles Kaelber, M.D.
Barbara Kamholz, M.D.
Gary Kaplan, M.D.
Fred Karlin, M.D.
Roger G. Kathol, M.D.
Sherry Katz-Bearnot, M.D.
David J. Knesper, M.D.
Bob G. Knight, Ph.D.
Ronald R. Koegler, M.D.
Sharon Levine, M.D.
Glenn Lippman, M.D.
Rex S. Lott, Pharm.D.
Velandy Manohar, M.D.
Peter J. Manos, M.D., Ph.D.
James R. McCartney, M.D.
Dinesh Mittel, M.D.
Kevin O'Connor, M.D.
Joseph F. O'Neill, M.D.
Edmond H. Pi, M.D.
Michael K. Popkin, M.D.
Peter V. Rabins, M.D.
Stephen R. Rapp, M.D.
Vaughn I. Rickert, Psy.D.
Jonathan Ritro, M.D.
Laura Roberts, M.D.
Stephen M. Saravay, M.D.
Marc A. Schuckit, M.D.
Ben Seltzer, M.D.
Todd Semla, Pharm.D.
David Servan-Schreiber, M.D., Ph.D.
Elisabeth J. Shakin Kunkel, M.D.
Winston W. Shen, M.D.

Edward Silberman, M.D.
Theodore A. Stern, M.D.
Janice Zalen Stiers
John Tanquary, M.D.
William R. Tatomer, M.D.
Larry E. Tripp, M.D.
Vera Trzepacz, M.D.
Gary J. Tucker, M.D.
Peter VanDyck, M.D.

John Wattis, M.D.
William Weddington, M.D.
Richard D. Weiner, M.D.
Joseph Westermeyer, M.D., M.P.H., Ph.D.
Donald Wexler, M.D.
Thomas N. Wise, M.D.
Linda Worley, M.D.
William Zurhellen, M.D.

Alabama Department of Mental Health and Mental Retardation
American Academy of Pediatrics
American College of Emergency Physicians
American Society of Health-System Pharmacists
Association for Academic Psychiatry
Association for the Advancement of Behavior Therapy
Association of Gay and Lesbian Psychiatrists
Group for the Advancement of Psychiatry
Michigan Psychiatric Society
National Institute on Alcohol Abuse and Alcoholism
Society of Adolescent Medicine
U.S. Department of Health and Human Services—HIV/AIDS Bureau

VII. REFERENCES

The following coding system is used to indicate the nature of the supporting evidence in the references:

[A]   *Randomized clinical trial.* A study of an intervention in which subjects are prospectively followed over time; there are treatment and control groups; subjects are randomly assigned to the two groups; both the subjects and the investigators are blind to the assignments.

[B]   *Clinical trial.* A prospective study in which an intervention is made and the results of that intervention are tracked longitudinally; study does not meet standards for a randomized clinical trial.

[C]   *Cohort or longitudinal study.* A study in which subjects are prospectively followed over time without any specific intervention.

[D]   *Case-control study.* A study in which a group of patients and a group of control subjects are identified in the present and information about them is pursued retrospectively or backward in time.

[E]   *Review with secondary data analysis.* A structured analytic review of existing data, e.g., a meta-analysis or a decision analysis.

[F]   *Review.* A qualitative review and discussion of previously published literature without a quantitative synthesis of the data.

[G]   *Other.* Textbooks, expert opinion, case reports, and other reports not included above.

1. American Psychiatric Association: Diagnostic and Statistical Manual of Mental Disorders, 4th ed (DSM-IV). Washington, DC, APA, 1994 [F]
2. Lipowski ZJ: Delirium (acute confusional states). JAMA 1987; 258:1789–1792 [F]
3. Lipowski ZJ: Delirium: Acute Confusional States. New York, Oxford University Press, 1990 [G]
4. Ross CA, Peyser CE, Shapiro I: Delirium: phenomenologic and etiologic subtypes. Int Psychogeriatr 1991; 3:135–147 [F]
5. Stiefel F, Holland J: Delirium in cancer patients. Int Psychogeriatr 1991; 3:333–336 [F]
6. Perry S: Organic mental disorders caused by HIV: update on early diagnosis and treatment. Am J Psychiatry 1990; 147:696–710 [F]
7. Tune LE: Post-operative delirium. Int Psychogeriatr 1991; 3:325–332 [F]
8. Massie MJ, Holland J, Glass E: Delirium in terminally ill cancer patients. Am J Psychiatry 1983; 140:1048–1050 [C, G]
9. Rockwood K: The occurrence and duration of symptoms in elderly patients with delirium. J Gerontol 1993; 48:M162–M166 [C]
10. Sirois F: Delirium: 100 cases. Can J Psychiatry 1988; 33:375–378 [D]
11. Koponen H, Stenback U, Mattila E: Delirium among elderly persons admitted to a psychiatric hospital: clinical course during the acute stage and one-year follow-up. Acta Psychiatr Scand 1989; 79:579–585 [D]
12. Koizumi J, Shiraishi H, Suzuki T: Duration of delirium shortened by the correction of electrolyte imbalance. Jpn J Psychiatry Neurol 1988; 42:81–88 [D]
13. Rockwood K: Acute confusion in elderly medical patients. J Am Geriatr Soc 1989; 37:150–154 [C]
14. Manos PJ, Wu R: The duration of delirium in medical and postoperative patients referred for psychiatric consultation. Ann Clin Psychiatry 1997; 9:219–226 [C]
15. Levkoff SE, Evans DA, Liptzin B, Cleary PD, Lipsitz LA, Wetle TT, Reilly CH, Pilgrim DM, Schor J, Rowe J: Delirium: the occurrence and persistence of symptoms among elderly hospitalized patients. Arch Intern Med 1992; 152:334–340 [C]
16. Fernandez F, Levy JK, Mansell PWA: Management of delirium in terminally ill AIDS patients. Int J Psychiatry Med 1989; 19:165–172 [C]
17. Inouye S, Horowitz R, Tinetti M, Berkman L: Acute confusional states in the hospitalized elderly: incidence, risk factors and complications (abstract). Clin Res 1989; 37:524A [C]
18. Cole MG, Primeau FJ: Prognosis of delirium in elderly hospital patients. Can Med Assoc J 1993; 149:41–46 [E]
19. Rogers M, Liang M, Daltroy L: Delirium after elective orthopedic surgery: risk factors and natural history. Int J Psychiatry Med 1989; 19:109–121 [C]
20. Gustafson Y, Berggren D, Brannstrom B, Bucht G, Norberg A, Hansson LI, Winblad B: Acute confusional states in elderly patients treated for femoral neck fracture. J Am Geriatr Soc 1988; 36:525–530 [C]
21. Antoon AY, Volpe JJ, Crawford JD: Burn encephalopathy in children. Pediatrics 1972; 50:609–616 [C]
22. Rabins PV, Folstein MF: Delirium and dementia: diagnostic criteria and fatality rates. Br J Psychiatry 1982; 140:149–153 [C]
23. Varsamis J, Zuchowski T, Maini KK: Survival rates and causes of death in geriatric psychiatric patients: a six-year follow-up study. Can Psychiatr Assoc J 1972; 17:17–22 [C]
24. Cameron DJ, Thomas RI, Mulvihill M, Bronheim H: Delirium: a test of the Diagnostic and Statistical Manual III criteria on medical inpatients. J Am Geriatr Soc 1987; 35:1007–1010 [C]
25. Trzepacz P, Teague G, Lipowski Z: Delirium and other organic mental disorders in a general hospital. Gen Hosp Psychiatry 1985; 7:101–106 [G]
26. Weddington WW: The mortality of delirium: an under-appreciated problem? Psychosomatics 1982; 23:1232–1235 [E, F]

27. Inouye SK: The dilemma of delirium: clinical and research controversies regarding diagnosis and evaluation of delirium in hospitalized elderly medical patients. Am J Med 1994; 97:278–288 [F]

28. Francis J, Kapoor WN: Delirium in hospitalized elderly. J Gen Intern Med 1990; 5:65–79 [F]

29. Smith MJ, Breitbart WS, Platt MM: A critique of instruments and methods to detect, diagnose, and rate delirium. J Pain Symptom Manage 1995; 10:35–77 [F]

30. Trzepacz PT: A review of delirium assessment instruments. Gen Hosp Psychiatry 1994; 16:397–405 [F]

31. Levkoff S, Liptzin B, Cleary P, Reilly CH, Evans D: Review of research instruments and techniques used to detect delirium. Int Psychogeriatr 1991; 3:253–271 [F]

32. Vermeersch PE: The Clinical Assessment of Confusion—A. Appl Nurs Res 1990; 3:128–133 [D]

33. Williams MA, Ward SE, Campbell EB: Confusion: testing versus observation. J Gerontol Nurs 1988; 14:25–30 [D]

34. Rutherford L, Sessler C, Levenson JL, Hart R, Best A: Prospective evaluation of delirium and agitation in a medical intensive care unit (abstract). Crit Care Med 1991; 19:S81 [C]

35. Neelon V, Champagne MT, Carlson JR, Funk SG: The NEECHAM Confusion Scale: construction, validation, and clinical testing. Nurs Res 1996; 45:324–330 [C]

36. Albert MS, Levkoff SE, Reilly C, Liptzin B, Pilgrim D, Cleary PD, Evans D, Rowe JW: The Delirium Symptom Interview: an interview for the detection of delirium symptoms in hospitalized patients. J Geriatr Psychiatry Neurol 1992; 5:14–21 [C]

37. Inouye SK, van Dyck CH, Alessi CA, Balkin S, Siegal AP, Horwitz RI: Clarifying confusion: the confusion assessment method, a new method for the detection of delirium. Ann Intern Med 1990; 113:941–948 [C]

38. Lowy F, Engelsmann F, Lipowski Z: Study of cognitive functioning in a medical population. Compr Psychiatry 1973; 14:331–338 [C]

39. Anthony JC, LeResche LA, Von Korff MR, Niaz U, Folstein MF: Screening for delirium on a general medical ward: the tachistoscope and a global accessibility rating. Gen Hosp Psychiatry 1985; 7:36–42 [C]

40. Gustafsson I, Lindgren M, Westling B: The OBS Scale: a new rating scale for evaluation of confusional states and other organic brain syndromes (abstract). Presented at the II International Congress on Psychogeriatric Medicine, Umeå, Sweden, Aug 28–31, 1985, abstract 128 [G]

41. Miller PS, Richardson JS, Jyu CA, Lemay JS, Hiscock M, Keegan DL: Association of low serum anticholinergic levels and cognitive impairment in elderly presurgical patients. Am J Psychiatry 1988; 145:342–345 [A]

42. Trzepacz P, Baker R, Greenhouse J: A symptom rating scale for delirium. Psychiatry Res 1988; 23:89–97 [C]

43. Breitbart W, Rosenfeld B, Roth F, Smith MJ, Cohen K, Passik S: The Memorial Delirium Assessment Scale. J Pain Symptom Manage 1997; 13:128–137 [C]

44. Engel G, Romano J: Delirium, a syndrome of cerebral insufficiency. J Chronic Dis 1959; 9:260–277 [G]

45. Pro J, Wells C: The use of the electroencephalogram in the diagnosis of delirium. Dis Nerv Syst 1977; 38:804–808 [D]

46. Tsai L, Tsuang MT: The Mini-Mental State test and computerized tomography. Am J Psychiatry 1979; 136:436–439 [C]

47. Hemmingsen R, Vorstrup S, Clemmesen L, Holm S, Tfelt-Hansen P, Sørensen AS, Hansen C, Sommer W, Bolwig TG: Cerebral blood flow during delirium tremens and related clinical states studied with xenon-133 inhalation tomography. Am J Psychiatry 1988; 145:1384–1390 [C]

48. Golinger RC, Peet T, Tune LE: Association of elevated plasma anticholinergic activity with delirium in surgical patients. Am J Psychiatry 1987; 144:1218–1220 [C]

49. Trzepacz PT, Wise MG: Neuropsychiatric aspects of delirium, in American Psychiatric Press Textbook of Neuropsychiatry. Edited by Yudofsky SC, Hales RE. Washington, DC, American Psychiatric Press, 1997, pp 447–470 [G]

50. Inouye SK, Charpentier PA: Precipitating factors for delirium in hospitalized elderly persons: predictive model and interrelationships with baseline vulnerability. JAMA 1996; 275:852–857 [C]

51. American Psychiatric Association: Seclusion and Restraint: Psychiatric Uses. Washington, DC, APA, 1984, addendum 1992 [G]

52. Joint Commission on Accreditation of Healthcare Organizations: 1998 Accreditation Manual for Hospitals. Oak Brook Terrace, Ill, JCAHO, 1998 [G]

53. Inouye SK, Viscoli CM, Horwitz RI: A predictive model for delirium in hospitalized elderly medical patients based on admission characteristics. Ann Intern Med 1993; 119:474–481 [C]

54. Hashimoto H, Yamashiro M: Postoperative delirium and abnormal behaviour related with preoperative quality of life in elderly patients. Nippon Ronen Igakkai Zasshi 1994; 31:633–638 [C]

55. Lazarus HR, Hagens JH: Prevention of psychosis following open-heart surgery. Am J Psychiatry 1968; 124:1190–1195 [B]

56. Budd S, Brown W: Effect of a reorientation technique on postcardiotomy delirium. Nurs Res 1974; 23:341–348 [B]

57. Williams MA, Campbell EB, Raynor WJ, Mlynarczyk SM, Ward SE: Reducing acute confusional states in elderly patients with hip fractures. Res Nurs Health 1985; 8:329–337 [B]

58. Cole MG, Primeau FJ, Bailey RF, Bonnycastle MJ, Masciarelli F, Engelsmann F, Pepin MJ, Ducic D: Systematic intervention for elderly inpatients with delirium: a randomized trial. Can Med Assoc J 1994; 151:965–970 [A]

59. Meagher DJ, O'Hanlon D, O'Mahony E, Casey PR: The use of environmental strategies and psychotropic medication in the management of delirium. Br J Psychiatry 1996; 168:512–515 [C]

60. Allen JG, Lewis L, Blum S, Voorhees S, Jernigan S, Peebles MJ: Informing psychiatric patients and their families about neuropsychological assessment findings. Bull Menninger Clin 1986; 50:64–74 [G]

61. Sipahimalani A, Masand PS: Use of risperidone in delirium: case reports. Ann Clin Psychiatry 1997; 9:105–107 [G]

62. Ravona-Springer R, Dolberg OT, Hirschmann S, Grunhaus L: Delirium in elderly patients treated with risperidone: a report of three cases (letter). J Clin Psychopharmacol 1998; 18:171–172 [G]

63. Adams F, Fernandez F, Andersson BS: Emergency pharmacotherapy of delirium in the critically ill cancer patient. Psychosomatics 1986; 27(suppl 1):33–38 [F]

64. Muskin P, Mellman L, Kornfeld D: A "new" drug for treating agitation and psychosis in the general hospital: chlorpromazine. Gen Hosp Psychiatry 1986; 8:404–410 [D]

65. Rosen H: Double-blind comparison of haloperidol and thioridazine in geriatric patients. J Clin Psychiatry 1979; 40:17–20 [A]

66. Smith G, Taylor C, Linkous P: Haloperidol versus thioridazine for the treatment of psychogeriatric patients: a double-blind clinical trial. Psychosomatics 1974; 15:134–138 [A]

67. Tsuang MM, Lu LM, Stotsky BA, Cole JO: Haloperidol versus thioridazine for hospitalized psychogeriatric patients: double-blind study. J Am Geriatr Soc 1971; 19:593–600 [A]

68. Kirven LE, Montero EF: Comparison of thioridazine and diazepam in the control of nonpsychotic symptoms associated with senility: double-blind study. J Am Geriatr Soc 1973; 12:546–551 [A]

69. Thomas H, Schwartz E, Petrilli R: Droperidol versus haloperidol for chemical restraint of agitated and combative patients. Ann Emerg Med 1992; 21:407–413 [A]

70. Breitbart W, Marotta R, Platt MM, Weisman H, Derevenco M, Grau C, Corbera K, Raymond S, Lund S, Jacobsen P: A double-blind trial of haloperidol, chlorpromazine, and lorazepam in the treatment of delirium in hospitalized AIDS patients. Am J Psychiatry 1996; 153:231–237 [A]

71. van Leeuwen A, Molders J, Sterkmans P, Mielants P, Martens C, Toussaint C, Hovent A, Desseilles M, Koch H, Devroye A, Parent M: Droperidol in acutely agitated patients. J Nerv Ment Dis 1977; 164:280–283 [B]

72. Resnick M, Burton B: Droperidol vs haloperidol in the initial management of acutely agitated patients. J Clin Psychiatry 1984; 45:298–299 [A]

73. Chen B, Cardasis W: Delirium induced by lithium and risperidone combination (letter). Am J Psychiatry 1996; 153:1233–1234 [D]

74. Sipahimalani A, Sime RM, Masand PS: Treatment of delirium with risperidone. Int J Geriatric Psychopharmacology 1997; 1:24–26 [G]

75. Frye MA, Coudreaut MF, Hakeman SM, Shah BG, Strouse TB, Skotzko CE: Continuous droperidol infusion for management of agitated delirium in an intensive care unit. Psychosomatics 1995; 36:301–305 [G]

76. Menza MA, Murray GB, Holmes VF, Rafuls WA: Decreased extrapyramidal symptoms with intravenous haloperidol. J Clin Psychiatry 1987; 48:278–280 [B]

77. Wilt JL, Minnema AM, Johnson RF, Rosenblum AM: Torsade de pointes associated with the use of intravenous haloperidol. Ann Intern Med 1993; 119:391–394 [G]

78. Sharma ND, Rosman HS, Padhi D, Tisdale JE: Torsades de pointes associated with intravenous haloperidol in critically ill patients. Am J Cardiol 1998; 81:238–240 [G]

79. Jackson T, Ditmanson L, Phibbs B: Torsades de pointes and low-dose oral haloperidol. Arch Intern Med 1997; 157:2013–2015 [G]

80. Tesar GE, Murray GB, Cassem NH: Use of high-dose intravenous haloperidol in the treatment of agitated cardiac patients. J Clin Psychopharmacol 1985; 5:344–347 [G]

81. Liptzin B: Delirium, in Comprehensive Review of Geriatric Psychiatry, 2nd ed. Edited by Sadavoy J, Lazarus LW, Jarvik LF, Grossberg GT. Washington, DC, American Psychiatric Press, 1996, pp 479–495 [G]

82. Stern TA: The management of depression and anxiety following myocardial infarction. Mt Sinai J Med 1985; 52:623–633 [G]

83. Levenson JL: High-dose intravenous haloperidol for agitated delirium following lung transplantation. Psychosomatics 1995; 36:66–68 [G]

84. Riker RR, Fraser GL, Cox PM: Continuous infusion of haloperidol controls agitation in critically ill patients. Crit Care Med 1994; 22:433–439 [D]

85. Metzger E, Friedman R: Prolongation of the corrected QT and torsades de pointes cardiac arrhythmia associated with intravenous haloperidol in the medically ill. J Clin Psychopharmacol 1993; 13:128–132 [G]

86. Hunt N, Stern TA: The association between intravenous haloperidol and torsades de pointes: three cases and a literature review. Psychosomatics 1995; 36:541–549 [F, G]

87. Lawrence KR, Nasraway SA: Conduction disturbances associated with administration of butyrophenone antipsychotics in the critically ill: a review of the literature. Pharmacotherapy 1997; 17:531–537 [F]

88. Menza MA, Murray GB, Holmes VF: Controlled study of extrapyramidal reactions in the management of delirious medically ill patients: intravenous haloperidol versus intravenous haloperidol plus benzodiazepines. Heart Lung 1988; 17:238–241 [B]

89. Marcantonio ER, Goldman L, Mangione CM, Ludwig LE, Muraca B, Haslauer CM, Donaldson MC, Whittemore AD, Sugarbaker DJ, Poss R, Haas S, Cook EF, Orav EJ, Lee TH: A clinical prediction rule for delirium after elective noncardiac surgery. JAMA 1994; 271:134–139 [C]

90. Coffey B, Shader RI, Greenblatt DJ: Pharmacokinetics of benzodiazepines and psychostimulants in children. J Clin Psychopharmacol 1983; 3:217–225 [F]

91. Reiter S, Kutcher SP: Disinhibition and anger outbursts in adolescents treated with clonazepam (letter). J Clin Psychopharmacol 1991; 11:268 [G]

92. Greene LT: Physostigmine treatment of anticholinergic-drug depression in postoperative patients. Anesth Analg 1971; 50:222–226 [C]

93. Goff DC, Garber HJ, Jenike MA: Partial resolution of ranitidine-associated delirium with physostigmine: case report. J Clin Psychiatry 1985; 46:400–401 [G]

94. Delberghe X, Zegers de Beyl D: Repeated delirium from homatropine eyedrops. Clin Neurol Neurosurg 1987; 89:53–54 [G]

95. Stern TA: Continuous infusion of physostigmine in anticholinergic delirium: case report. J Clin Psychiatry 1983; 44:463–464 [G]

96. Eisendrath SJ, Goldman B, Douglas J, Dimatteo L, Van Dyke C: Meperidine-induced delirium. Am J Psychiatry 1987; 144:1062–1065 [D]

97. Mendelson G: Pheniramine aminosalicylate overdosage: reversal of delirium and choreiform movements with tacrine treatment. Arch Neurol 1977; 34:313 [G]

98. Physicians Desk Reference, 52nd ed. Montvale, NJ, Medical Economics Co, 1998 [G]

99. Watkins PB, Zimmerman HJ, Knapp MJ, Gracon SI, Lewis KW: Hepatoxic effects of tacrine administration in patients with Alzheimer's disease. JAMA 1994; 271:992–998 [A]

100. Waterlot Y, Sabot JP, Marchal M, Vanherweghem JL: Pellagra: unusual cause of paranoid delirium in dialysis. Nephrol Dial Transplant 1986; 1:204–205 [G]

101. Bahr M, Sommer N, Petersen D, Wietholter H, Dichgans J: Central pontine myelinolysis associated with low potassium levels in alcoholism. J Neurol 1990; 237:275–276 [G]

102. O'Keeffe ST, Tormey WP, Glasgow R, Lavan JN: Thiamine deficiency in hospitalized elderly patients. Gerontology 1994; 40:18–24 [G]

103. Day JJ, Bayer AJ, McMahon M, Pathy MS, Spragg BP, Rolands DC: Thiamine status, vitamin supplements and postoperative confusion. Age Ageing 1988; 17:29–34 [A]

104. Shapiro BA, Warren J, Egol AB, Greenbaum DM, Jacobi J, Nasraway SA, Schein RM, Spevetz A, Stone JR: Practice parameters for intravenous analgesia and sedation for adult patients in the intensive care unit: an executive summary. Society of Critical Care Medicine. Crit Care Med 1995; 23:1596–1600 [F]

105. Stromgren LS: ECT in acute delirium and related clinical states. Convuls Ther 1997; 13:10–17 [G]

106. Kramp P, Bolwig TG: Electroconvulsive therapy in acute delirious states. Compr Psychiatry 1981; 22:368–371 [G]

107. Krystal AD, Coffey CE: Neuropsychiatric considerations in the use of electroconvulsive therapy. J Neuropsychiatry Clin Neurosci 1997; 9:283–292 [G]

108. Fink M: Convulsive therapy in delusional disorders. Psychiatr Clin North Am 1995; 18:393–406 [F]

109. Dudley WHC, Williams JG: Electroconvulsive therapy in delirium tremens. Compr Psychiatry 1972; 13:357–360 [F]

110. Zwil AS, Pelchat RJ: ECT in the treatment of patients with neurological and somatic disease. Int J Psychiatry Med 1994; 24:1–29 [F]

111. Roberts AH: The value of ECT in delirium. Br J Psychiatry 1963; 109:653–655 [G]

112. Davis JM, Janicak PJ, Sakkar P, Gilmore C, Wang Z: Electroconvulsive therapy in the treatment of the neuroleptic malignant syndrome. Convuls Ther 1991; 7:111–120 [E]

113. Shefner WA, Shulman RB: Treatment choice in neuroleptic malignant syndrome. Convuls Ther 1998; 8:267–279 [F, G]

114. Silverman M: Organic stupor subsequent to severe head injury treated with ECT. Br J Psychiatry 1964; 110:648–650 [G]

115. Kant R, Bogyi A, Carasella N, Fishman E, Kane V, Coffey E: ECT as a therapeutic option in severe brain injury. Convuls Ther 1995; 11:45–50 [G]

116. Burke WJ, Rubin EH, Zorumski CP, Wetzel RD: The safety of ECT in geriatric psychiatry. J Am Geriatr Soc 1987; 35:516–521 [B]

117. Calev A, Gaudino EA, Squires NK, Zervas IM, Fink M: ECT and non-memory cognition: a review. Br J Clin Psychol 1995; 34:505–515 [F]

118. Devanand DP, Fitzsimons L, Prudic J, Sackeim HA: Subjective side effects during electro-convulsive therapy. Convuls Ther 1995; 11:232–240 [A]

119. Fink M: Post-ECT delirium. Convuls Ther 1993; 9:326–330 [F]

120. Nelson JP, Rosenberg DR: ECT treatment of demented elderly patients with major depression: a retrospective study of efficacy and safety. Convuls Ther 1991; 7:157–165 [D]

121. Martin M, Figiel G, Mattingly G, Zorumski CF, Jarvis MR: ECT-induced interictal delirium in patients with a history of a CVA. J Geriatr Psychiatry Neurol 1992; 5:149–155 [B]

122. Figiel GS, Coffey CE, Djang WT, Hoffman G Jr, Doraiswamy PM: Brain magnetic resonance imaging findings in ECT-induced delirium. J Neuropsychiatry Clin Neurosci 1990; 2:53–58 [G]

123. Figiel GS, Krishnan KR, Doraiswamy PM: Subcortical structural changes in ECT-induced delirium. J Geriatr Psychiatry Neurol 1990; 3:172–176 [G]

124. Figiel GS, Hassen MA, Zorumski C, Krishnan KR, Doraiswamy PM, Jarvis MR, Smith DS: ECT-induced delirium in depressed patients with Parkinson's disease. J Neuropsychiatry Clin Neurosci 1991; 3:405–411 [G]

125. Zervas IM, Fink M: ECT and delirium in Parkinson's disease (letter). Am J Psychiatry 1992; 149:1758 [G]

126. Parry JW: In defense of lawyers. Hosp Community Psychiatry 1988; 39:1108–1109 [G]

127. Grossberg GT, Zimny GH: Medical-legal issues, in Comprehensive Review of Geriatric Psychiatry, 2nd ed. Edited by Sadavoy J, Lazarus LW, Jarvik LF, Grossberg GT. Washington, DC, American Psychiatric Press, 1996, pp 1037–1049 [G]

128. Goldstein R: Non compos mentis: the psychiatrist's role in guardianship and conservatorship proceedings involving the elderly, in Geriatric Psychiatry and the Law. Edited by Rosner R, Schwartz HI. New York, Plenum, 1987, pp 269–278 [G]

129. Fogel B, Mills M, Landen J: Legal aspects of the treatment of delirium. Hosp Community Psychiatry 1986; 37:154–158 [F]

130. Breitbart W, Marotta RF, Call P: AIDS and neuroleptic malignant syndrome. Lancet 1988; 2:1488–1489 [D]

131. Hriso E, Kuhn T, Masdeu JC, Grundman M: Extrapyramidal symptoms due to dopamine-blocking agents in patients with AIDS encephalopathy. Am J Psychiatry 1991; 148:1558–1561 [D]

132. Someya T, Shibasaki M, Noguchi T, Takahashi S, Inaba T: Haloperidol metabolism in psychiatric patients: importance of glucuronidation and carbamyl reduction. J Clin Psychopharmacol 1992; 12:169–174 [B]

133. Tune L, Carr S, Hoag E, Cooper T: Anticholinergic effects of drugs commonly prescribed for the elderly: potential means for assessing risk of delirium. Am J Psychiatry 1992; 149:1393–1394 [G]

134. Tune L, Carr S, Cooper T: Association of anticholinergic activity of prescribed medications with postoperative delirium. J Neuropsychiatry Clin Neurosci 1993; 5:208–210 [C]

135. Tune LE, Damlouji NF, Holland A, Gardner TJ, Folstein MF, Coyle JT: Association of postoperative delirium with raised serum levels of anticholinergic drugs. Lancet 1981; 2:651–653 [C]

PRACTICE GUIDELINE FOR THE
Treatment of Patients With Alzheimer's Disease and Other Dementias of Late Life

WORK GROUP ON ALZHEIMER'S DISEASE AND RELATED DEMENTIAS

Peter Rabins, M.D., M.P.H., Chair

Deborah Blacker, M.D., Sc.D. (Consultant)
Walter Bland, M.D.
Lory Bright-Long, M.D.
Eugene Cohen, M.D.
Ira Katz, M.D.
Barry Rovner, M.D.
Lon Schneider, M.D.

NOTE TO THE READER

In this practice guideline, treatment recommendations are discussed in sections IV and V and are summarized in section I. Data regarding the safety and efficacy of available treatments are reviewed in section III.

This practice guideline was approved in December 1996 and was published in *The American Journal of Psychiatry* in May 1997.

CONTENTS

INTRODUCTION

This guideline seeks to summarize data to inform the care of patients with dementia of the Alzheimer's type (referred to here as Alzheimer's disease) and other dementias associated with aging, including vascular dementia, Parkinson's disease, Lewy body disease, and Pick's and other frontal lobe dementias. The guideline does not purport to cover dementias associated with general medical conditions, such as human immunodeficiency virus (HIV) infection, Huntington's disease, head trauma, structural lesions, or endocrine and metabolic disturbances. However, while many of the research data on which the recommendations are based come from the study of Alzheimer's disease and to a lesser extent vascular dementia, many of the recommendations regarding the management of cognitive and functional changes and behavioral complications apply to dementia in general.

The guideline begins at the point where the psychiatrist has diagnosed a patient with a dementing disorder according to the criteria in DSM-IV (1) and has evaluated the patient for coexisting mental disorders, such as delirium, major depression, and substance use disorder. It also assumes that the psychiatrist, neurologist, or primary care physician has evaluated the patient for treatable factors that may be causing or exacerbating the dementia and for general medical or other conditions that may affect its treatment.

The purpose of this guideline is to assist the psychiatrist in caring for a demented patient. It should be noted that many patients have comorbid conditions that cannot be completely covered with one DSM diagnostic category. The guideline attempts to be inclusive and to cover the range of necessary treatments that might be used by a psychiatrist who provides or coordinates the overall care of the patient with dementia. The psychiatrist caring for a patient with dementia should consider, but not be limited to, the treatments recommended in this practice guideline. Psychiatrists care for patients with dementia in many different settings and serve a variety of functions. For some patients a psychiatrist will be the primary evaluator or treater, for some the psychiatrist will serve as a consultant to another physician regarding the care of psychiatric symptoms, and for other patients the psychiatrist will act as part of a multidisciplinary team.

Much of the emphasis of this practice guideline is on behavioral symptoms because most of the effective treatments available for dementing disorders are in this realm. The treatment of these symptoms is a role uniquely filled by a psychiatrist in the management of these disorders. Other key roles include administering treatments aimed at cognitive and functional deficits, which is expected to gain in importance over time as new treatments are developed, and providing support for family members and other caregivers, who will always remain critical to the care of patients with dementia.

DEVELOPMENT PROCESS

This practice guideline was developed under the auspices of the Steering Committee on Practice Guidelines. The process is detailed in the Appendix to this volume. Key features of the process include the following:

- initial drafting by a work group that included psychiatrists with clinical and research expertise in dementia;
- a comprehensive literature review (description follows);
- the production of multiple drafts with widespread review, in which 10 organizations and over 48 individuals submitted comments (see section VII);
- approval by the APA Assembly and Board of Trustees;
- planned revisions at 3- to 5-year intervals.

The following computerized searches of relevant literature were conducted by using Excerpta Medica and MEDLINE for the period 1966 to 1994. The primary search was done in three parts: 1) medication treatment of dementia and complications (except depression), 2) nonmedication treatment of dementia and complications (except depression), and 3) treatment of depression in dementia.

In addition to this primary search, additional searches were performed where there did not appear to be adequate coverage, as follows. The key words used in Excerpta Medica searches for the period 1991–1995 were all terms indexed under "dementia," "alzheimer's," "hydergine," and "tacrine." These terms resulted in 376 citations. The key words used in MEDLINE searches were "chloral hydrate in treatment for dementia," "valproic acid in treatment for agitation," "lithium in treatment for agitation," "carbamazepine in treatment for agitation," and "beta blockers in treatment for agitation" for the period 1966–1995; "driving and dementia" for the period 1990–1995; and "MAO-inhibitors" with all terms indexed under "dementia" and "alzheimer's," all terms indexed under "dihydroergotoxine," all terms relevant for "tacrine," "NSAIDS in treatment of cognition disturbance," "estrogen in the treatment of cognition disorders," "chelation therapy in the treatment of cognition disorders," "day care—respite care—non-institutional treatment in dementia," and "zolpidem in the treatment of dementia or cognition" for the period 1991–1995.

I. SUMMARY OF RECOMMENDATIONS

The following executive summary is intended to provide an overview of the organization and scope of recommendations in this practice guideline. The treatment of patients with Alzheimer's disease and related dementias requires the consideration of many factors and cannot adequately be reviewed in a brief summary. The reader is encouraged to consult the relevant portions of the guideline when specific treatment recommendations are sought. This summary is not intended to stand by itself.

▶ A. CODING SYSTEM

Each recommendation is identified as falling into one of these three categories of endorsement, indicated by a bracketed Roman numeral following the statement. The three categories represent varying levels of clinical confidence:

[I]   Recommended with substantial clinical confidence.
[II] Recommended with moderate clinical confidence.
[III] May be recommended on the basis of individual circumstances.

▶ B. GENERAL TREATMENT PRINCIPLES AND ALTERNATIVES

Patients with dementia display a broad range of cognitive impairments, behavioral symptoms, and mood changes. As a result, they require an individualized and multimodal treatment plan. Dementia is often progressive; thus, treatment must evolve with time in order to address newly emerging issues. At each stage the psychiatrist should be vigilant for symptoms likely to be present and should help the patient and family anticipate future symptoms and the care likely to be required [I].

1. Psychiatric management

The core of the treatment of demented patients is psychiatric management, which must be based on a solid alliance with the patient and family and thorough psychiatric, neurological, and general medical evaluations of the nature and cause of the cognitive deficits and associated noncognitive symptoms [I]. It is particularly critical to identify and treat general medical conditions that may be responsible for or contribute to the dementia or associated behavioral symptoms [I].

Ongoing assessment should include periodic monitoring of the development and evolution of cognitive and noncognitive psychiatric symptoms and their response to intervention [I]. In order to offer prompt treatment, assure safety, and provide timely advice to the patient and family, it is generally necessary to see patients in routine follow-up every 4–6 months [II]. More frequent visits (e.g., once or twice a week) may be required for patients with complex or potentially dangerous symptoms or during the administration of specific therapies [I]. Safety measures include evaluation of suicidality and the potential for violence; recommendations regarding adequate supervision, preventing falls, and limiting the hazards of wandering; vigilance regarding neglect or abuse; and restrictions on driving and use of other dangerous equipment [I]. Driving poses particular concern because of its public health impact. All patients and families should be informed that even mild dementia increases the risk of accidents [I]. Mildly impaired patients should be urged to stop driving or limit their driving to safer situations [II], and moderately and severely impaired patients should be advised not to drive [II]; in both cases, the advice should be given to the family as well as the patient [I]. Another critical aspect of psychiatric management is educating the patient and family about the illness, its treatment, and available sources of care and support (e.g., support groups, various types of respite care, nursing homes and other long-term care facilities, the Alzheimer's Association). It is also important to help patients and their families plan for financial and legal issues due to the patient's incapacity (e.g., power of attorney for medical and financial decisions, an up-to-date will, the cost of long-term care) [I].

2. Specific psychotherapies and other psychosocial treatments

In addition to the psychosocial interventions subsumed under psychiatric management, a number of specific interventions are appropriate for some patients with dementia. Few of these treatments have been subjected to double-blind, randomized evaluation, but some research, along with clinical practice, supports their effectiveness. Behavior-oriented treatments identify the antecedents and consequences of problem behaviors and institute changes in the environment that minimize precipitants and/or consequences. These approaches have not been subjected to randomized clinical trials but are supported by single-case studies and are in widespread clinical use [II]. Stimulation-oriented treatments, such as recreational activity, art therapy, and pet therapy, along with other formal and informal means of maximizing pleasurable activities for patients, have modest support from clinical trials for improving function and mood, and common sense supports their use as part of the humane care of patients with dementia [II]. Among the emotion-oriented treatments, supportive psychotherapy is used by some practitioners to address issues of loss in the early stages of dementia, reminiscence therapy has some modest research support for improvement of mood and behavior, while validation therapy and sensory integration have less research support; none of these modalities has been subjected to rigorous testing [III]. Cognition-oriented treatments, such as reality orientation, cognitive retraining, and skills training, are focused on specific cognitive deficits, are unlikely to be beneficial, and have been associated with frustration in some patients [III].

3. Special concerns regarding somatic treatments for elderly and demented patients

Psychoactive medications are effective in the management of some symptoms associated with dementia, but they must be used with caution [I]. Elderly individuals have decreased renal clearance and slowed hepatic metabolism of many medications, so lower starting doses, smaller increases in dose, and longer intervals between increments must be used [I]. General medical conditions and other medications may further alter the binding, metabolism, and excretion of many medications [I]. In addition, the elderly and patients with dementia are more sensitive to certain medication side effects, including anticholinergic effects, orthostasis, central nervous system (CNS) sedation, and parkinsonism [I]. For all of these reasons, medications should be used with considerable care, particularly when more than one agent is being used [I].

4. Treatment of cognitive symptoms

The available treatments for the cognitive symptoms of dementia are limited. Two cholinesterase inhibitors are available for Alzheimer's disease: tacrine and donepezil. Either may be offered to patients with mild to moderate Alzheimer's disease after a thorough discussion of its potential risks and benefits [I]. Tacrine has been shown to lead to modest improvements in cognition in a substantial minority of patients, but up to 30% of patients cannot tolerate the medication because of nausea and vomiting or substantial (but reversible) elevations in liver enzyme levels [I]. Donepezil has also been shown to lead to modest improvements in a substantial minority of patients, and it appears to have a similar propensity to cause nausea and vomiting [II]. Because donepezil does not share tacrine's risk for liver toxicity, and thus does not require frequent monitoring, it may prove preferable as a first-line treatment [III]. However, accumulated data from additional clinical trials and clinical practice will be necessary in order to establish a more complete picture of its efficacy and side effect profile.

Vitamin E may also be considered for patients with moderate Alzheimer's disease to prevent further decline [I], and might also be beneficial earlier or later in the course of the disease [III]. A single large well-conducted trial of vitamin E showed a significant delay in poor outcome over a 2-year period [I], and the agent appears to be very safe [I]. Thus, it might be considered alone or in combination with a cholinesterase inhibitor in the treatment of Alzheimer's disease [II]. Its role in the treatment of other dementing disorders is unknown.

Selegiline may also be considered for patients with moderate Alzheimer's disease to prevent further decline [II], and may possibly be beneficial earlier or later in the course of the disease [III]. A single large well-conducted trial showed a significant delay in poor outcome over a 2-year period [I]. However, selegiline is associated with orthostatic hypotension and a risk for medication interactions, so vitamin E, which appeared equally efficacious in a direct comparison, may be preferable [II]. However, because limited evidence suggests that selegiline may offer short-term improvement in dementia, it might be appropriate as an alternative to cholinesterase inhibitors in patients who are ineligible for, intolerant of, or unresponsive to these agents [III]. Because there was no evidence of an additive effect of vitamin E and selegiline, there is no empirical basis for using the two agents in combination [I]. The effect of selegiline in combination with cholinesterase inhibitors is unknown.

The mixture of ergot mesylates known by the trade name Hydergine cannot be recommended for the treatment of cognitive symptoms but may be offered to patients with vascular dementia and may be appropriately continued for patients who experience a benefit [III]. This agent has been assessed in a large number of studies with inconsistent findings, but there is a suggestion that it may have more benefit for patients with vascular dementia than those with degenerative dementias [III]. It has no significant side effects [I].

A variety of other agents have been suggested as possibly helpful in the treatment of cognitive symptoms, some of the most promising of which are under active study in clinical trials. Because these agents remain experimental, they are best taken in the context of a clinical trial. Such trials may be an appropriate option for some patients, since they offer the chance of clinical benefit while contributing to progress in treating dementia [III].

5. Treatment of psychosis and agitation

Psychosis and agitation are common in demented patients, often coexist, and may respond to similar therapies. In approaching any of these symptoms, it is critical to consider the safety of the patient and those around him or her [I]. The next step is a careful evaluation for a general medical, psychiatric, or psychosocial problem that may underlie the disturbance [I]. If attention to these issues does not resolve the problem and the symptoms do not cause undue distress to the patient or others, they are best treated with reassurance and distraction [I]. For agitation, some of the behavioral measures discussed in section I.B.2 may be helpful as well [II]. If other measures are unsuccessful, these symptoms may be treated judiciously with one of the agents discussed in the following paragraphs [II]. The use of such agents must be evaluated and documented on an ongoing basis [I].

Antipsychotics are the only documented pharmacologic treatment for psychosis in dementia [I] and are the best documented for agitation [II]. While they have been shown to provide modest improvement in behavioral symptoms in general [I], some research evidence, along with considerable anecdotal evidence, suggests that this improvement is greater for psychosis than for other symptoms [II]. There is no evidence of a difference in efficacy among antipsychotic agents [II]. The efficacy of these agents beyond 8 weeks has limited research support, but there is considerable clinical experience with this practice [II]. Antipsychotics have a number of potentially severe side effects, including sedation and worsening of cognition, and thus must be used at the lowest effective dose: extremely low starting doses are recommended for this population [I]. High-potency agents are more likely to cause akathisia and parkinsonian symptoms; low-potency agents are more likely to cause sedation, confusion, delirium, postural hypotension, and peripheral anticholinergic effects [I]. All conventional antipsychotic agents are also associated with more serious complications, including tardive dyskinesia (for which the elderly, women, and individuals with dementia are at greater risk) and neuroleptic malignant syndrome. Risperidone appears to share the risks associated with high-potency agents, although it may be somewhat less likely to cause extrapyramidal reactions [III]. Clozapine is much less likely to be associated with extrapyramidal reactions, but it is associated with sedation, postural hypotension, and an elevated seizure risk and carries a risk of agranulocytosis, so it requires regular monitoring of blood counts [I]. The decision of which antipsychotic to use is based on the relationship between the side effect profile and the characteristics of a given patient [I]. It is expected that in the near future new agents that may alter decision making in this area will be released, but they have not yet been tested with geriatric or demented populations, so they cannot be recommended at this time.

Benzodiazepines are most useful for treating patients with prominent anxiety or for giving on an as-needed basis to patients who have infrequent episodes of agitation or to individuals who need to be sedated for a procedure such as a tooth extraction [II]. Benzodiazepines appear to perform better than placebo but not as well as antipsychotics in treating behavioral symptoms, although the data are of limited quality [II]. They can have many side effects, including sedation, worsening cognition, delirium, an increase in the risk of falls, and worsening of sleep-disordered breathing [I]. It may be preferable to use lorazepam and oxazepam, which have no active metabolites and are not metabolized in the liver [III].

The anticonvulsant agents carbamazepine and valproate, the sedating antidepressant trazodone, the atypical anxiolytic buspirone, and possibly selective serotonin release inhibitors (SSRIs) are less well studied but may be appropriate for nonpsychotic patients with behavioral disorders, especially those with mild symptoms or sensitivity to antipsychotic medications. There is preliminary evidence to support their efficacy in the treatment of agitation [III]. Medroxyprogesterone and related hormones may have a role in the treatment of disinhibited sexual behavior in male patients with dementia [III]. Lithium and β blockers are not generally recommended: the few data supporting their use concern nondemented populations, and the potential side effects are serious [II].

6. Treatment of depression

Depression is common in patients with dementia. Patients with depression should be carefully evaluated for suicide potential [I]. Depressed mood may respond to improvements in the living situation or stimulation-oriented treatments [II], but patients with severe or persistent depressed mood with or without a full complement of neuro-vegetative signs should be treated with antidepressant medications [II]. Although formal evaluation of the efficacy of antidepressants for demented patients is limited, there is considerable clinical evidence supporting their use [II]. The choice among agents is based on the side effect profile and the characteristics of a given patient [I]. SSRIs are probably the first-line treatment, although one of the tricyclic antidepressants or newer agents, such as bupropion or venlafaxine, may be more appropriate for some patients [II]. Agents with significant anticholinergic effects (e.g., amitriptyline, imipramine) should be avoided [I]. Because of the elevated risk of dietary indiscretion in demented patients and the substantial risk of postural hypotension, monoamine oxidase inhibitors (MAOIs) are probably appropriate only for patients who have not responded to other treatments [II]. Although research data are limited, clinical experience suggests that electroconvulsive therapy (ECT) is effective in the treatment of patients who do not respond to other agents [II]. Twice- rather than thrice-weekly and unilateral rather than bilateral treatments may decrease the risk of delirium or memory loss associated with this modality [III].

Treatments for apathy are not well documented, but psychostimulants, bupropion, bromocriptine, and amantadine may be helpful [III]. Psychostimulants are also sometimes useful in the treatment of depression in patients with significant general medical illness [III].

7. Treatment of sleep disturbances

Sleep disturbances are common in patients with dementia. Pharmacologic intervention should be considered only when other interventions, including careful attention to sleep hygiene, have failed [I]. If a patient has a sleep disturbance and requires medication for another condition, an agent with sedating properties, given at bedtime, should be selected if possible [II]. If the sleep disturbance does not coexist with other problems, possibly effective agents include zolpidem and trazodone [II], but there are few data on the efficacy of specific agents for demented patients. Benzodiazepines and chloral hydrate are usually not recommended for other than brief use because of the risk of daytime sedation, tolerance, rebound insomnia, worsening cognition, disinhibition, and delirium [II]. Triazolam in particular is not recommended because of its association with amnesia [II]. Diphenhydramine is generally not recommended because of its anticholinergic properties [II].

8. Special issues for long-term care

Many patients with dementia eventually require placement in a nursing home or other long-term care facility, and approximately two-thirds of nursing home patients suffer from dementia. Facilities should be structured to meet the needs of patients with dementia, including those with behavioral problems [I], which are extremely common. Staff with knowledge and experience concerning dementia and the management of noncognitive symptoms appear to be important [II]. Special care units may offer a model of optimal care for patients with dementia, although there is no evidence that special care units achieve better outcomes than traditional units [III].

A particular concern is the use of physical restraints and antipsychotic medications. When used appropriately, antipsychotics can relieve symptoms and reduce distress for patients and can increase safety for patients, other residents, and staff [I]. However, overuse can lead to worsening of the dementia, oversedation, falls, and tardive dyskinesia. Thus, federal regulations and good clinical practice require careful consideration and documentation of the indications and available alternatives, both initially and over time [I]. A dose decrease or discontinuation should be considered periodically for all patients who receive antipsychotic medications [I]. A structured education program for staff may decrease the use of these medications in nursing homes [II]. Physical restraints should be used only for patients who pose an imminent risk of physical harm to themselves or others and only until more definitive treatment is provided or when other measures have been exhausted [I]. When restraints are used, the indications and alternatives should be carefully documented [I]. The need for restraints can be decreased by environmental changes that decrease the risk of falls or wandering and by careful assessment and treatment of possible causes of agitation [II].

II. DISEASE DEFINITION, NATURAL HISTORY, AND EPIDEMIOLOGY

Although there are many types of dementia, they have a number of features in common. This section contains a discussion of dementia in general and brief descriptions of some of its more common types.

▶ A. DEFINITION OF DEMENTIA

The essential features of a dementia are multiple cognitive deficits that include memory impairment and at least one of the following: aphasia, apraxia, agnosia, or a disturbance in executive functioning (the ability to think abstractly and to plan, initiate, sequence, monitor, and stop complex behavior). The order of onset and relative prominence of the cognitive disturbances and associated symptoms vary with the specific type of dementia, as discussed in the following.

Memory impairment is generally a prominent early symptom. Individuals with dementia have difficulty learning new material and may lose valuables, such as wallets and keys, or forget food cooking on the stove. In more severe dementia, individuals also forget previously learned material, including the names of loved ones. Individuals with dementia may have difficulty with spatial tasks, such as navigating around the house or in the immediate neighborhood (where difficulties with memory are unlikely to play a role). Poor judgment and poor insight are common as well. Individuals may exhibit little or no awareness of memory loss or other cognitive abnormalities. They may make unrealistic assessments of their abilities and make plans that are not congruent with their deficits and prognosis (e.g., planning to start a new business). They may underestimate the risks involved in activities (e.g., driving).

In order to make a diagnosis of dementia, the cognitive deficits must be sufficiently severe to cause impairment in occupational or social functioning and must represent a decline from a previous level of functioning. The nature and degree of impairment are variable and often depend on the particular social setting of the individual. For example, mild cognitive impairment may significantly impair an individual's ability to perform a complex job but not a less demanding one.

▶ B. ASSOCIATED FEATURES

Some individuals with dementia show disinhibited behavior, including making inappropriate jokes, neglecting personal hygiene, exhibiting undue familiarity with strangers, or disregarding conventional rules of social conduct. Occasionally, they may harm others by striking out. Suicidal behavior may occur, especially in mildly impaired individuals, who are more likely to have insight into their deficits and to be capable of formulating (and carrying out) a plan of action. Anxiety is fairly common, and some patients manifest "catastrophic reactions," overwhelming emotional responses to relatively minor stressors, such as changes in routine or environment. Depressed mood, with or without neurovegetative changes, is quite common, as are sleep disturbances independent of depression. Delusions can occur, especially those involving themes of persecution (e.g., the belief that misplaced possessions have been stolen). Misidentifications of familiar people as unfamiliar (or vice versa) frequently occur. Hallucinations can occur in all sensory modalities, but visual hallucinations are most common. Some patients exhibit a peak period of agitation (or other behavioral disturbances) during the evening hours, which is sometimes referred to as "sundowning."

Delirium is frequently superimposed on dementia because the underlying brain disease increases susceptibility to the effects of medications or concurrent general medical conditions. Individuals with dementia may also be especially vulnerable to psychosocial stressors (e.g., going to the hospital, bereavement), which may exacerbate their intellectual deficits and associated problems.

Dementia is sometimes accompanied by motor disturbances, which may include gait difficulties, slurred speech, and a variety of abnormal movements. Other neurological symptoms, such as myoclonus and seizures, may also occur.

C. DIFFERENTIAL DIAGNOSIS

The differential diagnosis of dementia is described in detail in DSM-IV (1) and is summarized only briefly here. Memory impairment occurs in both *delirium* and dementia. Delirium is also characterized by a reduced ability to maintain and shift attention appropriately, but the cognitive deficits tend to fluctuate, while those of dementia tend to be stable or progressive. An *amnestic disorder* is characterized by memory impairment without significant impairment in other cognitive domains. *Mental retardation* has an onset before age 18 and is characterized by significantly subaverage general intellectual functioning, which does not necessarily include memory impairment. *Schizophrenia* may be associated with multiple cognitive impairments and a decline in functioning, but the cognitive impairment tends to be less severe and occurs against a background of psychotic and behavioral symptoms meeting the established diagnostic criteria. Particularly in elderly persons, *major depressive disorder* may be associated with complaints of memory impairment, difficulty concentrating, and a reduction in intellectual abilities shown by history or mental status examination; this is sometimes referred to as *pseudodementia*. The two may sometimes be distinguished on the basis of an assessment of the course and onset of depressive and cognitive symptoms and by response to treatment of the depression. However, even when the onset of depressive symptoms precedes or coincides with the onset of cognitive symptoms and both resolve with antidepressant treatment, as many as one-half of patients go on to develop an irreversible dementia within 3 years (2). Dementia must be distinguished from *malingering* and *factitious disorder*, which generally manifest patterns of cognitive deficits that are inconsistent over time and are uncharacteristic of those typically seen in dementia. Dementia must also be distinguished from *age-related cognitive decline*, the mild decline in cognitive functioning that may occur with aging, which is nonprogressive and does not lead to functional impairment.

D. PREVALENCE AND COURSE

Exact estimates of the prevalence of dementia depend on the definition and specific threshold used, but it is clear that the prevalence increases dramatically with age. The syndrome affects approximately 5%–8% of individuals over age 65, 15%–20% of individuals over age 75, and 25%–50% of individuals over age 85. Alzheimer's disease is the most common dementia, accounting for 50%–75% of the total, with a greater proportion in the higher age ranges. Vascular dementia is probably next most common, but its prevalence is unknown. The remaining types of dementia account for a much smaller fraction of the total, although in the last few years it has been suggested that Lewy body disease may be more prevalent than previously realized (3).

The mode of onset and subsequent course of dementia depend on the underlying etiology. Classically, Alzheimer's disease has an insidious onset and gradual decline, while vascular dementia is characterized by a more acute onset and stepwise decline. However, since both disorders are common, the two frequently coexist, although only one diagnosis may be made during a person's life. Other dementias may be progressive, static, or remitting. The reversibility of a dementia is a function of the underlying pathology and of the availability and timely application of effective treatment.

E. STAGING OF DEMENTIA

Progressive dementias are generally staged according to the level of functional impairment, and the same categories may be used to describe the degree of severity of any dementia (4, 5). The ability to perform a specific function depends on baseline skills, deficits, and the social environment, so the severity of illness should be assessed in the context of past functioning in several domains. Individuals with *questionable* impairment show borderline functioning in several areas but definite impairment in none. Such individuals are not considered demented, but they should be evaluated over time: some may progress to a dementing disorder, some may return to normal functioning, and others may remain in a questionable state. Individuals with *mild* impairment are likely to have difficulties with balancing a checkbook, preparing a complex meal, or managing a difficult medication schedule. Those with *moderate* impairment also have difficulties with simpler food preparation, household cleanup, and yard work and may require assistance with some aspects of self-care (e.g., reminders to use the bathroom, help with fasteners or shaving). Those whose dementia is *severe* require considerable assistance with personal care, including feeding, grooming, and toileting. In *profound* dementia, the patients may become largely oblivious to their surroundings and are almost totally dependent on caregivers. In the *terminal* phase, patients are generally bed bound, require constant care, and may be susceptible to accidents and infectious diseases, which often prove fatal.

F. SPECIFIC DEMENTIAS

1. Dementia of the Alzheimer's type

Dementia of the Alzheimer's type, referred to here for brevity as Alzheimer's disease, is a dementia with an insidious onset and gradual progression. Various patterns of deficits are seen, but the disorder begins most commonly with deficits in recent memory, which are followed by aphasia, apraxia, and agnosia after several years. Deficits in executive function (e.g., performing tasks involving multiple steps, such as balancing a checkbook or preparing a meal) are also typically seen early in the course of the disease. Some individuals may show personality changes or increased irritability in the early stages. In the middle and later stages of the disease, psychotic symptoms are common. Patients also tend to develop incontinence and gait and motor disturbances, and eventually they become mute and bedridden. Seizures and myoclonus may also occur late in the disease.

The diagnosis of Alzheimer's disease should be made only when other etiologies for the dementia have been ruled out by careful history, physical and neurological examinations, and laboratory tests. A definitive diagnosis of Alzheimer's disease depends on microscopic examination of the brain (generally at autopsy), which reveals numerous characteristic senile plaques and neurofibrillary tangles widely distributed in the cerebral cortex. A clinical diagnosis of Alzheimer's disease conforms to the pathological diagnosis 70%–90% of the time.

Onset generally occurs in late life, most commonly in the 60s, 70s, and 80s and beyond, but in rare instances the disorder appears in the 40s and 50s. The incidence of Alzheimer's disease also increases with age, and it is estimated at 0.5% per year from age 65 to 69, 1% per year from age 70 to 74, 2% per year from age 75 to 79, 3% per year from 80 to 84, and 8% per year from age 85 onward (6). Progression is gradual but steadily downward, with an average duration from onset of symptoms to death of 8–10 years. Plateaus may occur, but progression generally resumes after 1 to several years.

DSM-IV subdivides Alzheimer's disease into the following subtypes, indicating the predominant feature of the current clinical presentation: With Delirium, With Delusions, With Depressed Mood (including but not limited to presentations that meet symptom criteria for a Major Depressive Episode), and Uncomplicated. In addition, the specifier "With Behavioral Disturbance" can also be used to indicate the presence of clinically significant difficulties, such as wandering or combativeness. DSM-IV further divides Alzheimer's disease arbitrarily into early onset, which is used if the symptoms of cognitive decline begin at or before age 65, and late onset, if they begin after age 65.

2. Vascular (multi-infarct) dementia

Vascular dementia is a dementia due to the effects of one or more strokes on cognitive function. Typically, it is characterized by an abrupt onset and stepwise course in the context of cerebrovascular disease documented by history, focal neurological signs and symptoms, and/or imaging studies. The pattern of cognitive deficits is often patchy, depending on which regions of the brain have been destroyed. Certain cognitive functions may be affected early, whereas others remain relatively unimpaired. Associated focal neurological signs and symptoms include extensor plantar response, pseudobulbar palsy, gait abnormalities, exaggeration of deep tendon reflexes, and weakness of an extremity. Structural imaging studies usually indicate multiple vascular lesions of the cerebral cortex and subcortical structures.

The onset of vascular dementia may occur any time in late life but becomes less common after age 75, while the incidence of Alzheimer's disease continues to rise. The relationship between Alzheimer's disease and vascular dementia is complex, in part because Alzheimer's disease and strokes are both common and frequently coexist (although generally only one diagnosis is recognized during a person's life), and because recent evidence suggests that small strokes may lead to increased clinical expression of Alzheimer's disease (7). The degree to which strokes alone are responsible for dementia is unclear. However, one study estimated that 8% of individuals over 60 who have a stroke develop dementia within the following year, compared to 1% of age-matched individuals without a history of stroke (8). Vascular dementia tends to progress in a stepwise fashion but can be static. Early treatment of hypertension and vascular disease may prevent further progression.

Like Alzheimer's disease, vascular dementia is subtyped in DSM-IV according to any prominent associated symptoms: With Delirium, With Delusions, With Depressed Mood, and Uncomplicated. The additional modifier "With Behavioral Disturbance" may also be used. No subtyping based on age of onset is used.

3. Dementia due to Parkinson's disease

Parkinson's disease is a slowly progressive neurological condition characterized by tremor, rigidity, bradykinesia, and postural instability; its onset is typically in middle to late life. In 20% to 60% of the cases, it is accompanied by a dementia, which is particularly common late in the course. The dementia associated with Parkinson's disease has an insidious onset and slow progression and is characterized by cognitive and motoric slowing, executive dysfunction, and impairment in memory retrieval. Parkinson's disease is important to psychiatrists because of the high prevalence of associated depression and the frequent occurrence of psychotic symptoms during pharmacologic treatment of the primary motor deficit.

4. Dementia due to Lewy body disease

Lewy body disease is a recently characterized disorder (9) that is clinically fairly similar to Alzheimer's disease but tends to have earlier and more prominent visual hallucinations and parkinsonian features and a somewhat more rapid evolution. Patients are notably sensitive to extrapyramidal effects of antipsychotic medications. Histopathologically, it is marked by the presence of Lewy inclusion bodies in the cerebral cortex. Recent studies suggest that Lewy body disease may account for many as 7%–26% of dementia cases, depending on the criteria used (3). The disorder is particularly likely to come to psychiatric attention because of the patients' prominent psychotic symptoms and sensitivity to antipsychotic medications.

5. Dementia due to Pick's disease and other frontal lobe dementias

Pick's disease and other frontal lobe dementias are characterized in their early stages by changes in personality, executive dysfunction, deterioration of social skills, emotional blunting, behavioral disinhibition, and prominent language abnormalities. Difficulties with memory, apraxia, and other features of dementia usually follow later in the course. Prominent primitive reflexes (snout, suck, grasp) may be present. As the dementia progresses, it may be accompanied by either apathy or extreme agitation. Individuals may develop such severe problems with language, attention, or behavior that it may be difficult to assess the degree of cognitive impairment. The diagnosis is difficult to make clinically, and it is especially difficult to distinguish from atypical Alzheimer's disease. In Pick's disease, structural brain imaging typically reveals prominent frontal and/or temporal atrophy, with relative sparing of the parietal and occipital lobes. The diagnosis of Pick's disease must be confirmed by the autopsy finding of characteristic Pick inclusion bodies. Other frontal lobe dementias tend to have more nonspecific histopathology. The disorder most commonly manifests itself in individuals between the ages of 50 and 60 years, although it can occur among older individuals. The course is progressive and tends to be more rapid than that of Alzheimer's disease. These disorders are fairly rare but are important for psychiatrists because they often present with psychiatric symptoms.

6. Other progressive dementing disorders

A number of other disorders can lead to progressive dementia. These include Huntington's disease—an autosomal dominant disorder that affects the basal ganglia and other subcortical structures and includes motor, behavioral, and cognitive symptoms—and Creutzfeldt-Jakob disease—a rapidly progressive spongiform encephalopathy associated with a slow virus or a prion (proteinaceous infectious particle).

7. Dementia due to other causes

In addition to the preceding categories, a number of general medical conditions can cause dementia. These conditions include structural lesions (primary or secondary brain tumor, subdural hematoma, slowly progressive or normal-pressure hydrocephalus), head trauma, endocrine conditions (hypothyroidism, hypercalcemia, hypoglycemia), nutritional conditions (deficiency of thiamin, niacin, or vitamin B_{12}), other infectious conditions (HIV, neurosyphilis, *Cryptococcus*), derangements of renal and hepatic function, neurological conditions (e.g., multiple sclerosis), effects of medications (e.g., benzodiazepines, β blockers, diphenhydramine), and the toxic effect of long-standing substance abuse, especially alcohol abuse. It is critical that psychiatrists caring for demented individuals be familiar with the general medical and neurological causes of dementia in order to assure that the diagnosis is accurate and, in particular, that potentially treatable conditions are not missed.

III. TREATMENT PRINCIPLES AND ALTERNATIVES

The treatment of Alzheimer's disease and related dementias is multimodal. It is guided by the stage of illness and is focused on the specific symptoms manifested by the patient. This discussion begins with psychiatric management, the cornerstone of the treatment of the demented patient, and then goes on to review specific treatments, first the broad range of psychosocial interventions used with dementia and then the pharmacologic options organized by target symptom.

A. DETERMINING THE SITE OF TREATMENT AND FREQUENCY OF VISITS

As for all patients, the site of treatment for an individual with dementia is determined by the need to provide safe and effective treatment in the least restrictive setting. Individuals with dementia may need to be admitted to an inpatient facility for the treatment of psychotic, affective, or behavioral symptoms. In addition, they may need to be admitted for treatment of comorbid general medical conditions or for psychiatric comorbidity. For patients who are very frail or who have significant medical illnesses, a geriatric psychiatry or medical psychiatric unit may be helpful when available. Indications for hospitalization include factors based on illness (e.g., threats of harm to self or others, violent or uncontrollable behavior) and those based on the intensity of services needed (e.g., the need for continuous skilled observation, ECT, or a medication or test that cannot be performed on an outpatient basis) (10, 11). The length of stay is similarly determined by the ability of the patient to safely receive the needed care in a less intensive setting.

Decisions regarding the need for placement in a long-term care facility often depend on the degree to which the patient's needs can be met in the home, by either relatives or other potential caregivers. The decision to remain at home should be reassessed regularly, with consideration of the patient's clinical status and the continued ability of the patient's caregivers to supervise the patient and manage the burden of care.

The necessary frequency of visits is determined by a number of factors, including the patient's clinical status and the likely rate of change, the current treatment plan and the need for any specific monitoring of treatment effects, and the reliability and skill of the patient's caregivers, particularly regarding the likelihood of their notifying the psychiatrist if a clinically important change occurs. In order to be able to offer prompt treatment, assure safety, and provide timely advice to the patient and family, it is generally, but not always, necessary to see patients in follow-up at least every 3 to 6 months. More frequent visits are likely to be required for patients with complex, distressing, or potentially dangerous symptoms or during the administration of specific therapies. For example, outpatients who present with or experience acute exacerbations of depressive or psychotic symptoms may need to be seen as frequently as once or twice a week.

▶ B. PSYCHIATRIC MANAGEMENT; PSYCHOTHERAPY AND OTHER PSYCHOSOCIAL TREATMENTS

Successful management of patients with dementia requires a broad range of tasks, which are grouped under the term "psychiatric management." These tasks help to maximize the patient's level of function and to assure the safety and comfort of patients and their families in the context of living with a difficult disease. In some cases, psychiatrists perform all or most of these tasks themselves. In others, they are part of multidisciplinary teams. In either case, they must be aware of the full range of available treatments and take steps to assure that any necessary treatments are administered.

1. Establish and maintain an alliance with the patient and family

As with any psychiatric care, a solid alliance is critical to taking care of the demented patient. The care of a demented patient requires an alliance with the family and other caregivers, as well as the patient. Family members and other caregivers are a critical source of information, as the patient is frequently unable to give a reliable history, they are generally responsible for implementing and monitoring treatment plans, their own attitudes and behaviors have a profound effect on the patient, and they often need the treating psychiatrist's compassion and concern.

2. Perform a diagnostic evaluation and refer the patient for any needed general medical care

Patients with dementia need a thorough diagnostic evaluation. This serves to identify a diagnosis that may guide specific treatment decisions and to reveal any treatable psychiatric or general medical conditions (e.g., major depression, thyroid disease, B_{12} deficiency, tertiary syphilis, hydrocephalus, or structural brain lesion) that might be causing or exacerbating the dementia. The details of this evaluation are beyond the scope of this guideline: the reader is referred to the Consensus Conference on the Differential Diagnosis of Dementing Disorders of the National Institute on Aging, National Institute of Neurological and Communication Disorders and Stroke, National Institute of Mental Health, and National Institutes of Health (12), the practice guideline on the diagnosis and evaluation of dementia of the American Academy of Neurology (13), and the Agency for Health Care Policy and Research's clinical practice guideline *Recognition and Initial Assessment of Alzheimer's Disease and Related Dementias* (14) for more-complete descriptions of the evaluation of patients with dementia. A brief summary follows.

The general principles of a complete psychiatric evaluation are outlined in the American Psychiatric Association's *Practice Guideline for Psychiatric Evaluation of Adults* (15; included in this volume). Evaluation of a patient with dementia frequently involves a number of physicians. The psychiatrist who has overall responsibility for the care of the patient oversees the evaluation, which should at a minimum include a clear history of the onset and progression of symptoms; a complete physical and neurological examination; a psychiatric examination, including a cognitive evaluation, e.g., the Mini-Mental State examination (16); a review of the patient's medications; and laboratory studies, i.e., complete blood count (CBC), blood chemistry battery (including glucose, electrolytes, calcium, and kidney and liver function tests), measurement of vitamin B_{12} level, syphilis serology, thyroid function tests, and determination of erythrocyte sedimentation rate. An assessment for past or current psychiatric illness, such as schizophrenia or major depression, that might mimic or exacerbate the dementia is also critical. For some patients, toxicology studies, HIV testing, a lumbar puncture, or an electroencephalogram may be indicated. If the history and neurological examination suggest a possible focal lesion, a structural imaging study, with computerized tomography (CT) or magnetic resonance imaging (MRI), should be obtained. Functional imaging techniques, such as positron emission tomography (PET) and single photon emission computed tomography (SPECT), have not yet shown clinical utility but are the focus of current study. Neuropsychological testing may be helpful in deciding whether a patient is actually demented or for more thoroughly characterizing an unusual symptom picture. It may also help identify strengths and weaknesses that might guide expectations for the patient and suggest interventions to improve overall function. Testing for the apolipoprotein E-4 gene (APOE-4), one form of a gene on chromosome 19 that is more common in individuals with Alzheimer's disease than in age-matched individuals without dementia, is not currently recommended for use in diagnosis because it is found in many undemented elderly and is not found in many patients with dementia (17, 18).

3. Assess and monitor psychiatric status

The psychiatrist must periodically assess the patient for the presence of noncognitive psychiatric symptoms and progression of cognitive symptoms.

Both cognitive and noncognitive symptoms of dementia tend to evolve over time, so regular monitoring allows adaptation of treatment strategies to current needs. For example, among the behavioral disturbances common in Alzheimer's disease, depression is more common early in the illness, while delusions and hallucinations are more common in the middle and later stages. Among the cognitive deficits, memory loss is a common early symptom, while language and spatial dysfunction tend to occur later.

Behavioral issues to be addressed include major depression and other depressive syndromes, suicidal ideation or behavior, hallucinations, delusions, agitation, aggressive behavior, disinhibition, anxiety, apathy, and sleep disturbances. Cognitive symptoms to address include memory, executive function, language, judgment, and spatial abilities. It is often helpful to track cognitive status with a simple examination such as the Mini-Mental State (16). A detailed assessment of functional status may also aid the clinician in documenting and tracking changes over time. These assessments of recent cognitive and functional status provide a baseline for assessing the effect of any intervention, and they improve the recognition and treatment of acute problems, such as delirium.

Whenever there is an acute worsening of cognition, functioning, behavior, or mood, the clinician should bear in mind that the elderly in general and demented patients in particular are at high risk for delirium associated with general medical problems, medications, and surgery. Newly developing or acutely worsening agitation in particular can be a sign of an occult general medical condition, untreated or undertreated pain, or physical or emotional discomfort. Thus, a thoughtful assessment of the patient's overall status and a general medical evaluation must precede any intervention with psychotropic medications or physical restraint except in an emergency.

Before undertaking an intervention, the psychiatrist should enlist the help of caregivers in carefully characterizing the target symptoms. Their nature, intensity, frequency, precipitants, and consequences should be reviewed and documented. This process is critical to monitoring the impact of any intervention and helps caregivers begin to achieve some mastery over the problem. It is also helpful if clinicians explicitly review their own, the patient's, and caregivers' expectations before embarking on any intervention.

4. Monitor safety and intervene when required

The psychiatrist treating demented patients must be vigilant regarding assessment of cognitive deficits or behavioral difficulties that might lead such patients to pose a danger to themselves or others. The psychiatrist should a) assess suicidality, b) assess violence potential, c) make recommendations regarding adequate supervision, d) make recommendations regarding the prevention of falls, and e) be vigilant regarding neglect or abuse. Other important safety issues in managing patients with dementia include interventions to decrease the hazards of wandering and recommendations concerning driving and other use of hazardous equipment, which will be discussed separately.

If suicidal ideation occurs in patients with Alzheimer's disease or others with dementia, it tends to be when the disease is mild—when depressive symptoms are common and insight is more likely to be preserved. It is a particular concern in patients who are clinically depressed but can occur in the absence of major depression. The elderly in general and elderly men in particular are at high risk for suicide, although the diagnosis of dementia confers no special risk. Interventions are similar to those for nondemented patients and may include, depending on the nature and intensity of the suicidal ideation or behavior and capacity and support system of the patient, psychotherapy; pharmacotherapy; removal of potentially dangerous items, such as medications, guns, or vehicles; increased supervision; and hospitalization.

Threats, combativeness, and physical violence are more likely to occur later in the illness and are often associated with frustration, misinterpretations, delusions, or hallucinations. These behaviors pose a particular problem for patients cared for at home, especially by frail spouses. If such behavior cannot be brought under control rapidly, hospitalization and/or nursing home placement must be considered.

The patient should be adequately supervised in the context of his or her cognitive abilities and the risk of dangerous activities. For instance, a patient with significant cognitive impairment may not be safe alone at home: he or she might improperly administer medications, be unable to cope with a household emergency, or use the stove, power tools, or other equipment in a dangerous manner.

Psychiatrists caring for demented patients should be aware that falls are a common and potentially serious problem for all elderly patients and especially those with dementia. They can lead to hip fracture, head trauma, and a variety of other injuries. In order to prevent falls, every effort should be made to minimize orthostatic hypotension. Medications associated with CNS sedation should also be kept to a minimum. If gait disturbances are present, canes, walkers, or other supports may be helpful if not contraindicated by the symptoms of the dementia. Patients at high risk for falling may need to be closely supervised while walking. The removal of loose rugs, low tables, and other obstacles can diminish risk. The use of lower beds, night-lights, and bedside commodes and/or frequent toileting may help prevent falls at night. Bed rails may also help prevent a patient from rolling out of bed but, for patients who tend to climb, may actually increase the risk of falls.

The psychiatrist should be vigilant regarding the possibility of elder abuse or neglect. Demented individuals are at particular risk for abuse because of their limited ability to protest and the added demands and emotional strain on caregivers, and those whose caregivers appear angry or frustrated may be at still higher risk. Any concern, especially one raised by the patient, must be thoroughly evaluated. However, corroborating evidence (e.g., from physical examination) should be sought in order to distinguish delusions, hallucinations, and misinterpretations from actual abuse. In most states, if neglect or abuse is suspected, the psychiatrist may be required to make a report to the appropriate local agency responsible for investigating elder abuse.

5. Intervene to decrease the hazards of wandering

Families should be advised that patients with dementia sometimes wander away from home and that wandering may be dangerous to patients who cannot find their way back or lack the judgment to recognize and deal with a dangerous situation. Since walking may be beneficial, both as stimulation and exercise, it should not be limited unnecessarily. A large, safe area for walking or an opportunity for supervised walks is ideal. When this cannot be made available to a patient who tends to wander, adequate supervision is important in order to prevent wandering into risky situations and to locate missing patients promptly. It may also be necessary to structure the environment to prevent unsupervised departures. At home, the addition of a more complex or less accessible door latch may be helpful. In institutional settings, electronic locks may be used or a high-risk patient may be fitted with an electronic Wanderguard, which triggers an alarm when the patient tries to leave. In addition, there is weak evidence that interventions such as floor grids, mirrors, and covers designed to disguise exits and doorknobs may decrease wandering (19–21), at least in institutional settings. If patients are prevented from leaving on their own, adequate supervision must be provided in order to assure egress in an emergency.

In addition, provision should be made for locating a patient should wandering occur. Such measures include sewing or pinning identifying information onto clothes, placing medical-alert bracelets on patients, and filing photographs with local police departments. Referrals to the Safe Return Program of the Alzheimer's Association (1-800-621-0379) or similar options provided by local police departments or other organizations are appropriate for many families.

6. Advise the patient and family concerning driving (and other activities that put other people at risk)

Most of the available evidence suggests that dementia, even when mild, impairs driving performance to some extent and that the risk of accidents increases with increasing severity of the dementia (22–28). The issue raises significant public health concerns, since extensive data document that individuals with dementia, even some with fairly serious impairment, continue to drive (29–33).

There is a strong consensus that demented patients with moderate impairment (e.g., those who cannot perform moderately complex tasks, such as preparing simple meals, household chores, yard work, or simple home repairs) pose an unacceptable risk and should not drive. Those with severe impairment are generally unable to drive and certainly should not do so. However, there is no consensus regarding the threshold level of dementia at which driving should be permanently curtailed (25, 34). Some clinicians argue that in mild dementia the benefits to the patient of continued independence and access to needed services outweigh the risk of an accident and that, while the risk is greater than for age-matched nondemented individuals, it is less than that for cognitively intact young drivers (e.g., under age 25). Others argue that no patient with dementia should drive because the risk of an accident is elevated even in mildly demented patients and that it is impossible to say at what point the risk becomes unacceptable. Many clinicians believe that the risk of driving is greater for patients with mild dementia whose deficits include substantial impairment in judgment, spatial function, or praxis, although research studies have been unable to confirm this (22, 26, 33). Increased risk may also be associated with concomitant motor deficits (e.g., due to stroke or a parkinsonian syndrome), sensory deficits (e.g., neglect, visual loss, deafness), general medical problems (e.g., symptomatic cardiac arrhythmia, syncope, seizures, poorly controlled diabetes), or the use of sedative-hypnotic or other sedating medications.

Psychiatrists should discuss the risks of driving with all demented patients and their families, and these discussions should be carefully documented. They should include an exploration of the patient's current driving patterns, transportation needs, and potential alternatives. The psychiatrist should ask the family about any history of getting lost or traffic accidents. For demented patients who continue to drive, the issue should be raised repeatedly and reassessed over time. This is especially true for patients with Alzheimer's disease or other progressive dementias. Eventually the point will be reached where the danger is undeniable, so patients and their families need to make plans for alternative modes of transportation. A social service referral may be helpful for some families to help with transportation arrangements and costs.

Patients with moderate to severe impairment should be strongly advised not to drive. This recommendation may also be appropriate for patients with mild dementia who have significant deficits in judgment, spatial function, or praxis or a history of at-fault traffic incidents. This advice should be communicated to family members, as well as to the patient, since the burden of the decision often falls on families. The psychiatrist can also lend moral authority and support to family members who wish to restrict driving but are reluctant to take responsibility for the decision (e.g., write on a prescription pad, "DO NOT DRIVE"). In addition, the psychiatrist can provide concrete advice regarding how best to accomplish this goal (e.g., confrontation regarding risks to grandchildren, discussion of the impact on insurance coverage and rates, removing the car from view, hiding the keys, removing ignition wires).

Patients with milder impairment should be urged to consider giving up driving. For those who are unwilling to do so, it may be helpful to advise them to consider the use of a spouse navigator and to begin limiting their driving to conditions likely to be less risky (e.g., familiar locations, modest speeds, good visibility, clear roads) (35). Mildly impaired patients who wish an independent assessment of their driving skills may be referred to an occupational therapist, rehabilitation center, driving school, or local department of motor vehicles, but the predictive value of these assessments for behind-the-wheel performance is not established.

Psychiatrists caring for demented patients should familiarize themselves with state regulations. In some states, disclosure is forbidden. In others, a diagnosis of dementia or Alzheimer's disease must be reported to the state department of motor vehicles, and the patient and family should be so informed. In most states, the physician may breach confidentiality to inform the state motor vehicle department of a patient who is judged to be a dangerous driver: on rare occasions this option is appropriate for patients with significant dementia who refuse to stop driving and whose families are unwilling or unable to stop them.

Although the data and recommendations just described refer to the operation of motor vehicles, similar principles apply to the operation of other equipment that puts the patient and others at risk. Thus, patients whose leisure or work activities involve firearms, heavy machinery, or other dangerous equipment or material may need to have these activities limited.

7. Educate the patient and family regarding the illness and available treatments

An important role of the psychiatrist caring for an individual with dementia is educating the patient and family regarding the illness and its natural history. Often the first step is to communicate the diagnosis of dementia or a specific dementing illness, such as Alzheimer's disease. Patients themselves vary in their awareness of and ability to discuss their diagnoses. Most mildly and some moderately impaired individuals are able to discuss the matter at some level, but the discussion must be adapted to the specific concerns and abilities of the patient; it may be helpful to seek the family's input regarding the nature and timing of any discussion with the patient (36). In most cases, the psychiatrist will have an explicit discussion with family members regarding the diagnosis, prognosis, and options for intervention, but this too must be adapted to the concerns and abilities of the patient and family. Recent work suggests that certain specific symptoms (e.g., psychosis, extrapyramidal symptoms) are predictive of more rapid decline, and thus may be used in tandem with other features to assess prognosis (37).

One critical part of educating the patient and family is help with the recognition of current symptoms and anticipation of future manifestations. This allows them to plan for the future and to recognize emergent symptoms that should be brought to medical attention. Family members and other caregivers may be particularly concerned about behavioral symptoms, which they often associate with a loss of dignity, social stigma, and an increased caregiving burden. It may be helpful to reassure patients and their families that these symptoms are part of the illness and are direct consequences of the damage to the brain. Moreover, they may be relieved to know that, while cognitive losses themselves may not be reversible much of the time, many symptoms, especially the more disruptive ones, can be alleviated or even eliminated with treatment, resulting in an overall increase in functional status and comfort.

It is also helpful to educate the family regarding basic principles of care. These include: a) keeping requests and demands relatively simple and avoiding overly complex tasks that might lead to frustration; b) avoiding confrontation and deferring requests if the patient becomes angered; c) remaining calm, firm, and supportive if the patient becomes upset; d) being consistent and avoiding unnecessary change; e) providing frequent reminders, explanations, and orientation cues; f) recognizing declines in capacity and adjusting expectations appropriately; and g) bringing sudden declines in function and the emergence of new symptoms to professional attention. In addition, the psychiatrist can offer more specific behaviorally or psychodynamically informed suggestions for techniques that caregivers can use to avoid or deal with difficult behaviors.

Last, many patients and families are interested in understanding what is known regarding the pathophysiology and etiology of the disorder. The local chapter and national office of the Alzheimer's Association (1-800-621-0379) are often very helpful resources: they distribute a number of pamphlets written for patients, caregivers, and health professionals and operate hotlines staffed by well-informed volunteers. Many clinicians also recommend that families read articles or books written specifically for lay readers interested in understanding dementia and its care, e.g., *The Thirty-Six Hour Day: A Family Guide to Caring for Persons With Alzheimer's Disease, Related Dementing Illness, and Memory Loss in Later Life* (38), or view informational videotapes that may be available from the local Alzheimer's Association chapter or public library.

One issue that comes up frequently is the etiology of dementia. The risk factors for vascular dementia and Alzheimer's disease are probably the best characterized. The principal risk factors for vascular dementia are the same as those for stroke: advanced age, hypertension, diabetes, and hyperlipidemia. Risk factors for Alzheimer's disease include increased age, female gender, head trauma, family history, and Down's syndrome. Apparent protective factors include education, use of nonsteroidal anti-inflammatory drugs (NSAIDs), estrogen replacement therapy, and possibly smoking. Aside from age, the best-studied risk factors are genetic. Abnormal genes on chromosomes 21, 14, and 1 appear to account for the vast majority of cases of the early-onset familial form of the illness (39–41), and one form of the apolipoprotein gene (APOE-4) on chromosome 19 has been shown to carry an increased, but not definite, risk of Alzheimer's disease (42–44). Testing for APOE-4 has been suggested by some as a potential predictive test for Alzheimer's disease, but two independent expert panels (17, 18) strongly recommended against such testing because its predictive value is unknown, especially in the context of other risk factors for Alzheimer's disease and for mortality.

8. Advise the family regarding sources of care and support

Family members often feel overwhelmed by the combination of hard work and personal loss associated with caring for a demented individual. The caring attitude of the psychiatrist may provide a critical piece of support. This may include thoughtful inquiries about current needs and how they are being met; advice about available sources of help, both moral and practical; and more-extensive supportive psychotherapy. It also may include referrals to a variety of community resources.

A substantial literature, along with extensive practical experience, reinforces the value of support groups, especially those combining information with emotional support (45, 46). Support groups conforming to this general pattern are available in many localities through local chapters of the Alzheimer's Association and/or hospitals, community organizations, and religious groups. These groups may vary widely in their approaches, and caregivers may elect to try several before finding one that suits them. In addition to providing helpful information about the disease, how to care for it, and ways to decrease caregiver burden, these groups may enhance the quality of life of patients and spouses or other caregivers and may delay nursing home placement (46, 47). Other programs have been developed and may be appropriate for reducing the

92

burden and relieving the stress and depression associated with long-term caregiving; these interventions include psychoeducational programs for coping with frustration or depression and workshops in stress management techniques (48, 49).

With or without such support, caregivers frequently become frustrated, over-whelmed, or clinically depressed. Psychiatrists caring for demented patients should be vigilant for these conditions in caregivers, which increase the risk of substandard care, neglect, or abuse of patients and are a sign that the caregivers themselves are in need of care. When caregivers are in significant distress, prompt treatment should be rec-ommended; such treatment could be provided (according to the preference of psy-chiatrist, patient, and caregiver) by the patient's psychiatrist or through a referral.

As for the logistical aspects of care, many resources provide valuable help for those trying to care for demented individuals at home. Respite care allows the caregiver pe-riods of relief from the responsibilities of caring for a demented individual. It provides essential physical and emotional support, serving the dual purposes of decreasing the burden of care and allowing caregivers to continue to work or fulfill other respon-sibilities. Respite care may last for hours to weeks and may be provided through com-panions, home health aides, visiting nurses, day care programs, and brief nursing home stays or other temporary overnight care. Depending on the local and individual circumstances, these types of care may be available from local senior services agen-cies, from the local chapter of the Alzheimer's Association, religious groups, or other community organizations. Although there is little documentation of improvement in patient variables, these programs may lead to a delay in institutionalization (50–53). In addition, clinical experience suggests that, by decreasing caregiver burden, these programs may also improve the quality of life for patients and their families. Other re-sources that might be helpful include social service agencies, community-based social workers, home health agencies, cleaning services, Meals on Wheels, transportation programs, geriatric law specialists, and financial planners.

When families feel that they are no longer able to care for patients at home, they may need both logistical and emotional support in placing the patient in a long-term care facility (e.g., continuing care retirement community, group home, or nursing home). The psychiatrist can be a valuable resource in informing families about the available options and helping them evaluate and anticipate their needs in the context of their values, priorities, and other responsibilities. The question of placement in a long-term care facility should be raised well before it becomes an immediate necessity so that families who wish to pursue this option have time to select and apply for a suit-able home, to plan for paying for long-term care, and to make needed emotional ad-justments. A referral to a social service agency, private social worker, or the local chapter of the Alzheimer's Association may assist with this transition. Some social ser-vice agencies provide comprehensive home service assessment, which may help fam-ilies recognize and address their needs.

9. Guide the family in financial and legal issues

Patients with dementia often lose their ability to make medical, legal, and financial de-cisions as the disorder progresses, and these functions must be taken over by others (54). In the case of a progressive dementing illness, such as Alzheimer's disease, if family members act while the patient is still able to participate, they can seek his or her guidance regarding long-term plans. In addition, documents such as durable pow-ers of attorney for health care and for financial matters can help families avoid the dif-ficulty and expense of petitioning the courts for guardianship or conservatorship should this become necessary later on in the illness. The specific rules vary from state to state, but the basic principles are the same.

Patients and family members should be advised about the opportunity to discuss preferences about medical treatment early in the course of the illness, while the patient is still able to make his or her wishes known. Issues that might be raised about care in the later stages of the illness include the use of feeding tubes, the care desired for infections and other potentially life-threatening medical conditions, and artificial life support. In most locales, medical decision making can be transferred to a trusted family member (or friend) in the form of a durable power of attorney for health care. For some patients, a living will or advance directive may also be appropriate, but which document is used and its specific features depend on the prevailing state law.

Patients may also pass authority for legal and financial decision making in the form of a durable power of attorney for financial matters. At a minimum, it is generally wise to include a trusted family member as a cosigner on any bank accounts so that payment of expenses can proceed smoothly even when the patient is no longer able to complete the task himself or herself. In some instances, it may be a good idea to warn families about the vulnerability of demented individuals to unscrupulous individuals seeking "charitable" contributions or selling inappropriate goods. If need be, the family can ask the patient to give up charge cards and checkbooks to prevent the loss of the patient's resources.

Patients and families should also be advised of the importance of financial planning early in the illness. This advice may include a frank discussion regarding the financing of home health care and/or institutional care. Unfortunately, once the patient is clearly demented it is too late to purchase long-term care insurance, but careful planning in the early stages may help to lessen the burden of nursing home care or home health services later in the disease.

Patients should also be advised to complete or update their wills while they are able to make and express decisions (55). A patient with more complex financial issues should be referred to an attorney or financial planner to establish any appropriate trusts, plan for transfer of assets, and so on.

C. SPECIFIC PSYCHOTHERAPIES/PSYCHOSOCIAL TREATMENTS

The psychiatric care of patients with dementia involves a broad range of psychosocial treatments for the patient and his or her family, as already described. In addition, some patients may benefit from more specific psychosocial interventions. These more specific psychosocial treatments for dementia can be divided into four broad groups: behavior oriented, emotion oriented, cognition oriented, and stimulation oriented.

Although few of these treatments have been subjected to rigorous double-blind, randomized controlled trials, some are supported by research findings and practice. The studies were generally small, and many of the reports failed to fully characterize the intervention, the nature of the subjects' dementia or their baseline status, or the posttreatment outcome. Nonetheless, a review of the literature reveals modest efficacy of such treatments (although the limited available follow-up data suggest that the benefits of most do not persist beyond the duration of the interventions).

1. Goals

While these treatments differ in philosophy, focus, and methods, they have the broadly overlapping goals of improving quality of life and maximizing function in the context of existing deficits. Many have as an additional goal the improvement of cognitive skills, mood, or behavior. They are discussed together here because of their overlapping goals and apparent nonspecificity of action.

2. Types of psychotherapies/treatments and their efficacy

a) Behavior-oriented approaches

Although there are limited data from formal assessments of these treatments, there is widespread agreement that behavioral approaches (56, 57) can be effective in lessening or abolishing problem behaviors (e.g., aggression, screaming, incontinence) (58). The first step is a careful description of the behavior in question, including where it occurs, when it occurs, and how often it occurs. The next step is an assessment of the specific antecedents and consequences of each problem behavior, which will often suggest specific strategies for intervention. Activities that consistently precede the problem behavior may be acting as precipitants and should be avoided whenever possible. If the activity is a necessary one, such as bathing, it may be helpful to decrease its frequency or alter the environment so that the negative consequences are minimized (e.g., switch bath time to allow a home health aid to supervise, or change the location of baths to decrease the impact of aggressive outbursts on family members or other patients). When multistep activities, such as dressing and eating, precipitate problem behaviors, such as aggression, it often helps to simplify them or break them into parts (e.g., using clothing with Velcro closures, serving several simple snacks instead of a large meal). Whatever the intervention, it is critical to match the level of demand on the patient with his or her current capacities, avoiding both infantilization and frustration, and to modify the environment insofar as possible to compensate for deficits and capitalize on the patient's strengths.

b) Emotion-oriented approaches

These interventions include supportive psychotherapy (59), reminiscence therapy (reviewed by Burnside and Haight [60]), validation therapy (61, 62), sensory integration (63), and simulated presence therapy (64).

Reminiscence therapy, which aims to stimulate memory and mood in the context of the patient's life history, has been shown in three studies of "confused" elderly persons (65–67) to be associated with modest short-lived gains in mood, behavior, and cognition. In a single small study (68), the effects of validation therapy, which aims to restore self-worth and reduce stress by validating emotional ties to the past, on cognitive, functional, and mood measures were not significantly different from the effects of reality orientation or no intervention. Preliminary evidence from one small study (64) suggests that simulated presence therapy may be helpful in diminishing problem behaviors associated with social isolation. In another small study (63), sensory integration showed no difference from no intervention in effects on cognitive, behavioral, and functional measures. Supportive psychotherapy also falls under this rubric. It has received little or no formal assessment, but some clinicians find it useful in helping mildly impaired patients adjust to their illness.

c) Cognition-oriented approaches

These techniques include reality orientation (reviewed by Powell-Proctor and Miller [69]) and skills training (70). The aim of these treatments is to redress cognitive deficits, often in a classroom setting. In a number of studies of both institutionalized and noninstitutionalized patients, reality orientation has produced modest transient improvement in verbal orientation (65, 71–80). Some studies have also demonstrated slight transient improvement in other measures of cognition, function, behavior, and social interaction. Of note, there have been case reports of anger, frustration, and depression precipitated by reality orientation (81). There is also some evidence for transient benefit from cognitive remediation and from skills (or memory) training (70, 82–86) but there have been reports of frustration in patients and depression in caregivers associated with this type of intervention (47). The slight improvements observed with some of these treatments have not lasted beyond the treatment sessions and thus do not appear to warrant the risk of adverse effects.

d) Stimulation-oriented approaches

These treatments include activities or recreational therapies (e.g., crafts, games, pets) and art therapies (e.g., music, dance, art). They provide stimulation and enrichment and thus mobilize the patient's available cognitive resources. There is some evidence that, while they are in use, these interventions decrease behavioral problems and improve mood (79, 87, 88). Although the data supporting efficacy are limited either by small number of subjects (79, 87) or multiple interventions (87), there is anecdotal and common sense support for their inclusion as part of the humane care of patients with dementia. Additional support for this approach comes from the work of Teri et al. (89, 90), who have developed a behavioral protocol for managing Alzheimer's disease that includes a number of interventions. The core of this protocol is identifying and increasing the number of pleasant activities, which has been shown in preliminary studies to improve the mood of patients and caregivers alike.

3. Side effects

Short-term adverse emotional consequences have been reported with psychosocial treatments. This is especially true of the cognitively oriented treatments, during which frustration, catastrophic reactions, agitation, and depression have been reported. Thus, treatment regimens must be tailored to the cognitive abilities and frustration tolerance of each patient.

4. Implementation

Behavioral interventions have strong support in clinical practice and deserve careful trials with patients who have behavioral problems that are difficult to manage. Many stimulation treatments provide the kind of environmental stimulation that is recognized as part of the humane care of patients, and thus such treatments are often included in the care of patients with dementia. Beyond this, the choice of therapy is generally based on patient characteristics and preference, availability, and cost. For instance, some approaches are available only in institutional settings, such as nursing homes or day care centers, while others can be used at home. In many cases, several modalities will be selected at the same time. Because these treatments generally do not provide lasting effects, those that can be offered regularly may be the most practical and beneficial. These treatments are generally delivered daily or weekly.

Rates of short-term response to emotion-oriented treatments are consistent with modest efficacy on a wide variety of outcome measures, and thus these treatments may be helpful for some patients. Cognition-oriented treatments are not supported by efficacy data and also have the potential to produce adverse effects.

▶ D. SOMATIC TREATMENTS

The sections that follow describe medications (and for depression, ECT) used for the purpose of treating the cognitive and functional losses associated with dementia; psychosis, anxiety, and agitation; depression and apathy; and sleep disturbances. Although the sections are organized by these target symptoms, many medications have broader impact in actual practice.

1. Special considerations for elderly and demented populations

Certain principles underlie the pharmacologic treatment of elderly and demented patients. They will be discussed in more detail in the APA practice guideline for geriatric psychiatry (in preparation) and can be summarized as follows. First, it must be remembered that elderly individuals may have decreased renal clearance and slowed hepatic metabolism, so lower starting doses, smaller increases in dose, and longer intervals between increments must be used (this practice is sometimes referred to as "start low and go slow"). Because elderly individuals are more likely to have a variety of general medical problems and take multiple medications, one must be alert to general medical conditions and medication interactions that may further alter the serum binding, metabolism, and excretion of the medication. In addition, certain medication side effects pose particular problems for elderly and demented patients, so medications with these effects must be used especially judiciously. Anticholinergic side effects may be more burdensome in the elderly owing to coexisting cardiovascular disease, prostate or bladder disease, or other general medical conditions. Especially in demented elderly persons, these medications may also lead to worsening cognitive impairment, confusion, or even delirium (91). Elderly individuals have decreased vascular tone, are more likely to be taking other medications that cause orthostasis, and, especially if they are demented, are also more prone to falls and associated injuries. Medications associated with CNS sedation may worsen cognition, increase the risk of falls, and put patients with sleep apnea at risk of additional respiratory depression. Last, the elderly, especially those with Alzheimer's or Parkinson's disease, are especially susceptible to extrapyramidal side effects.

For all these reasons, medications should be used with considerable care. The use of multiple agents (sometimes referred to as "polypharmacy") should be avoided if possible. However, as elderly demented individuals frequently manifest multiple behavioral symptoms that do not respond to psychosocial interventions, and multiple general medical problems as well, some patients benefit from the use of several medications at once.

2. Treatments for cognitive and functional losses

a) Goals

There are a number of psychoactive medications that are used for the purposes of restoring cognitive abilities, preventing further decline, and increasing functional status in patients with dementia. These include cholinesterase inhibitors (tacrine and donepezil); α-tocopherol (vitamin E); selegiline (deprenyl), approved for Parkinson's disease but studied and used in demented populations; and ergoloid mesylates (Hydergine), which are approved for nonspecific cognitive decline. In addition, a number of other medications have been proposed for the treatment of cognitive decline, including NSAIDs, estrogen supplementation, melatonin, botanical agents (e.g., ginkgo biloba), and chelating agents. Many additional agents are currently being tested; for patients who have access to academic medical centers, participation in clinical trials is another option. Interventions for specific medical conditions, such as blood pressure control and use of aspirin to prevent further strokes, and prescription of L-dopa as a general treatment of Parkinson's disease, are beyond the purview of this guideline.

b) Cholinesterase inhibitors

In 1993 tacrine became the first agent approved specifically for the treatment of cognitive symptoms in Alzheimer's disease. Tacrine is a reversible cholinesterase inhibitor and is thought to work by increasing the availability of intrasynaptic acetylcholine in the brains of Alzheimer's disease patients. The medication may also have other actions. Donepezil, another reversible cholinesterase inhibitor, is now available for treatment of Alzheimer's disease. Additional agents that increase cholinergic function are in development.

(1) Efficacy

The efficacy of tacrine in mild to moderate Alzheimer's disease has been extensively studied. At least five double-blind, placebo-controlled trials with parallel group comparisons including a total of over 2,000 patients have been reported (92–96). Overall, these clinical trials consistently demonstrated differences between tacrine and placebo: approximately 30 to 40% of patients taking tacrine who were able to complete the trials showed modest improvements in cognitive and functional measures over study periods ranging from 6 to 30 weeks, compared to up to 10% of those taking placebo. Modest improvement in these studies corresponds to maintaining or improving function by an amount typically lost over 6 months in untreated groups of similar Alzheimer's disease patients. Response appeared to be related to dose, at least in the largest clinical trial (94), in which patients who could tolerate 120 to 160 mg/day were more likely to respond. Only approximately 60% of the patients overall completed the tacrine trials even at moderate doses; 30% of subjects were dropped from these trials prior to completion because of elevation in hepatic transaminases, as specified in the protocols (i.e., more than three times the upper limit of normal, a lower threshold than the current prescribing guidelines, described in the section on implementation), and another 10% had to leave because of other adverse effects, mainly cholinergic effects (e.g., nausea and vomiting). The benefits and adverse effects of administration beyond 30 weeks are unknown. However, one observational study suggests that continued use of tacrine at doses above 120 mg/day was associated with delay in nursing home placement compared with patients who used daily doses below 120 mg (97). Anecdotal reports suggest that individuals who respond to the medication and then stop taking it may have a significant decline. The effects of tacrine on individuals with more severe or very mild Alzheimer's disease or with other dementing illnesses have not been assessed.

The efficacy of donepezil has been reported in three trials (98; Aricept package insert). A 12-week double-blind, randomized parallel group trial (99) included 160 patients with mild to moderate Alzheimer's disease randomized to receive placebo or 1, 3, or 5 mg/day of donepezil. Modest improvements in neuropsychological test results and clinicians' impressions were reported for higher doses. In another 12-week double-blind, parallel group trial (Aricept package insert), approximately 450 patients were randomized to receive placebo, 5 mg/day, or 10 mg/day of donepezil (after 5 mg/day for 1 week). A third trial (Aricept package insert), this one for 24 weeks, involved 473 patients similarly randomized to placebo, 5 mg, or 10 mg. In both of the latter two trials, the treatment groups showed modest improvement in neuropsychological test performance, clinician's impression of change, and Mini-Mental State examination scores with a trend for a somewhat greater response for the 10-mg dose during the course of the trial. Consistent with observations of tacrine, patients discontinued from donepezil after 12 or 24 weeks of treatment returned to the cognitive level of the placebo treated patients within 3-6 weeks. In long-term observations over 2 years, patients continued on doses of 5 mg or greater of donepezil overall maintained their performance at or above baseline for an average of 40 weeks and deteriorated less when compared to a historical comparison group (100).

(2) Side effects and toxicity

As would be expected with cholinesterase inhibitors, side effects associated with cholinergic excess, particularly nausea and vomiting, are common, but tend to be mild to moderate for both agents. Observed rates are on the order of 10%–20% of patients. Additional cholinergic side effects include bradycardia, which can be dangerous in individuals with cardiac conduction problems, and increased gastrointestinal acid, a particular concern in those with a history of ulcer and those taking NSAIDs. However, these effects appear to occur infrequently with these agents. In general, cholinergic effects tend to wane within 2 to 4 days, so if patients can tolerate unpleasant effects in the early days of treatment, they may be more comfortable later on.

A unique property of tacrine is direct medication-induced hepatocellular injury. Approximately 30% of patients develop significant (e.g., three times the upper limit of normal) but reversible and asymptomatic elevations in liver enzyme levels, and for 5%–10% of patients the medication must be stopped owing to more marked elevations (e.g., 10 times the upper limit of normal). However, perhaps 80% of patients who initially develop elevations in liver enzyme levels can be successfully rechallenged with more-gradual increases in dose, as described in the following section. The hepatotoxicity is more common in women and tends to occur about 6 to 8 weeks into treatment. It has thus far proved to be reversible with discontinuation of the medication (101). No additional toxicities with donepezil have been reported, but the experience with this agent is limited.

(3) Implementation

Given the evidence for modest improvement in some patients and the lack of established alternatives, it is appropriate to consider a trial of one of these agents for mildly or moderately impaired patients with Alzheimer's disease for whom the medication is not contraindicated (e.g., in the case of tacrine, because of liver disease). Patients and their families should be apprised of the limited potential benefits and potential costs (including, in the case of tacrine, risk of hepatotoxicity) (102). Although the currently available data do not allow a direct comparison, they suggest similar degrees of efficacy for the two medications. However, donepezil has the advantage of greater ease of use because it can be given once instead of four times per day and does not require regular liver function tests. Thus, donepezil may prove preferable as a first-line treatment. However, accumulated data from clinical practice with typical Alzheimer's disease patients, along with the outcome of additional clinical trials, will be critical in developing a more complete picture of donepezil's efficacy and adverse effects. Because the efficacy of these two agents is modest, it is also appropriate to discuss alternative options, including vitamin E or possibly selegiline, psychosocial interventions, participation in a trial of an experimental treatment (if available locally), or no treatment.

For tacrine, the starting dose is currently 10 mg q.i.d. The dose may be increased by 10 mg q.i.d. (40 mg/day) every 6 weeks up to a maximum dose of 40 mg q.i.d. The highest tolerated dose (up to 160 mg/day) should be administered, since cognitive improvement is more likely to occur at higher doses. If there is no improvement in clinical status after 3–6 months, most clinicians would stop the medication.

Because of hepatotoxicity, the patient's baseline level of alanine aminotransferase (ALT) should be measured before tacrine treatment is begun; patients with elevations should not receive the medication. Once the medication is begun, ALT should be measured every 2 weeks for approximately 3 months after each dose increase, and once the dose has been stable for 3 months, ALT may be measured every 3 months. If the ALT level is three to five times the upper limit of normal, the dose should be decreased to the prior dose. A later repeat trial at the higher dose can often be accomplished without a significant increase in ALT. If it is five to 10 times the upper limit of normal, the medication should be temporarily discontinued, with a rechallenge considered after the ALT level returns to baseline. A later repeat trial can sometimes be accomplished without a significant increase in ALT. If the ALT level is more than 10 times the upper limit of normal, the medication should be discontinued. These recommendations are currently under review and may change in the near future. In addition, a trial of sustained-release tacrine is underway, so the frequency of administration may change and four-times-per-day dosing may no longer be necessary.

For donepezil, the currently recommended starting dose is 5 mg/day. After 1 week, the dose may be increased to 10 mg/day. The higher dose should be used if tolerated, as it is associated with greater efficacy; however, it has a greater tendency to cause cholinergic side effects. It should be noted that dosing and other aspects of administration may evolve as clinical experience with this medication accumulates.

c) Vitamin E

There has been considerable interest in vitamin E (α-tocopherol) as a treatment for Alzheimer's disease and other dementias because of its antioxidant properties. Vitamin E has been shown to slow nerve cell damage and death in animal models and cell culture (including damage associated with amyloid deposition, and thus possibly relevant to the development and progression of Alzheimer's disease) (103–106).

(1) Efficacy

A single clinical trial has been conducted concerning vitamin E in Alzheimer's disease (106). This placebo-controlled, double-blind, multicenter trial included 341 moderately impaired patients randomized to receive either 1000 IU b.i.d. of vitamin E alone, 5 mg b.i.d. of selegiline alone, both, or placebo, and found that vitamin E alone and selegiline alone were equivalently helpful in delaying the advent of a poor outcome (defined as death, institutionalization, or significant functional decline). Combined treatment performed somewhat worse than either agent alone, but the difference was not statistically significant. The benefit observed among individuals treated with vitamin E or selegiline alone was equivalent to approximately 7 months delay in reaching any of the endpoints designated as a poor functional outcome. It should be noted that there was no evidence of *improvement* in function compared to baseline, but only of *decreased rates of functional decline* on active treatment compared to on placebo. Despite the evidence for a better *functional* outcome in the treatment groups compared to the placebo group, all groups showed similar rates of *cognitive* decline during the 2-year study period. There are no data concerning the role of vitamin E in Alzheimer's disease with mild or severe impairment, or in other dementing illnesses. There are also no data concerning the effect of vitamin E in combination with medications other than selegiline.

(2) Side effects and toxicity

Vitamin E has been widely used clinically, has been observed in many clinical trials for other indications, and is considered to have low toxicity. Doses between 200–3000

IU/day have been shown to be safe and well-tolerated in many studies (107). At high doses, it has sometimes been noted to worsen blood coagulation defects in patients with vitamin K deficiency (107).

In the trial described above (106), the vitamin E group showed an elevated rate of falls and syncope compared to placebo, but the difference was not statistically significant and did not lead to attrition from the study. Vitamin E has not been associated with this effect in trials for other indications (107).

(3) Implementation

On the basis of these data, vitamin E may be used in moderately impaired patients with Alzheimer's disease in order to delay the progression of disease. Vitamin E has not been studied in Alzheimer's disease with mild or severe impairment, but, given its lack of toxicity (and possible other health benefits), some physicians might consider the medication for patients at these stages of disease as well. Vitamin E has not been studied in combination with cholinesterase inhibitors, and there is no clinical experience with this combination. However, given vitamin E's lack of medication interactions, it might be considered for use in combination with a cholinesterase inhibitor. Available evidence suggests that there is no benefit to giving vitamin E in combination with selegiline, since the combination treatment performed no better than either agent alone in the large clinical trial described above (106).

The efficacy data reported here are for a fairly high dose of 2000 IU/day. There are no data concerning other doses. Because of the association of vitamin E and worsening of coagulation defects in patients with vitamin K deficiency, vitamin E should be limited to conventional doses (200–800 IU/day) in this population.

d) Selegiline

Selegiline (also known as l-deprenyl) is a selective MAO-B inhibitor licensed in the United States for the treatment of Parkinson's disease. It is approved as a dementia medication in some European countries and is used by some clinicians in the United States for this indication. It has been suggested that selegiline may act as an antioxidant or neuroprotective agent and slow the progression of Alzheimer's disease, although, because of its effects on catecholamine metabolism, it could also act in a variety of other ways (106).

(1) Efficacy

Selegiline has been studied in six double-blind, randomized clinical trials involving over 500 patients with dementia followed over periods ranging from 1 month to 2 years (106, 108–115). The largest and most methodologically rigorous of these trials was the comparison of selegiline and vitamin E to placebo, described in section III.D.2.c.1., in which selegiline appeared similar to vitamin E and both were superior to placebo in delaying poor outcome, and combined treatment appeared similar but somewhat worse than either agent alone.

The remaining five double-blind, randomized trials (108–115) were generally smaller, briefer (1–3 months), and had methodologic limitations. Nonetheless, all but one (110, 111) showed statistically significant or nearly significant improvements in a variety of measures across multiple domains, both cognitive and noncognitive. In addition there were five small, within-subject crossover studies of similar durations that supported a beneficial effect of selegiline (116–120).

(2) Side effects and toxicity

Selegiline's principal side effect is orthostatic hypotension, which has been reported to interfere with some patients' tolerance of the medication. However, this may be more common in patients with Parkinson's disease, since it was not observed in the large Alzheimer's disease trial reported above (106). The investigators reported that the agent was well-tolerated, and, although a somewhat higher rate of falls and syncope were reported with selegiline than with placebo, the differences were not statistically significant and did not lead to drop-out from the study.

Beyond these effects, selegiline is reported to be quite activating, which is helpful for some patients but may lead to anxiety and/or irritability in others (118). The 5- to 10-mg/day dose used in the treatment of dementia is relatively selective for MAO-B and does not fully inhibit MAO-A, so a tyramine-free diet and avoidance of sympathomimetic agents are not required. However, patients and caregivers should be warned about the symptoms of hypertensive crisis and the critical nature of the 10-mg dose ceiling. More critical, adverse effects of medication interactions, including changes in mental status, seizures, and even death have been observed with meperidine, SSRIs, and tricyclic antidepressants, although there are also reports of patients who have tolerated these combinations. Selegiline is generally considered contraindicated for patients who are taking any of these agents.

(3) Implementation

The recent large study confirms the efficacy of selegiline in delaying the progression of Alzheimer's disease with moderate impairment. However, in the same study, vitamin E, which is generally less expensive and has a more favorable side effect profile and less potential for medication interactions, had approximately equal efficacy, and thus might appear preferable to selegiline. On the other hand, there is also modest support for cognitive and functional improvement with selegiline, rather than simply the prevention of functional decline, so a trial of selegiline might be considered, especially for those patients who cannot take cholinesterase inhibitors. There are limited data concerning the role of selegiline at other stages of Alzheimer's disease, but it is possible that it would offer a benefit to either milder or more severely impaired patients. Last, if the side effects and medication interactions do not pose a problem, selegiline may be continued in patients whose families report a benefit. The standard dose of selegiline for dementia is 5–10 mg/day. In the largest trial (106), which was reported above, 10 mg was used.

e) Ergoloid mesylates

(1) Efficacy

A mixture of ergoloid mesylates, known by the trade name Hydergine, is currently marketed for the treatment of nonspecific cognitive impairment. It has been available for at least 40 years and has been studied in at least 150 clinical trials. Of these, seven were double-blind, placebo-controlled, randomized trials with a parallel group design involving a total of 297 patients with diagnoses consistent with Alzheimer's disease (84, 121–126). A recent meta-analysis (116) suggested that there might have been improvements in some neuropsychological and behavioral measures, but the overall effect sizes were not statistically significant. There was a general impression that any improvement observed was in behavioral rather than cognitive measures. In seven trials involving a total of 140 patients with vascular dementia (123, 125, 127–131), there was somewhat more compelling evidence of modest improvement on neuropsychological and behavioral measures.

(2) Side effects and toxicity

Ergoloid mesylates occasionally cause mild nausea or gastrointestinal distress, but no significant side effects or toxicity have emerged during long-term use. However, the medication is contraindicated for patients with psychosis.

(3) Implementation

The questionable efficacy of ergoloid mesylates suggested by extensive study argues against routine use of this medication in the treatment of dementia. However, under some circumstances it may be appropriate to offer a trial of this agent for vascular dementia. For Alzheimer's disease, a trial of a cholinesterase inhibitor, vitamin E, or selegiline is probably preferable, and for some patients participation in a clinical trial at an academic medical center may also be preferable. However, when these options are inappropriate or unsuccessful, a trial of ergoloid mesylates may be appropriate for patients with a strong interest in pharmacologic therapy. In addition, use of the medication may be safely continued for patients whose families report a benefit. The manufacturer's recommended dose is 3 mg/day, but studies using 4 or more (up to 9) mg/day were more likely to show significant improvements in patient outcomes.

f) Other agents

A number of additional medications marketed for other indications have been proposed for the treatment of dementia on the basis of epidemiologic data or pilot studies, but they cannot be recommended for use at this time. Aspirin and other NSAIDs have been proposed because of epidemiologic data suggesting that they protect against the development of the disease (132–135) and because of hypotheses regarding the involvement of inflammatory mechanisms (136). In a single small treatment trial for patients with Alzheimer's disease, patients receiving indomethacin, 100 to 150 mg/day, experienced less decline over 6 months than did a matched control group (134). Patients using or considering these agents for other indications (e.g., arthritis treatment) might consider this preliminary evidence when weighing the risks and benefits of nonsteroidal therapy.

Estrogen replacement therapy, which is known to affect cognitive function (137), has been shown to be beneficial in the treatment of dementia in at least two case series (138, 139), and it has been associated with later onset and/or decreased risk of cognitive decline in at least two observational studies of postmenopausal women (140, 141). A clinical trial of estrogen in the treatment of postmenopausal women with Alzheimer's disease is in progress. In the meantime, postmenopausal women weighing the risks and benefits of estrogen replacement might consider this preliminary evidence (142).

There is also interest in the hormone melatonin and in botanical agents, such as ginkgo biloba, which are available without a prescription. Because some of these agents are quite popular, psychiatrists should routinely inquire about their use and should advise patients and their families that these agents are marketed with limited quality control and have not been subjected to efficacy evaluations.

The chelating agent desferrioxamine has also been studied as a possible treatment for Alzheimer's disease on the basis of hypotheses regarding heavy metals in the pathogenesis of the disease. In one small single-blind trial, there was some evidence of a decrease in cognitive decline over 2 years (143). Study of another chelating agent has failed to confirm this finding (144). Because chelating agents are quite toxic and support for them is so weak, they cannot be recommended for the treatment of dementia.

3. Treatments for psychosis and agitation

a) Goals

Use of such treatments is intended to decrease psychotic symptoms (including paranoia, delusions, and hallucinations) and associated or independent agitation, screaming, combativeness, or violence and thereby increase the comfort and safety of patients and their families and caregivers. Although DSM-IV defines one subtype of Alzheimer's disease (and other dementias) on the basis of delusions and another subtype by behavioral disturbances, this section covers both, along with hallucinations, paranoia, and suspiciousness. This section also briefly addresses the treatment of anxiety in demented individuals.

In the consideration of an intervention, it is critical to be specific in describing target symptoms, both to select the optimal treatment and to monitor the effect of that treatment (145–147). However, the treatments used for this broad group of symptoms overlap to a considerable extent, so they are discussed together here.

b) General principles

Interventions for psychosis should be guided by the patient's level of distress and the risk to the patient or caregivers. If there is little distress or danger, reassurance and distraction are often all that is required. If the patient is distressed or if accompanying agitation, combativeness, or violent behavior put the patient or others in danger, psychopharmacologic treatment is indicated. The principles for anxiety are similar, although it is less commonly associated with dangerous behavior.

"Agitation" is an umbrella term that can refer to a range of behavioral disturbances, including aggression, combativeness, hyperactivity, and disinhibition. The first priority in treating such conditions is a careful medical evaluation. Agitation can result from an occult general medical problem, untreated or undertreated pain, depression, sleep loss, or delirium. The agitation will often resolve with treatment of the underlying condition. The next step is an assessment of the patient's overall situation: agitation can also result from physical discomfort, such as hunger, constipation, or sleep deprivation; an interpersonal issue, such as a change in living situation or a new caregiver or roommate; or an emotional difficulty, such as frustration, boredom, or loneliness. Attending to unmet needs, providing reassurance, or redirecting activities may resolve the problem. If the agitation occurs repeatedly, it is often helpful to institute the behavioral measures discussed in section III.C.2.a. If these measures are unsuccessful, then pharmacologic treatment should be considered, especially if the agitation puts the patient or others in danger.

If the psychosis and/or agitation is deemed dangerous to the patient and caregiver, the psychiatrist must undertake the measures necessary to assure safety, in addition to pharmacologic intervention. Such additional measures may include hospitalization, one-on-one care, or physical restraint.

Whatever agent is used in the treatment of behavioral disturbances, its continued use must be evaluated and justified on an ongoing basis. As a dementing illness evolves, psychosis and agitation may wax and wane or may change in character: more or less of a medication, a change in medications, or no medication at all may be indicated in response to these changes.

c) Antipsychotics

(1) Efficacy

Antipsychotic medications have been extensively studied in the treatment of psychosis and agitation in demented individuals. For example, a 1990 review (148) identified seven double-blind, placebo-controlled, randomized parallel group clinical trials including 252 patients studied over 3 to 8 weeks (149–155). Despite some methodologic flaws, notably small numbers of subjects and a lack of diagnostic specificity, taken together these studies constitute solid evidence for a modest improvement in behavioral symptoms with antipsychotic treatment. A meta-analysis of these seven trials (148), using clinician assessment of improvement in a variety of behavioral symptoms as the primary outcome, showed improvement in 59% of the subjects taking antipsychotics and 41% of those taking placebo. The studies varied widely in dose, ranging from 66 to 267 mg/day in chlorpromazine equivalents, and efficacy for behavioral symptoms was not correlated with standardized dose. Adverse effects were common, but specific rates are not available. Dropout rates were also high, whether associated with side effects or poor efficacy. Of note, one study suggested that antipsychotic agents are most effective specifically for psychotic symptoms (149). The available studies comparing antipsychotics to one another are of limited power but suggest no difference in efficacy (147, 148). Of note, there are limited data on the efficacy of antipsychotic medications for demented individuals beyond 8 weeks of follow-up, although extensive clinical experience suggests that they are helpful for longer periods of time.

Newer agents, such as risperidone and clozapine, have not been studied for demented populations in well-controlled trials. However, risperidone was effective in several case series of geriatric patients, including those with dementia (156), and also has support from some geriatric clinicians, who report that it is effective against agitation and psychosis in geriatric patients even at very low doses (i.e., 0.5–2.0 mg/day), which may limit extrapyramidal side effects. Clozapine has been found to be useful in controlling psychotic symptoms in Parkinson's disease (157) and Lewy body disease (158) and may also be useful for patients with Alzheimer's disease who are sensitive to the extrapyramidal effects of conventional antipsychotic agents (159). Olanzapine was released in 1996, and sertindole and quetiapine are due to be released in the near future. Early data suggest that their efficacy is similar to that of conventional antipsychotic agents, but they have not yet been tested in geriatric or demented populations.

(2) Side effects and toxicity
Antipsychotic agents have a broad range of common side effects that tend to vary with medication potency, although any effect can be seen with any agent. High-potency agents (e.g., haloperidol, fluphenazine) are most strongly associated with akathisia (which can worsen the target behaviors) and parkinsonian symptoms. Low-potency agents (e.g., thioridazine, chlorpromazine) are associated with sedation (which can lead to worsening cognition or falls), confusion, delirium, postural hypotension (which can also lead to falls), and a variety of peripheral anticholinergic effects (e.g., dry mouth, constipation). Risperidone shares many features with high-potency antipsychotic agents, although some clinicians feel that it has a somewhat lower risk of extrapyramidal effects, especially if low doses (0.5–2.0 mg/day) are used. Unfortunately, there are few data from direct comparisons of risperidone and conventional antipsychotics using equivalent doses, especially for elderly patients. Clozapine is less commonly associated with extrapyramidal side effects but is associated with sedation, postural hypotension, and an elevated risk of seizures. Early trials of the newer agents—olanzapine, sertindole, and quetiapine—suggest that they carry little or no risk of extrapyramidal effects for general psychiatric patients, but additional research and clinical experience will be necessary to characterize their performance for elderly and demented patients in general practice.

All of these side effects can be minimized by using the lowest effective dose. This principle is particularly important in order to minimize sedation and akathisia, both of which can actually worsen target behaviors and may thus make antipsychotics less effective (160). It may also be helpful to select an agent with the side effect profile most suited to a given patient. Anticholinergic agents may be effective in the treatment of parkinsonian side effects, but the high risk of associated cognitive decline, delirium, and other anticholinergic effects suggests that they should be used only with extreme caution for elderly and demented patients.

In addition to these common side effects, antipsychotic agents are associated with a risk of more serious complications that must be considered in weighing the risks and benefits of antipsychotic treatment. The first is tardive dyskinesia, which is more likely with increasing dose and duration of treatment and occurs more commonly in women, demented individuals, and the elderly in general. The risk may be as high as 30% for elderly patients with significant exposure (161–163). The second additional possible complication is neuroleptic malignant syndrome, which is rare but potentially lethal. Both of these complications have been reported with risperidone, although they may occur at lower frequencies. Clozapine appears less likely to be associated with these two complications, although they have been described with clozapine treatment. Clozapine has a significant risk of agranulocytosis, which is more common in the elderly than in younger patients (159), and regular monitoring of blood counts is required. Olanzapine, sertindole, and quetiapine have not been associated with these complications, although additional research data and practice experience will be needed to identify and characterize their effects on demented and geriatric patients in general practice.

(3) Implementation

Antipsychotics are the only pharmacologic treatment available for psychotic symptoms in dementia. They are also the most commonly used and best-studied pharmacologic treatment for agitation, and there is considerable evidence for their efficacy. However, there are a number of nonpharmacologic interventions that can be used before a trial of an antipsychotic or other medication is begun, as already outlined. Use of nonpharmacologic treatments is particularly critical given the large number and potential severity of side effects and more serious complications associated with antipsychotic medications.

There are no efficacy data to guide the choice among antipsychotic agents. Instead, the choice is based on the side effect profile. Some clinicians recommend agents that fall between the extremes of side effect profiles (e.g., perphenazine), but there are no data to support the contention that these agents have fewer adverse effects. It generally makes sense to select an agent whose most typical side effects are least likely to cause problems for a given patient (for instance, a higher-potency agent, e.g., haloperidol, might be selected if the patient is likely to be sensitive to anticholinergic effects, or a lower-potency agent, e.g., thioridazine, might be chosen if the patient has parkinsonian symptoms) or might actually be beneficial (e.g., a more sedating medication, given at bedtime, for a patient with difficulty falling asleep). Some clinicians believe that risperidone also poses a lower risk of extrapyramidal symptoms when used at doses of 2 mg/day or lower (164), but others disagree (165). Clozapine may be a good choice for individuals with Parkinson's disease (157) or Lewy body disease (158) and possibly for others who cannot tolerate extrapyramidal side effects (156). Olanzapine and the two novel agents due to be released soon (sertindole and quetiapine) may prove to be good choices for geriatric and demented patients, especially those who are sensitive to extrapyramidal side effects, but insufficient data are available to recommend them at this time.

Antipsychotics are most commonly administered in the evening, so that maximum blood levels occur when they will help foster sleep and treat behavioral problems that peak in the evening hours (sometimes called "sundowning"). Most of these medications have long half-lives, so once-a-day dosing is generally sufficient. However, morning doses or twice-a-day doses may be helpful for patients with different symptom patterns.

On the whole, antipsychotic agents are given as standing doses rather than as needed, although as-needed doses may be appropriate for symptoms that occur infrequently. Oral administration is generally preferred, although an intramuscular injection may sometimes be used in an emergency or when a patient is unable to take medications by mouth (e.g., for a surgical procedure). Very low doses of depot antipsychotic medications (e.g., 1.25–3.75 mg/month of fluphenazine decanoate) were shown in a small open study to be effective in managing chronic behavioral problems in this population (166).

Low starting doses are recommended, e.g., 0.5 mg/day of haloperidol, 10–25 mg/day of thioridazine, 2 mg/day of perphenazine, 1 mg/day of thiothixene, 0.5–1.0 mg/day of risperidone, 12.5 mg/day of clozapine. The dose can be increased on the basis of the response of the target symptom(s). The usual maximum doses of these agents for demented elderly patients are 2–5 mg/day of haloperidol, 10–15 mg/day of thiothixene, 10–15 mg/day of trifluoperazine, 16–24 mg/day of perphenazine, 50–100 mg/day of thioridazine, 4–6 mg/day of risperidone, and 75–100 mg/day of clozapine. Most patients with dementia do best with doses below these maxima, but younger and less frail individuals may tolerate and respond to somewhat higher doses.

Given their side effects and potential toxicity, the risks and benefits of antipsychotic agents must be reassessed on an ongoing basis. The lowest effective dose should be sought, and emergent side effects should first be treated by dose reduction. The routine prescribing of anticholinergic agents is to be avoided. In addition, periodic attempts (e.g., every several months) to reduce or withdraw antipsychotic medications should be considered for all patients in the context of the probability of a relapse and the dangerousness of the target behavior(s).

d) Benzodiazepines

(1) Efficacy

The use of benzodiazepines in the treatment of behavioral symptoms in dementia has been studied in at least seven randomized clinical trials. Five studies including a total of 825 patients compared benzodiazepines to antipsychotics (167–171), and two studies compared benzodiazepines to placebo (172, 173). These studies are limited by poorly specified diagnosis, a mixture of target symptoms, limited outcome measures, and, in most cases, high doses of long-acting agents. Nonetheless, they show fairly consistently that benzodiazepines perform better than placebo but not as well as antipsychotics in reducing behavior problems. However, it is somewhat difficult to extrapolate these results, most of which are based on substantial doses of long-acting agents (e.g., 12 mg/day of diazepam), to the lower doses or the shorter-acting agents more commonly used today. There are no data concerning the efficacy of benzodiazepines after 8 weeks or whether one benzodiazepine is more effective than another.

(2) Side effects and toxicity

The most commonly reported side effects are sedation, ataxia, amnesia, confusion (even delirium), and paradoxical anxiety. These can lead to worsening cognition and behavior and can also contribute to the risk of falls (174). They also carry a risk of respiratory suppression in patients with sleep-related breathing disorders. Because all of these effects are dose related, the minimum effective dose should be used. Agents with long half-lives and long-lived metabolites can take weeks to reach steady-state levels, especially in elderly patients, so these agents must be used with particular caution. There is some evidence that elderly patients taking long-acting benzodiazepines are more likely to fall, and to suffer hip fractures, than those taking short-acting agents (175), although it is possible that the total dose, and not the duration of action, is the culprit (176). Clinical experience suggests that, like alcohol, benzodiazepines may lead to disinhibition, although there are few data to support this. The risk of medication dependence (and withdrawal, if the medication is stopped abruptly) is also a concern for some patients.

(3) Implementation

Although benzodiazepines may have a higher likelihood of side effects and a lower likelihood of benefit than antipsychotics, they can be useful in treating agitation in some patients with dementia, particularly those in whom anxiety is prominent. They may be particularly useful on an as-needed basis for patients who have only rare episodes of agitation or those who need to be sedated for a particular procedure, such as a tooth extraction. However, given the risk of disinhibition (and thus worsening of the target behaviors), oversedation, falls (and associated injuries), and delirium, their use should be kept to a minimum.

Among the benzodiazepines, many clinicians favor agents such as oxazepam and lorazepam that do not require oxidative metabolism in the liver and have no active metabolites. Temazepam shares these characteristics but is more problematic because of its long half-life. Lorazepam may be given on an as-needed basis in doses from 0.5 to 1.0 mg every 4–6 hours. Standing doses of 0.5 to 1.0 mg may be given from one to four times per day. Oxazepam is absorbed more slowly, so it is less useful on an as-needed basis. Standing doses of 7.5 to 15.0 mg may be given one to four times per day. Some clinicians prefer long-acting agents, such as clonazepam (starting at 0.5 mg/day with increases up to 2 mg/day) (177). However, such agents must be used with caution: dose increases must be made very gradually, as the medication can continue to accumulate over a substantial period, and vigilance concerning the increased risk of falls must be exercised. If benzodiazepines are used for an extended period (e.g., a month), they should be tapered rather than stopped abruptly owing to the risk of withdrawal.

e) Anticonvulsants

(1) Efficacy

Use of carbamazepine has support from several case series (178), a small open trial (179), a double-blind, nonrandomized trial (180), and one randomized trial (181) in which it was associated with nonsignificant decreases in behavioral measures.

Several favorable case reports and open trials have been reported for the anticonvulsant valproate (182, 183).

(2) Side effects and toxicity

The principal side effects of carbamazepine include ataxia, sedation, and confusion, which are particular concerns for elderly and demented patients. In addition, in rare instances carbamazepine can lead to bone marrow suppression or hyponatremia.

Valproate's principal side effects are gastrointestinal disturbances and ataxia. In addition, in rare instances it can lead to bone marrow suppression or hepatic toxicity.

(3) Implementation

Given the sparse data on these agents, they cannot be recommended with confidence for the treatment of agitation in demented patients. Nonetheless, a therapeutic trial of one of these agents (especially carbamazepine, for which the data are somewhat stronger at this point) may be appropriate for some nonpsychotic patients, especially those who are mildly agitated or are sensitive or unresponsive to antipsychotics. Given the potential toxicity of these anticonvulsant agents, it is particularly critical to identify and monitor target symptoms and to stop administering the medication if no improvement is observed.

Carbamazepine may be given in two to four doses per day, started at a dose of 100 mg/day, and increased gradually as warranted by behavioral response and side effects or until blood levels reach 8–12 ng/ml. Valproate is given in two or three doses per day and should be started at 125 to 250 mg/day, with gradual increases based on behavioral response and side effects or until blood levels reach 50–60 ng/ml (or, for rare patients in this population, 100 ng/ml).

Many clinicians recommend monitoring CBC and electrolyte levels in patients taking carbamazepine and monitoring CBC and liver function values in patients taking valproate, owing to the possibility of bone marrow suppression, hyponatremia, and liver toxicity. However, this practice is not uniform. For details concerning the assessment and monitoring necessary during use of these agents, along with their side effects and potential toxicities, the reader is referred to the American Psychiatric Association's *Practice Guideline for the Treatment of Patients With Bipolar Disorder* (184; included in this volume). However, a particularly cautious approach is warranted when treating elderly and demented patients, who may be more vulnerable to adverse effects, particularly CNS effects, and yet less likely to be able to report warning symptoms.

f) Other agents

A number of other agents have been proposed for the treatment of agitation in patients with dementia (reviewed in references 148, 185, and 186). Efficacy data for these agents generally come from case reports or small open trials, often of mixed populations.

Data on trazodone have been provided by a few favorable case reports and case series (187–189), one small open trial (190), and one small double-blind, randomized clinical trial (191). Postural hypotension, sedation, and dry mouth are the principal side effects. Trazodone is generally given before bed but can be given in two or three divided doses per day. It can be started at 25 to 50 mg/day and gradually increased up to a maximum dose of 150 to 250 mg/day. Preliminary data suggest that SSRIs may also be useful in the treatment of agitation (190, 192, 193).

There have been at least two case reports (194, 195) and one open trial (196) concerning buspirone as a treatment for agitation or anxiety in elderly patients with dementia. Buspirone is generally well tolerated by elderly individuals but is sometimes associated with nausea, headache, dizziness, light-headedness, and fatigue. It is not associated with psychomotor impairment or tolerance and dependence. It is given in up to four doses per day and can be started at 5 mg/day and increased up to a total

daily dose of 60 mg. There have been case reports of serotonin syndrome when buspirone is combined with SSRIs, so it should be used with SSRIs or other serotonergic
agents only with cautious monitoring.

Given the limited efficacy data, none of these less-well-studied agents can be recommended with any confidence for the treatment of agitation and psychosis in patients with dementia. Nonetheless, a therapeutic trial of trazodone, buspirone, or
perhaps an SSRI may be appropriate for some nonpsychotic patients, especially those
with relatively mild symptoms or those who are intolerant of or unresponsive to antipsychotics.

When male patients display intrusive disinhibited sexual behavior, a particular
problem in patients with frontal lobe dementias, medroxyprogesterone and related
hormonal agents are sometimes recommended (197–199), but only case series support this recommendation at present.

Lithium carbonate has also been suggested because of its occasional utility for mentally retarded patients, but support for it is quite limited and side effects (including a
considerable risk of delirium) are common (148).

Beta blockers, notably propranolol, metoprolol, and pindolol, have also been reported to be helpful for some agitated patients with dementia (200). However, most
of the patients included in the case reports had unusual illnesses. In addition, large
doses (e.g., 200–300 mg/day of propranolol) were used, and such doses create a considerable risk of bradycardia, hypotension, and delirium for elderly patients.

4. Treatments for depression

a) Goals

Somatic treatments for depression in demented patients are used to improve mood,
functional status, and quality of life. Even patients with depressed mood who do not
meet the diagnostic criteria for major depression should be considered for treatment.
This is in keeping with the subtypes of Alzheimer's disease and other dementias included in DSM-IV, which are diagnosed when a patient with dementia has a depressed
mood *with* or *without* the full depressive syndrome. However, patients should be
carefully evaluated for neurovegetative signs, suicidal ideation, and other indicators
of major depression, since these may indicate a need for safety measures (e.g., hospitalization for suicidality) or more vigorous and aggressive therapies (such as higher
medication doses, multiple medication trials, or ECT).

One goal of treating depression in dementia is to improve cognitive symptoms.
Sometimes cognitive deficits partially or even fully resolve with successful treatment
of the depression. Individuals whose cognitive symptoms recover fully with treatment
of the depression are considered not to have been demented (this condition is sometimes referred to as "pseudodementia"); however, as many as one-half of such persons
develop dementia within 5 years (2). Thus, caution is urged in ruling out an underlying early dementia in patients with both mood and cognitive impairment.

A related goal in the treatment of patients with dementia is diminishing apathy,
which is common in Alzheimer's disease and many other dementing illnesses, especially those affecting the frontal lobes, and may occur even in the absence of depression. The treatments for apathy overlap those for depression, so they are reviewed
here as well.

Before any treatment is instituted, patients should be evaluated for general medical
problems (e.g., hypo- or hyperthyroidism, electrolyte imbalance), substance abuse,
and medications (e.g., β blockers, corticosteroids, benzodiazepines) that may be caus-

ing or contributing to the depression. Correctable general medical problems should be addressed, and potentially offending medications should be discontinued (with appropriate substitutions as necessary).

b) Antidepressants

(1) Efficacy

The evidence for the efficacy of antidepressants for demented patients is limited. There have been five small placebo-controlled studies (192, 193, 201–203) and an additional two studies using a within-subject design (204, 205). These studies are limited by small number of subjects, mixed and poorly characterized dementia syndromes, mixed and poorly characterized depressive symptoms (defined variously by mood alone, by diagnosis, or by symptom severity threshold), lack of randomization, and the use of uncommon agents (including many not available in the United States). However, the available evidence suggests that depressive symptoms (including depressed mood alone and with neurovegetative changes) in dementia are responsive to antidepressant therapy. Cognitive symptoms beyond the impairment induced by the depression do not appear to respond to antidepressant treatment. Indeed, one imipramine trial suggested that antidepressant treatment might exert a *negative* effect on cognition, but this observation might have been due to the medication's anticholinergic properties (201).

Although the data from the best-designed trials concern unusual agents, they document that depression in patients with dementia is responsive to treatment. This, along with extensive clinical experience in using more-typical antidepressants for this population (206), suggests that the more substantial efficacy literature concerning pharmacologic treatment of depression may be cautiously applied to patients with dementia. The reader is referred to the *Practice Guideline for Major Depressive Disorder in Adults* (207; included in this volume) for a summary of this literature.

The literature concerning the treatment of apathy is much sparser. There is minimal evidence that dopaminergic agents, such as psychostimulants (*d*-amphetamine, methylphenidate), amantadine, bromocriptine, and bupropion, are helpful in the treatment of severe apathy, but promising case reports suggest that efficacy studies are warranted (208). Psychostimulants have also received some support for the treatment of depression in elderly individuals with severe general medical disorders (209–211).

(2) Side effects and toxicity

The reader is referred to the practice guideline on major depression (207) for a more detailed discussion of the side effects of antidepressant agents and to the forthcoming practice guideline on geriatric psychiatry for a discussion of the particular issues for the elderly. These effects, divided by medication class, are summarized briefly here.

SSRIs, including fluoxetine, paroxetine, and sertraline, tend to have a more favorable side effect profile than do cyclic agents. However, any SSRI can produce nausea and vomiting, agitation and akathisia, parkinsonian side effects, sexual dysfunction, and weight loss, although some of these effects are more common with one agent than another. In addition, physicians prescribing SSRIs should be aware of the many possible medication interactions.

The structurally unique agent bupropion is associated with a risk of seizures, especially at high doses. Venlafaxine is associated with elevations in blood pressure, which sometimes diminish over time.

Cyclic antidepressants generally have significant cardiovascular effects, including orthostatic hypotension and delays in cardiac conduction. Their effects on conduction make these agents dangerous in overdose, so they should be used only for patients who are adequately supervised to guard against accidental or purposeful overdose. Most cyclic antidepressants have anticholinergic properties to some degree, including blurred vision, tachycardia, dry mouth, urinary retention, constipation, sedation, impaired cognition, and delirium. These effects are most marked for amitriptyline and imipramine and least so for nortriptyline and desipramine, but there is considerable variation from patient to patient. Trazodone has minimal cardiac conduction or anticholinergic effects but is associated with postural hypotension, sedation, and a risk of priapism. Nefazodone is most commonly associated with sedation.

MAOIs, including tranylcypromine and phenelzine, can lead to postural hypotension, a particular concern with the elderly because of the risk of falls. In addition, they have complex medication interactions (sympathomimetic agents, narcotics, especially meperidine, and serotonergic agents must be avoided) and require dietary modifications (tyramine-containing foods, such as cheeses, preserved meat, and red wine, must be avoided), which may make them potentially dangerous for poorly supervised individuals with dementia.

Psychostimulants (*d*-amphetamine, methylphenidate) are associated with tachycardia, restlessness, agitation, sleep disturbances, and appetite suppression. Bromocriptine is associated with psychosis, confusion, and dyskinesias. Amantadine is sometimes associated with anticholinergic effects, including delirium.

(3) Implementation

There are no efficacy data on which to base the selection of one antidepressant over another. Thus, the choice of an antidepressant is generally based on the side effect profile and the general medical and psychiatric status of each patient. For example, if sedation is desired, trazodone or perhaps nortriptyline may be selected. If activation is desired, fluoxetine, bupropion, or desipramine may be selected. If the patient has urinary outflow obstruction, even agents with modest anticholinergic effects should be avoided. If the patient has a prolonged Q-T interval or A-V block, fascicular block, or significant coronary artery disease, cyclic antidepressants should be avoided if possible. These and other implementation issues are discussed in greater detail in the practice guidelines on depression and on geriatric psychiatry and are only briefly summarized here.

Many clinicians choose SSRIs as the initial treatment because of their better side effect profiles. Once-a-day dosing is appropriate. Fluoxetine should be started at 5–10 mg/day and increased at several-week intervals to a maximum of 40–60 mg/day. Paroxetine has the same dosing, but the dose can be increased every 1–2 weeks because of its shorter half-life. Sertraline may be started at 25 mg/day and increased at 1–2-week intervals up to a maximum dose of 150–200 mg/day.

Some clinicians favor bupropion. However, it appears to decrease the seizure threshold, so it should not be the first choice for individuals with a high risk of seizures. It is started at 37.5 mg b.i.d. and increased every 5 to 7 days as tolerated up to a maximum of 350–450 mg/day in divided doses. No more than 150 mg should be given within any 4-hour period because of the risk of seizures. Venlafaxine should be avoided for individuals with hypertension if good alternatives are available; if it is used, careful monitoring of blood pressure and adjustment of antihypertensive medication are required. It is started at 18.75 to 37.50 mg b.i.d. and may be increased at approximately weekly intervals up to a maximum dose of 300–375 mg/day. If elevations in blood pressure occur and do not diminish over time and venlafaxine is effective in treating depression in an individual who has not responded to trials of other agents, the medication may be continued and the hypertension may be treated.

Among the tricyclic and heterocyclic agents, theoretical reasoning and clinical experience suggest avoiding agents with prominent anticholinergic activity (e.g., amitriptyline, imipramine). Among the remaining agents, sample dosing strategies are given here for nortriptyline, desipramine, and trazodone. Nortriptyline may be started at 10 to 25 mg/day, with increases at 5–7-day intervals up to a maximum daily dose of 100–150 mg. Dosing is guided by clinical response and side effects. Blood levels, which should not exceed 100–150 ng/ml, may also be helpful. For desipramine, the starting dose is 25 to 50 mg/day, with increases at 5–7-day intervals up to a maximum daily dose of 200 mg. Blood levels should not exceed 150–250 ng/ml. For trazodone, the starting dose is 25–50 mg/day, with increases at 5–7-day intervals up to a maximum daily dose of 300–400 mg.

Because of their side effects and the extra monitoring required, MAOIs should be considered only for individuals who are unresponsive to or unable to take other agents. The MAOIs tranylcypromine and phenelzine may be used at starting doses of 10 mg/day and 15 mg/day, respectively, with monitoring of orthostatic blood pressure, and increased at weekly intervals to maximum doses of 40 and 60 mg/day (in divided doses), respectively. Patients and caregivers must be advised in detail about dietary and medication restrictions. They should also be educated about the symptoms of hypertensive crisis and advised to seek medical attention immediately if these symptoms arise. It is important to inform caregivers that dietary supervision is necessary, since demented patients are unlikely to remember dietary restrictions on their own.

Stimulants are sometimes used in the treatment of apathy or of depression in individuals with serious general medical illness. Dextroamphetamine and methylphenidate are started at 2.5 to 5.0 mg in the morning. They can be increased by 2.5 mg every 2 or 3 days to a maximum of 30 to 40 mg/day. As they are controlled substances, adequate steps to avoid abuse should be taken. Amantadine is sometimes used in the treatment of apathy as well. It may be started at 100 mg/day and increased to a maximum of 200 mg/day. Bromocriptine may be started at 1.25 mg b.i.d. and gradually increased; few patients tolerate more than 2.50 mg b.i.d.

Most patients with dementia will not tolerate the higher maxima given for antidepressant agents, but younger and less frail individuals may tolerate and respond to somewhat higher doses. When a rapid response is not critical, a still more gradual increase may increase the likelihood that a therapeutic dose will be tolerated.

c) Electroconvulsive therapy

There is no substantial literature on the efficacy of ECT in the treatment of depression in dementia. However, considerable clinical experience suggests that ECT may be beneficial for patients with severe major depression who are ineligible for, cannot tolerate, or do not respond to other agents (212). Dementia increases the likelihood of delirium and of memory loss following ECT, but these effects are generally of short duration: delirium tends to resolve within days and memory loss within weeks. Twice-weekly rather than thrice-weekly and unilateral rather than bilateral ECT may decrease the risk of cognitive side effects after ECT.

5. Treatments for sleep disturbance

a) Goals

Treatment of sleep disturbance in dementia is aimed at decreasing the frequency and severity of insomnia, interrupted sleep, and nocturnal confusion in patients with dementia. The goals are to increase patient comfort and to decrease the disruption to families and caregivers. Sleep disorder is common in dementia (213, 214) and is not always so disruptive that the risk of medication side effects is outweighed by the need for a pharmacologic trial. Thus, the psychiatrist assessing a patient for a sleep disorder should first consider whether treatment is needed and then whether appropriate sleep hygiene—including regular sleep and waking times, limited daytime sleeping, avoidance of fluid intake in the evening, calming bedtime rituals, and adequate daytime physical and mental activities (215)—has been tried. If the patient lives in a setting that can provide adequate supervision without undue disruption to others, permitting daytime sleep and nocturnal awakening may provide an alternative to pharmacologic intervention. Pharmacologic treatment should be instituted only after other measures have been unsuccessful. In addition, the clinician should consider whether the sleep disorder could be due to an underlying condition. It is particularly important to be aware of sleep apnea (216), which is relatively common in elderly individuals and contraindicates the use of benzodiazepines or other agents that suppress respiratory drive.

b) Efficacy

There are no available reports of studies that have assessed the efficacy of pharmacologic treatment for sleep disturbances specifically in individuals with dementia or that have compared pharmacologic to nonpharmacologic therapies. However, there are some data concerning use of various agents for mixed elderly populations. Reports of two small studies of chloral hydrate use with the elderly (217, 218) are available. Piccione et al. (217) found chloral hydrate to be better than placebo but not as good as triazolam in the short-term treatment of insomnia in elderly individuals. Linnoila et al. (218) found chloral hydrate to be superior to both tryptophan and placebo in the treatment of sleep disturbances in elderly psychiatric patients. Zolpidem was studied in 119 elderly psychiatric inpatients (219), of whom 50% suffered from dementia. In a double-blind, randomized parallel group clinical trial, zolpidem was superior to placebo on multiple sleep outcomes. A dose of 10 mg appeared to be superior to 20 mg: it was equally effective in promoting sleep and lacked the daytime sleepiness and ataxia sometimes observed at the higher dose. The impact of benzodiazepines and antipsychotics on sleep has not been studied systematically in demented elderly patients. Clinical experience suggests that low-dose antipsychotics (e.g., haloperidol, 0.5–1.0 mg) can be helpful in managing sleep problems in patients with dementia. Clinical experience with benzodiazepines is less favorable, although short- to medium-acting agents at low to moderate doses (e.g., lorazepam, 0.5–1.0 mg; oxazepam, 7.5–15.0 mg) are sometimes helpful for short-term disturbances (e.g., after a change in caregivers).

In addition to pharmacologic agents, there is preliminary evidence from three small open trials for elderly subjects with dementia (220–222) that early morning or evening bright light therapy may improve sleep (and possibly behavior as well). Others have reported preliminary evidence that the hormone melatonin may also be beneficial in the treatment of sleep disturbances in elderly individuals (223, 224), but the agent has not yet been subjected to controlled trials with demented individuals. In addition, it should be noted that such agents lack the quality controls of pharmaceutical agents.

c) Implementation

Given the sparse efficacy data, the choice of pharmacologic agents is generally guided by the presence of other symptoms. For instance, if the patient has psychotic symptoms and sleep disturbance, antipsychotics will generally be given at bedtime, and a relatively sedating antipsychotic (e.g., thioridazine, mesoridazine) may be chosen if not otherwise contraindicated. If the patient is depressed and has a sleep disturbance, an antidepressant with sedative properties (e.g., trazodone, nortriptyline) will be given at bedtime. When anxiety is prominent, a benzodiazepine (e.g., lorazepam) may be selected.

When sleep disturbances occur without other psychiatric symptoms beyond the dementia itself, there is little to guide the choice among agents. Some clinicians prefer trazodone at 25–100 mg h.s. for sleep disturbances. Some prefer zolpidem, 5–10 mg h.s. Benzodiazepines (e.g., lorazepam, 0.5–1.0 mg; oxazepam, 7.5–15.0 mg) and chloral hydrate (250–500 mg) may be used but are generally not recommended for other than short-term sleep problems because of the possibility of tolerance, daytime sleepiness, rebound insomnia, worsening cognition, disinhibition, and even delirium. Triazolam in particular is not recommended for individuals with dementia because of its association with amnesia. Diphenhydramine, which is found in most over-the-counter sleep preparations, is used by some clinicians, but its anticholinergic properties make it suboptimal for the treatment of demented patients.

IV. DEVELOPMENT OF A TREATMENT PLAN

When choosing specific treatments for a demented patient, one begins from the assessment of symptoms. A multimodal approach is often used, combining, for instance, a behavioral and a psychopharmacologic intervention as available and appropriate. When multiple agents or approaches are being used and problems persist (or new problems develop), it is advisable, if possible, to make one change at a time so that the effect of each change can be assessed; this is particularly critical when unusual treatments are being tried. Whatever interventions are implemented, their continuing utility must be periodically reevaluated.

The treatment of dementia varies through the course of the illness, as symptoms evolve over time. Although many symptoms can and do occur throughout the illness, certain symptoms are typical of the various stages, as outlined in section II.E. At each stage of the illness, the psychiatrist should be vigilant for cognitive and noncognitive symptoms likely to be present and should help the patient and family anticipate future symptoms. The family may also benefit from a reminder to plan for the care likely to be necessary at later stages.

▶ A. MILDLY IMPAIRED PATIENTS

At the early stages of a dementing illness, patients and their families are often dealing with recognition of the illness and associated limitations, and they may appreciate suggestions for how to cope with these limitations (e.g., making lists, using a calendar). It may be helpful to identify specific impairments and highlight remaining abilities. Families and patients may also suffer from a sense of loss and from a perceived stigma associated with the illness. Mildly impaired patients should also be advised about the risk of driving. Although there is no consensus on this issue, a review of the data coupled with a concern for the safety of the patient and others suggest that patients with mild impairment should be urged to stop driving or to limit their driving to familiar routes and less challenging situations (e.g., good road conditions, low speeds, spouse or other navigator in the car). At this stage of the illness, the patient should also be advised to draw up a power of attorney for medical and financial decision making, an advance directive, and/or a living will. Patients may also wish to revise their wills and to make the necessary financial arrangements to plan for long-term care. Caregivers should be made aware of the availability of support groups and social agencies.

Patients with Alzheimer's disease seen in the early stages may be offered a trial of tacrine or donepezil for cognitive impairment. Although available data are limited to moderately impaired patients, it is possible that vitamin E might also delay progression of Alzheimer's disease in patients with mild impairment. Thus, physicians might consider vitamin E alone or possibly in combination with a cholinesterase inhibitor at this stage. Selegiline, which also delayed progression in moderately impaired patients, might also be considered, although vitamin E may be preferable because of its more favorable side effect profile and lack of drug interactions. Mildly impaired patients might also be interested in referrals to local research centers for participation in clinical trials of experimental agents for the treatment of Alzheimer's disease. Additional information regarding such trials may be obtained from the local or national chapter of the Alzheimer's Association or from the National Institute on Aging.

Mildly impaired patients also deserve a careful evaluation for depressed mood or major depression, which suggests the need for pharmacologic intervention, as reviewed in section III.D.4.b. Patients with moderate to severe major depression who do not respond to or cannot tolerate antidepressant medications should be considered for ECT. Particularly—but not only—if they are depressed, mildly impaired patients should also be carefully assessed for suicidality.

B. MODERATELY IMPAIRED PATIENTS

As patients become more impaired, they are likely to require more supervision to remain safe. Families should be advised regarding the possibility of accidents due to forgetfulness (e.g., fires while cooking), of difficulties coping with household emergencies, and of the possibility of wandering. Family members should be advised to determine whether the patient is handling finances appropriately and to consider taking over the paying of bills and other responsibilities. At this stage of the disease, patients should be strongly urged not to drive, and families should be urged to undertake measures (such as taking away the car keys) to prevent patients from driving.

As patients' dependency increases, caregivers may begin to feel more burdened. A referral for some form of respite care (e.g., home health aid, day care, or brief nursing home stay) may be helpful. At this stage, families should begin to consider and plan for additional support at home or possible transfer to a long-term care facility.

Treatment for cognitive symptoms should also be considered at this stage. For patients with Alzheimer's disease, currently available data suggest that a trial of tacrine or donepezil is the intervention most likely to lead to improvement in cognitive function. In addition, vitamin E or selegiline, which have been shown to delay progression in Alzheimer's disease patients with moderate impairment, may be offered to patients at this stage. Vitamin E appears preferable because of its low toxicity and lack of drug interactions. It may be appropriate to offer vitamin E in combination with a cholinesterase inhibitor.

Delusions and hallucinations often develop in moderately impaired patients. The patient and family may be troubled and fearful about these symptoms, and it may be helpful to reassure them that the symptoms are part of the illness and are often treatable. If these symptoms cause no distress to the patient and are unaccompanied by agitation or combativeness, they are probably best treated with reassurance and distraction. If they do cause distress or are associated with behavior that may place the patient or others at risk, they should be treated with low doses of antipsychotic medications. If a patient is agitated or combative in the absence of psychosis, treatment with an antipsychotic medication has the most support in the literature, but carbamazepine, valproate, trazodone, buspirone, or possibly an SSRI may be used in a careful therapeutic trial. If behavioral symptoms are time limited, a benzodiazepine may also prove useful. Depression often remains part of the picture at this stage and should be treated vigorously.

▶ C. SEVERELY AND PROFOUNDLY IMPAIRED PATIENTS

At this stage of the illness, patients are severely incapacitated and are almost completely dependent on others for help with basic functions, such as dressing, bathing, and feeding. Families are often struggling with a combined sense of burden and loss and may benefit from a frank exploration of these feelings and any associated resentment or feelings of guilt. They may also need encouragement to get additional help at home or to consider nursing home placement.

There are no data available to guide decisions about the use of cognition-enhancing medications for the severely impaired: use of these medications may be continued, or a medication-free trial may be used to assess whether the medication is still providing a benefit.

Similarly, there are no data available about whether vitamin E or selegiline retards the progression at this stage, and, for patients who reach this stage of illness already taking one of these agents, even a medication-free interval may not clarify the picture, since the expected benefit is slower progression rather than frank improvement.

Depression is somewhat less likely to be present at this stage but should be treated vigorously if it is. Psychotic symptoms and agitation are often present and should be treated pharmacologically if they cause distress to the patient or significant danger or disruption to caregivers.

At this stage, it is important to ensure adequate nursing care, including measures to prevent bed sores and contractures. The psychiatrist should help the family prepare for the patient's death. Ideally, discussions about feeding tube placement, treatment of infection, and cardiopulmonary resuscitation and intubation will have taken place when the patient could also participate, but in any case it is important to raise these issues with the family before a decision about one of these options becomes urgent.

Hospice care is an underused resource for patients with end-stage dementia (225). It provides physical support for the patient (with an emphasis on attentive nursing care rather than medical intervention) and emotional support for the family during the last months of life. In most settings, a physician must certify that the patient is within 6 months of death; the use of a formal rating scale (226) may help in this determination.

V. FACTORS MODIFYING TREATMENT DECISIONS

A. COMORBID CONDITIONS

1. General medical conditions

The likelihood of chronic general medical illnesses and the likelihood of dementia both increase with age, so the two commonly coexist. The assessment and treatment of general medical comorbidity are complicated by memory impairment and aphasia, both of which interfere with the patient's ability to provide a reliable description of symptoms. Resistance to physical examination, laboratory testing, and radiologic procedures can also complicate assessment. The involvement of family members and other caregivers in gathering a history and completing an evaluation is essential.

2. Delirium

Dementia predisposes to the development of delirium (227, 228), especially in the presence of general medical and neurological illnesses. In addition, medications needed to treat comorbid general medical disorders can lead to further cognitive impairment or to delirium, even when doses are appropriate and blood levels are in the nontoxic range. Compounds with anticholinergic effects (e.g., tricyclic antidepressants, low-potency antipsychotics, diphenhydramine, disopyramide phosphate) or histamine-2 activity (cimetidine, ranitidine) are particularly likely to cause delirium, but many classes of medications can do so (229). Of particular relevance to psychiatrists, delirium has been associated with virtually all psychotropic medications, including lithium, other mood stabilizers, tricyclic antidepressants, SSRIs, and benzodiazepines. Avoidance of unnecessary medications, use of the lowest effective dose, vigilant monitoring aimed at early recognition, a thorough search for causes, and prompt treatment may diminish the prevalence and morbidity of delirium.

3. Parkinson's disease

Cognitive impairment coexisting with Parkinson's disease requires a broad treatment approach. First, mild cognitive impairment may be partially ameliorated by dopaminergic agents prescribed for the treatment of motor symptoms, so both cognitive and motor symptoms should be carefully monitored, especially after any intervention. Second, the use of dopaminergic agents predisposes to the development of visual hallucinations and other psychotic phenomena, especially in patients with coexisting dementia, so these agents must be used with particular care, and the minimal dose needed to control the motor symptoms should be used. In addition, these patients, like other elderly and demented patients, are vulnerable to delirium due to medications and concomitant general medical conditions, so the development of these symptoms deserves a thorough evaluation. Third, if psychotic symptoms result in distress or dangerousness, the judicious use of an antipsychotic agent is indicated. Some clinicians prefer the use of low-potency antipsychotic agents (e.g., thioridazine). Others now favor clozapine, but it has received limited study (157). Fourth, the patient must be carefully assessed and treated for depression, which is common in Parkinson's disease and may exacerbate or even be misinterpreted as dementia.

4. Stroke

For patients with dementia and a history of stroke, whether or not the strokes are responsible for or contribute to the dementia, it is critical to conduct a careful evaluation to determine the etiology of the strokes (e.g., atrial fibrillation, valvular disease) and to make any needed referrals for further evaluation and treatment. Beyond this, good control of blood pressure, and perhaps low-dose aspirin, may help to prevent further strokes. In addition, a trial of Hydergine, which appears to be possibly effective in dementia due to vascular disease, may be appropriate. Some clinicians favor pentoxifylline, alleged to improve cognition after stroke by increasing cerebral blood flow (230–232), but this treatment has limited support.

▶ B. SITE-SPECIFIC ISSUES

The care of patients with dementia should be adapted not only to the patient's symptoms and associated general medical problems, but also to his or her environment. Certain issues arise frequently in particular care settings.

1. Home

Of the 3 to 4.5 million Americans with dementia in the United States, only about 1 million reside in nursing homes, leaving over 2 million individuals with dementia who reside at home (233). Psychosocial problems include the need for family care providers to work at jobs outside the home during the day and the adverse emotional impact on caregivers and children or grandchildren. Particularly difficult behavior problems for patients with dementia living at home include poor sleep, wandering, accusations directed toward caregivers, threatening or combative behavior, and reluctance to accept help; all of these are potentially solvable. Interventions with the family that focus on the specific behavior problem and, where appropriate, carefully monitored pharmacologic treatment of behavioral symptoms can be helpful. In addition, the use of home health aides, day care, and respite care may provide stimulation for patients and needed relief for caregivers. The psychological stress on families from Alzheimer's disease appears to be more complex than simply the burden of caring for a disabled family member (234). It has been estimated that 30% of spousal caregivers experience a depressive disorder while providing care for a husband or wife with Alzheimer's disease (235). The prevalence of depressive disorders among adult children caring for a parent with Alzheimer's disease ranges from 22%, among those with no prior history of affective disorder, to 37%, among those with a prior history of depression (235).

2. Day care

Ideally, day care provides a protected environment and appropriate stimulation to patients during the day and gives caregivers a needed break to attend to other responsibilities. Some centers specialize in the care of individuals with dementia and may thus offer more appropriate activities and supervision. Anecdotal reports and practice support the benefit to patients of scheduled activities. However, behavioral symptoms can be precipitated by overstimulation as well as understimulation, so activities must be selected with care and participation should be adjusted according to each patient's response. Of note, problems can arise when patients with different levels of severity are expected to participate together in the same activities.

3. Long-term care

A high proportion of patients with dementia eventually require placement in nursing homes or other long-term care facilities (e.g., assisted living, group home) because of the progression of the illness, the emergence of behavioral problems, the development of intercurrent illness, or the loss of social support. Approximately two-thirds of the residents of long-term care facilities suffer from dementia (233, 236), and as many as 90% of them have behavioral symptoms. Thus, these facilities should be tailored to meet the needs of patients with dementia and to adequately address behavioral symptoms (88, 237).

Research data on the optimum care of individuals with dementia in nursing homes are sparse. One important element is staff who are committed to working with demented patients and knowledgeable about dementia and the management of its noncognitive symptoms. Structured activity programs can improve both behavior and mood (88). Other factors valued in nursing homes include privacy, adequate stimulation, maximization of autonomy, and adaptation to change with the progression of the disease (see references 238, 239). Use of design features such as particular colors for walls, doors, and door frames is widely touted but lacks scientific support.

In recent years special care units have been specifically developed for persons with Alzheimer's disease or other dementing disorders. There are few data to demonstrate that these units are more effective than traditional nursing home units (237), and clinical experience suggests that they vary a great deal in quality. However, the better ones may offer a model for the optimal care of demented patients in any nursing home setting.

A particular concern regarding nursing homes is the use of physical restraints and antipsychotic medications. The Omnibus Budget Reconciliation Act of 1987 (OBRA) regulates the use of physical restraints and many psychotropic medications in nursing homes. Psychiatrists practicing in nursing homes must be familiar with these regulations, which can generally be obtained from the nursing home administrator, local public library, or regional office of the Health Care Financing Administration.

Antipsychotic medications are used in nursing homes, as elsewhere, for the treatment of behavioral and psychotic symptoms. When used appropriately, these medications can be effective in reducing patient distress and increasing safety for the demented patient, other residents, and staff. Overuse, on the other hand, can lead to worsening cognition, oversedation, falls, and numerous other complications and can place patients at risk of tardive dyskinesia. Thus, the OBRA regulations and good clinical practice require careful documentation of the indications for antipsychotic medication treatment and available alternatives and outcomes. In the context of these regulations, a clinical strategy of carefully considering which patients may be appropriate for withdrawal of antipsychotic medications and being prepared to maintain use of the medications in some cases and reinstate them in others, as deemed clinically necessary, may be optimal (240). Of note, a structured education program for nursing and medical staff has been shown to decrease antipsychotic usage in the nursing home setting without adverse outcomes (240). Ongoing use of antipsychotic medication requires regular reassessment of medication response, monitoring for adverse effects, and thorough documentation. Tardive dyskinesia, for which older age, female gender, and brain injury are risk factors, deserves particular attention.

Physical restraints (e.g., Posey restraints, geri-chairs) are sometimes used to treat agitation or combativeness that puts the patient, other residents, or staff at risk. Use of restraints is fairly common in nursing homes (241). However, regulations and humane care support keeping the use of restraints to a minimum, and there is even a suggestion that restraints may increase the risk of falls and contribute to cognitive decline (242, 243).

Although few studies are available to guide the appropriate use of restraints in nursing homes, clinical experience suggests that restraint use can be decreased by environmental changes that reduce the risk of falls or wandering and by careful assessment and treatment of possible causes of agitation. Chest or wrist restraints are appropriately used during a wait for more-definitive treatment for patients who pose an imminent risk of physical harm to themselves or others (e.g., during evaluation of a delirium or during an acute-care hospitalization for an intercurrent illness). For long-term care facilities, geri-chairs may have a place in the care of patients at extreme risk of falling. In any case, regular use of restraints is not recommended unless alternatives have been exhausted. When they are used, they require periodic reassessment and careful documentation.

Documentation of the need for temporary use of restraints should discuss the other measures that were tried and failed to bring the behavior under control. Such measures include a) routine assessment to identify risk factors for falls that would, if addressed, obviate the need for restraints; b) bed and chair monitors that alert nursing staff when patients may be climbing out of bed or leaving a chair; and c) prompted voiding schedules through the day and night in order to decrease the urge for unsupervised trips to the bathroom.

4. Inpatient general medical or surgical services

Patients with dementia on general medical and surgical services are at particular risk for three problems, all of which can lead to aggressive behavior, wandering, climbing over bed rails, removal of intravenous lines, and resistance to needed medical procedures. First, cognitive impairment makes demented individuals vulnerable to behavioral problems owing to fear, lack of comprehension, and lack of memory of what they have been told. No data are available to guide treatment recommendations, but general practice supports having family members or aides stay with the patient as one preventive approach. Frequent reorientation and explanation of hospital procedures and plans, adequate light, and avoidance of overstimulation may also be useful. Second, persons with dementia are at high risk for delirium (227, 228). Prevention of delirium by judicious use of any necessary medications and elimination of any unnecessary ones, attention to fluid and electrolyte status, and prompt treatment of infectious diseases can also diminish morbidity. Occasionally, psychopharmacologic treatment, generally with a high-potency antipsychotic such as haloperidol, is necessary. Third, patients with dementia may have difficulty understanding and communicating pain, hunger, and other troublesome states. For this reason, the development of irritability and/or agitation should prompt a thorough evaluation to identify an occult medical problem or a possible source of discomfort. A significant part of the psychiatrist's role in this setting is educating other physicians and hospital staff regarding the diagnosis and management of dementia and its behavioral manifestations.

5. General psychiatric inpatient units

Individuals with dementia may be admitted to psychiatric units for the treatment of psychotic, affective, or behavioral symptoms. For patients who are very frail or who have significant general medical illnesses, a geriatric psychiatry or medical psychiatric unit may be helpful when available. Indications for hospitalization include those based on severity of illness (e.g., threats of harm to self or others, violent or uncontrollable behavior) and those based on the intensity of services (e.g., need for continuous skilled observation, need for ECT or a medication or test that cannot be performed on an outpatient basis) (10, 11).

A thorough search for psychosocial, general medical, or noncognitive psychiatric difficulties that may be leading to the disturbance will often reveal a treatable problem. If it is reasonably safe, patients should be encouraged to walk freely. Both non-pharmacologic and pharmacologic interventions can be tried more readily and aggressively on inpatient units than in outpatient settings.

C. DEMOGRAPHIC AND SOCIAL FACTORS

1. Age

Because most dementias occur in the elderly, age is the major psychosocial factor affecting treatment. Individuals with dementia occurring in middle age (e.g., early-onset Alzheimer's disease) are likely to have particular difficulty coping with the diagnosis and its impact on their lives. In addition, they may require assistance with problems not generally seen with older patients, such as relinquishing work responsibilities (particularly if their jobs are such that their dementia may put others at risk), obtaining disability benefits, and arranging care for minor children. On the other hand, extremely old patients may be frail and have multiple other general medical problems that lead to more difficult diagnosis and treatment and much greater disability for a given level of dementia.

2. Gender

Another critical area affecting treatment is gender. Dementia, particularly Alzheimer's disease, is more common in women, partly because of greater longevity but possibly also because of other risk factors not yet identified. In addition, because of their greater life expectancy (and tendency to marry men older than themselves), women with dementia are more likely to have an adult child rather than a spouse as caregiver. Unlike an elderly spouse caregiver, who is more likely to be retired, adult child caregivers (most often daughters or daughters-in-law) are more likely to have jobs outside the home and/or to be raising children. These additional responsibilities of caregivers may contribute to earlier institutionalization for elderly women with dementia.

3. Other demographic factors

Perhaps the most critical demographic factor affecting the care of patients with dementia is social support. The availability of a spouse, adult child, or other loved one with the physical and emotional ability to supervise and care for the patient and communicate with treating physicians is critical in both the quality of life and need for institutionalization. In addition, a network of friends, neighbors, and community may play a key role in supporting the patient and primary caregivers.

Another factor is resource availability, which varies widely by geographic region and socioeconomic status. These issues need to be considered for all treatment decisions, but they have a particular impact on decisions about long-term care. A referral to the local chapter of the Alzheimer's Association or a social worker or other individual knowledgeable about local resources, treatment centers, and Medicaid laws can be important in helping families find local treatment options that fit their needs and their budget.

Ethnic background also has an impact on caregiving style, symptom presentation, and acceptance of behavioral disorder. This needs to be taken into account in assessment and treatment planning.

4. Family history

When there are other cases of Alzheimer's disease in the family of a patient with the disease, families may be particularly concerned about the risk to other family members. Such concern is warranted, as first-degree relatives of Alzheimer's disease patients have a risk for the disease that is two to four times that for the general population, and four genes associated with Alzheimer's disease have been identified (see section III.B.7). Families with multiple cases of early-onset (before age 60 or 65) Alzheimer's disease may carry one of the known genes on chromosome 21, 14, or 1 (39–41). Even so, there are currently no associated genetic tests for the disease because it is not possible to screen for the specific mutations, which are often found in only a single family. However, it may be appropriate to refer such families to genetic counselors to help family members further characterize their risk and ensure that they receive up-to-date information on genetic testing and related issues. Late-onset Alzheimer's disease can also run in families, but the only identified gene associated with this pattern is APOE-4, which also confers increased risk in early-onset and nonfamilial disease (42–44). Because APOE-4 is not found in many demented individuals and is found in many nondemented elderly individuals, it too is not considered appropriate for predictive testing for the illness (17, 18). However, information on the genetics of both early- and late-onset Alzheimer's disease is evolving rapidly, so it may be appropriate to refer interested families to a local academic medical center or to the national information number (1-800-621-0379) of the Alzheimer's Association for up-to-date information.

VI. RESEARCH DIRECTIONS

A review of currently available treatments suggests a number of areas for further study. Several of these are in the realm of evaluation and assessment. The first is better detection and evaluation of dementia, especially in the prodromal and early stages, when treatment that slows progression would be more likely to be beneficial. Another is earlier and more accurate detection of noncognitive problems, so as to facilitate optimal intervention. The next is better assessment of dangerous symptoms, especially impaired driving ability. The last is the development of a consensus on clinically meaningful outcome measures, including neuropsychological testing, functional assessment, and "hard" end points, such as institutionalization and mortality.

In the realm of pharmacologic treatments, there is a critical need for medications with greater ability to improve cognition or at least halt the progression of dementia. Promising leads being actively studied for patients with Alzheimer's disease include additional cholinergic agents, further work on vitamin E (especially for mildly impaired patients) and other antioxidants, NSAIDs, and estrogen supplementation. In addition, medication development needs to go beyond these areas to identify and test new cognition-enhancing medications based on the pathophysiological picture of dementia emerging from neuroscience and molecular genetics. For example, pharmacologic agents that prevent or slow down amyloid deposition or remove precipitated amyloid might function as preventive or reversing therapies for Alzheimer's disease. As the understanding of other dementing disorders advances, targeted therapies must be developed and tested for these illnesses as well. Efforts to prevent stroke and to decrease its destructive effect on brain tissue are particularly important avenues for dementia prevention.

Another arena is the optimal pharmacologic treatment of noncognitive symptoms, including psychosis, agitation, depression, and sleep disturbance. Many current recommendations are extrapolated from small uncontrolled studies of agents no longer in common use and/or at doses well above those used in current practice. There is a critical need for randomized controlled studies of up-to-date treatments for psychosis, agitation, depression, and sleep disturbance in dementia.

Further research into nonpharmacologic interventions, such as behavioral and environmental modification, is also needed. One aspect of dementia care that deserves further study is the rehabilitation model, which focuses on identifying and maximizing remaining abilities as a way to maximize function. Further research into this and other strategies may help to identify specific aspects of these therapies that benefit persons with dementia or specific types of dementia. Similarly, research is needed to better characterize the aspects of nursing homes and other environments most likely to improve patient outcomes.

In the health services arena, managed care organizations are beginning to enroll large numbers of elderly individuals. It will be critical to study the impact of this major shift in payment for health services on the care of individuals with dementia so that any needed changes in policy can be made in a timely fashion.

Research is also needed to identify which patients will benefit from alternative forms of living environments and supplemental caregiving. The identification of sites that are more comfortable, less costly, and equally safe and effective for the care of individuals with moderate to severe dementia would have enormous benefits for patients, their families, and society.

VII. INDIVIDUALS AND ORGANIZATIONS THAT SUBMITTED COMMENTS

Marilyn Albert, Ph.D.
Leonard Berg, M.D.
Charles H. Blackington, M.D., P.A.
Dan G. Blazer, M.D., Ph.D.
Carlos A. Cabán, M.D.
Jeffrey L. Cummings, M.D.
Kenneth L. Davis, M.D.
D.P. Devanand, M.D.
Leah Dickstein, M.D.
George Dyck, M.D.
David V. Espino, M.D.
Laura Fachtmann, M.D.
William E. Falk, M.D.
Sanford Finkel, M.D.

Lois T. Flaherty, M.D.
Dolores Gallagher-Thompson, Ph.D.
Larry S. Goldman, M.D.
Marion Z. Goldstein, M.D.
Kevin Gray, M.D.
Sheila Hafter Gray, M.D.
William M. Greenberg, M.D.
George Grossberg, M.D.
Edward Hanin, M.D.
Hugh C. Hendrie, M.D.
Claudia Kawas, M.D.
Lawrence Y. Kline, M.D.
Ronald R. Koegler, M.D.
Rosalie J. Landy

VIII. REFERENCES

The following coding system is used to indicate the nature of the supporting evidence in the summary recommendations and references:

[A]   *Randomized clinical trial.* A study of an intervention in which subjects are pro-spectively followed over time; there are treatment and control groups; subjects are randomly assigned to the two groups; both the subjects and the investigators are blind to the assignments.

[B]   *Clinical trial.* A prospective study in which an intervention is made and the re-sults of that intervention are tracked longitudinally; study does not meet stan-dards for a randomized clinical trial.

[C]   *Cohort or longitudinal study.* A study in which subjects are prospectively fol-lowed over time without any specific intervention.

[D]   *Case-control study.* A study in which a group of patients is identified in the present and information about them is pursued retrospectively or backward in time.

[E]   *Review with secondary data analysis.* A structured analytic review of existing data, e.g., a meta-analysis or a decision analysis.

[F]   *Review.* A qualitative review and discussion of previously published literature without a quantitative synthesis of the data.

[G]   *Other.* Textbooks, expert opinion, case reports, and other reports not included above.

1. American Psychiatric Association: Diagnostic and Statistical Manual of Mental Disorders, 4th ed (DSM-IV). Washington, DC, APA, 1994 [G]

2. Alexopoulos G, Meyers BS, Young RC, Mattis S, Kakuma T: The course of geriatric depression with "reversible dementia": a controlled study. Am J Psychiatry 1993; 150:1693–1699 [C]

3. Shergill S, Mullan E, D'Ath P, Katona C: What is the clinical prevalence of Lewy body dementia? Int J Geriatr Psychiatry 1994; 9:907–912 [G]

4. Reisberg B, Ferris SH, de Leon MJ, Crook T: The Global Deterioration Scale for assessment of primary degenerative dementia. Am J Psychiatry 1982; 139:1136–1139 [G]

5. Hughes CP, Berg L, Danziger WL, Coben LA, Martin RL: A new clinical scale for the staging of dementia. Br J Psychiatry 1982; 140:566–572 [G]

6. Hebert LE, Scherr PA, Beckett LA, Albert MS, Pilgrim DM, Chown MJ, Funkenstein HH, Evans DA: Age-specific incidence of Alzheimer's disease in a community population. JAMA 1995; 273:1354–1359 [C]

7. Snowdon DA, Greiner LH, Mortimer JA, Riley KP, Greiner PA, Markesbery WR: Brain infarction and the clinical expression of Alzheimer disease. JAMA 1997; 277:813–817 [C]

8. Tatemichi TK, Paik M, Bagiella E, Desmond DW, Stern Y, Sano M, Hauser WA, Mayeux R: Risk of dementia after stroke in a hospitalized cohort: results of a longitudinal study. Neurology 1994; 44:1885–1891 [C]

9. McKeith IG, Fairbairn AF, Perry RH, Thompson P: The clinical diagnosis and misdiagnosis of senile dementia of Lewy body type (SDLT). Br J Psychiatry 1994; 165:324–332 [G]

10. Rabins P, Nicholson M: Acute psychiatric hospitalization for patients with irreversible dementia. Int J Geriatr Psychiatry 1991; 6:209–211 [G]

11. Zubenko GS, Rosen J, Sweet RA, Mulsant BH, Rifai AH: Impact of psychiatric hospitalization on behavioral complications of Alzheimer's disease. Am J Psychiatry 1992; 149:1484–1491 [B]

12. NIH Consensus Development Panel on the Differential Diagnosis of Dementing Diseases: Differential diagnosis of dementing diseases. JAMA 1987; 258:3411–3416 [G]

13. Okagaki JF, Alter M, Byrne TN, Daube JR, Franklin G, Frishberg BM, Goldstein ML, Greenberg MK, Lanska DJ, Mishra S, Odenheimer GL, Paulson G, Pearl RA, Rosenberg JH, Sila C, Stevens JC: Practice parameter for diagnosis and evaluation of dementia. Neurology 1994; 44:2203–2206 [G]

14. Recognition and Initial Assessment of Alzheimer's Disease and Related Dementias: Clinical Practice Guideline, vol 19. Washington, DC, US Department of Health and Human Services, Agency for Health Care Policy and Research, 1996 [G]

15. American Psychiatric Association: Practice Guideline for Psychiatric Evaluation of Adults. Am J Psychiatry 1995; 152(Nov suppl):63–80 [G]

16. Folstein MF, Folstein SE, McHugh PR: "Mini-Mental State": a practical method for grading the cognitive state of patients for the clinician. J Psychiatr Res 1975; 12:189–198 [G]

17. American College of Medical Genetics/American Society of Human Genetics Working Group on ApoE and Alzheimer's Disease: Statement on use of apolipoprotein E testing for Alzheimer's disease. JAMA 1995; 274:1627–1629 [G]

18. National Institute on Aging/Alzheimer's Association Working Group: Apolipoprotein E genotyping in Alzheimer's disease. Lancet 1996; 347:1091–1095 [G]

19. Hussian RA, Brown DC: Use of two-dimensional grid patterns to limit hazardous ambulation in demented patients. J Gerontol 1987; 42:558–560 [B]

20. Namazi KH, Rosner TT, Calkins MP: Visual barriers to prevent ambulatory Alzheimer's patients from exiting through an emergency door. Gerontologist 1989; 29:699–702 [B]

21. Mayer R, Darby SJ: Does a mirror deter wandering in demented older people? Int J Geriatr Psychiatry 1991; 6:607–609 [B]

22. Hunt L, Morris JC, Edwards D, Wilson BA: Driving performance in persons with mild senile dementia of the Alzheimer type. J Am Geriatr Soc 1993; 41:747–753 [B]

23. Friedland RP, Koss E, Kumar A, Gaine S, Metzler D, Haxby J, Moore A: Motor vehicle crashes in dementia of the Alzheimer type. Ann Neurol 1988; 24:782–786 [C]

24. Dubinsky RM, Williamson A, Gray CS, Glatt SL: Driving in Alzheimer's disease. J Am Geriatr Soc 1992; 40:1112–1116 [G]

25. Drachman DA, Swearer JM: Driving and Alzheimer's disease: the risk of crashes. Neurology 1993; 43:2448–2456 [D]

26. Fitten LJ, Perryman KM, Wilkinson CJ, Little RJ, Burns MM, Pachana N, Mervis JR, Malmgren R, Siembieda DW, Ganzell S: Alzheimer and vascular dementias and driving: a prospective road and laboratory study. JAMA 1995; 273:1360–1365 [C]

27. Tuokko H, Tallman K, Beatti BL, Cooper P, Weir J: An examination of driving records in a dementia clinic. J Gerontol 1995; 50:S173–S181 [G]

28. Trobe JD, Waller PF, Cook-Flannagan CA, Teshima SM, Bieliauskas LA: Crashes and violations among drivers with Alzheimer disease. Arch Neurol 1996; 53:411–416 [D]

29. Lucas-Blaustein MJ, Filipp L, Dungan C, Tune L: Driving in patients with dementia. J Am Geriatr Soc 1988; 36:1087–1091 [G]

30. Gilley DW, Wilson RS, Bennett DA, Stebbins GT, Bernard BA, Whalen ME, Fox JH: Cessation of driving and unsafe motor vehicle operation by dementia patients. Arch Intern Med 1991; 151:941–946 [G]

31. Carr D, Jackson T, Alquire P: Characteristics of an elderly driving population referred to a geriatric assessment center. J Am Geriatr Soc 1990; 38:1145–1150 [D]

32. O'Neill D, Neubauer K, Boyle M, Gerrard J, Surmon D, Wilcock GK: Dementia and driving. J R Soc Med 1992; 85:199–202 [G]

33. Odenheimer GL, Beaudet M, Jette AM, Albert MS, Grande L, Minaker KL: Performance-based driving evaluation of the elderly driver: safety, reliability, and validity. J Gerontol 1994; 49(4):M153–M159 [G]

34. Adler G, Rottunda SJ, Dysken MW: The driver with dementia: a review of the literature. Am J Geriatr Psychiatry 1996; 4:110–120 [F]

35. Shua-Haim JR, Gross JS: The co-pilot driver syndrome. J Am Geriatr Soc 1996; 44:815–817 [G]

36. Drickamer MA, Lachs MS: Should patients with Alzheimer's disease be told their diagnosis? N Engl J Med 1992; 326:947–951 [G]

37. Stern Y, Tang M-X, Albert MS, Brandt J, Jacobs DM, Bell K, Marder K, Sano M, Devanand D, Albert SM, Bylsma F, Tsai W-Y: Predicting time to nursing home care and death in individuals with Alzheimer disease. JAMA 1997; 277:806–812 [C]

38. Mace NL, Rabins PV: The Thirty-Six Hour Day: A Family Guide to Caring for Persons With Alzheimer's Disease, Related Dementing Illness, and Memory Loss in Later Life, 2nd revised ed. New York, Warner Books, 1992 [G]

39. Goate A, Chartier-Harlin MC, Mullan M, Brown J, Crawford F, Fidani L, Giuffra L, Haynes A, Irving N, James L, Mant R, Newton P, Rooke K, Roques P, Talbot C, Pericak-Vance M, Roses A, Williamson R, Rossor M, Owen M, Hardy J: Segregation of a missense mutation in the amyloid precursor protein gene with familial Alzheimer's disease. Nature 1991; 349:704–706 [G]

40. Sherrington R, Rogaev EI, Liang Y, Rogaeva EA, Levesque G, Ikeda M, Chi H, Lin C, Li G, Holman K, Tsuda T, Mar L, Foncin J-F, Bruni AC, Montesi MP, Sorbi S, Rainero I, Pinessi L, Nee L, Chumakov I, Po D, Brookes A, Sanseau P, Polinsky RJ, Wasco W, Da Silva HAR, Hai JL, Pericak-Vance MA, Tanzi RE, Roses AD, Fraser PE, Rommens JM, George-Hyslop PH: Cloning of a gene bearing missense mutations in early-onset familial Alzheimer's disease. Nature 1995; 375:754–760 [G]

41. Levy-Lahad E, Wasco W, Poorkaj P, Romano DM, Oshima J, Pettingell WH, Yu CE, Jondro PD, Schmidt SD, Wang K, Crowley AC, Fu YH, Guenette SY, Galas D, Nemens E, Wijsman

EM, Bird TD, Schellenberg GD, Tanzi RE: Candidate gene for the chromosome 1 familial Alzheimer's disease locus. Science 1995; 269:973–977 [G]

42. Strittmatter WJ, Saunders AM, Schmechel D, Pericak-Vance M, Enghild J, Salvesen GS, Roses AD: Apolipoprotein E: high-avidity binding to β-amyloid and increased frequency of type 4 allele in late-onset familial Alzheimer's disease. Proc Natl Acad Sci USA 1993; 90:1977–1981 [G]

43. Saunders AM, Strittmatter WJ, Schmechel D, George-Hyslop PH, Pericak-Vance MA, Joo SH, Rosi BL, Gusella JF, Crapper-MacLachlan DR, Alberts MJ: Association of apolipoprotein E allele ε4 with late-onset familial and sporadic Alzheimer's disease. Neurology 1993; 43:1467–1472 [G]

44. Locke PA, Conneally PM, Tanzi RE, Gusella JF, Haines JL: Apolipoprotein E4 allele and Alzheimer disease: examination of allelic association and effect on age at onset in both early- and late-onset cases. Genet Epidemiol 1995; 12:83–92 [G]

45. Chiverton P, Caine ED: Education to assist spouses in coping with Alzheimer's disease. J Am Geriatr Soc 1989; 37:593–598 [C]

46. Mittelman MS, Ferris SH, Steinberg G, Shulman E, Mackell JA, Ambinder A, Cohen J: An intervention that delays institutionalization of Alzheimer's disease patients: treatment of spouse-caregivers. Gerontologist 1993; 33:730–740 [Λ]

47. Brodaty H, Peters KE: Cost effectiveness of a training program for dementia carers. Int Psychogeriatr 1991; 3:11–22 [G]

48. Lovett S, Gallagher D: Psychoeducational interventions for family caregivers: preliminary efficacy data. Behav Ther 1988; 19:321–330 [B]

49. Gallagher-Thompson D: Direct services and interventions for caregivers: a review and critique of extant programs and a look ahead to the future, in Family Caregiving: Agenda for the Future. Edited by Cantor MM. San Francisco, American Society on Aging, 1994, pp 102–122 [G]

50. Flint AJ: Effects of respite care on patients with dementia and their caregivers. Int J Psychogeriatr 1995; 7:505–517 [F]

51. Burdz M, Eaton W, Bond J: Effect of respite care on dementia and nondementia patients and their caregivers. Psychol Aging 1988; 3:38–42 [G]

52. Conlin MM, Caranasos GJ, Davidson RA: Reduction of caregiver stress by respite care: a pilot study. South Med J 1992; 85:1096–1100 [B]

53. Wimo A, Mattsson B, Adolfsson R, Eriksson T, Nelvig A: Dementia day care and its effects on symptoms and institutionalization—a controlled Swedish study. Scand J Prim Health Care 1993; 11:117–123 [B]

54. Overman W Jr, Stoudemire A: Guidelines for legal and financial counseling of Alzheimer's disease patients and their families. Am J Psychiatry 1988; 145:1495–1500 [G]

55. Spar JE, Garb AS: Assessing competency to make a will. Am J Psychiatry 1992; 149:169–174 [G]

56. Robinson A, Spencer W, White L: Understanding Difficult Behaviors. Lansing, Mich, Geriatric Education Center of Michigan, 1988 [G]

57. Mintzer JE, Lewis L, Pennypacker L, Simpson W, Bachman D, Wohlreich G, Meeks A, Hunt S, Sampson R: Behavioral intensive care unit (BICU): a new concept in the management of acute agitated behavior in elderly demented patients. Gerontologist 1993; 33:801–806 [G]

58. Burgio LD, Engel BT, Hawkins AM, McCormick KA, Scheve A, Jones LT: A staff management system for maintaining improvements in continence with elderly nursing home residents. J Appl Behav Anal 1990; 23:111–118 [G]

59. Group for the Advancement of Psychiatry Committee on Aging: The Psychiatric Treatment of Alzheimer's Disease: Report 125. New York, Brunner/Mazel, 1988 [G]

60. Burnside I, Haight B: Reminiscence and life review: therapeutic interventions for older people. Nurse Pract 1994; 19(4):55–61 [F]

61. Jones GM: Validation therapy: a companion to reality orientation. Can Nurse 1985; 81(3):20–23 [G]

62. Feil N: The Feil Method—How to Help Disoriented Old-Old. Cleveland, Edward Feil Productions, 1992 [G]

63. Robichaud L, Hebert R, Desrosiers J: Efficacy of a sensory integration program on behaviors of inpatients with dementia. Am J Occup Ther 1994; 48:355–360 [A]

64. Woods P, Ashley J: Simulated presence therapy: using selected memories to manage problem behaviors in Alzheimer's disease patients. Geriatr Nurs 1995; 16(1):9–14 [B]

65. Baines S, Saxby P, Ehlert K: Reality orientation and reminiscence therapy: a controlled crossover study of elderly confused people. Br J Psychiatry 1987; 151:222–231 [A]

66. Kiernat JM: The use of life review activity with confused nursing home residents. Am J Occup Ther 1979; 33:306–310 [B]

67. Cook J: Reminiscing: how can it help confused nursing home residents? Social Casework 1984; 65:90–93 [G]

68. Scanland SG, Emershaw LE: Reality orientation and validation therapy: dementia, depression, and functional status. J Gerontol Nurs 1993; 19:7–11 [B]

69. Powell-Proctor L, Miller E: Reality orientation: a critical appraisal. Br J Psychiatry 1982; 140:457–463 [F]

70. Tappen RM: The effect of skill training on functional abilities of nursing home residents with dementia. Res Nurs Health 1994; 17:159–165 [B]

71. Hanley IG, McGuire RJ, Boyd WD: Reality orientation and dementia: a controlled trial of two approaches. Br J Psychiatry 1981; 138:10–14 [A]

72. Koh K, Ray R, Lee J, Nair A, Ho T, Ang P: Dementia in elderly patients: can the 3R mental stimulation programme improve mental status? Age Aging 1994; 23:195–199 [B]

73. Johnson CH, McLaren SM, McPherson FM: The comparative effectiveness of three versions of "classroom" reality orientation. Age Aging 1981; 10:33–35 [B]

74. Woods RT: Reality orientation and staff attention: a controlled study. Br J Psychiatry 1979; 134:502–507 [A]

75. Brook P, Degun G, Mather M: Reality orientation, a therapy for psychogeriatric patients: a controlled study. Br J Psychiatry 1975; 127:42–45 [B]

76. Greene JG, Timbury GC, Smith R: Reality orientation with elderly patients in the community: an empirical evaluation. Age Ageing 1983; 12:38–43 [B]

77. Reeve W, Ivison D: Use of environmental manipulation and classroom and modified informal reality orientation with institutionalized, confused elderly patients. Age Ageing 1985; 14:119–121 [B]

78. Williams R, Reeve W, Ivison D, Kavanagh D: Use of environmental manipulation and modified informal reality orientation with institutionalized, confused, elderly subjects: a replication. Age Ageing 1987; 16:315–318 [B]

79. Gerber GJ, Prince PN, Snider HG, Atchinson K, Dubois L, Kilgour JA: Group activity and cognitive improvement among patients with Alzheimer's disease. Hosp Community Psychiatry 1991; 42:843–845 [A]

80. Baldelli MV, Pirani A, Motta M, Abati E, Mariani E, Manzi V: Effects of reality orientation therapy on elderly patients in the community. Arch Gerontol Geriatr 1993; 7:211–218 [B]

81. Dietch JT, Hewett LJ, Jones S: Adverse effects of reality orientation. J Am Geriatr Soc 1989; 37:974–976 [B]

82. Beck C, Heacock P, Mercer S, Thatcher R, Sparkman C: The impact of cognitive skills remediation training on persons with Alzheimer's disease or mixed dementia. J Geriatr Psychiatry 1988; 21:73–88 [A]

83. Zarit SH, Zarit JM, Reever KE: Memory training for severe memory loss: effects on senile dementia patients and their families. Gerontologist 1982; 22:373–377 [A]

84. Yesavage JA, Westphal J, Rush L: Senile dementia: combined pharmacologic and psychologic treatment. J Am Geriatr Soc 1981; 29:164–171 [A]

85. McEvoy CL, Patterson RL: Behavioral treatment of deficit skills in dementia patients. Gerontologist 1986; 26:475–478 [B]

86. Abraham IL, Reel SJ: Cognitive nursing interventions with long-term care residents: effects on neurocognitive dimensions. Arch Psychiatr Nurs 1992; 6:356–365 [B]

87. Karlsson I, Brane G, Melin E, Nyth AI, Rybo E: Effects of environmental stimulation on biochemical and psychological variables in dementia. Acta Psychiatr Scand 1988; 77:207–213 [B]

88. Rovner BW, Steel CD, Shmuely Y, Folstein MF: A randomized trial of dementia care in nursing homes. J Am Geriatr Soc 1996; 44:7–13 [B]

89. Teri L: Behavioral treatment of depression in patients with dementia. Alzheimer Dis Assoc Disord 1994; 8(3):66–74 [B]

90. Teri L, Logsdon RG: Identifying pleasant activities for Alzheimer's disease patients: the Pleasant Events Schedule-AD. Gerontologist 1991; 31:124–127 [G]

91. Sunderland T, Weingartner H, Cohen RM, Tariot PN, Newhouse PA, Thompson KE, Lawlor BA, Mueller EA: Low-dose oral lorazepam administration in Alzheimer subjects and age-matched controls. Psychopharmacology (Berl) 1989; 99:129–133 [D]

92. Davis KL, Thal LJ, Gamzu ER, Davis CS, Woolson RF, Gracon SI, Drachman DA, Schneider LS, Whitehouse PJ, Hoover TM, Morris JC, Kawas CH, Knopman DS, Earl NL, Kumar V, Doody RS, Tacrine Collaborative Study Group: A double-blind, placebo-controlled multicenter study of tacrine for Alzheimer's disease. N Engl J Med 1992; 327:1253–1259 [A]

93. Farlow M, Gracon SI, Hershey LA, Lewis KW, Sadowsky CH, Dolan-Ureno J: A controlled trial of tacrine in Alzheimer's disease. JAMA 1992; 268:2523–2529 [A]

94. Knapp MJ, Knopman DS, Solomon PR, Pendlebury WW, Davis CS, Gracon SI: A 30-week randomized controlled trial of high-dose tacrine in patients with Alzheimer's disease. JAMA 1994; 271:985–991 [A]

95. Forette F, Hoover T, Gracon S, de Rotrou J, Hervy MP: A double-blind, placebo-controlled, enriched population study of tacrine in patients with Alzheimer's disease. Eur J Neurology 1995; 2:1–10 [A]

96. Foster NL, Petersen RC, Gracon SI, Lewis K, Tacrine 970-6 Study Group: An enriched-population, double-blind, placebo-controlled, crossover study of tacrine and lecithin in Alzheimer's disease. Dementia 1996; 7:260–266 [A]

97. Knopman D, Schneider L, Davis K, Talwalker S, Smith F, Hoover T, Gracon S: Long-term tacrine (Cognex) treatment: effects on nursing home placement and mortality. Neurology 1996; 47:166–177 [C]

98. Rogers SL, Doody R, Mohs R, Friedhoff LT: E2020 produces both clinical global and cognitive test improvement in patients with mild to moderately severe Alzheimer's disease: results of a 30-week phase III trial (abstract). Neurology 1996; 46:A217 [A]

99. Rogers SL, Friedhoff LT, Apter JT, Richter RW, Hartford JT, Walshe TM, Baumel B, Linden RD, Kinney FC, Doody RS, Borison RL, Ahem GL: The efficacy and safety of donepezil in patients with Alzheimer's disease: results of a US multicentre, randomized, double-blind, placebo-controlled trial. Dementia 1996; 7:293–303 [A]

100. Rogers SL, Friedhoff LT: Donepezil (E2020) produces long-term clinical improvement in Alzheimer's disease. Presented at the 4th International Nice/Springfield Symposium on Advances in Alzheimer Therapy, April 10–14, 1996 [A]

101. Watkins PB, Zimmerman HJ, Knapp MJ, Gracon SI, Lewis KW: Hepatotoxic effects of tacrine administration in patients with Alzheimer's disease. JAMA 1994; 271:992–998 [C]

102. Lyketsos CG, Corazzini K, Steele CD, Kraus MF: Guidelines for the use of tacrine in Alzheimer's disease: clinical application and effectiveness. J Neuropsychiatry Clin Neurosci 1996; 8:67–73 [F]

103. Halliwell B, Gutteridge JMC: Oxygen radicals in the nervous system. Trends Neurosci 1985; 8:22–26 [G]

104. Behl C, Davis J, Cole G, Shubert D: Vitamin E protects nerve cells from beta-amyloid protein toxicity. Biochem Biophys Res Commun 1992; 186:944–950 [G]

105. Sano M, Ernesto C, Klauber MR, Schafer K, Woodbury P, Thomas R, Grundman F, Growdon S, Thal LJ: Rationale and design of a multicenter study of selegiline and α-tocopherol in the treatment of Alzheimer disease using novel clinical outcomes. Alzheimer Dis Assoc Disord 1996; 10:132–140 [G]

106. Sano M, Ernesto C, Thomas RG, Klauber MR, Schafer K, Grundman M, Woodbury P, Growdon J, Cotman CW, Pfeiffer E, Schneider LS, Thal LJ: A two-year, double blind randomized multicenter trial of selegeline and α-tocopherol in the treatment of Alzheimer's disease. N Engl J Med (in press) [A]

107. Kappus H, Diplock AT: Tolerance and safety of vitamin E: a toxicological position report. Free Radic Biol Med 1992; 13:55–74 [G]

108. Tatton WG, Greenwood CE: Rescue of dying neurons: a new action for deprenyl in MPTP parkinsonism. J Neurosci Res 1991; 30:666–672 [G]

109. Mangoni A, Grassi MP, Frattola L, Piolti R, Bassi S, Motta A, Marcone A, Smirne S: Effects of a MAO-B inhibitor in the treatment of Alzheimer disease. Eur Neurol 1991; 31:100–107; correction 31:433 [A]

110. Burke WJ, Roccaforte WH, Wengel SP, Bayer BL, Ranno AE, Willcockson NK: L-deprenyl in the treatment of mild dementia of the Alzheimer type: results of a 15-month trial. J Am Geriatr Soc 1993; 41:1219–1225 [A]

111. Burke WJ, Ranno AE, Roccaforte WH, Wengel SP, Bayer BL, Willcockson NK: L-deprenyl in the treatment of mild dementia of the Alzheimer type: preliminary results. J Am Geriatr Soc 1993; 41:367–370 [A]

112. Agnoli A, Martucci N, Fabbrini G, Buckley AE, Fioravanti M: Monoamine oxidase and dementia: treatment with an inhibitor of MAO-B activity. Dementia 1990; 1:109–114 [A]

113. Filip V, Kolibas E, Ceskova E, Hronek J, Novotna D, Novotny V: Selegiline in mild SDAT: results of a multi-center, double-blind, placebo-controlled trial (abstract). Neuropsychopharmacol 1991 [A]

114. Loeb C, Albano C: Selegiline: a new approach to DAT treatment (abstract). Presented at the European Conference on Parkinson's Disease and Extrapyramidal Disorders, Rome, July 1990 [A]

115. Martucci N, Fabbrini G, Fioravanti M: Monoaminossidasi e demenza: trattamento con un inibitore dell'attivita MAO-B. Giornale di Neuropsicofarmacologia 1989; 11:265–269 [A]

116. Schneider LS, Olin JT: Overview of clinical trials of Hydergine in dementia. Arch Neurol 1994; 51:787–798 [E]

117. Tariot PN, Cohen RM, Sunderland T, Newhouse PA, Yount D, Mellow AM, Weingartner H, Mueller EA, Murphy DL: L-Deprenyl in Alzheimer's disease: preliminary evidence for behavioral change with monoamine oxidase B inhibition. Arch Gen Psychiatry 1987; 44:427–433 [A]

118. Piccinin GL, Finali G, Piccirilli M: Neuropsychological effects of L-deprenyl in Alzheimer's type dementia. Clin Neuropharmacol 1990; 13:147–163 [A]

119. Finali G, Piccirilli M, Oliani C, Piccinin GL: L-deprenyl therapy improves verbal memory in amnesic Alzheimer patients. Clin Neuropharmacol 1991; 14:523–536 [B]

120. Schneider LS, Olin JT, Pawluczyk S: A double-blind crossover pilot study of l-deprenyl (selegiline) combined with cholinesterase inhibitor in Alzheimer's disease. Am J Psychiatry 1993; 150:321–323 [A]

121. Thompson TL II, Filley CM, Mitchell WD, Culig KM, LoVerde M, Byyny RL: Lack of efficacy of hydergine in patients with Alzheimer's disease. N Engl J Med 1990; 323:445–448; correction 323:691 [A]

122. McDonald WM, Krishnan KR: Pharmacologic management of the symptoms of dementia. Am Fam Physician 1990; 42:123–132 [A]

123. Irfan S, Linder L: The effect of dihydrogenated ergot alkaloids in the treatment of geriatric patients suffering from senile mental deterioration, in XIth International Congress of Gerontology. Tokyo, SCIMED, 1978, p 142 [A]

124. Puxty J: Community screening for dementia and evaluation of treatment, in Proceedings of the Basel Symposium (CH). Edited by Carlsson A, Kanowski S, Allain H, Spiegel R. Pearl River, NY, Parthenon Publishing Group, 1989, p 211–230 [A]

125. Soni SD, Soni SS: Dihydrogenated alkaloids of ergotoxine in nonhospitalised elderly patients. Curr Med Res Opin 1975; 3:464–468 [A]

126. Thienhaus OJ, Wheeler BG, Simon S, Zemlan FP, Hartford JT: A controlled double-blind study of high-dose dihydroergotoxine mesylate (Hydergine) in mild dementia. J Am Geriatr Soc 1987; 35:219–223 [A]

127. Rao DB, Norris JR: A double-blind investigation of hydergine in the treatment of cerebrovascular insufficiency in the elderly. Johns Hopkins Med J 1972; 130:317–324 [B]

128. Winslow IE: Clinical evaluation of hydergine. Unpublished manuscript, 1972 [A]

129. Lazzari R, Passeri M, Chierichetti SM: Le mésylate de dihydroergotoxine dans le traitement de l'insuffisance cérébrale sénile. Le Presse Médicale 1983; 12:3179–3185 [A]

130. Martucci N, Manna V: EEG-pharmacological and neuropsychological study of dihydroergocristine mesylate in patients with chronic cerebrovascular disease. Advances in Therapy 1986; 3:210–223 [A]

131. Moglia A, Bono G, Sinforiani E, Alfonsi E, Zandrini C, Pistarini C, Arrigo A, Franch F: La diidroergotossina mesilato dell'insufficienza cerebrovasculare cronica: analisi spettrale dell'EEG e correlati neuropsicologici. Farmaco 1983; 38:97–102 [A]

132. Breitner JCS, Gau BA, Welsh KA, Plassman BL, McDonald WM, Helm MJ, Anthony JC: Inverse association of anti-inflammatory treatments and Alzheimer's disease: initial results of a co-twin control study. Neurology 1994; 44:227–232 [D]

133. McGeer PL, Rogers J: Anti-inflammatory agents as a therapeutic approach to Alzheimer's disease. Neurology 1992; 42:447–448 [G]

134. Rogers J, Kirby LC, Hempelman SR, Berry DL, McGeer PL, Kaszniak AW, Zalinski J, Cofield M, Mansukhani L, Willson P, Kogan F: Clinical trial of indomethacin in Alzheimer's disease. Neurology 1993; 43:1609–1611 [A]

135. Stewart WF, Kawas C, Corrada M, Metter EJ: Risk of Alzheimer's disease and duration of NSAID use. Neurology 1997; 48:626–632 [C]

136. Aisen PS, Davis KL: Inflammatory mechanisms in Alzheimer's disease: implications for therapy. Am J Psychiatry 1994; 151:1105–1113 [G]

137. Sherwin BB: Estrogenic effects on memory in women. Ann NY Acad Sci 1994; 743:213–230 [G]

138. Fillit H, Weinreb H, Cholst I, Luine V, McEwen B, Amador R, Zabriskie J: Observations in a preliminary open trial of estradiol therapy for senile dementia-Alzheimer's type. Psychoneuroendocrinology 1986; 11:337–345 [B]

139. Ohkura T, Isse K, Akazawa K, Hamamoto M, Yaoi Y, Hagino N: Long-term estrogen replacement therapy in female patients with dementia of the Alzheimer type: 7 case reports. Dementia 1995; 6(2):99–107 [G]

140. Henderson VW, Paganini-Hill A, Emanuel CK, Dunn ME, Buckwalter JG: Estrogen replacement therapy in older women: comparisons between Alzheimer's disease cases and nondemented control subjects. Arch Neurol 1994; 51:896–900 [D]

141. Tang MX, Jacobs D, Stern Y, Marder K, Schofield P, Gurland B, Andrews H, Mayeux R: Effect of oestrogen during menopause on risk and age at onset of Alzheimer's disease. Lancet 1996; 348:429–432 [C]

142. Burns A, Murphy D: Protection against Alzheimer's disease? Lancet 1996; 348:420–421 [G]

143. Crapper-McLachlan DR, Dalton AJ, Kruck TPA, Bell MY, Smith WL, Kalow W, Andrews DF: Intramuscular desferrioxamine in patients with Alzheimer's disease. Lancet 1991; 337:1304–1308; correction 337:1618 [B]

144. Cardelli MB, Russell M, Bagne CA, Pomara N: Chelation therapy: unproved modality in the treatment of Alzheimer-type dementia. J Am Geriatr Soc 1985; 33:548–551 [G]

145. Leibovici A, Tariot PN: Agitation associated with dementia: a systematic approach to treatment. Psychopharmacol Bull 1988; 24:49–53 [G]

146. Reisberg B, Borenstein J, Salob SP, Ferris SH, Franssen E, Georgotas A: Behavioral symptoms in Alzheimer's disease: phenomenology and treatment. J Clin Psychiatry 1987; 48(May suppl):9–15 [G]

147. Devanand DP, Sackeim HA, Brown RP, Mayeux R: Psychosis, behavioral disturbance, and the use of neuroleptics in dementia. Compr Psychiatry 1988; 29:387–401 [F]

148. Schneider LS, Pollack VE, Lyness SA: A metaanalysis of controlled trials of neuroleptic treatment in dementia. J Am Geriatr Soc 1990; 38:553–563 [E]

149. Rada RT, Kellner R: Thiothixene in the treatment of geriatric patients with chronic organic brain syndrome. J Am Geriatr Soc 1976; 24:105–107 [A]

150. Barnes R, Veith R, Okimoto J, Raskind M, Gumbrecht G: Efficacy of antipsychotic medications in behaviorally disturbed dementia patients. Am J Psychiatry 1982; 139:1170–1174 [A]

151. Sugarman AA, Williams BH, Adlerstein AM: Haloperidol in the psychiatric disorders of old age. Am J Psychiatry 1964; 120:1190–1192 [A]

152. Petrie WM, Ban TA, Berney S, Fujimori M, Guy W, Ragheb M, Wilson WH, Schaffer JD: Loxapine in psychogeriatrics: a placebo- and standard-controlled clinical investigation. J Clin Psychopharmacol 1982; 2:122–126 [A]

153. Hamilton LD, Bennett JL: The use of trifluoperazine in geriatric patients with chronic brain syndrome. J Am Geriatr Soc 1962; 10:140–147 [A]

154. Hamilton LD, Bennett JL: Acetophenazine for hyperactive geriatric patients. Geriatrics 1962; 17:596–601 [A]

155. Abse DW, Dahlstrom WG, Hill C: The value of chemotherapy in senile mental disturbance. JAMA 1960; 174:2036–2042 [A]

156. Madhusoodanan S, Brenner R, Araujo L, Abaza A: Efficacy of risperidone treatment for psychoses associated with schizophrenia, schizoaffective disorder, bipolar disorder, or senile dementia in 11 geriatric patients: a case series. J Clin Psychiatry 1995; 56:514–518 [G]

157. Friedman JH, Lannon MC: Clozapine in the treatment of psychosis in Parkinson's disease. Neurology 1989; 39:1219–1221 [G]

158. Chacko R, Hurley R, Jankovic J: Clozapine use in diffuse Lewy body disease. J Neuropsychiatry Clin Neurosci 1993; 5:206–208 [G]

159. Salzman C, Vaccaro B, Lieff J, Weiner A: Clozapine in older patients with psychosis and behavioral disturbances. Am J Geriatr Psychiatry 1995; 3:26–33 [G]

160. Devanand DP, Sackeim HA, Brown RP, Mayeux R: A pilot study of haloperidol treatment of psychosis and behavioral disturbance in Alzheimer's disease. Arch Neurol 1989; 46:854–857 [B]

161. Woerner MG, Alvir JMJ, Kane JM, Saltz BL, Lieberman JA: Neuroleptic treatment of elderly patients. Psychopharmacol Bull 1995; 31:333–337 [B]

162. Jeste DV, Caliguiri MP, Paulsen JS, Heaton RK, Lacro JP, Harris M, Bailey A, Fell RL, McAdams LA: Risk of tardive dyskinesia in older patients: a prospective longitudinal study of 266 outpatients. Arch Gen Psychiatry 1995; 52:756–765 [B]

163. Salzman C: Treatment of the elderly agitated patient. J Clin Psychiatry 1987; 48(May suppl):19–22 [G]

164. Allen RL, Walker Z, D'Ath PJ, Katona CLE: Risperidone for psychotic and behavioural symptoms in Lewy body dementia (letter). Lancet 1995; 346:185 [G]

165. McKeith IG, Ballard CG, Harrison RW: Neuroleptic sensitivity to risperidone in Lewy body dementia (letter). Lancet 1995; 346:699 [G]

166. Gottlieb G, McAllister T, Gur R: Depot neuroleptics in the treatment of behavioral disorders in patients with Alzheimer's disease. J Am Geriatr Soc 1988; 36:619–621 [G]

167. Kirven LE, Montero EF: Comparison of thioridazine and diazepam in the control of non-psychotic symptoms associated with senility: double-blind study. J Am Geriatr Soc 1973; 21:546–551 [A]

168. Covington J: Alleviating agitation, apprehension and related symptoms in geriatric patients. South Med J 1975; 68:719–724 [G]

169. Stotsky B: Multicenter study comparing thioridazine with diazepam and placebo in elderly nonpsychotic patients with emotional and behavioral disorders. Clin Ther 1984; 6:546–559 [A]

170. Coccaro EF, Kramer E, Zemishlany Z, Thorne A, Rice CM III, Giordani B, Duvvi K, Patel BM, Torres J, Nora R, Neufeld R, Mohs RC, Davis KL: Pharmacologic treatment of noncognitive behavioral disturbances in elderly demented patients. Am J Psychiatry 1990; 147:1640–1645 [G]

171. Cevera AA: Psychoactive drug therapy in the senile patient: controlled comparison of thioridazine and diazepam. Psychiatry Digest 1974: pp 15–21 [A]

172. Beber CR: Management of behavior in the institutionalized aged. Dis Nerv Syst 1965; 26:591–595 [A]

173. Lemos GP, Clement MA, Nickels E: Effects of diazepam suspension in geriatric patients hospitalized for psychiatric illnesses. J Am Geriatr Soc 1965; 13:355–359 [A]

174. Salzman C: Clinical Geriatric Psychopharmacology, 2nd ed. Baltimore, Williams & Wilkins, 1992 [G]

175. Grad R: Benzodiazepines for insomnia in community-dwelling elderly: a review of benefit and risk. J Fam Pract 1995; 41:473–481 [F]

176. Herings RM, Stricker BH, de Boer A, Bakker A, Sturmans F: Benzodiazepines and the risk of falling leading to femur fractures: dosage more important than elimination half-life. Arch Intern Med 1995; 155:1801–1807 [D]

177. Ashton H: Guidelines for the rational use of benzodiazepines: when and what to use. Drugs 1994; 48:25–40 [G]

178. Gleason RP, Schneider LS: Carbamazepine treatment of agitation in Alzheimer's outpatients refractory to neuroleptics. J Clin Psychiatry 1990; 51:115–118 [G]

179. Lemke MR: Effect of carbamazepine on agitation in Alzheimer's inpatients refractory to neuroleptics. J Clin Psychiatry 1995; 56:354–357 [B]

180. Tariot PN, Erb R, Leibovici A, Podgorski CA, Cox C, Asnis J, Kolassa J, Irvine C: Carbamazepine treatment of agitation in nursing home patients with dementia: a preliminary study. J Am Geriatr Soc 1994; 42:1160–1166 [B]

181. Chambers CA, Bain J, Rosbottom R, Ballinger BR, McLaren S: Carbamazepine in senile dementia and overactivity: a placebo controlled double blind trial. IRCS Med Sci 1982; 10:505–506 [A]

182. Lott AD, McElroy SL, Keys MA: Valproate in the treatment of behavioral agitation in elderly patients with dementia. J Neuropsychiatry Clin Neurosci 1995; 7:314–319 [G]

183. Mellow AM, Solano-Lopez C, Davis S: Sodium valproate in the treatment of behavioral disturbance in dementia. J Geriatr Psychiatry Neurol 1993; 6:205–209 [G]

184. American Psychiatric Association: Practice Guideline for the Treatment of Patients With Bipolar Disorder. Am J Psychiatry 1994; 151 (Dec suppl)[G]

185. Risse SC, Barnes R: Pharmacologic treatment of agitation associated with dementia. J Am Geriatr Soc 1986; 34:368–376 [A]

186. Kunik ME, Yudofsky SC, Silver JM, Hales RE: Pharmacologic approach to management of agitation associated with dementia. J Clin Psychiatry 1994; 55(Feb suppl):13–17 [G]

187. Simpson DM, Foster D: Improvement in organically disturbed behavior with trazodone treatment. J Clin Psychiatry 1986; 47:191–193 [G]

188. Nair NP, Ban TA, Hontela S, Clarke R: Trazodone in the treatment of organic brain syndromes, with special reference to psychogeriatrics. Curr Ther Res 1973; 15:769–775 [G]

189. Houlihan DJ, Mulsant BH, Sweet RA, Rifai AH, Pasternak R, Rosen J, Zubenko GS: A naturalistic study of trazodone in the treatment of behavioral complications of dementia. Am J Geriatr Psychiatry 1994; 2:78–85 [G]

190. Lebert F, Pasquier F, Petit H: Behavioral effects of trazodone in Alzheimer's disease. J Clin Psychiatry 1994; 55:536–538 [B]

191. Sultzer D, Gray KF, Gunay I, Berisford MA, Mahler ME: A double-blind comparison of trazodone and haloperidol for treatment of agitation in patients with dementia. Am J Geriatr Psychiatry 1997; 5:60–69 [A]

192. Nyth AL, Gottfries CG: The clinical efficacy of citalopram in treatment of emotional disturbances in dementia disorders: a Nordic multicentre study. Br J Psychiatry 1990; 157:894–901 [B]

193. Nyth AL, Gottfries CG, Lyby K, Smedegaard-Andersen L, Gylding-Sabroe J, Kristensen M, Refsum HE, Ofsti E, Eriksson S, Syversen S: A controlled multicenter clinical study of citalopram and placebo in elderly depressed patients with and without concomitant dementia. Acta Psychiatr Scand 1992; 86:138–145 [B]

194. Colenda CC III: Buspirone in treatment of agitated demented patient (letter). Lancet 1988; 1:1169; correction 1988; 2:754 [G]

195. Tiller JW, Dakis JA, Shaw JM: Short-term buspirone treatment in disinhibition with dementia (letter). Lancet 1988; 2:510 [G]

196. Sakauye KM, Camp CJ, Ford PA: Effects of buspirone on agitation associated with dementia. Am J Geriatr Psychiatry 1993; 1:82–84 [B]

197. Weiner MF, Denke M, Williams K, Guzman R: Intramuscular medroxyprogesterone acetate for sexual aggression in elderly men. Lancet 1992; 339:1121–1122 [G]

198. Kyomen H, Nobel K, Wet J: The use of estrogen to decrease aggressive physical behavior in elderly men with dementia. J Am Geriatr Soc 1991; 39:1110–1112 [G]

199. Rich SS, Ovsiew F: Leuprolide acetate for exhibitionism in Huntington's disease. Mov Disord 1994; 9:353–357 [G]

200. Weiler PG, Mungas D, Bernick C: Propranolol for the control of disruptive behavior in senile dementia. J Geriatr Psychiatry Neurol 1988; 1:226–230 [G]

201. Reifler BV, Teri L, Raskind M, Veith R, Barnes R, White E, McLean P: Double-blind trial of imipramine in Alzheimer's disease patients with and without depression. Am J Psychiatry 1989; 146:45–49 [A]

202. Passeri M, Cucinotta D, DeMello M, Biziere K: Comparison of minaprine and placebo in the treatment of Alzheimer's disease and multi-infarct dementia. Int J Geriatr Psychiatry 1987; 2:97–103 [B]

203. Fuchs A, Henke U, Erhart DH, Schell CH, Pramshohler B, Danninger B, Schautzer F: Video rating analysis of effect of maprotiline in patients with dementia and depression. Pharmacopsychiatry 1993; 26:37–41 [B]

204. Conti L, Fosca RE, Lazzerini F, Morey LC, Ban TA, Santini V, Modafferi A, Postiglione A: Glycosaminoglycan polysulfate (Ateroid) in old-age dementias: effects upon depressive symptomatology in geriatric patients. Prog Neuropsychopharmacol Biol Psychiatry 1989; 13:977–981 [B]

205. Passeri M, Cucinotta D, Abate G, Senin U, Ventura A, Badiale MS, Diana R, La Greca P, Le Grazie C: Oral 5'-methyltetrahydrofolic acid in senile organic mental disorders with depression: results of a double-blind multicenter study. Aging 1993; 5:63–71 [B]

206. NIH Consensus Development Panel on Depression in Late Life: Diagnosis and treatment of depression in late life. JAMA 1992; 268:1018–1024 [G]

207. American Psychiatric Association: Practice Guideline for Major Depressive Disorder in Adults. Am J Psychiatry 1993; 150 (April suppl)[G]

208. Marin RS, Fogel BS, Hawkins J, Duffy J, Krupp B: Apathy: a treatable syndrome. Clin Neuroscience 1995; 7(1):23–30 [G]

209. Wallace AE, Kofoed LL, West AN: Double-blind, placebo-controlled trial of methylphenidate in older, depressed, medically ill patients. Am J Psychiatry 1995; 152:929–931 [A]

210. Pickett P, Masand P, Murray G: Psychostimulant treatment of geriatric depressive disorders secondary to medical illness. J Geriatr Psychiatry Neurol 1990; 3:146–151 [G]

211. Lazarus LW, Moberg PJ, Langsley PR, Lingam VR: Methylphenidate and nortriptyline in the treatment of poststroke depression: a retrospective comparison. Arch Phys Med Rehabil 1994; 75:403–406 [G]

212. Price TR, McAllister TW: Safety and efficacy of ECT in depressed patients with dementia: a review of clinical experience. Convulsive Ther 1989; 5:1–74 [G]

213. Aharon-Peretz J, Masiah A, Pillar T, Epstein R, Tzischinsky O, Lavie P: Sleep-wake cycles in multi-infarct dementia and dementia of the Alzheimer type. Neurology 1991; 41:1616–1619 [G]

214. Satlin A: Sleep disorders in dementia. Psychiatr Ann 1994; 24:186–190 [G]

215. Hoch CC, Reynolds CF III, Houck PR: Sleep patterns in Alzheimer, depressed, and healthy elderly. West J Nurs Res 1988; 10:239–256 [G]

216. Strollo P, Rogers R: Obstructive sleep apnea. N Engl J Med 1996; 334:99–104 [G]

217. Piccione P, Zorick F, Lutz T, Grissom T, Kramer M, Roth T: The efficacy of triazolam and chloral hydrate in geriatric insomniacs. J Int Med Res 1980; 8:361–367 [B]

218. Linnoila M, Viukari M, Numminen A, Auvinen J: Efficacy and side effects of chloral hydrate and tryptophan as sleeping aids in psychogeriatric patients. Int Pharmacopsychiatry 1980; 15:124–128 [B]

219. Shaw SH, Curson H, Coquelin JP: A double-blind, comparative study of zolpidem and placebo in the treatment of insomnia in elderly psychiatric in-patients. J Int Med Res 1992; 20:150–161; correction 20:494 [A]

220. Satlin A, Volicer L, Ross V, Herz L, Campbell S: Bright light treatment of behavioral and sleep disturbances in patients with Alzheimer's disease. Am J Psychiatry 1992; 149:1028–1032 [B]

221. Okawa M, Mishima K, Nanami T, Shimizu T, Iijima S, Hishikawa Y, Takahashi K: Vitamin B12 treatment for sleep-wake rhythm disorders. Sleep 1990; 13(1):15–23 [A]

222. Mishima K, Okawa M, Hishikawa Y, Hozumi S, Hori H, Takahashi K: Morning bright light therapy for sleep and behavior disorders in elderly patients with dementia. Acta Psychiatr Scand 1994; 89:1–7 [B]

223. Maurizi CP: The therapeutic potential for tryptophan and melatonin: possible roles in depression, sleep, Alzheimer's disease and abnormal aging. Med Hypotheses 1990; 31:233–242 [E]

224. Singer C, McArthur A, Hughes R, Sack R, Kaye J, Lewy A: High dose melatonin administration and sleep in the elderly. Sleep Res 1995; 24A:151 [G]

225. Volicer L, Volicer BJ, Hurley AC: Is hospice care appropriate for Alzheimer patients? Caring 1993; 12(11):50–55 [G]

226. Volicer L, Hurley AC, Lathi DC, Kowall NW: Measurement of severity in advanced Alzheimer's disease. J Gerontol 1994; 49(5):M223–M226 [G]

227. Levkoff SE, Evans DA, Liptzin B, Wetle T, Reilly C, Pilgrim D, Schor J, Rowe J: Delirium: the occurrence and persistence of symptoms among elderly hospitalized patients. Arch Intern Med 1992; 152:334–340 [G]

228. Erkinjuntti T, Wikstrom J, Palo J, Autio L: Dementia among medical inpatients. Arch Intern Med 1986; 146:1923–1926 [C]

229. Tune L, Carr S, Hoag E, Cooper T: Anticholinergic effects of drugs commonly prescribed for the elderly: potential means for assessing risk of delirium. Am J Psychiatry 1992; 149:1393–1394 [G]

230. Torigoe R, Hayashi T, Anegawa S, Harada K, Toda K, Maeda K, Katsuragi M: Effect of propentofylline and pentoxifylline on cerebral blood flow using ^{123}I-IMP SPECT in patients with cerebral arteriosclerosis. Clin Ther 1994; 16:65–73 [G]

231. Blume J, Ruhlmann KU, de la Haye R, Rettig K: Treatment of chronic cerebrovascular disease in elderly patients with pentoxifylline. J Med 1992; 23:417–432 [A]

232. Black RS, Barclay LL, Nolan KA, Thaler HT, Hardiman ST, Blass JP: Pentoxifylline in cerebrovascular dementia. J Am Geriatr Soc 1992; 40:237–244 [A]

233. Rovner BW, Kafonek S, Filipp L, Lucas MJ, Folstein MF: Prevalence of mental illness in a community nursing home. Am J Psychiatry 1986; 143:1446–1449 [G]

234. Boss P, Caron W, Horbal J, Mortimer J: Predictors of depression in caregivers of dementia patients: boundary ambiguity and mastery. Fam Process 1990; 29:245–254 [G]

235. Dura JR, Stukenberg KW, Kiecolt-Glaser JK: Chronic stress and depressive disorders in older adults. J Abnorm Psychol 1990; 99:284–290 [D]

236. Tariot PN, Podgorski CA, Blazina L, Leibovici A: Mental disorders in the nursing home: another perspective. Am J Psychiatry 1993; 150:1063–1069 [G]

237. Sloane PD, Barrick AL: Improving long-term care for persons with Alzheimer's disease (editorial). J Am Geriatr Soc 1996; 44:91–92 [G]

238. Lawton MP, Brody EM, Saperstein AR: A controlled study of respite service for caregivers of Alzheimer's patients. Gerontologist 1989; 29:8–16 [B]

239. Pynoos J, Regnier V: Improving residential environments for frail elderly: bridging the gap between theory and application, in The Concept and Measurement of Quality of Life in the Frail Elderly. Edited by Birren JE, Lubben JE, Rowe JC, Deutchman DE. San Diego, Academic Press, 1991, pp 91–119 [G]

240. Horwitz GJ, Tariot PN, Mead K, Cox C: Discontinuation of antipsychotics in nursing home patients with dementia. Am J Geriatr Psychiatry 1995; 3:290–299 [C]

241. Tinetti ME, Liu WL, Marottoli RA, Ginter SF: Mechanical restraint use among residents of skilled nursing facilities. JAMA 1991; 265:468–471 [G]

242. Burton LC, German PS, Rovner BW, Brant LJ: Physical restraint use and cognitive decline among nursing home residents. J Am Geriatr Soc 1992; 40:811–816 [C]

243. Capezuti E, Evans L, Strumpf N, Maislin G: Physical restraint use and falls in nursing home residents. J Am Geriatr Soc 1996; 44:627–633 [D]

PRACTICE GUIDELINE FOR THE
Treatment of Patients With Substance Use Disorders: Alcohol, Cocaine, Opioids

WORK GROUP ON SUBSTANCE USE DISORDERS

Steven M. Mirin, M.D., Chair

Steven L. Batki, M.D.
Oscar Bukstein, M.D.
Patricia Gonzales Isbell, M.D.
Herbert Kleber, M.D.
Richard S. Schottenfeld, M.D.
Roger D. Weiss, M.D.
Valery W. Yandow, M.D.

This practice guideline is organized as follows: sections I, II, and III include information of relevance to all patients with a substance use disorder. These sections include a review of available safety and efficacy data, as well as treatment recommendations. Section IV includes information of relevance to patients with alcohol use disorders, section V includes information of relevance to patients with cocaine use disorders, and section VI includes information of relevance to patients with opioid use disorders.

This practice guideline was approved in July 1995 and was published in *The American Journal of Psychiatry* in November 1995.

CONTENTS

INTRODUCTION

This guideline seeks to provide guidance to psychiatrists who care for patients with substance use disorders. It summarizes somatic and psychosocial treatments that are used for such patients, as well as the data relevant to the choice of treatments, and is applicable to psychiatrists in any treatment setting who make treatment decisions with their patients. Psychiatrists care for such patients in a variety of practice settings and frequently work in collaboration with other professionals. The psychiatrist's precise role varies, depending on the specific clinical situation. The psychiatrist may provide all of the care or may work as part of a treatment team with other professionals: it is understood that in some situations the psychiatrist will not be directly providing all of the treatments recommended in this guideline.

The guideline is divided into four main sections. Section III provides an overview of the principles of treatment, and the evidence underlying them, that are broadly applicable to patients with all forms of substance use disorders. Sections IV, V, and VI discuss the treatment of patients with alcohol, cocaine, and opioid use disorders, respectively; these sections build on the general discussion in section III and are not intended to stand alone. Although some of the treatment principles discussed in each of these three sections may apply to a broader group of substances (e.g., there is an area of overlap between the treatment of patients with alcohol use disorders and treatment of patients with other sedative/hypnotic use disorders), the basis of the discussion and the resulting recommendations are based on data relevant to alcohol, cocaine, and opioids. These three substances were chosen because of their public health importance, the availability of a base of treatment research, and their utility in illustrating a variety of treatment modalities. A practice guideline on the treatment of patients with nicotine dependence is also included in this volume. The treatment of patients with other substance use disorders will be addressed in future guidelines.

The degree of specificity of recommendations in this guideline depends on the quality of available research and the degree of consensus among expert clinicians. By providing guidance in choosing among available treatment options and making specific recommendations whenever possible, the guideline reflects the variability in the availability of relevant research data and in the extent of clinical consensus. In section I, recommendations are summarized and coded according to their degree of clinical confidence.

The use of terminology in this guideline is consistent with DSM-IV. The term "substance-related disorders" encompasses substance use disorders and substance-induced disorders. The focus of this guideline is on the treatment of patients with substance use disorders, which include substance abuse and substance dependence. Many of these patients have coexisting conditions; psychiatrists should therefore consider, but not be limited to, the practice guidelines applicable to both substance use disorders and other comorbid disorders that may be present.

I. SUMMARY OF RECOMMENDATIONS

The following executive summary is intended to provide an overview of the organization and scope of recommendations in this practice guideline. The treatment of patients with substance use disorders requires the consideration of many factors and cannot adequately be reviewed in a brief summary. The reader is encouraged to consult the relevant portions of the guideline when specific treatment recommendations are sought. This summary is not intended to stand by itself. Unless otherwise noted, the principles and recommendations set forth under general substance use disorders (section III) apply to the treatment of patients with alcohol (section IV), cocaine (section V), and opioid (section VI) use disorders.

▶ A. CODING SYSTEM

Each recommendation is identified as falling into one of three categories of endorsement, indicated by a bracketed Roman numeral following the statement. The three categories represent varying levels of clinical confidence:

[I] Recommended with substantial clinical confidence.
[II] Recommended with moderate clinical confidence.
[III] May be recommended on the basis of individual circumstances.

▶ B. SUBSTANCE USE DISORDERS: GENERAL TREATMENT PRINCIPLES AND ALTERNATIVES

Substance use disorders constitute a major public health problem, costing our society in excess of $300 billion annually, including direct and indirect costs.

Individuals with substance use disorders are heterogeneous with regard to a number of clinically important features. Treatment for individuals with substance use disorders includes an assessment phase, the treatment of intoxication and withdrawal when necessary, and the development and implementation of an overall treatment strategy. Two general treatment strategies are used, depending on the clinical circumstances: drug free and substitution.

Substance use disorders may affect many domains of an individual's functioning and frequently require multimodal treatment. Goals of treatment include reduction in the use and effects of substances or achievement of abstinence, reduction in the frequency and severity of relapse, and improvement in psychological and social functioning.

1. Assessment

A comprehensive psychiatric evaluation is essential to guide the treatment of a patient with a substance use disorder (I). The assessment includes a) a detailed history of the patient's past and present substance use and its effects on cognitive, psychological, behavioral, and physiologic functioning; b) a general medical and psychiatric history and examination; c) a history of prior psychiatric treatments and outcomes; d) a family and social history; e) screening of blood, breath, or urine for abused substances; and

f) other laboratory tests to help confirm the presence or absence of comorbid conditions frequently associated with substance use disorders.

2. Psychiatric management

Psychiatric management is the foundation of treatment for patients with substance use disorders (I). Psychiatric management has the following specific objectives: establishing and maintaining a therapeutic alliance, monitoring the patient's clinical status, managing intoxication and withdrawal states, developing and facilitating adherence to a treatment plan, preventing relapse, providing education about substance use disorders, and reducing the morbidity and sequelae of substance use disorders. Generally, psychiatric management is combined with specific treatments carried out in a collaborative fashion with professionals of various disciplines at a variety of sites, including community-based agencies, clinics, hospitals, detoxification programs, and residential treatment facilities.

3. Specific treatments

The specific pharmacologic and psychosocial treatments for patients with substance use disorders are reviewed separately, although they are generally studied and applied in the context of treatment programs that combine a number of different treatment modalities. It is uncommon for a single treatment to be effective when used in isolation.

4. Pharmacologic treatments

Pharmacologic treatments are beneficial for selected patients with substance use disorders (I). The categories of pharmacologic treatments are a) medications to treat intoxication and withdrawal states; b) medications to decrease the reinforcing effects of abused substances; c) medications that discourage the use of substances by inducing unpleasant consequences through a drug-drug interaction or by coupling substance use with an unpleasant, drug-induced condition; d) agonist substitution therapy; and e) medications to treat comorbid psychiatric conditions.

5. Psychosocial treatments

Psychosocial treatments are essential components of a comprehensive treatment program (I). Although controlled studies are few in number and many have major design limitations, the available data, along with clinical experience, indicate that the following forms of treatment are effective for selected patients with substance use disorders: cognitive behavioral therapies, behavioral therapies, psychodynamic/interpersonal therapies, group and family therapies, and participation in self-help groups.

6. Formulation and implementation of a treatment plan

The goals of treatment and the specific choice of treatments needed to achieve these goals may vary among different patients and for the same patient at different phases of the illness. Since many substance use disorders are chronic, patients usually require long-term treatment, although the intensity and specific components may vary over time. A treatment plan is developed that includes the following components: a) psychiatric management; b) a strategy for achieving abstinence or reducing the effects or use of illicit substances; c) efforts to enhance ongoing compliance with the treatment program, prevent relapse, and improve functioning; and d) additional treatments necessary for patients with comorbid conditions.

7. Treatment settings

Treatment settings vary with regard to the availability of specific treatment modalities, the degree of restriction on access to substances that are likely to be abused, the availability of general medical and psychiatric care, and the overall milieu and treatment philosophy.

Patients should be treated in the least restrictive setting that is likely to be safe and effective (I). Decisions regarding the site of care should be based on patients' ability to cooperate with and benefit from the treatment offered, the need for structure and support, patients' ability to refrain from illicit use of substances, their ability to avoid high-risk behaviors, and the need for particular treatments that may be available only in certain settings (I). Patients move from one level of care to another on the basis of these factors and an assessment of their ability to safely benefit from a different level of care (I).

Commonly available treatment settings include hospitals, residential treatment facilities, partial hospital care, and outpatient programs. Hospitalization is appropriate for a) patients with a drug overdose that cannot be safely treated in an outpatient or emergency room setting; b) patients at risk for severe or medically complicated withdrawal syndromes; c) patients with comorbid general medical conditions that make ambulatory detoxification unsafe; d) patients with a documented history of not engaging in or benefiting from treatment in a less intensive setting (e.g., residential or outpatient); e) patients with a level of psychiatric comorbidity that would markedly impair their ability to participate in, comply with, or benefit from treatment or whose comorbid disorder would by itself require hospital-level care (e.g., depression with suicidal thoughts, acute psychosis); f) patients manifesting substance use or other behaviors that constitute an acute danger to themselves or others; or g) patients who have not responded to less intensive treatment efforts and whose substance use disorder(s) poses an ongoing threat to their physical and mental health (I).

Residential treatment is indicated for patients who do not meet the clinical criteria for hospitalization but whose lives and social interactions have come to focus predominantly on substance use, and who lack sufficient social and vocational skills and drug-free social supports to maintain abstinence in an outpatient setting (II). Residential treatment of 3 months or more is associated with better long-term outcome in such patients (II).

Partial hospital care should be considered for patients who require intensive care but have a reasonable probability of refraining from illicit use of substances outside a restricted setting (II). Partial hospital settings are frequently used for patients leaving hospitals or residential settings who remain at high risk for relapse. The latter include patients who are thought to lack sufficient motivation to continue in treatment, patients with severe psychiatric comorbidity and/or a history of relapse to substance use in the immediate posthospital or postresidential period, and those returning to high-risk environments who have limited psychosocial supports for remaining drug free. Partial hospital programs are also indicated for patients who are doing poorly in intensive outpatient treatment (II).

Outpatient treatment of substance use disorders is appropriate for patients whose clinical condition or environmental circumstances do not require a more intensive level of care (I). As in other treatment settings, a comprehensive approach using, where indicated, a variety of psychotherapeutic and pharmacologic interventions, along with behavioral monitoring, is optimal.

The duration of treatment should be tailored to individual needs and may vary from a few months to several years (I). Monitoring for substance use should be intensified during periods of high risk of relapse, including the early stages of treatment, times of transition to less intensive levels of care, and the first year following cessation of active treatment (I).

8. Clinical features influencing treatment

Treatment planning and implementation should reflect consideration of comorbid psychiatric and general medical conditions, gender-related factors (including the possibility of pregnancy), age (e.g., for children, adolescents, and the elderly), social milieu and living environment, cultural factors, and family characteristics. The high prevalence of comorbid psychiatric disorders and the diagnostic distinction between substance use symptoms and other disorders should receive particular attention, and specific treatment for comorbid disorders should be provided (I).

▶ C. ALCOHOL USE DISORDERS: TREATMENT PRINCIPLES AND ALTERNATIVES

Psychiatric management (section III.C) forms the basis for the treatment of patients with alcohol use disorders.

1. Treatment settings

Patients with alcohol withdrawal must be detoxified in a setting that provides for frequent clinical assessment and the provision of any necessary treatments (I). Some outpatient settings can accommodate these requirements and may be appropriate for patients deemed to be at low risk of a complicated withdrawal syndrome. However, those who have a prior history of delirium tremens, whose documented history of very heavy alcohol use and high tolerance places them at risk for a complicated withdrawal syndrome, who are concurrently abusing other drugs, who have a severe comorbid general medical or psychiatric disorder, or who repeatedly fail to cooperate with or benefit from outpatient detoxification are more likely to require a residential or hospital setting that can safely provide the necessary care (I). Patients in severe withdrawal (i.e., delirium tremens) require treatment in a hospital setting (I).

Most treatments for patients with alcohol dependence or abuse can be successfully conducted outside of the hospital (e.g., in outpatient, day hospital, or partial hospital settings) (II). However, patients who are unlikely to benefit from less intensive and less restrictive alternatives may need to be hospitalized at times during their treatment. The general criteria for hospitalization are summarized in sections III.G.1 and IV.B.

2. Pharmacologic treatments

The effectiveness of specific pharmacotherapies for alcohol-dependent patients is not well established. Naltrexone may attenuate some of the reinforcing effects of alcohol, but there are limited data regarding the long-term efficacy for patients with alcohol use disorders (II). Disulfiram is an effective adjunct to a comprehensive treatment program in reliable, motivated patients whose drinking may be triggered by events that suddenly increase alcohol craving (II). Patients with impulsive behavior, psychotic symptoms, or suicidal thoughts are poor candidates for disulfiram treatment (I).

In patients with clearly established comorbid psychiatric disorders, treatment specifically directed at these disorders is indicated (I). Such treatment must be coordinated with other treatments for the substance use disorder.

3. Psychosocial treatments

Psychosocial treatments found effective for selected patients with alcohol use disorders include cognitive behavioral therapies (II), behavioral therapies (I), psychodynamic/interpersonal therapy (III), brief interventions (II), marital and family therapy (II), and group therapies (II). Patient participation in self-help groups, such as Alcoholics Anonymous, is frequently helpful (II).

4. Management of alcohol intoxication and withdrawal

The acutely intoxicated patient should be monitored and maintained in a safe environment (II).

Symptoms of alcohol withdrawal typically begin within 4–12 hours after cessation or reduction of alcohol use, peak in intensity during the second day of abstinence, and generally resolve within 4–5 days. Serious complications include seizures, hallucinations, and delirium.

Clinical assessment of intoxicated patients and those manifesting signs and symptoms of withdrawal should include laboratory determination of the presence of other substances (I). The treatment of patients in moderate to severe withdrawal includes efforts to reduce central nervous system (CNS) irritability and restore physiologic homeostasis (I), and it requires the use of thiamine and fluids (I), benzodiazepines (II), and, in selected patients, other medications (II). Once clinical stability is achieved, the tapering of benzodiazepines and other medications should be carried out as necessary, and the patient should be observed for the re-emergence of withdrawal symptoms and the emergence of signs and symptoms suggestive of a comorbid psychiatric disorder (I).

5. Other clinical features influencing treatment

In addition to the considerations addressed in section III.H.3, the treatment of pregnant women with alcohol use disorders is complicated by the risk of fetal alcohol syndrome and the corresponding urgency of minimizing the intake of alcohol (I).

▶ D. COCAINE USE DISORDERS: TREATMENT PRINCIPLES AND ALTERNATIVES

Psychiatric management (section III.C) forms the basis for the treatment of patients with cocaine use disorders.

1. Treatment settings

Clinical and research experience suggests that intensive (i.e., more than twice a week) outpatient treatment, in which a variety of treatment modalities are simultaneously used and in which the focus is the maintenance of abstinence, is effective for most patients with cocaine use disorders (II).

2. Pharmacologic treatments

Pharmacologic treatment is not ordinarily indicated as an initial treatment for patients with cocaine dependence. However, patients with more severe dependence or individuals who fail to respond to psychosocial treatment should be considered for treatment with dopaminergic medications (III).

3. Psychosocial treatments

Psychosocial treatments focusing on abstinence are effective for most patients with cocaine use disorders (II). The following specific types of psychotherapies have been evaluated and have been shown to have variable efficacy with different groups of patients: cognitive behavioral therapies (II), behavioral therapies (II), and psychodynamic psychotherapy (III). In addition, regular participation in self-help groups may improve the outcome for selected patients with cocaine use disorders (III).

4. Management of cocaine intoxication and withdrawal

Cocaine intoxication can produce hypertension, tachycardia, seizures, and paranoid delusions. The syndrome is usually self-limited and typically requires only supportive care (II). Acutely agitated patients may benefit from sedation with benzodiazepines (III).

Following cessation of cocaine use, anhedonia and craving are common. Most patients will not benefit from any currently available pharmacotherapy for withdrawal symptoms. The efficacy of dopamine agonists (e.g., amantadine, bromocriptine) in the treatment of acute cocaine withdrawal has not been clearly demonstrated (III).

5. Other clinical features influencing treatment

In addition to the considerations discussed in section III.H.3, the treatment of pregnant women with cocaine use disorders is complicated by the increased risk of prematurity, low birth weight, stillbirth, and sudden infant death syndrome and the corresponding urgency of minimizing the intake of cocaine (I).

E. OPIOID USE DISORDERS: TREATMENT PRINCIPLES AND ALTERNATIVES

Psychiatric management (section III.C) forms the basis for the treatment of patients with opioid use disorders (I). Some opioid-dependent patients will be able to achieve abstinence from all opioid drugs; many others will require long-term maintenance with opioid agonists (e.g., methadone or LAAM [L-α-acetylmethadol or levomethadyl acetate]).

1. Treatment settings

In addition to the standard treatment settings described in section III.G, therapeutic communities have been found effective in the treatment of patients with opioid use disorders (II).

2. Pharmacologic treatments

Maintenance on methadone or LAAM is appropriate for patients with a prolonged history (>1 year) of opioid dependence and has been shown to reduce the morbidity associated with opioid dependence (I). The goals of treatment are to achieve a stable maintenance dose and to facilitate engagement in a comprehensive program of rehabilitation (I).

Maintenance on naltrexone is an alternative treatment strategy whose utility is often limited by lack of patient compliance and low treatment retention (II).

For some patients, abstinence can never be achieved, but important reductions in morbidity and mortality can be achieved through efforts to reduce the effects of opioid use.

3. Psychosocial treatments

Psychosocial treatments are effective components of a comprehensive treatment plan for patients with opioid use disorders (II). Cognitive behavioral therapies (II), behavioral therapies (II), psychodynamic psychotherapy (III), group and family therapies (III), and self-help groups (III) have been found effective for some patients with opioid use disorders. The choice of treatment should be made after consideration of the patient's preferences, the clinical issues to be addressed, associated comorbid psychopathology, and past response to various treatment modalities.

4. Management of opioid intoxication and withdrawal

Acute opioid intoxication of mild to moderate degree usually does not require specific treatment (II). However, severe opioid overdose, marked by respiratory depression, may be fatal and requires treatment in a hospital emergency room or inpatient setting (I). Naloxone will reverse respiratory depression and other manifestations of opioid overdose (I).

The treatment of opioid withdrawal is directed at safely ameliorating acute symptoms and facilitating entry into a long-term treatment program for opioid use disorders (I). Strategies found to be effective include methadone or LAAM substitution with gradual tapering (I); abrupt discontinuation of opioids, with the use of clonidine to suppress withdrawal symptoms (II); and clonidine-naltrexone detoxification (II). Buprenorphine substitution followed by abrupt discontinuation of buprenorphine (II) has also been found to be effective in laboratory settings but is not yet approved for use in clinical practice. Monitoring for the presence of other substances (particularly alcohol, benzodiazepines, or other anxiolytic or sedative agents) is essential because the concurrent use of or withdrawal from other substances can complicate the treatment of opioid withdrawal (I).

5. Other clinical features influencing treatment

A substantial number of opioid-dependent patients have comorbid psychiatric disorders that must be identified and treated concurrently with the patients' substance use disorders (I).

The use of opioids by injection is associated with high risk of general medical complications, such as bacterial endocarditis, hepatitis, HIV infection, and tuberculosis.

In addition to the considerations discussed in section III.H.3, the treatment of pregnant women with opioid use disorders is complicated by the increased risk of low birth weight, prematurity, neonatal abstinence syndrome, stillbirth, and sudden infant death syndrome and the corresponding urgency of minimizing the intake of opioids (I).

II. DISEASE DEFINITION, EPIDEMIOLOGY, AND NATURAL HISTORY

By any measure, substance use disorders constitute a major public health problem, costing our society in excess of $300 billion annually, including the costs of treatment, related health problems, absenteeism, lost productivity, drug-related crime and incarceration, and efforts in education and prevention (1). (The issues raised by nicotine use disorders are sufficiently different to warrant a separate guideline and are not included in this discussion unless specifically mentioned.)

The motivation for using any psychoactive substance is, in part, related to the acute and chronic effects of these agents on mood, cognition, and behavior. In some individuals the subjective changes (e.g., euphoria, tension relief) that accompany substance intoxication are experienced as highly pleasurable and lead to repetitive use. About 15% of regular users become psychologically dependent in that they come to believe that they are unable to function optimally in social, work, or other settings without experiencing some degree of substance intoxication. These individuals, in turn, are at high risk of developing one or more substance use disorders as defined in the DSM-IV criteria (2).

A. DSM-IV CRITERIA FOR SUBSTANCE DEPENDENCE AND ABUSE

1. Criteria for substance dependence

A maladaptive pattern of substance use, leading to clinically significant impairment or distress, as manifested by three (or more) of the following, occurring at any time in the same 12-month period:

1) tolerance, as defined by either of the following:
   a) a need for markedly increased amounts of the substance to achieve intoxication or desired effect
   b) markedly diminished effect with continued use of the same amount of the substance
2) withdrawal, as manifested by either of the following:
   a) the characteristic withdrawal syndrome for the substance . . .
   b) the same (or a closely related) substance is taken to relieve or avoid withdrawal symptoms
3) the substance is often taken in larger amounts or over a longer period than was intended
4) there is a persistent desire or unsuccessful efforts to cut down or control substance use
5) a great deal of time is spent in activities necessary to obtain the substance (e.g., visiting multiple doctors or driving long distances), use the substance (e.g., chain-smoking), or recover from its effects
6) important social, occupational, or recreational activities are given up or reduced because of substance use
7) the substance use is continued despite knowledge of having a persistent or recurrent physical or psychological problem that is likely to have been caused or exacerbated by the substance (e.g., current cocaine use despite recognition of cocaine-induced depression, or continued drinking despite recognition that an ulcer was made worse by alcohol consumption)

2. Criteria for substance abuse

A. A maladaptive pattern of substance use leading to clinically significant impairment or distress, as manifested by one (or more) of the following, occurring within a 12-month period:

1) recurrent substance use resulting in a failure to fulfill major role obligations at work, school, or home (e.g., repeated absences or poor work performance related to substance use; substance-related absences, suspensions, or expulsions from school; neglect of children or household)

2) recurrent substance use in situations in which it is physically hazardous (e.g., driving an automobile or operating a machine when impaired by substance use)

3) recurrent substance-related legal problems (e.g., arrests for substance-related disorderly conduct)

4) continued substance use despite having persistent or recurrent social or interpersonal problems caused or exacerbated by the effects of the substance (e.g., arguments with spouse about consequences of intoxication, physical fights)

B. The symptoms have never met the criteria for substance dependence for this class of substance.

In using the DSM-IV criteria, one should specify whether substance dependence is *with* physiologic dependence (i.e., there is evidence of tolerance or withdrawal) or *without* physiologic dependence (i.e., no evidence of tolerance or withdrawal). In addition, patients may be variously classified as currently manifesting a pattern of abuse or dependence or as in remission. Those in remission can be divided into four subtypes—full, early partial, sustained, and sustained partial—on the basis of whether any of the criteria for abuse or dependence have been met and over what time frame. The remission category can also be used for patients receiving agonist therapy (e.g., methadone maintenance) or for those living in a controlled drug-free environment.

B. DISEASE DEFINITION AND DIAGNOSTIC FEATURES

1. Cross-sectional features

Patients presenting for treatment of a substance use disorder frequently manifest signs and symptoms of substance-induced intoxication or withdrawal. The clinical picture varies with the substance used, its dosage, the duration of action, the time elapsed since the last dose, the presence or absence of tolerance, and/or psychiatric or general medical comorbidity. The expectations of the patient, his or her style of responding to states of intoxication or physical discomfort, and the setting in which intoxication or withdrawal is taking place also play a role.

Patients experiencing substance-induced intoxication generally manifest changes in mood, cognition, and/or behavior. Mood-related changes may range from euphoria to depression, with considerable lability in response to, or independent of, external events. Cognitive changes may include shortened attention span, impaired concentration, and disturbances of thinking (e.g., delusions) and/or perception (e.g., hallucinations). Behavioral changes may include wakefulness or somnolence, lethargy or hyperactivity. Impairment in social and occupational functioning is also common in intoxicated individuals.

Other cross-sectional diagnostic features commonly found in patients with substance use disorders include those related to any comorbid psychiatric or general medical disorders that may be present. Psychiatric disorders commonly found in such patients include conduct disorder (particularly the aggressive subtype) in children and adolescents (3, 4), depression, bipolar disorder, schizophrenia, anxiety disorders, eating disorders, pathological gambling, antisocial personality disorder, and other personality disorders (5–13).

Examples of general medical problems that may be directly related to substance use include cardiac toxicity resulting from acute cocaine intoxication, respiratory depression and coma in severe opioid overdose, and hepatic cirrhosis after prolonged heavy drinking (14). Examples of general medical conditions frequently associated with opioid-dependent individuals who administer opioids by injection include subacute bacterial endocarditis, HIV infection, and hepatitis. Patients whose substance dependence is accompanied by diminished self-care and/or high levels of risk-taking behavior are at increased risk of experiencing malnutrition, physical trauma, and HIV infection (15).

2. Longitudinal features

Patients with substance use disorders frequently present with a long history of repeated episodes of intoxication and withdrawal, interspersed with attempts to remain substance free. In patients who meet the DSM-IV criteria for substance abuse, episodes of intoxication may be sporadic and brief, rarely requiring general medical or psychiatric intervention. Patients who meet the DSM-IV criteria for dependence often experience repeated episodes of intoxication that may last for weeks or months, interrupted by voluntary or involuntary periods of self-managed, or medically managed, withdrawal. Partial or complete withdrawal from abused substances may be followed by variable periods of self-imposed or involuntary (e.g., during periods of incarceration) abstinence, often ending in relapse to substance use and, eventually, resumption of dependence.

In some patients, dependence on a single substance may lead to use of, and ultimately dependence on, another substance (e.g., the development of alcohol dependence in patients already dependent on opioids or cocaine) (16). In such patients, replacement of one form of substance dependence by another may occur.

Although many individuals who abuse alcohol or illicit substances maintain their ability to function in interpersonal relationships and in the work setting, substance-dependent patients presenting for treatment often manifest profound psychological, social, general medical, legal, and financial problems. These may include disrupted interpersonal (particularly family) relationships, absenteeism, job loss, criminal behavior, poor academic or work performance, failure to develop adaptive coping skills, and a general constriction of normal life activities. Peer relationships often focus extensively on obtaining and using illicit drugs or alcohol. The risk of accidents, violence, and suicide is significantly greater than for the general population (17).

C. NATURAL HISTORY AND COURSE

Not uncommonly, initial experiences with substance use take place before puberty. At the earliest stages of use, experimenters or casual users who go on to develop a substance use disorder are generally indistinguishable from their peers with respect to the type and frequency of substance use. However, early onset and/or regular use of "gateway" drugs, such as alcohol, marijuana, or nicotine, and early evidence of aggressive behavior, intrafamilial disturbances, and associating with substance-using peers contribute to, and predict, continued substance use and the subsequent development of abuse and dependence (18, 19).

In adolescents, growing preoccupation with substance use, frequent episodes of intoxication, use of drugs with greater dependence liability (e.g., opioids, cocaine), and a preference for routes of administration that result in quicker onset of drug effects (e.g., by injection, freebasing) and for more rapidly acting preparations (e.g., methamphetamine) presage the development of substance dependence. Although in most cases the onset of substance use disorders occurs in the late teens and early 20s, some individuals begin abusing substances in mid to late adulthood (20, 21).

Although experience with multiple substances often continues throughout adolescence, some individuals settle on a "drug of choice" early on. Drug preference is shaped by a variety of factors, including current fashion, availability, peer influences, and individual biological and psychological factors. Gender-specific differences in drug preference (e.g., heroin use in males, sedative/hypnotic and benzodiazepine use in females) have diminished somewhat over the last two decades. Although substance abuse and dependence appear to aggregate in families, some of this effect may be explained by the concurrent familial distribution of antisocial personality disorder, which may predispose individuals to the development of these disorders. On the other hand, genetic factors do affect the risk of developing alcoholism, particularly in males with biological male relatives who are also alcoholic (22, 23) and, to a lesser extent, in females with strong family histories of the disorder (24, 25). Finally, some clinicians have suggested, on the basis of retrospective reports from patients, that drug preference is also shaped by the "fit" between specific drug effects and the psychological needs of the user (26). However, there are no controlled studies to support this "self-medication" paradigm.

While there is considerable heterogeneity, for many patients substance dependence has a chronic course, often lasting for years. Periods of sustained use are interrupted by periods of partial or complete remission. Although some individuals are able to achieve prolonged periods of abstinence without formal treatment, abstinence or periods of greatly reduced substance use are more likely to be sustained by patients who are able to maintain active participation in formalized treatment and/or self-help groups (e.g., Alcoholics Anonymous) (27–30). Patients who experience a severe life crisis (e.g., loss of an important relationship, incarceration, or serious general medical sequelae of substance use) are generally more motivated to seek treatment, but most still require external support to maintain their motivation to continue in treatment beyond the initial stages (e.g., detoxification).

During the first several years of treatment, most substance-dependent patients continue to relapse, although with decreasing frequency. Risk of relapse is higher in the first 12 months after the onset of a remission. Many patients experience several cycles of remission and relapse before they conclude that a return to "controlled" substance use is not possible for them. Regardless of the treatment site or the modalities employed, the frequency, intensity, and duration of treatment participation are positively correlated with improved outcome (31).

The majority of patients treated for substance dependence (up to 70% in some studies) are eventually able to stop compulsive use and either abstain from abused substances entirely or experience only brief episodes of substance use that do not progress to abuse or dependence; only a minority of patients (15%–20%) exhibit a pattern of chronic relapse (i.e., over 10–20 years) requiring repetitive intervention. Of those who remain abstinent for 2 years, almost 90% are substance free at 10 years, and those who remain substance free for 10 years have a very high likelihood (i.e., >90%) of being substance free at 20 years (30, 32, 33). Prolonged abstinence, accompanied by improvement in social and occupational functioning, is more apt to occur in those who have lower levels of premorbid psychopathology, demonstrate the ability to develop new relationships, and consistently make use of self-help groups (e.g., Alcoholics Anonymous) (28, 34).

D. EPIDEMIOLOGY

Estimates developed by the Institute of Medicine (35) suggest that there are approximately 5.5 million individuals, or about 2.7% of the U.S. population over age 12, who clearly (2.4 million) or probably (3.1 million) need treatment for drug use disorders and an additional 13 million who clearly or probably need treatment for alcohol use disorders. Of these, approximately two-thirds are men and approximately one-third concurrently have more than one substance use disorder (36).

Substance use disorders are associated with a significant increase in morbidity and mortality, particularly among men. Each year nonnicotine substance dependence is, directly or indirectly, responsible for at least 40% of all hospital admissions and approximately 25% of all deaths (500,000 per year) (37, 38). Approximately 100,000 deaths per year result directly from the use of illicit drugs or alcohol. Two-thirds of these deaths occur in individuals who are dependent on heroin or cocaine; nearly 40% occur in individuals between the ages of 30 and 39. Black men and women appear to be at much higher risk of drug-related mortality than their white counterparts. More than one-third of all new AIDS cases occur among users of intravenous drugs or individuals who have had sexual contact with such individuals, and AIDS-related illnesses account for about 8,000 deaths per year among intravenous drug users (39).

Substance use disorders also exert a profound impact on those who come in contact with these individuals. For example, approximately one-half of all highway fatalities involve either a driver or pedestrian who is intoxicated, and more than 50% of all cases of domestic violence occur under the influence of illicit drugs or alcohol (40). In addition, estimates based on urine testing in general populations suggest that between 7.5% and 15.0% of all pregnant women have had recent exposure to drugs of abuse (excluding alcohol) at the time they first seek prenatal care (41, 42).

Finally, substance use disorders are frequently associated with other forms of psychopathology. The lifetime prevalence of comorbid axis I psychiatric disorders in individuals with substance use disorders (including those with alcohol dependence or abuse) is between 20% and 90%, depending on the population screened and the rigor of the diagnostic criteria used, with treatment-seeking patients being at the higher end of the range (43–50). Approximately one-third of hospitalized psychiatric patients manifest comorbid nonnicotine substance use disorders (51, 52).

III. GENERAL TREATMENT PRINCIPLES AND ALTERNATIVES

Individuals with substance use disorders are heterogeneous with regard to a number of clinically important features:

- the number and type of substances used;
- the severity of the disorder and the degree of associated functional impairment;
- the associated general medical and psychiatric conditions;
- the patient's strengths (protective/resiliency factors) and vulnerabilities; and
- the social/environmental context in which the individual lives and will be treated.

Although the full spectrum of substance use disorders includes conditions that have a narrow impact on an individual's health and functioning, many patients have more severe conditions that broadly affect their health and functioning and that are long-term and/or relapsing in nature. Individuals with more severe conditions, which are less responsive to low-intensity treatments, are the focus of much of this guideline.

Treatment for individuals with substance use disorders may be thought of as occurring in phases:

- assessment phase, during which information on the aforementioned cross-sectional and longitudinal features, as well as other critical information, is obtained and integrated;
- treatment of intoxication/withdrawal, as necessary; and
- development and implementation of an overall treatment strategy.

Depending on the clinical circumstances, the treatment strategy may emphasize the individual's need to remain drug free or it may entail substitution of one presumably safer drug (e.g., methadone) for another (e.g., heroin). Substance use disorders may affect many domains of an individual's functioning, and they frequently require multimodal treatment. Some components of treatment may be focused directly on the substance use, and others may be focused on the associated conditions that have contributed to or resulted from the substance use disorder.

The specific pharmacologic and psychosocial treatments for patients with substance use disorders are reviewed separately, although they are generally studied and applied in the context of treatment programs that combine a number of different treatment modalities. It is uncommon for a single treatment to be effective when used in isolation.

▶ A. GOALS OF TREATMENT

Long-range goals of treatment for patients with substance use disorders include reduction in the use and effects of abused substances, the achievement of abstinence, reduction in the frequency of relapses, and rehabilitation. For some patients, abstinence can never be achieved or can be achieved only after many years of either continuous or episodic treatment. However, even in the absence of complete abstinence, important reductions in morbidity and mortality can be achieved through reduction in the frequency and intensity of substance use and its associated sequels.

1. Abstinence or reduction in the use and effects of substances

The ideal outcome for patients with substance use disorders is total cessation of substance use. However, many patients are unable or unmotivated to reach this goal, particularly in the early phases of treatment. Such patients can still be helped to minimize the direct and indirect effects of substance use. Interventions discussed in this guideline may result in substantial reductions in the general medical, psychiatric, interpersonal, familial/parental, occupational, and other difficulties commonly associated with substance abuse or dependence. Reductions in the amount or frequency of substance use, substitution of a less risky substance, and reduction of high-risk behavior may also be achieved. Engagement of the patient in a long-term treatment that may eventually lead to further reductions in substance use and its associated morbidity is an important goal of early treatment.

Psychiatrists frequently encounter patients who wish to reduce their substance use to a "controlled" level. Some of these patients may be helped to reach a stable level of use (e.g., controlled drinking) that does not cause morbidity (53), while patients who cannot achieve this outcome (the majority) may subsequently be more motivated to accept a goal of total abstinence. For some patients, achieving sustained abstinence is a long-term goal, but the psychiatrist and patient may, for clinical reasons, decide that reduction in the use and/or the harmful consequences of substance use (without total abstinence) is a reasonable intermediate goal. On the other hand, a goal of "controlled" substance use may be unattainable for many patients, may dissuade some from working toward abstinence, and is inappropriate when the psychiatrist believes that any substance use carries a risk of acute or chronic risk (e.g., high-risk behaviors that could be harmful to the patient or others).

Patients who achieve total abstinence from abused substances have the best long-term prognosis, and many experienced psychiatrists feel that since substance use by these patients may be accompanied by disinhibition, increased craving for other drugs, poor judgment, and an increased risk of relapse, patients should be abstinent from all potential drugs of abuse, including alcohol (49, 54, 55).

Patients who agree to pursue a goal of achieving and maintaining abstinence should be advised about the possibility of relapse and participate in developing a treatment plan that includes methods for early detection of and intervention in episodes of relapse.

2. Reduction in the frequency and severity of relapse

Reduction in the frequency and severity of relapse is a critical goal of treatment (56). A major focus of relapse prevention is helping patients to identify situations that place them at high risk for relapse and to develop alternative responses other than substance use. High-risk situations may include craving, a complex phenomenon resulting from patients' acute or chronic physiologic responses to substance withdrawal or their classically conditioned responses to cues associated with substance availability or withdrawal (57–59). For some patients, interpersonal or social situations constitute risk factors for relapse.

It is important for psychiatrists and their patients to understand the chronic, relapsing nature of these disorders for many patients. A reduction in the frequency and severity of relapses may often be a more realistic goal than the complete prevention of any further episodes.

3. Improvement in psychological and social/adaptive functioning

Substance use disorders are associated with problems in psychological development and social adjustment, alienation from friends and family, impaired school or work performance, financial and legal problems, and deterioration of patients' general health (60). Substance dependence is associated with failure to develop age-appropriate interpersonal or coping skills or gradual atrophy of such skills (61). A substantial minority of substance-dependent individuals lack the educational, social, or vocational skills necessary to succeed in our society. Treatment specifically directed toward repairing disrupted relationships, reducing impulsivity, developing social and vocational skills, and obtaining and maintaining employment is important in itself, as well as in helping to maximize the patient's chances of remaining substance free.

B. ASSESSMENT

In evaluating a patient with a suspected or confirmed substance use disorder, a comprehensive psychiatric evaluation is essential. Information should be sought from the patient and, with the patient's consent, available family members and peers, current and past treaters, employers, and others as appropriate. The assessment may include the following:

1. A systematic inquiry into the degree of associated intoxication; the severity of associated withdrawal syndromes; most recent dose and time elapsed since most recent use; the mode of onset, quantity, frequency, and duration of use; and subjective effects of all substances used, including drugs other than the patient's "drug of choice."

2. A comprehensive general medical and psychiatric history, including a complete physical and mental status examination, to ascertain the presence or absence of comorbid general medical or psychiatric disorders, as well as signs and symptoms of intoxication or withdrawal. In some cases, psychological or neuropsychological testing may be indicated.

3. A history of any prior treatment for substance use disorders, including the following characteristics: setting, context (e.g., voluntary or involuntary), modalities used, compliance, duration, and short- (3-month), intermediate- (1-year), and longer-term outcome as measured by subsequent substance use, the level of social and occupational functioning achieved, and other outcome variables. Prior efforts to control or stop substance use outside of a formal treatment setting should be discussed, as well as the patient's attitudes toward his or her previous treatment and nontreatment experiences.

4. A complete family, social, and substance use history, including information on familial substance use disorders or other psychiatric disorders; familial factors contributing to the development or perpetuation of substance use disorders (e.g., enabling behaviors); school or vocational adjustment, peer relationships, and financial or legal problems; the impact of the patient's current living environment on his or her ability to comply with treatment and remain abstinent in the community; and the specific circumstances of the patient's substance use (where, with whom, how much, and by what route of administration).

5. Qualitative and quantitative blood and urine screening for drugs of abuse and laboratory tests for abnormalities that may accompany acute or chronic substance use. These tests may also be used during treatment to monitor for potential relapse.

6. Screening for infectious and other diseases often found in substance-dependent persons (e.g., HIV, tuberculosis, hepatitis). Such individuals, particularly those with evidence of compromised immune function, are felt to be at high risk for these disorders. For example, patients exposed to social or environmental conditions conducive to the spread of tuberculosis should be routinely screened for this disorder.

C. PSYCHIATRIC MANAGEMENT

Successful treatment of substance use disorders may involve the use of multiple specific treatments, which may vary for any one individual, may change over time, and may involve more than one clinician. Psychiatric management is crucial in the ongoing process of choosing among various treatments, monitoring the patient's clinical status, and coordinating different treatment components. Psychiatric management has the following specific objectives: establishing and maintaining a therapeutic alliance, monitoring the patient's clinical status, managing intoxication and withdrawal states, developing and facilitating adherence to a treatment plan, preventing relapse, providing education about substance use disorders, and reducing the morbidity and sequelae of substance use disorders.

The frequency, intensity, and focus of psychiatric management must be tailored to meet each patient's needs, and the type of management is likely to vary over time, depending on the patient's clinical status. In each of these endeavors the psychiatrist should, when appropriate, work collaboratively with members of other professional disciplines, community-based agencies, treatment programs, and lay organizations to coordinate and integrate the patient's care and to address his or her social, vocational, educational, and rehabilitative needs.

1. Establishing and maintaining a therapeutic alliance

An essential feature of psychiatric management of patients with substance use disorders is the establishment and maintenance of a therapeutic alliance wherein the psychiatrist empathically obtains necessary diagnostic and treatment-related information, gains the confidence of the patient and significant others, and is available in times of crisis. The frequency and duration of treatment contacts should be sufficient to engage the patient and, where appropriate, significant others in a sustained effort to participate in all relevant treatment modalities and, where appropriate, self-help groups. Within the context of this alliance, learning, practicing, and internalizing changes in attitudes and behavior conducive to relapse prevention are the primary goal of treatment (62, 63). The strength of the therapeutic alliance has been found to be a significant predictor of psychotherapy outcome (64). For example, in a sample of persons with substance use disorders (65), a stronger alliance predicted less drug use and better psychological functioning during follow-up.

2. Monitoring the patient's clinical status

The ongoing evaluation of the patient's safety is critical, because the patient's clinical status may change over time. It is particularly important to monitor patients for the potential emergence of suicidal or homicidal thoughts or of treatment-emergent side effects.

The ongoing assessment of the patient's psychiatric status is also necessary, to ensure that the patient is receiving the appropriate treatment(s) and to monitor the patient's response to treatment (e.g., determining the optimal dose of a drug and evaluating its efficacy).

Because relapse is common and is inconsistently self-reported by patients (particularly when use is met with negative consequences or a judgmental response), laboratory monitoring through breath, blood, saliva, and urine testing for drugs of abuse may be helpful in the early detection of relapse. Such monitoring is often initially conducted on a frequent and random schedule, since many drugs and their metabolites may be detected for only a few days after use. Random urine screening for recent (i.e., within the last 1–3 days) substance use should be supplemented by nonrandom testing when recent substance use is suspected.

Methods of urine screening vary as to levels of sensitivity, specificity, and cost. The psychiatrist should be familiar with the applicability and sensitivity of the available analytic methods and collection procedures used in local laboratories, and he or she should specify the type of drug use suspected. Direct supervision of patient voiding and other "chain of custody" procedures will help to ensure the validity and reliability of the test results.

The decision whether to test a patient's breath, blood, or urine depends on the type of drug use suspected, the drug's duration of action, the sensitivity of the test employed, and the clinical setting in which care is being rendered. For example, serum testing is useful for assessing very recent substance use (since it reflects current serum levels). Alcohol can be detected for up to 24 hours in urine, but breath testing is frequently preferred because of the immediacy of the results, noninvasiveness of the procedure, and low cost. Finally, there is some evidence that elevation of certain state markers, such as mean corpuscular volume (MCV) or γ-glutamyl transpeptidase (GGT), may indicate that a patient has recently returned to drinking.

3. Managing intoxication and withdrawal states

In general, acutely intoxicated patients require reassurance and maintenance in a safe and monitored environment, with efforts to decrease external stimulation and provide orientation and reality testing. Clinical assessment is directed toward ascertaining which substances have been used, the route of administration, dose, time since the last dose, whether the level of intoxication is waxing or waning, and other diagnostic information as already described. Management of acute intoxication is also directed toward hastening the removal of substances from the body, which may be accomplished through gastric lavage, in the case of substances that have been recently ingested, or through techniques that increase the rate of excretion of drugs or their active metabolites. Drug effects may also be reversed by administering drugs that antagonize the effects of abused substances. Examples include the administration of naloxone to patients who have overdosed with heroin or other opioids.

Not all intoxicated individuals will develop withdrawal symptoms. Withdrawal syndromes usually occur in tolerant and/or physically dependent individuals who discontinue or reduce their substance use after a period of heavy and prolonged use. The specific signs and symptoms of withdrawal vary according to the substance used, the time elapsed since the last dose, the rate of elimination and duration of action of the substance in question, the concomitant use of other prescribed or nonprescribed drugs, the presence or absence of concurrent general medical or psychiatric disorders, and individual biological and psychosocial variables.

Many patients use multiple substances simultaneously to enhance, ameliorate, or otherwise modify the degree or nature of their intoxication or to relieve withdrawal symptoms. Intoxication with alcohol and cocaine, use of heroin and cocaine ("speedball"), and the combined use of alcohol, marijuana, and/or benzodiazepines by opioid-dependent patients are particularly frequent. Patients using multiple substances (including alcohol) are at risk for withdrawal from each of these.

4. Reducing the morbidity and sequelae of substance use disorders

The psychiatrist should engage the patient and significant others in developing a comprehensive treatment plan that addresses all areas of biological, psychological, and social functioning, the patient's vocational, educational, or recreational needs, and the treatment of any coexisting general medical or psychiatric disorders, including other substance use disorders, that may be present.

5. Facilitating adherence to a treatment plan and preventing relapse

Since substance-dependent patients are often highly ambivalent about giving up substance use, psychiatrists must monitor, throughout all phases of treatment, patient attitudes about participating in treatment and complying with specific recommendations. Barriers to treatment participation include denial of the problem by the patient and the patient's family or social network; patterns of behavior that facilitate substance use (e.g., criminal activity or continued contact with drug-using peers); the likely re-emergence of craving for abused substances; unproductive attitudes about the value of work, treatment, or interpersonal relationships; continued psychosocial or vocational dysfunction; and comorbid psychiatric or general medical problems. These barriers should be discussed at the beginning and throughout the course of treatment.

The psychiatrist may address these barriers by actively attempting to increase motivation through specific enhancing techniques (66), encouraging the patient to participate in self-help or professionally led groups that include recovering individuals; encouraging the development of a substance-free peer group and lifestyle; helping the patient develop techniques to improve interpersonal relationships in family, work, and social settings; encouraging the patient to seek new experiences and roles consistent with a substance-free existence (e.g., greater involvement in vocational, social, and religious activities); discouraging the patient from instituting major life changes that might increase the risk of relapse; and providing, or arranging for, treatment of comorbid psychiatric and general medical conditions (67, 68).

Relapse prevention efforts may include helping patients anticipate and avoid drug-related cues (e.g., instructing the patient to avoid drug-using peers), training patients in self-monitoring affective or cognitive states associated with increased craving and substance use, contingency contracting, teaching desensitization and relaxation techniques to reduce the potency of drug-related stimuli and modulate craving intensity, helping patients develop alternative, nonchemical coping responses to uncomfortable feelings and situations, and providing coping and social skills training to help patients become involved in satisfying drug-free alternative activities (69). Behavioral techniques to enhance the availability and perceived value of social reinforcement as an alternative to drug use or reward for remaining drug free have also been used (70).

A mutually acceptable therapeutic plan for intervening in situations in which there is a high likelihood of relapse to substance use should be developed in the early stages (e.g., first few weeks) of treatment and reviewed on a regular basis (e.g., monthly or more frequently) for patients for whom relapse is an immediate concern. It is frequently helpful to obtain the patient's agreement to 1) predetermined guidelines for obtaining information from family, friends, and employers with which to assess the patient's ability to remain substance free and 2) the clinical criteria for altering the type, intensity, or site of treatment.

6. Providing education about substance use disorders and their treatments

Patients with substance use disorders should receive some education and feedback in regard to their illness, prognosis, and treatment. The psychiatrist should educate patients and, where appropriate, significant others regarding the etiology and course of the disorder, the need for abstinence, the risk of switching addictions, the identification of relapse triggers, available treatments, and the role of family and friends in aiding or impeding recovery. Where appropriate, the psychiatrist should also provide education about associated general medical problems (e.g., HIV infection, the effects of alcohol and other drugs on the fetus), the advantages of using sterile needles, procedures for safer sex, birth control, and the availability of treatment services for drug-affected newborns. Educational efforts should be geared to the developmental and cognitive level of the patient.

7. Diagnosing and treating associated psychiatric disorders

An ongoing, longitudinal assessment of the patient may be critical to the accurate diagnosis of a comorbid condition (see section III.H.1). Comorbid psychiatric conditions may complicate the substance use treatment and may require the addition of specific treatments (e.g., an antidepressant medication for a patient with comorbid major depressive disorder).

D. PHARMACOLOGIC TREATMENTS

Pharmacotherapy for patients with substance use disorders may be used 1) to ameliorate the signs and symptoms of drug intoxication or withdrawal; 2) to decrease the effect of an abused substance and, more specifically, to decrease its subjective reinforcing effects; 3) to make the use of an abused substance aversive by a) inducing unpleasant consequences through a drug-drug interaction or b) coupling substance use with an unpleasant drug-induced condition; 4) to use an agonist substitution strategy to promote abstinence from a more dangerous illicit substance (e.g., the use of methadone for individuals with opioid use disorders); and 5) to treat comorbid psychiatric or general medical conditions.

1. Medications to treat intoxication or withdrawal states

Patients who develop tolerance to a particular drug also develop cross-tolerance to other drugs in the same pharmacologic class. As a result, one can take advantage of cross-tolerance in the treatment of withdrawal states by replacing the abused drug with a drug in the same general class but with a longer duration of action and then slowly tapering the longer-acting drug in a way that allows time for the restoration of physiologic homeostasis. Examples include the use of methadone in the treatment of heroin withdrawal and benzodiazepines in the treatment of alcohol withdrawal (71–73). Clonidine is an example of an agent that ameliorates abstinence-related symptoms in patients withdrawing from opioids but is not a competitive agonist (74).

2. Medications to decrease the reinforcing effects of abused substances

A variety of medications have been used to block or otherwise counteract the physiologic and/or subjective reinforcing effects of abused substances. For example, the narcotic antagonist naltrexone blocks the subjective and physiologic effects of subsequently administered opioid drugs (e.g., heroin) (75, 76). Repetitive testing of antagonist-induced "blockade" of opioid effects theoretically leads to extinction of conditioned craving for opioids (77).

Because of their strong affinity for and binding to opioid receptor sites, the narcotic antagonists also displace opioid agonists from neuronal and other receptors and can, therefore, be used to treat acute opioid intoxication. Abstinence symptoms precipitated by narcotic antagonists have also been used as a provocative test for the presence of opioid dependence (71).

3. Medications that discourage the use of substances

The most prominent example within this category is disulfiram (Antabuse), a drug that inhibits the activity of aldehyde dehydrogenase, the enzyme that metabolizes acetaldehyde, the first metabolic breakdown product of alcohol. In the presence of disulfiram pretreatment, alcohol use results in the accumulation of toxic levels of acetaldehyde, accompanied by a host of unpleasant, potentially dangerous, and rarely lethal signs and symptoms (78–80).

Medications have also been used as part of a chemical aversion treatment in which conditioned stimuli signaling drug availability, or the abused substance itself, are coupled with drugs that produce highly unpleasant effects, such as succinylcholine, which interferes with respiratory function, or emetine, which induces vomiting. The use of aversive medications for this purpose has been tried with patients who have alcohol use disorders (81) and or cocaine use disorders (82) with some success, but it is not recommended outside of specialized treatment settings.

4. Agonist substitution therapy

The use of agonist medications may help some patients to reduce illicit drug use by reducing or eliminating symptoms of withdrawal and by decreasing craving for that particular class of substances. An example is the use of methadone or LAAM in the treatment of opioid-dependent patients (section VI.C.1).

5. Medications to treat comorbid psychiatric conditions

Also refer to section III.B for important diagnostic considerations. The high prevalence of comorbid psychiatric disorders in substance-dependent patients implies that many such patients will require specific pharmacotherapy directed at their comorbid disorders. Examples include the use of lithium or other mood stabilizers for substance-dependent patients with bipolar disorder, the use of neuroleptics for patients with schizophrenia, and the use of antidepressants for patients with major or atypical depressive disorder.

Potential problems for substance-dependent patients receiving pharmacotherapy for comorbid psychiatric illnesses include potentiation of acute drug effects (e.g., in combining antidepressants and alcohol) and intentional or unintentional overdose. Certain drugs used to treat comorbid psychiatric illnesses may themselves be abused. For example, patients with comorbid alcohol dependence and panic disorder may abuse benzodiazepines, and patients with comorbid schizophrenia and neuroleptic-induced parkinsonism may abuse anticholinergics. Whenever possible, medications with low abuse potential and relative safety in overdose should be chosen, e.g., selective serotonin reuptake inhibitors for depression.

E. PSYCHOSOCIAL TREATMENTS

The major psychotherapeutic orientations that have been studied in patients with substance use disorders are cognitive behavioral and psychodynamic/interpersonal therapies. Although controlled studies often have major design limitations, the available data, along with clinical experience, suggest that psychosocial interventions can be useful when adapted for the special needs of this patient population. In many cases, however, treatment effects may not be apparent until the patient has been consistently in treatment for 3 months or more (83). This section will review the treatment approaches, the principles underlying their use, and their application in the treatment of patients with substance use disorders. Studies of the efficacy of psychosocial treatments for alcohol, cocaine, and opioid disorders are discussed in sections IV.D, V.D, and VI.D. Two terms, "psychotherapy" and "drug counseling," are used by clinicians and in the literature to describe some of the treatments described in this section. In general, the term "drug counseling" is applied to treatment that is given by a nonprofessional and that narrowly focuses on specific strategies for avoiding drug use.

"Drug counseling" in this sense may be accompanied by other specific treatments, including psychotherapy.

1. Cognitive behavioral therapies

Cognitive behavioral therapies focus on a) altering the cognitive processes that lead to maladaptive behaviors in substance users, b) intervening in the behavioral chain of events that lead to substance use, c) helping patients deal successfully with acute or chronic drug craving, and d) promoting and reinforcing the development of social skills and behaviors compatible with remaining drug free.

a) Cognitive therapy

Cognitive therapy, initially developed by Beck et al. (84) for the treatment of depression and anxiety, has been modified by that group for the treatment of patients with substance use disorders (85). The foundation of cognitive therapy is the belief that by identifying and subsequently modifying maladaptive thinking patterns, patients can reduce or eliminate negative feelings and behavior (e.g., substance use).

b) Relapse prevention

"Relapse prevention" is an approach to treatment in which cognitive behavioral techniques are used in an attempt to help patients develop greater self-control in order to avoid relapse (56, 86). Specific relapse prevention strategies include discussing ambivalence, identifying emotional and environmental triggers of craving and substance use, developing and reviewing specific coping strategies to deal with internal or external stressors, exploring the decision chain leading to resumption of substance use, and learning from brief episodes of relapse ("slips") about triggers leading to relapse and developing effective techniques for early intervention (56, 87).

In controlled studies, relapse prevention has generally been found over time to be as effective as other psychosocial treatments (53, 88), and it may be more effective than other psychosocial treatments for patients who are more severely dependent and those with concurrent sociopathy or high levels of psychiatric symptoms (89–91).

c) Motivational enhancement therapy

Motivational enhancement therapy, based on cognitive behavioral, client-centered, systems, and social-psychological persuasion techniques, was shown to have positive effects in eight of nine controlled studies (92–94). This brief treatment modality is characterized by an empathic approach in which the therapist helps to motivate the patient by asking about the pros and cons of specific behaviors, by exploring the patient's goals and associated ambivalence about reaching these goals, and by listening reflectively. Motivational enhancement therapy has demonstrated substantial efficacy in the treatment of substance-dependent patients (92).

2. Behavioral therapies

Operant behavioral therapy involves operant rewarding or punishing of patients for desirable (e.g., demonstrating treatment compliance) or undesirable (e.g., associated with relapse) behaviors (95–97). Rewards have included vouchers, awarded for producing drug-free urine samples, that can be exchanged for mutually agreed on items (e.g., movie tickets) or "community reinforcement," in which family members or peers reinforce behaviors that demonstrate or facilitate abstinence (e.g., participation in positive activities) (98).

Contingency management is a behavioral treatment based on the use of predetermined positive or negative consequences to reward abstinence or punish (and thus deter) drug-related behaviors. Negative consequences for returning to substance use may include notification of courts, employers, or family members. The effectiveness of contingency management depends heavily on the concurrent use of frequent, random, supervised urine monitoring for substance use. When negative contingencies are based on the anticipated response of others (e.g., spouses, employers), one should obtain the written informed consent of the patient at the time the contract is initiated (99).

Cue exposure treatment based on a Pavlovian extinction paradigm involves exposure of the patient to cues that induce drug craving while preventing actual drug use and, therefore, the experience of drug-related reinforcement (100). Cue exposure can also be paired with relaxation techniques and drug refusal training to facilitate extinction of classically conditioned craving (101, 102). Although two studies (103, 104) of cue exposure treatment showed encouraging results in laboratory settings, further studies are necessary before it can be recommended for general use.

Aversion therapy, which involves coupling drug or alcohol use with an unpleasant experience (e.g., mild electric shock or pharmacologically induced vomiting), is used in certain specialized facilities. Controlled trials of such treatment have had mixed results (105, 106).

3. Individual psychodynamic/interpersonal therapies

a) Individual psychodynamic psychotherapy

Systematic investigations have examined the efficacy of specially adapted forms of psychotherapy when combined with other treatment modalities (e.g., pharmacotherapies and self-help groups). For example, Woody et al. found that psychodynamic psychotherapy facilitated continued abstinence in patients with a baseline period of sustained abstinence (i.e., 1 to 2 years) (107, 108). Patients with comorbid antisocial personality disorder and high levels of sociopathy have been found to be poor candidates for psychodynamic psychotherapy (107, 109). The efficacy of psychodynamic psychotherapy when used as the sole treatment modality has not been demonstrated by controlled studies.

A number of structured short-term psychodynamic treatments have recently been developed. Supportive-expressive therapy (110) is a modification of psychodynamically oriented treatment based on creating a safe and supportive therapeutic relationship in which patients are encouraged to deal with negative patterns in other relationships. The largest study of supportive-expressive therapy (107) was described in the preceding paragraph. When supportive-expressive therapy was compared to multimodal behavior therapy for alcohol use disorders, subjects in the former group had somewhat better outcomes (i.e., less drinking) than the latter group at 2-year follow-up but similar drinking outcomes at 3-year follow-up (111). However, because of the small number of subjects in the study and a higher follow-up rate among patients in the multimodal behavior therapy group, these results need to be replicated in carefully controlled trials. A multisite clinical trial of supportive-expressive therapy for cocaine dependence, funded by the National Institute on Drug Abuse (NIDA), is currently underway (section V.D.4).

The efficacy of psychodynamic psychotherapy and psychoanalysis has been suggested by case reports and other reports of clinical experience.

b) Individual interpersonal therapy

Interpersonal therapy, described in detail by Klerman et al. (112), focuses on difficulties in current interpersonal functioning by using psychodynamic principles and techniques with some modifications, such as including limit setting and using advice and suggestions. Interpersonal therapy has been shown to be useful in the treatment of both opioid users and cocaine users with low levels of dependence (113). Neither interpersonal therapy nor psychodynamically oriented psychotherapy is indicated for patients with profound cognitive deficits resulting from heavy drinking or other causes.

4. Group therapies

Group therapies are regarded by some psychiatrists as the preferred mode of psychotherapeutic treatment for substance-dependent patients. Many types of group therapy have been used with this population, including modified psychodynamic, interpersonal, interactive, rational emotive, Gestalt, and psychodrama (114, 115). For patients able to tolerate the dynamics of group interaction, including group confrontation of their denial, dealing with issues of interpersonal conflict or closeness, and the sharing of painful experiences or affects, group therapy can be a supportive, therapeutic, and educational experience that can motivate and sustain patients struggling to cope with life stresses and drug craving while remaining drug free (116–118).

Group therapy offers patients opportunities to identify with others who are going through similar problems, to understand the impact of substance use on their lives, to learn more about their own and others' feelings and reactions, and to learn to communicate needs and feelings more adaptively. Group therapy can also be useful in providing a forum for discussing and updating the treatment plan and for developing and monitoring specific behavioral contracts that help prevent relapse (and re-establish abstinence when relapse occurs). Even when the patient is not in immediate danger with regard to substance use, attendance at a weekly therapy group and the opportunity to hear other people's concerns about abstinence underscore the need for constant vigilance. While for many patients regular attendance at 12-step meetings can serve a similar function, often patients slip away from Alcoholics Anonymous (AA) and Narcotics Anonymous when they are in the greatest difficulty. Participation in a therapy group increases accountability by providing opportunities for the therapist and other group members to note and respond to early warning signs of relapse.

5. Family therapies

Dysfunctional families, characterized by impaired communication among family members and an inability to set appropriate limits or maintain standards of behavior, are associated with poor short- and long-term treatment outcome for patients with substance use disorders (119). The goals of family therapy, in a formalized ongoing therapeutic relationship or through periodic contact, include encouraging family support for abstinence; providing information about the patient's current attitudes toward drug use, treatment compliance, social and vocational adjustment, level of contact with drug-using peers, and degree of abstinence; maintaining marital relationships; and improving treatment compliance and long-term outcome (120, 121). Controlled studies have shown family therapy to be effective for adolescents, patients on methadone maintenance, and patients with alcohol dependence.

Different theoretical orientations of family therapy include structural, strategic, psychodynamic, systems, and behavioral approaches. Family interventions include those focused on the nuclear family; on the patient and his or her spouse; on concurrent treatment for patients, spouses, and siblings; on multifamily groups; and on social networks (68, 122, 123).

Family interventions are indicated in circumstances in which a patient's abstinence upsets a previously well-established but maladaptive style of family interaction (121, 124) and in which other family members need help in adjusting to a new set of individual and familial goals, attitudes, and behaviors. Family therapy that addresses interpersonal and family interactions leading to conflict or enabling behaviors can reduce the risk of relapse for patients with high levels of family involvement. Structured family intervention techniques are often effective in breaking through denial and resistance to treatment and are appropriate when less confrontive measures fail. Similarly, coercion exerted by family members, employers, or courts is an effective and appropriate means of engaging otherwise noncompliant patients in treatment. The use of coercion per se does not adversely affect the long-term prognosis for such patients.

Couple and family therapy are also useful for promoting psychological differentiation of family members, providing a forum for the exchange of information and ideas about the treatment plan, developing behavioral management contracts and ground rules for continued family support, and reinforcing behaviors that help prevent relapse and enhance the prospects for recovery.

The duration of family therapy is determined by progress in addressing and altering patterns of family interaction that may have contributed to substance abuse in the index patient, as well as interpersonal or systemic difficulties that may arise as a consequence of the patient's remaining abstinent and that may increase the risk of relapse. Other important considerations include meeting with sufficient frequency so as to maintain open lines of communication and a therapeutic focus on family issues, the coordination of family therapy with other ongoing treatment interventions, referral of family members for individual or group treatment where necessary, defining the role of family members in monitoring compliance with medication regimens, and contingency contracts or participation in other treatment-related activities. In the case of adolescents or patients under guardianship, the roles of responsible family members in decisions about pharmacologic treatment, drug testing, hospitalization, financing of treatment, maintenance of confidentiality, requirements for living at home, and the sharing of parental responsibilities, particularly when the parents are separated or divorced, are among the important issues addressed by family therapy (125).

In many instances, formal termination of family treatment should be followed by renewed contact at times when the patient, the psychiatrist, or family members feel the need to reassess progress in treatment, intervene in behaviors that may ultimately lead to relapse, or reinforce familial interactions that enhance the patient's ability to remain substance free (126).

6. Self-help groups

Although there is little empirical evidence to support their efficacy, clinical experience suggests that participation in self-help groups can be an important adjunct to treatment for many patients with substance use disorders. Referral is appropriate at all stages in the treatment process, even for patients who may still be active substance users. These groups, which are generally based on the 12-step approach of AA and related groups, such as Narcotics Anonymous and Cocaine Anonymous, can provide critical support for patients in recovery. Patients who attend AA or Narcotics Anonymous regularly receive group support and repeated reminders of the disastrous consequences of alcohol or other drug use and the benefits of abstinence and sobriety. Straightforward advice and encouragement about avoiding relapse, the personalized support of a recovering sponsor, and opportunities for both structured and unstructured substance-free social events and interactions are important features of self-help groups. In addition, the process of working through the 12 steps with a sponsor provides a structured opportunity to re-assess the role of past life experiences and personal identity in the development and maintenance of substance use disorders.

Members of self-help groups can attend meetings on a self-determined or prescribed schedule, every day if necessary. Periods associated with high risk for relapse (e.g., weekends, holidays, and evenings) are particularly appropriate for attendance. A sponsor who is compatible with the patient can provide important guidance and support during the recovery process, particularly during periods of emotional distress and increased craving. Patients being treated with medication for comorbid psychiatric disorders should be referred to self-help groups in which such treatment is supported.

Self-help groups are useful for many, but not all, patients. The refusal to participate in self-help groups is not synonymous with resistance to treatment in general. Some self-help groups (e.g., Rational Recovery) do not follow the abstinence-oriented, 12-step approach of AA and related groups and are alternatives for patients who do not accept the philosophy and spiritual focus of AA. Young people generally do better in groups that include age-appropriate peers in addition to some older recovering members. Patients who require psychoactive medications (e.g., lithium, antidepressants) for comorbid psychiatric illness should be directed to groups in which this activity is recognized and supported as useful treatment, rather than another form of substance abuse. Self-help groups based on the 12-step model are also available for family members and friends (e.g., Al-Anon, Alateen, Nar-Anon). They provide group support and education about the illness, and they function to reduce maladaptive enabling behavior in family and friends.

F. FORMULATING AND IMPLEMENTING A TREATMENT PLAN

The goals of treatment and the specific choice of treatments needed to achieve those goals (section III.A) vary among patients and, for the same patient, among different phases of the illness. Since many substance use disorders are chronic, patients may require long-term treatment, although the intensity and specific components may vary over time.

Decisions regarding the site and components of treatment depend on individual patient factors, with the least restrictive setting that is likely to be safe and effective generally being preferable (section III.G).

On the basis of the assessment (section III.B), a treatment plan is developed. The components of a treatment plan and the factors that go into their choice are summarized in the following list. It must be kept in mind, however, that the separation of components is done for heuristic reasons: in practice, the components, and the factors that underlie their potential utility, overlap considerably.

1) Psychiatric management (section III.C) is crucial to coordinating the use of multiple modalities applied in individual, group, family, and self-help settings. It includes the following elements: establishment and maintenance of a therapeutic alliance, monitoring of the patient's clinical status, management of intoxication and withdrawal states, reduction in the morbidity and sequelae of substance use disorders, facilitation of adherence to a treatment plan and prevention of relapse, education about substance use disorders, and diagnosis and treatment of associated psychiatric disorders.

In addition to psychiatric management, a treatment plan must include specific interventions that address the objectives listed in items 2, 3, and 4. These interventions may include specific pharmacologic treatments, specific psychosocial treatments, or a combination of these.

2) A strategy for achieving abstinence or reducing the effects or use of illicit substances (or nonillicit substances that exacerbate the substance use disorder) must be developed and implemented. The range of available strategies depends, in part, on the severity of the disorder and the availability of an effective pharmacologic treatment (e.g., an antagonist to block the effects of the substance or an agonist to reduce craving).

3) Efforts to enhance ongoing compliance with the treatment program and prevent relapse (section III.C.5) and improve functioning (III.A.3) are critical. The likelihood of success in continued treatment compliance is improved by decreasing the patient's access to abusable substance(s); optimizing the use of any specific pharmacologic treatments; addressing factors that help precipitate and/or perpetuate substance use, including both external factors (e.g., living/social environment) and internal factors (e.g., other psychopathology); providing disincentives for substance use (e.g., through the use of monitoring or pharmacologic strategies); and helping the patient develop cognitive and behavioral strategies to support a substance-free lifestyle (97). Referral to self-help groups is frequently helpful during this phase of treatment. Specific rehabilitative interventions to improve functioning may be necessary for patients whose functional level is impaired to the extent that it interferes with their ability to comply with treatment or is not expected to improve satisfactorily with cessation of substance use.

4) Patients with comorbid conditions generally require additional treatments (e.g., a specific psychotherapy, an antidepressant medication) in order to achieve optimal outcomes.

A growing body of research has addressed the issue of "patient-treatment matching," especially for psychosocial treatments. Clinical features such as age at onset, severity of dependence, presence of polydrug use, level of social/occupational impairment, level and nature of additional psychopathology, the quality of relationships, spiritual experience or religious affiliation, and the presence of neuropsychological impairments have all been studied (31, 53, 86, 90, 91, 127–144). Although these studies have generated findings that may eventually have implications for clinical practice, most had relatively small numbers of subjects and many of the findings have not been replicated. In addition, many of these studies, particularly psychotherapy studies, employed highly trained, experienced therapists who were closely supervised and monitored throughout with regard to their adherence to the treatment model that they were using. It is also not known to what degree the findings from these studies will generalize to other settings and other clinicians. A large-scale, multisite patient-treatment matching study currently under way may help determine whether patient factors can be used to predict response to various psychosocial treatments and, if so, at what stage in the cycle of recovery and relapse (145). The choice of treatments for patients with substance use disorders depends on the patient's clinical status and preferences: patient preferences are particularly important since adherence to a treatment plan over time is a powerful predictor of its effectiveness. In general, clinical features that guide the choice of psychosocial treatment for non-substance-using populations are also helpful guides for patients with substance use disorders (e.g., patients with antisocial personality disorder tend to do better in structured behavioral or cognitive behavioral treatments (91, 127).

A number of studies have shown that the amount and quality of treatment services received by individuals with substance use disorders are strong predictors of substance use outcome (146–150). There is also evidence that patients who receive more psychiatric services have better social adjustment outcomes (150), which might promote more abstinence over time.

G. TREATMENT SETTINGS

Patients with substance use disorders may receive their care in a variety of settings. The choice of setting should be guided by the demands of the treatment plan (as described in section III.F and as determined by the patient's clinical status) and the characteristics of available settings. Treatment settings vary with regard to the availability of various treatment capacities (e.g., general medical care, psychotherapy), the relative restrictiveness with respect to access to substances or involvement in other high-risk behaviors, hours of operation, and overall milieu and treatment philosophy (e.g., the use of psychotropic medications for comorbid conditions).

1. Factors affecting choice of treatment setting

Patients should be treated in the least restrictive setting that is likely to prove safe and effective. Decisions regarding the site of care should be based on the patient's a) capacity and willingness to cooperate with treatment; b) capacity to care for himself or herself; c) need for structure, support, and supervision in order to remain safe and pursue treatment away from environments and activities that promote substance use; d) need for specific treatments for comorbid general medical or psychiatric conditions; e) need for particular treatments or an intensity of treatment that may be available only in certain settings; and f) preference for a particular treatment setting.

Patients should be moved from one level of care to another on the basis of these factors and the clinician's assessment of patients' readiness and ability to benefit from a less intensive level of care.

Studies comparing the short-, intermediate-, and long-term benefits of treatment in various settings (i.e., inpatient, residential, partial hospital, outpatient) suffer from a variety of methodologic problems, including heterogeneity of patient populations, high dropout rates, and reliance on patient self-reports uncorroborated by data from collateral sources. Stated treatment goals, program features, and outcome measures also vary across studies (151).

2. Commonly available treatment settings

The availability of different settings varies among communities. The settings described may be considered as points along a continuum of care. Key characteristics of settings that are not described in this section can be used to determine where, along this continuum, they would fit.

a) Hospitals

The range of services available in hospital-based programs typically includes detoxification; assessment and treatment of general medical and psychiatric conditions; group, individual, and family therapies; psychoeducation; and motivational counseling. Other important components of hospital-based treatment programs include the willingness and ability to introduce patients to self-help groups and to develop a plan for posthospital care that includes strategies for relapse prevention and, where appropriate, rehabilitation (152).

Hospital-based treatment settings may be secure (i.e., locked) or permit patients and visitors to come and go in a monitored but generally less restricted fashion. Secure hospital settings should be considered for patients with comorbid psychiatric conditions whose clinical state would ordinarily require such a unit (e.g., actively suicidal patients). Patients with poor impulse control and judgment who in the presence of an "open door" are likely to leave the program or obtain or receive drugs on the unit are also candidates for a secure unit. In some states patients can reside on a secure unit in "conditional voluntary" status, which requires written notice and a time delay (e.g., 3 days) before a patient-initiated request for discharge must be acted on or another disposition (e.g., commitment) is implemented. Such restrictions can provide a useful period of delay in which poorly motivated patients can reconsider their wish to leave the program prematurely.

Available data do not support the notion that hospitalization per se has specific benefits over other treatment settings beyond the ability to address treatment objectives that require a medically monitored environment (70, 153). Nonetheless, patients in one or more of the specific following groups may require hospital-level care:

1. Patients with drug overdoses that cannot be safely treated in an outpatient or emergency room setting (e.g., patients with severe respiratory depression or coma).
2. Patients in withdrawal who are either at risk for a severe or complicated withdrawal syndrome (e.g., patients dependent on multiple drugs, patients with a past history of delirium tremens) or who cannot receive the necessary assessment, monitoring, or treatment in an alternative setting.
3. Patients with acute or chronic general medical conditions that make detoxification in a residential or ambulatory setting unsafe (e.g., patients with severe cardiac disease).
4. Patients with a documented history of not engaging in, or benefiting from, treatment in a less intensive setting (i.e., residential or outpatient).
5. Patients with marked psychiatric comorbidity who are an acute danger to themselves or others (e.g., patients who have depression with suicidal thoughts, acute psychosis).
6. Patients manifesting substance use or other behaviors that constitute an acute danger to themselves or others.
7. Patients who have not responded to less intensive treatment efforts and whose substance use disorder(s) poses an ongoing threat to their physical and mental health.

In general, the duration of hospital-based treatment should be dictated by the current need of the patient to receive treatment in a restrictive setting and by the patient's capacity to safely participate in, and benefit from, treatment in a less restrictive setting.

b) Residential treatment

(1) Generic residential facilities
Residential treatment is primarily indicated for patients whose lives and social interactions have come to focus exclusively on substance use and who currently lack sufficient motivation and/or drug-free social supports to remain abstinent in an ambulatory setting but who do not meet clinical criteria for hospitalization. For such patients, residential facilities provide a safe and drug-free environment in which residents learn individual and group living skills. As in the case of hospital-based pro-

grams, residential treatment programs should, at a minimum, also provide psychosocial, occupational, and family assessments; psychoeducation; an introduction to self-help groups; and referral for social or vocational rehabilitative services where necessary (154).

Many residential programs provide their own individual, group, and vocational counseling programs but rely on affiliated partial hospital or outpatient programs to supply the psychosocial and psychopharmacologic treatment components of their programs. Residential treatment settings should provide general medical and psychiatric care that is required to meet patient needs.

The duration of residential treatment should be dictated by the time necessary to achieve specific utilization criteria that would predict a successful transition to a less structured, less restrictive treatment setting (e.g., outpatient care); these may include demonstrated motivation to continue in outpatient treatment, the ability to remain abstinent even in situations where drugs are potentially available, the availability of a living situation and associated support system conducive to remaining drug free (e.g., family, drug-free peers), stabilization of any comorbid general medical or psychiatric disorder to the point where treatment can take place in an outpatient setting, and the availability of adequate follow-up care, including partial hospitalization and respite care if needed.

In some areas, residential treatment programs specifically designed for adolescents, pregnant or postpartum women, and women with young children are available, and such programs are preferred for these patient populations.

(2) Therapeutic communities

Patients with opioid, cocaine, or polysubstance use disorders may benefit from referral to a long-term residential therapeutic community. These programs are generally reserved for patients with a low likelihood of benefiting from outpatient treatment (e.g., those with multiple prior treatment failures or profound characterologic problems that make treatment compliance unlikely) (155). The therapeutic community provides a secure, drug-free environment in which behavioral modeling and peer pressure are used to 1) shape residents' ability to modulate emotional distress without resorting to substance use and 2) resocialize them to pursue a drug-free lifestyle (156).

Characteristically, therapeutic communities are organized along strict hierarchies, with newcomers assigned to the most menial social status and work tasks. Residents achieve higher status and take on increasing responsibility as they demonstrate that they can remain drug free and conform to community rules. Confrontation, individually and in groups, is used to break through denial about the role of substance use in one's life, identify maladaptive behaviors and coping styles that lead to interpersonal conflict and vocational failure, suggest alternative ways of handling disturbing affects, and encourage the development of attitudes and beliefs that are incompatible with continued substance use.

Data regarding the effectiveness of therapeutic communities are confounded by the fact that only 15%–25% of patients admitted voluntarily complete the program, with maximum attrition occurring in the first 3 months (157). Follow-up studies of patients who continue in the treatment program suggest that a minimum of 3 months of treatment is necessary to demonstrate benefit and that the optimal length of stay may be considerably longer (i.e., 6 to 12 months). Therapeutic community program graduates have lower rates of relapse and better outcomes at 1-year follow-up than do patients entering outpatient treatment, although the clinical circumstances may have biased the findings (158, 159).

Reasonable candidates for treatment in a therapeutic community include 1) patients who need a highly structured setting in which to initiate treatment and 2) patients whose level of denial is such that interpersonal and group confrontation is deemed an important part of the initial approach to treatment. In choosing a therapeutic community, a program's ability to treat comorbid psychopathology should be carefully considered.

c) Partial hospitalization

Partial hospital care can provide an intensive and structured treatment experience for patients with substance dependence who require more services than those generally available in traditional outpatient settings. Randomized controlled trials have demonstrated that some patients who would ordinarily be referred for residential or hospital level care do just as well in partial hospital care (160).

Partial hospital programs should also be considered for patients leaving hospital or residential settings who are at high risk for relapse. The latter include patients in the early stages of treatment with questionable motivation to remain drug free, those with a history of past failure in the immediate posthospital or postresidential period, patients living in or returning to environments characterized by high drug availability or low levels of social support for remaining drug free, and those with severe psychiatric comorbidity.

The treatment components of partial hospital programs usually include individual, group, and family therapy; vocational and educational counseling; medically supervised use of adjunctive medications (e.g., narcotic antagonists, methadone); random urine screening for drugs of abuse; and treatment for any comorbid psychiatric disorders that may be present. As in other treatment settings, partial hospital programs should provide opportunities for patients to learn and practice coping strategies to reduce drug craving and avoid relapse. Patient and family education about substance use disorders and the opportunity to confront patient or family denial are also important program components. Partial hospital programs for adolescents should be affiliated or work closely with school-based counseling programs.

The duration of outpatient treatment should be tailored to individual patient needs and may vary from a few months to several years. Patients in partial hospital care typically begin by attending 4–12 hours per day, 3–7 days per week. The availability of evening and weekend care is particularly desirable. The duration or frequency of partial hospital visits should be tapered as patients demonstrate that they can remain substance free and make progress toward rehabilitation. The availability of community-based supports (e.g., non-drug-using friends or family), a job, and a living situation conducive to remaining abstinent are also important considerations in deciding when to decrease or discontinue partial hospital care.

d) Outpatient settings

Outpatient treatment of substance use disorders is appropriate for those whose clinical condition or environmental circumstances do not require a more intensive level of care. As in other treatment settings, a comprehensive approach using, where indicated, a variety of psychotherapeutic and pharmacologic interventions, along with behavioral monitoring, is optimal. Treatment should encourage and be integrated with patient participation in self-help programs where appropriate (section III.E.6) (161).

As in the case of residential and partial hospital programs, high rates of attrition are a problem in outpatient settings, particularly in the early phase (i.e., first 6 months).

Since intermediate- and long-term outcomes are highly correlated with retention in treatment, specific efforts should be directed toward motivating patients to remain in treatment (162); such efforts may include the use of legal, family, or employer-generated pressure where available (see sections III.H.6, III.H.8, and III.I.1).

▶ H. CLINICAL FEATURES INFLUENCING TREATMENT

Because of the chronic and relapsing nature of these conditions, the psychiatrist will often need to manage patients in intoxication and withdrawal states. These issues are discussed in sections III.D.1, IV.E.1, IV.E.2, V.E.1, V.E.2, VI.E.1, and VI.E.2.

1. Psychiatric factors

a) Risk of suicide or homicide

The frequency of both suicide attempts and completed suicides is substantially higher among patients with substance use disorders than in the general population (163–168). The incidence of completed suicide is approximately 3–4 times that found in the general population (167), with a lifetime mortality of approximately 15% (166). The presence of major depressive disorder substantially increases the suicide risk of these patients (169).

Substance use disorders are also associated with greater than average risk for other forms of violence, including homicide (170, 171). Anxiety, irritability, increased aggressivity, impaired impulse control, and impaired reality testing may be due either to the direct effects of the substance(s) or to a withdrawal syndrome. Substances whose use may be associated with aggression include cocaine, hallucinogens, phencyclidine (PCP), and alcohol (72, 172, 173). Substances that lead to withdrawal syndromes associated with a risk of violence include alcohol, opioids, and hypnotic sedatives (72). Patients intoxicated on marijuana or hallucinogens may inadvertently commit violent acts on the basis of their faulty perception of reality coupled with high levels of anxiety and paranoia (174–176).

An additional implication of these findings is the need to consider the diagnosis of substance use disorder in all individuals who present with a history of suicide or other form of violence.

b) Comorbid psychiatric disorders

The presence of psychiatric comorbidity affects the onset, clinical course, treatment compliance, and prognosis for patients with substance use disorders (29, 137, 148, 177, 178). Penick et al. (179) studied a Department of Veterans Affairs (VA) hospital outpatient population of patients with alcohol dependence or abuse; of these, 56% reported psychiatric comorbidity. High rates of personality disorders have been reported in patients with substance use disorders (12, 44, 180, 181). Patients with comorbid borderline or antisocial personality disorder appear to have a poorer response to treatment (182) and a greater risk of suicide (183).

All patients with substance use disorders should be carefully assessed for the presence of psychiatric comorbidity (184). In a study by McLellan et al. (31), patients with no comorbid psychiatric illness did well in all types of treatment settings, whereas patients with more severe psychiatric symptoms did poorly. Rounsaville et al. (185) found that patients with comorbidities benefit from specific treatment for their comorbid mental disorders.

Conversely, patients with identified psychiatric disorders should be routinely assessed for the presence of comorbid substance use disorders. In so doing, it is important to establish the chronology of symptom development (i.e., whether the signs and symptoms predate or follow the onset of repetitive substance use), whether symptoms were present during extended drug-free periods (e.g., of 3 months or more), and the impact of each disorder on the presentation, clinical course, and outcome of the other(s).

The probability that the patient has a comorbid psychiatric disorder is increased if 1) there is a clear history of similar signs and symptoms preceding the onset of the substance use disorder or evident during previous extended drug-free periods or 2) at least one first-degree biological relative has a documented history of similar illness (2).

In many cases, it is necessary to observe patients during a substance-free period before concluding that there is a comorbid psychiatric disorder and/or instituting specific treatment for that disorder. The length of the observation period is generally determined by balancing the following considerations: the degree of diagnostic certainty, the severity of the patient's condition, and the anticipated benefits and risks of the proposed treatment. For patients with a comorbid disorder, initial treatment efforts should be directed toward any substance-induced disorder (i.e., intoxication or withdrawal) that may be present. Once patients are stable, treatment for substance abuse or dependence, as well as any other disorder present, should proceed concurrently in the context of an integrated treatment program. However, a patient who is psychotic, suicidal, or homicidal may require intensive psychiatric treatment to stabilize the condition before he or she can be integrated into ongoing rehabilitative treatment for the substance use disorder(s).

Finally, it is incorrect to assume that treatment of a comorbid non-substance-related psychiatric disorder will by itself assure that the substance use disorder will also resolve. Even when a substance use disorder arises in the context of another psychiatric disorder, over time it often takes on a life of its own and usually requires specific treatment (186).

c) Use of multiple substances

A number of studies have shown that many patients entering treatment for a substance use disorder are abusing more than one substance. For some patients, there is a "drug of choice" and other substances serve as substitutes when the primary substance is unavailable. For others, multiple drugs are routinely used simultaneously. Concurrent use of two or more drugs may be motivated by the patient's wish to modify the effects of the primary drug of choice and/or to prevent or relieve withdrawal symptoms. In addition, many patients use multiple substances largely on the basis of their availability. Frequent drug combinations include cocaine and alcohol, cocaine and heroin, and heroin and benzodiazepines.

The assessment of patients with substance use disorder should routinely include questions about polydrug use. Treatment is most successful when it is directed toward establishing and maintaining abstinence or reduced use of all abused substances (including, for many patients, the use of nicotine) (187). Treatment may be complicated by 1) simultaneous intoxication or withdrawal from two or more drugs, 2) varying time frames for experiencing withdrawal symptoms in patients using multiple drugs, 3) the need to detoxify the patient from more than one drug, and 4) potential interactions between an abused substance and medications used to treat a comorbid substance use disorder (e.g., inadvertent precipitation of opioid withdrawal in patients treated with naltrexone for alcohol dependence).

2. Comorbid general medical disorders

Concurrent general medical conditions frequently complicate the treatment of substance use disorders. Many patients with these disorders do not seek or receive adequate general medical care for a variety of reasons, including the chaotic and disorganized lifestyles often associated with substance abuse and lack of access to health care. Thus, the substance abuse treatment encounter may be the first opportunity to address the general medical care needs of these patients.

Because of their high prevalence, alcohol use disorders account for the majority of substance use problems encountered in general medical settings. Conversely, general medical problems related to alcohol dependence are frequently encountered in substance abuse treatment programs. Alcohol-related problems can affect almost all organ systems, most prominently the gastrointestinal and central nervous systems (188). Some of the more severe forms of alcohol-related injury to the CNS clearly have lasting effects on cognition, behavior, and the ability to comply with treatment. For example, the anterograde amnestic disorder found in patients with Korsakoff's syndrome dramatically limits the utility of treatment approaches that require the development of insight and/or the learning of new behaviors, such as maintaining abstinence. See also section V.E.3.

The following conditions contribute to an increased risk of death and disability in patients with substance use disorders: hepatitis, tuberculosis, motor vehicle accidents, falls, suicide, and homicide. Among injecting drug users, infectious diseases are the most common type of general medical comorbidity. From a public health standpoint, the most important of these are infection with HIV, tuberculosis, and sexually transmitted diseases. Approximately 30%–40% of inner-city intravenous drug users test positive for HIV (14, 189). The adoption of universal precautions against body contamination by infectious agents is a necessary part of protecting staff and patients against the spread of HIV (190). Sexually active patients should be specifically counseled in the use of safe sex practices. Needle exchange programs and effective treatment also reduce the spread of HIV infection (191).

The rise of treatment-resistant tuberculosis among patients with substance use disorders suggests the need to consider periodic tuberculosis screening for both patients and staff, along with efforts to reduce the spread of tuberculosis in treatment environments. Supervised on-site chemoprophylaxis or treatment for tuberculosis within substance abuse treatment programs is also strongly recommended (192, 193).

3. Pregnancy

Substance use during pregnancy has the following implications for both the mother and the developing fetus.

a) The health of the pregnant woman

Pregnant women with substance use disorders are at high risk for sexually transmitted diseases (e.g., HIV infection), hepatitis, anemia, tuberculosis, hypertension, and preeclampsia. In addition, the presence of a substance use disorder may affect the woman's ability to maintain a healthy lifestyle, including proper nutrition, and obtain needed health care (e.g., prenatal care).

b) The course of the pregnancy

Women with substance use disorders (depending on the substance) may be at greater than average risk for spontaneous abortions, preeclampsia, abruptio placentae, and early and prolonged labor, in addition to complications of other general medical conditions that may be due to the substance use (e.g., hypertension in cocaine users [194]).

c) Fetal development
Some abused substances, including opiates, cocaine, and alcohol, are known to pass through the placenta and directly affect the fetus (195–197). This may happen at any stage of development but is particularly likely during the third trimester, when maternal fetal blood flow and rates of placental transport are increased. Fetal concentrations of abused substances average 50%–100% of maternal blood levels and in some instances are higher (196). The circulation of active drug metabolites is another source of fetal exposure to potentially toxic substances.

The fetus may be at higher than average risk of birth defects, cardiovascular problems, impaired growth and development, prematurity, low birth weight, and stillbirth (198–203). After delivery, the neonate may suffer from withdrawal of the substance, which may be difficult to recognize, particularly if the mother's diagnosis is not known by the pediatrician.

d) Child development
Some substances (e.g., alcohol) are associated with long-term negative effects on physical and cognitive development (204).

e) Parenting behavior
In addition to ongoing treatment for the substance use disorder, mothers with substance use disorders are frequently in need of education and training in parenting skills, social services, nutritional counseling, assistance in obtaining health and welfare entitlements, and other interventions aimed at reducing the likelihood of child abuse or neglect.

Goals of treatment of pregnant substance-using women include eliminating all alcohol and drug use, treating any comorbid general medical or psychiatric disorders, guiding the patient safely through the pregnancy, facilitating appropriate parenting behavior, and motivating the patient to remain in treatment after delivery to minimize the risk of relapse.

The optimal therapeutic approach is nonpunitive and maintains patient confidentiality. Education and counseling to help women make an informed decision about continuing or terminating a pregnancy should be made available to those who want it. Sexually active women and men likely to return to a drug-abusing subculture should be advised about reliable contraceptive techniques.

4. Gender-related factors
Information on the natural history, clinical presentation, physiology, and treatment of substance use disorders in women is limited. Although women are estimated to comprise 34% of all persons with substance use disorders in the United States (205), psychosocial and financial barriers (e.g., lack of child care) prevent many women from seeking treatment. Other explanations for women's underuse of alcohol and drug treatment services may include women's perception of greater social stigma associated with their abuse of drugs and alcohol (206, 207). Once in treatment, women have been found to have a higher prevalence of primary comorbid depressive and anxiety disorders that require specific treatment, compared to men (207). Many women with substance use disorders have a history of physical and/or sexual abuse (both as children and as adults), which may also influence treatment planning, participation, and

outcome (208). Female patients also tend to have more family responsibilities and may need more help with family-related problems. There is evidence that increasing the focus of treatment on concerns specific to women, such as adding treatment components that specifically address women's issues and increasing female staff, improves treatment outcomes for women (209, 210).

5. Age

a) Children and adolescents

Children and adolescents are generally more likely to have abuse rather than dependence disorders and are less likely to appreciate the need for entering and remaining in treatment. Assessment and treatment must take into account the cognitive, social, and psychological developmental levels of the patient and the possible role of substance use disorders in impeding the successful attainment of developmental milestones, including a sense of autonomy, the ability to form interpersonal relationships, and general integration into society. The assessment should also place particular emphasis on evaluating areas of the adolescent's adaptive functioning, such as academic progress, school behavior and attendance, and social functioning with peers and family members. Adolescents' typical position as dependent members of family systems, their desire to attain an independent identity, their general ambivalence about authority, their need to develop social skills and appropriate peer relationships, and their need for education or vocational training require specific treatment attention. Treatment should also address the ability of parents to communicate and set appropriate behavioral limits.

Some adolescents with substance use disorders also have comorbid psychiatric disorders, including conduct disorder, attention deficit hyperactivity disorder (ADHD), anxiety disorders (including social phobia and posttraumatic stress disorder), affective disorders, learning disabilities, and eating disorders (6). In addition, children reared in family environments in which other family members abuse or are dependent on alcohol or other substances are also at higher risk of physical or sexual abuse and may exhibit psychological and behavioral sequelae (including substance abuse) as a result (211, 212).

The clinical manifestations of comorbid psychiatric disorders in adolescents often vary from those noted in similarly diagnosed adults. Thus, assessment for and treatment of these disorders require professionals and staff who are familiar with their manifestations in children and adolescents and the use of specific psychosocial (i.e., individual, group, family) therapies, age-appropriate psychosocial treatments (including individual, group, and family psychotherapies), and medication when needed. Lack of attention to coexisting psychiatric disorders may impede progress in treatment and result in further impairment in adaptive functioning. Many adolescents with substance use disorders have preexisting and concurrent impulsive, oppositional, and conduct-disordered behaviors. Treatment should address these problems and the conduct-disordered behavior as well as focusing on the substance abuse itself. Treatment and assessment of adolescents may be further compromised by questions about whether diagnostic criteria developed for adults are appropriate for adolescents (6).

Generally, the range of treatment modalities used with adults can be used with adolescents as well. These modalities include cognitive behavioral approaches, psychodynamic/interpersonal approaches (individual, group, and family), self-help groups (213), and medications. Treatment is often delivered in a group therapy format. Although research data establishing the efficacy of specific treatment modalities for adolescent substance use disorders are sparse, program outcomes for adolescents appear to be enhanced by the availability of treatment that is developmentally appropriate, peer oriented, and setting specific; includes educational, vocational, and recreational services; and emphasizes family involvement in both treatment planning and the treatment itself (213).

b) The elderly

Substance use disorders in elderly populations are an underrecognized and undertreated problem (214, 215). Abuse and dependence on prescribed medications, particularly benzodiazepines, hypnotic sedatives, and opioids, can contribute to excessive confusion and sedation in elderly patients, poor compliance with prescribed treatment regimens, and inadvertent overdose, particularly when these drugs are combined with alcohol (216). In addition, alcohol use disorders, as an extension of a longstanding disorder or of later onset, are a major problem among the elderly, particularly those living alone (217). Alcohol-related cognitive impairment, comorbid depressive disorder, dementia, poststroke syndromes, and other conditions common among the elderly may impair their ability to obtain or comply with treatment for substance abuse or for other general medical and psychiatric disorders (218).

6. Social milieu or living environment

The patient's overall social milieu has an important impact on both the development of and recovery from substance dependence. The social milieu shapes attitudes about the appropriate context for substance use (e.g., the difference between social drinking on family occasions and recreational drinking to achieve intoxication). Role models among one's family or peers influence the social and psychological context for substance use, the choice of drug, and the degree of control exerted over substance-using behaviors.

Once a pattern of dependence or abuse has developed, motivation and ability to comply with treatment are influenced by the degree of support within the patient's immediate peer group and social environment for remaining abstinent. Continued involvement with a substance-abusing peer group or enabling family members and residence in an environment in which there is a high level of drug availability predict a poor outcome. Thus, addressing these issues is an important component of any treatment plan. Patients with high levels of psychosocial and environmental stressors need correspondingly high levels of community-based support or, in some cases, temporary relief from these stressors through treatment in a residential setting until the patient is able to develop specific relapse-prevention strategies that can be applied in a community setting. Sexually active individuals should be educated about the prevalence and prevention of HIV infection and other sexually transmitted diseases.

7. Cultural factors

Current research suggests poorer prognoses for ethnic and racial minorities in conventional treatment programs, although this may be accounted for by social class differences (219–221). Although there is a paucity of research on the efficacy of culturally specific programming, treatment services that are culturally sensitive and address the special concerns of ethnic minority groups may improve acceptance of, compliance with, and, ultimately, the outcome of treatment. Training of staff and efforts to incorporate culture-specific beliefs about healing and recovery should be part of a comprehensive treatment program that serves different minority and ethnic groups (222).

8. Family characteristics

Substance use disorders exact an enormous toll on family members. High levels of interpersonal conflict, domestic violence, inadequate parenting, child abuse and neglect, separation and divorce, financial and legal difficulties, and drug-related general medical problems (e.g., AIDS, tuberculosis) all add to the family burden. In addition, children reared in family environments in which other family members abuse or are dependent on alcohol or other substances are also at increased risk of physical or sexual abuse (223).

Families with one or more members who have substance use disorders often display a multigenerational pattern of transmission of both substance abuse and other frequently associated psychiatric disorders (e.g., antisocial personality disorder, pathological gambling) (224). The impact of maternal substance use on both fetal development and childhood cognitive and emotional adjustment, coupled with the influence of genetically inherited risk factors (e.g., high genetic loading for alcoholism in males) and negative role models, all play a role in the development of substance use disorders across generational lines. In addition, pathological "enabling" behavior, the existence of psychiatric and general medical problems in parents and siblings, and high levels of social and/or transcultural stress also play a role in the development and perpetuation of substance use disorders.

The substantial burden imposed on families containing one or more members with substance use disorders, and the impact of family interactions in perpetuating or ameliorating these problems, affect the initiation of, perpetuation of, and recovery from the substance use disorders; the patient's motivation and ability to comply with treatment; and the patient's clinical course and outcome. These relationships, coupled with the high prevalence of substance use disorders, comorbid general medical and psychiatric disorders, psychosocial disability, and family burden, make family interventions extremely important in the treatment of these patients (120, 225).

I. LEGAL AND CONFIDENTIALITY ISSUES

1. Effect of legal pressure on treatment participation and outcome

Many patients with substance use disorders seek treatment in response to pressure from family members, employers, legal authorities, or other sources. While motivation for treatment is often regarded as a good prognostic sign, outcome studies of patients in therapeutic communities have shown that individuals who enter treatment under legal compulsion (e.g., a judge has made treatment a condition of probation or a mandatory alternative to incarceration) stay longer and do as well as comparable patients who enter treatment voluntarily (226, 227). Similarly, higher rates of compliance in treatment with the narcotic antagonist naltrexone have been reported for court-mandated patients and for physicians or other professionals who are at risk of losing their professional licenses should they fail to comply. Similar findings have been reported for professionals being treated for substance use problems by means of contingency contracting approaches in which the contingency for noncompliance with treatment is being reported to a professional board of registration (228).

2. Confidentiality and reporting of treatment information

To protect patients' privacy and encourage their entry into treatment, federal law and regulations mandate strict confidentiality for information about patients being treated for substance use disorders (i.e., 42 USC Section 290dd-3, ee-3; 42 C.F.R. Part 2). Disclosure of information from treatment records is prohibited unless the patient has given written consent, the disclosure is in response to a medical emergency, or there is a court order authorizing disclosure. Other instances in which patient confidentiality may be abrogated include disclosure in response to a crime committed at the treatment program or against program staff, and compliance with state laws addressing the psychiatrist's "duty to warn" third parties of a potential harm (by the patient); the initial reporting of child abuse or neglect may also abrogate confidentiality requirements. With regard to the last situation, psychiatrists should be familiar with reporting laws concerning the possible abuse and neglect of children and other dependents who may be at risk in the families of both male and female substance users.

Generally, federal law does not make specific reference to the confidentiality of information pertaining to the HIV/AIDS status of a patient in alcohol or drug treatment, but there are many different state laws restricting disclosure of such status.

3. Legal requirements for pharmacotherapy with opioids

Federal and state regulations govern the use of methadone and LAAM, the only two opioids approved by the Food and Drug Administration (FDA) for treating patients with opioid-related disorders. Federal law (P.L. 93-281) requires special registration of each physician using methadone or LAAM for maintenance or detoxification. The Drug Enforcement Administration will not register physicians without prior approval by the FDA and the state drug authority. FDA approval is contingent on practitioner willingness to comply with federal narcotic treatment regulations (229).

IV. ALCOHOL-RELATED DISORDERS: TREATMENT PRINCIPLES AND ALTERNATIVES

▶ A. OVERVIEW

The focus of this section is on the treatment of patients with alcohol dependence or abuse. Treatment of these disorders may be complicated by episodes of intoxication and withdrawal, the treatment of which is discussed in sections IV.E.1 and IV.E.2.

The Epidemiologic Catchment Area (ECA) studies indicate that 13.8% of American adults have had either alcohol dependence or abuse sometime in their lives (230).

Alcohol use disorders have a variable course that is frequently characterized by periods of remission and relapse. The first episode of alcohol intoxication is likely to occur in the midteens, and the age at onset of alcohol dependence peaks in the 20s to 30s. The first evidence of withdrawal is not likely to appear until after many other aspects of dependence have developed. Although some individuals with alcohol dependence achieve long-term sobriety without active treatment, many need treatment to stop the cycles of remission and relapse.

The relationship between alcohol dependence and abuse is also variable. In one study (231), only 30% of male subjects with alcohol abuse at baseline met criteria for alcohol dependence 4 years later. The other 70% met criteria for either alcohol abuse or alcohol abuse in remission.

The long-term goals of treatment for patients with alcohol use disorders are identical to those for patients with any type of substance use disorder; these are discussed in section III.A and include abstinence (or reduction in use and effects), relapse prevention, and rehabilitation. There is some controversy in the literature, however, regarding the possible benefits of striving for a reduction in alcohol intake, as opposed to total abstinence, for those who are unlikely to achieve the latter. In a comprehensive review of the issue (232), Rosenberg concluded that a lower severity of pretreatment alcohol dependence and the belief that controlled drinking is possible were associated with the achievement of controlled drinking after treatment. Interventions aimed at achieving moderate drinking have also been used with patients in the early stages of alcohol abuse (see, e.g., references 233 and 234). Controlled drinking may be an acceptable outcome of treatment, for a select group of patients, when accompanied by substantial improvements in morbidity and psychosocial functioning. For most patients with alcohol dependence or abuse, however, abstinence is the optimal goal.

Numerous studies have documented the efficacy of alcoholism treatment; approximately 70% of all patients manifest a reduction in the number of days of drinking and improved health status within 6 months (151, 235).

The majority of patients who are treated for alcohol use disorders have at least one relapse episode during the first year following treatment. However, there is now considerable evidence that most individuals with alcohol use disorders drink less frequently and consume less alcohol after receiving alcoholism treatment, compared to their pretreatment drinking behavior (138, 236–238). For example, patients typically report drinking heavily on 75% of the days during a 3-month period before treatment. During posttreatment follow-ups patients are often abstinent on 70%–90% of the days, and they engage in heavy drinking on 5%–10% of the days (119).

Treatment also has been shown to bring about improvements in family functioning, marital satisfaction, and psychiatric impairments (137, 239, 240). Although improvements following alcoholism treatment are at least in part attributable to nontreatment factors, such as patient motivation (93), it is generally accepted that treatment does make a difference, at least in the short run.

Psychiatric management (section III.C) is the key component of a successful treatment plan.

B. CHOICE OF TREATMENT SETTING

The range of available settings and the general criteria for choosing among them are described in section III.G. In general, the choice of a setting depends on the clinical characteristics of the patient, the preferences of the patient, the treatment needs, and the available alternatives. As in the treatment of all patients with substance-related disorders, the least restrictive setting that is likely to facilitate safe and effective treatment is preferred.

Most treatments for patients with alcohol dependence or abuse can be successfully conducted outside of the hospital (e.g., in outpatient, day hospital, or partial hospital settings) (138, 160). However, patients unlikely to benefit from less intensive and less restrictive alternatives may need to be hospitalized at times during their treatment. The general criteria for hospitalization are summarized in section III.G.2.a.

A large-scale epidemiologic study (241) showed that the mortality rates for male veterans with alcohol use disorders 3 years after discharge varied with the initial treatment setting. Veterans who completed inpatient rehabilitation had the lowest mortality rate, while the other groups, in order of increasing mortality rate, were 1) those who had at least 6 days of inpatient treatment (but did not complete the program),

2) those who were admitted for brief detoxification lasting less than 5 days, and 3) those who received no specific treatment for alcohol use disorders. Patients in this study were not randomly assigned to treatment conditions, so it is possible that self-selection influenced the results. However, the study provides preliminary evidence that more intensive treatment may lower the mortality associated with chronic alcohol use disorders.

With one exception (242), studies that have randomly assigned patients to different levels of treatment have generally not found an advantage for inpatient care over less restrictive settings (243–246). However, these studies have limited generalizability due to such problems as exclusion of patients who would ordinarily be considered to require inpatient treatment (140).

There is considerable evidence that longer treatment stays and treatment completion are associated with better outcomes (238, 247). This probably reflects the fact that better-motivated patients are more likely to stay in treatment and have better outcomes. However, patients randomly assigned to longer treatments typically do not have better outcomes than those randomly assigned to shorter treatments (138, 160).

Patients with alcohol withdrawal must be detoxified in a setting that provides for frequent clinical assessment and the provision of any necessary treatments. Some outpatient settings can accommodate these requirements and may be appropriate for patients deemed to be at low risk of a complicated withdrawal syndrome. However, those who have a prior history of delirium tremens, whose documented history of very heavy alcohol use and high tolerance places them at risk for a complicated withdrawal syndrome, who are concurrently abusing other drugs, who have a severe comorbid general medical or psychiatric disorder, or who repeatedly fail to cooperate with or benefit from outpatient detoxification are more likely to require a residential or hospital setting that can safely provide the necessary care. Patients in severe withdrawal (i.e., delirium tremens) require treatment in a hospital setting.

▶ C. PHARMACOLOGIC TREATMENTS FOR DEPENDENCE AND ABUSE

1. Naltrexone

Two independent double-blind, placebo-controlled studies (248, 249) have documented the efficacy of the narcotic antagonist naltrexone for the treatment of alcohol dependence. The study by O'Malley et al. (249) showed that naltrexone in doses of 50 mg/day was superior to placebo in terms of reduced drinking and the resolution of alcohol-related problems. Patients who received both naltrexone and coping skills training were the most successful at avoiding full relapse. These studies suggest the potential utility of this agent, particularly when combined with other therapeutic approaches, in preventing relapse. The mechanism by which naltrexone exerts its therapeutic effects is not adequately known but may involve blocking the primary subjective effects of a first drink. Animal studies suggest that part of alcohol's reinforcing effects relate to release of endogenous opioids, which are then blocked by naltrexone (250–252).

2. Disulfiram (Antabuse)

Pretreatment with disulfiram establishes conditions in which the subsequent use of alcohol results in a toxic and highly aversive reaction. Disulfiram inhibits the activity of aldehyde dehydrogenase, the enzyme that metabolizes acetaldehyde, a major metabolite of alcohol. The usual therapeutic dose is 250 mg/day, although some patients achieve optimal benefit at either a higher or a lower dose (range, 125–500 mg/day). In the presence of disulfiram, alcohol consumption results in the accumulation of toxic levels of acetaldehyde, which in turn produce a host of unpleasant signs and symptoms, including a sensation of heat in the face and neck, headache, flushing, nausea, vomiting, hypotension, and anxiety. Chest pain, seizures, liver dysfunction, respiratory depression, cardiac arrhythmias, myocardial infarction, and death have also been reported. Understanding and explaining disulfiram's toxic, or lethal, effects to patients is a prerequisite for its use (253–255), so it should never be used without the patient's knowledge and consent.

Controlled trials have not demonstrated any advantage of disulfiram over placebo in achieving total abstinence, in delaying relapse, or in improving employment status or social stability (256, 257). However, some clinicians believe that this medication, when combined with other therapeutic interventions, has some benefit for selected individuals who remain employed and socially stable (80, 257–260). Treatment effectiveness is enhanced when compliance is encouraged through frequent behavioral monitoring (e.g., breath tests), group support for remaining abstinent (e.g., in group therapy or AA) (261), contingency contracting, or, where feasible, supervised administration of disulfiram. Patients who are intelligent, motivated, and not impulsive and whose drinking is often triggered by unanticipated internal or external cues that increase alcohol craving are the best candidates for disulfiram treatment. Poor candidates include patients who are impulsive, have poor judgment, or are suffering from a comorbid psychiatric illness (e.g., schizophrenia, major depression) whose severity makes them unreliable or self-destructive (79, 262).

Patients taking disulfiram must be advised to avoid all forms of ethanol (including, for example, that found in cough syrup). In addition, disulfiram interferes with the metabolism of many medications, including tricyclic antidepressants, so that care must be taken to avoid toxicity (263). Disulfiram can cause a variety of adverse effects; hepatotoxicity and neuropathies are rare but potentially severe. The medication should be avoided for patients with moderate to severe hepatic dysfunction, peripheral neuropathies, pregnancy, renal failure, or cardiac disease (257).

3. Lithium

The use of lithium to treat patients with alcohol use disorders not comorbid with bipolar disorder was supported by some early anecdotal reports and by a small double-blind, placebo-controlled study (264). However, a large VA collaborative study (265) showed no benefits of lithium over placebo for patients with or without depressive symptoms.

4. Antidepressants

Although past evidence regarding the efficacy of tricyclic antidepressants for depression associated with alcohol use disorders is equivocal (72), two studies showed improved mood and reduced alcohol consumption in open and double-blind placebo-controlled trials with desipramine (266, 267). Preliminary data indicate that selective serotonin reuptake inhibitors may significantly reduce problem drinking in nondepressed social drinkers (268) and in those with alcohol abuse or dependence (269, 270).

▶ D. PSYCHOSOCIAL TREATMENTS

The psychotherapies described in section III.E have all been used in the treatment of alcohol use disorders (271). Several authors have reviewed the efficacy of various psychotherapies for alcohol use disorders (106, 135, 138). This section reviews the outcomes literature on cognitive behavioral therapies, behavioral therapies, psychodynamic/interpersonal therapies, brief interventions, marital and family therapy, group therapy, aftercare, and self-help groups.

1. Cognitive behavioral therapies

There is abundant evidence that cognitive behavioral treatments aimed at improving self-control and social skills consistently lead to reduced drinking (106, 272, 273). Self-control strategies include goal setting, self-monitoring, functional analysis of drinking antecedents, and learning alternative coping skills. Social skills training focuses on learning skills for forming and maintaining interpersonal relationships, assertiveness, and drink refusal. Holder et al. (106) found that self-control training produced better outcomes than control treatments in 12 of 17 studies and that social skills training was more effective than the control condition in 10 of 10 studies. Two studies have demonstrated that patients with sociopathic features do better in cognitive behavioral treatment than in interactional treatment (91, 274). Longabaugh et al. found that patients with antisocial personality disorder who received cognitive behavioral treatment had better drinking outcomes at 18-month follow-up than those who received relationship-enhancing treatment.

Holder et al. (106) found that cognitive behavioral stress management interventions were effective in six of 10 studies reviewed. Monti et al. (103) found that inpatients who received cue exposure treatment paired with coping skills training had better outcomes than those who received only standard inpatient treatment. Cognitive therapy interventions that are focused on identifying and modifying maladaptive thoughts but do not include a behavioral component have not been as effective as cognitive behavioral treatments (106).

Behavioral self-control training consists of cognitive and behavioral strategies, including self-monitoring, goal setting, rewards for goal attainment, functional analysis of drinking situations, and the learning of alternative coping skills (275, 276). Although some studies of behavioral self-control training have included controlled drinking, as well as abstinence, as a goal for treatment, behavioral self-control techniques should be used with the explicit long-term goal of abstinence.

In several studies, increases in coping responses or "self-efficacy" (277) at the end of treatment predicted better drinking outcomes during follow-up (56, 134, 278). Individuals who report more frequent use of cognitive or behavioral strategies aimed at problem solving or mastery ("approach coping") typically have better drinking outcomes than those who rely on staying away from high-risk situations ("avoidant coping") (238, 279).

2. Behavioral therapies

Individual behavior therapy and behavioral marital therapy have been found to be effective treatments for patients with alcohol use disorders (95, 106, 138). The most well-studied behavioral approach to the treatment of patients with alcohol use disorders is the community reinforcement approach, which uses behavioral principles and usually includes conjoint therapy, training in job finding, counseling focused on alcohol-free social and recreational activities, monitoring of disulfiram, and an alcohol-free social club (280). Using random assignment to community reinforcement or standard hospital treatments, Azrin (98) found that patients in the community reinforcement group drank less, spent fewer days away from home, worked more days, and were institutionalized less over a 24-month follow-up. A second controlled study comparing

a) the community reinforcement approach, b) disulfiram plus a behavioral compliance program, and c) regular outpatient treatment showed that patients treated with community reinforcement did substantially better on all outcome measures than those in the other treatment conditions (98).

3. Psychodynamic/interpersonal therapies

Holder et al. (106) concluded that there was little empirical evidence from controlled studies that either insight-oriented psychotherapy or counseling is an effective treatment for alcoholism. Individual psychotherapy produced better outcomes than a control condition in two of eight studies reviewed, and psychodynamically oriented group psychotherapy produced better outcomes in two of 11 studies. Generic counseling approaches (characterized as primarily directive and supportive) produced better outcomes than controls in one of eight studies reviewed. Existing studies of this modality may be limited by their short-term approaches.

4. Brief interventions

Brief interventions generally delivered over one to three sessions include an abbreviated assessment of drinking severity and related problems and the provision of motivational feedback and advice. In eight of nine controlled treatment trials reviewed by Holder et al. (106), brief interventions were found to be effective, although Chick et al. (281) reported negative results. Reviews by Babor (282) and Bien et al. (283) concluded that brief interventions a) are typically more effective (in terms of alcohol use, general health, or social functioning) than no intervention; b) often have efficacy comparable to that of traditional more intense, longer-term programs; and c) increase the effectiveness of later treatment. Even interventions that are very brief (i.e., a few hours) may have some positive effect (284). Brief interventions are typically used (and are most successful) for less severely affected patients who have not received previous treatment for an alcohol disorder. Further research is needed to determine which patients are optimally served by receiving a brief intervention.

5. Marital and family therapy

The state of the patient's relationship with family members or significant others can be a critical factor in the posttreatment environment for patients who are married or living with family members (106, 285). O'Farrell et al. (240) contrasted behavioral marital therapy and interactional marital therapy with a no-treatment control group. Both treatment groups showed greater improvement in marital adjustment, and the behavioral marital therapy groups showed a greater degree of sobriety over a short-term follow-up period. Two other studies (244, 286) showed that patients who received behavioral marital therapy began to have better drinking outcomes than those who did not at 1-year follow-up. Studies also have indicated that spousal involvement in treatment leads to improved marital and alcohol use outcomes early in the posttreatment period (287), that patients in conjoint therapy are less likely to drop out of treatment (288), and that therapy aimed at improving the marriage as a whole seems to work better than couples therapy focused strictly on alcohol-related problems (e.g., therapy with minimal or only alcohol-focused spouse involvement) (239).

6. Group therapy

Outcome studies have typically supported the efficacy of behavioral and cognitive behavioral group treatments, including group marital therapy. While research data regarding the efficacy of dynamically oriented group psychotherapy are limited and there are no empirical data to support the effectiveness of group psychotherapy for all alcohol-dependent patients, there are considerable data suggesting effectiveness for some patients (106, 138). The results of patient-matching studies in which patients were randomly assigned to cognitive behaviorally oriented treatment groups or interactional therapy groups suggest that patients with less sociopathy and those with neurological impairment fare better in interactional therapy; those with higher levels of sociopathy and psychopathology fare better in cognitive behavioral groups (90, 91). Litt et al. (289), in a randomized controlled study, also found a patient-treatment matching effect.

7. Aftercare

Aftercare may be defined as the period following an intense treatment intervention (e.g., hospital or residential care) and may include partial hospital care, outpatient care, or involvement in self-help approaches, alone or in combination. Patients frequently report that aftercare is helpful in maintaining abstinence following primary treatment (290). Walker et al. (291) found that involvement in aftercare was a stronger predictor of outcome than length of hospitalization, neuropsychological functioning, or pretreatment drinking and social stability measures. McLatchie and Lomp (292) randomly assigned patients to mandatory, voluntary, or no aftercare for a 12-week period and found that aftercare completers had the lowest relapse rate, with no difference between the mandatory and voluntary groups. Gilbert (293) randomly assigned patients to one of three aftercare conditions that varied in the degree of therapists' efforts to maintain patients in aftercare over 30 appointments. Patients in the maximal effort group were the most likely to complete aftercare, and aftercare completers in all groups had better outcomes than noncompleters. Studies that did not include random assignment suggest that greater participation in aftercare is generally associated with lower severity (e.g., fewer drinks on drinking days) but not with diminished frequency of drinking (294). A controlled study by O'Farrell et al. (295) showed that a version of behavioral marital therapy that included relapse prevention techniques (56) and was delivered as an aftercare intervention led to better drinking outcomes. Cooney et al. (90) and Kadden et al. (91) compared 3-week inpatient aftercare programs consisting of a) cognitive behavioral therapy and coping skills training and b) insight-oriented, interactional group therapy, and they reported similar outcomes in the two groups.

8. Self-help groups

See also section III.E.6. "AA is a fellowship of men and women who share their experience, strength and hope with each other that they may solve their common problem and help others to recover from alcoholism. The only requirement for membership is a desire to stop drinking" (296). AA provides tools for its participants to maintain sobriety, including the Twelve Steps, group identification, and mutual help. It is a spiritual (not religious) program requiring belief in something beyond oneself (297). Al-Anon (spouses), Alateen (teenagers and children of alcoholics), and Adult Children of Alcoholics help family members and friends of alcoholics focus on the need to avoid enabling behaviors and care for oneself whether a loved one is drinking or not. Other mutual-help programs include Women for Sobriety, Rational Recovery, Double Trouble (for patients with alcohol dependence comorbid with other psychiatric disorders), and Mentally Ill Chemical/Substance Abusers.

While the effectiveness of AA has not been evaluated in randomized studies because of a host of ethical and practical problems associated with attempting to assign patients not to go to AA, several studies have suggested that AA can be an important support for promoting an alcohol-free lifestyle in patients who are willing to attend (138, 237, 238). A number of studies have examined the relationship between degree of participation in AA and drinking outcomes (29, 298, 299). There is some evidence that patients with greater severity of drinking problems, an affective rather than cognitive focus, a concern about purpose and meaning in life, better interpersonal skills, and a high need for affiliation are good candidates for AA (300, 301).

Patients are more likely to benefit from AA groups composed of individuals of similar age and cultural and occupational status. All patients should be encouraged to attend a minimum number of AA meetings (i.e., five to 10) to ascertain the appropriateness and utility of AA in helping them remain alcohol free.

E. CLINICAL FEATURES INFLUENCING TREATMENT

The treatment implications of various clinical features are summarized in section III.H. In addition to these considerations, specific patterns of comorbidities and sequelae need to be considered for patients with alcohol use disorders, including the management of intoxication and withdrawal states.

1. Management of intoxication

In general, the acutely intoxicated patient requires reassurance and maintenance in a safe and monitored environment, with efforts to decrease external stimulation and provide orientation and reality testing. Adequate hydration and nutrition are also essential. Clinical assessment should follow the guidelines previously described, with particular emphasis on the patient's general medical and mental status, substance use history, and any associated social problems. Patients presenting with signs of intoxication should also be assessed for the possibility of recent use of other substances that could complicate the clinical course. Patients with a history of prolonged or heavy drinking or a past history of withdrawal symptoms are at particular risk for medically complicated withdrawal syndromes, which may require hospitalization.

2. Management of withdrawal

The syndrome of mild to moderate alcohol withdrawal generally occurs within the first several hours after cessation or reduction of heavy, prolonged ingestion of alcohol; it includes such signs and symptoms as gastrointestinal distress, anxiety, irritability, elevated blood pressure, tachycardia, and autonomic hyperactivity (2). The syndrome of severe alcohol withdrawal especially occurs within the first several days after cessation or reduction of heavy, prolonged ingestion of alcohol; the syndrome includes such signs and symptoms as clouding of consciousness, difficulty in sustaining attention, disorientation, grand mal seizures, respiratory alkalosis, and fever (2).

Fewer than 5% of individuals with alcohol withdrawal develop severe symptoms, and fewer than 3% develop grand mal seizures (2, 204). In the past, the mortality rate for patients experiencing alcohol withdrawal delirium was as high as 20%, but currently it is closer to 1% because of improved diagnosis and medical treatment of such patients (204).

Thiamin should be given routinely to all patients receiving treatment for moderate to severe alcohol use disorders to treat or prevent common neurologic sequelae of chronic alcohol use (302–304) (see section IV.E.3).

Although pharmacotherapeutic agents are often used to ameliorate the signs and symptoms of alcohol withdrawal and to prevent a major abstinence syndrome, the relative importance of supportive and pharmacologic treatment for these patients is not well established (305, 306). Generalized support, reassurance, and frequent monitoring is sufficient treatment for approximately two-thirds of the patients with mild to moderate withdrawal symptoms (307). In one case-controlled study (305), 74% of hospitalized alcohol-dependent patients without serious comorbid general medical problems responded to supportive treatment for alcohol withdrawal. Patients in more severe withdrawal and those who developed hallucinations required pharmacologic treatment.

There are numerous reviews of the pharmacologic treatment of moderate to severe withdrawal (308–310). The pharmacotherapy is directed toward reducing CNS irritability and restoring physiologic homeostasis. This often requires use of fluids, benzodiazepines, and, in selected cases, other medications (72). Most patients should be monitored by using breath and/or urine testing to ensure that they have not resumed alcohol use.

Many authors (e.g., Ciraulo and Shader [204]) recommend use of benzodiazepines to control abstinence symptoms, which takes advantage of the cross-tolerance between alcohol and this class of drugs. A single oral loading dose of chlordiazepoxide, 200–400 mg, or diazepam, 20–40 mg or as needed, may be used. Orally administered chlordiazepoxide (50 mg every 2–4 hours), diazepam (10 mg every 2–4 hours), oxazepam (60 mg every 2 hours), and lorazepam (1 mg every 2 hours) are commonly used (306, 311). The total dose necessary to suppress CNS irritability and autonomic hyperactivity in the first 24 hours (i.e., the stabilization dose) is then given in four divided doses the following day, after which the dose can usually be tapered over 3–5 days, with monitoring for reemergence of symptoms (312). For most patients, the equivalent of 600 mg/day of chlordiazepoxide is the maximum dose, and many patients require less; a few, however, may require substantially more (313). Patients in severe withdrawal and those with a history of withdrawal-related symptoms may require up to 10 days before benzodiazepines are completely withdrawn. Benzodiazepine administration should be discontinued once detoxification is completed.

For patients with severe hepatic disease, the elderly, and patients with delirium, dementia, or other cognitive disorders, short-acting benzodiazepines such as oxazepam or lorazepam are preferred by some clinicians. These agents have the advantage of being metabolized and excreted principally through the kidneys and may be more suitable for patients with poor hepatic function; they also do not have active intermediary metabolites that may accumulate. Unlike the longer-acting preparations, they can also be administered intramuscularly or intravenously. Because of their brief half-lives, the short-acting benzodiazepines need to be given more frequently (314–317).

Beta blockers (e.g., propranolol, 10 mg p.o. every 6 hours) have been used to reduce signs of autonomic nervous system hyperactivity (e.g., tremor, tachycardia, elevated blood pressure, diaphoresis) and, at higher doses, arrhythmias (318–320). Atenolol has been used for a similar purpose, usually combined with benzodiazepines (321), thus allowing use of lower doses of benzodiazepines and thereby reducing the sedation and cognitive impairment often associated with benzodiazepine use.

Clonidine, an α-adrenergic agonist (0.5 mg p.o., b.i.d., or t.i.d.) has been shown to reduce tremor, heart rate, and blood pressure (322, 323).

However, the use of either β blockers or clonidine alone for the treatment of alcohol withdrawal is not recommended, because of their lack of efficacy in preventing seizures.

Barbiturates (e.g., pentobarbital, phenobarbital, and secobarbital) may be useful in reducing withdrawal symptoms in patients refractory to benzodiazepines (324).

For patients manifesting delirium, delusions, or hallucinations, neuroleptics may be used, particularly haloperidol (0.5–2.0 mg i.m. every 2 hours as needed), in most cases less than 10 mg per 24 hours, although some patients may require considerably more. In such cases, neuroleptics are an adjunct to the benzodiazepines, since the former are not effective for treating the underlying withdrawal state.

The use of anticonvulsants to prevent seizures in patients with alcohol withdrawal syndromes is controversial (325, 326). For patients with a prior history of withdrawal-related seizures, benzodiazepines are generally effective for this purpose. For patients with a history of non-withdrawal-related seizures, their anticonvulsant medication should be continued or restarted. Patients currently taking phenytoin should have their dose increased to a minimum of 300 mg/day (327). Oral as well as intravenous loading doses of 10 mg/kg, not to exceed an administration rate of 50 mg/min, should be given to patients who have discontinued phenytoin during a drinking spree (328). The prophylactic use of phenytoin to prevent seizures during alcohol withdrawal is not indicated (329, 330). Carbamazepine (600–800 mg/day for the first 48 hours, then tapered by 200 mg/day) has also been demonstrated to be effective in preventing withdrawal-related seizures, although its tendency to lower white blood cell counts in some patients may pose an added risk of infection (331–335). Intramuscular magnesium sulfate has also been used for preventing withdrawal seizures (336).

3. Comorbid psychiatric and general medical disorders

Many patients with alcohol dependence present with signs and symptoms suggestive of dysthymia, major depression, or anxiety disorder and, if a comorbid diagnosis is made, may require pharmacotherapy. Given the propensity of these patients to misuse prescribed medications, one should give preference to drugs that have low abuse potential. Patients with a high level of depression, impulsivity, poor judgment, or the potential for making a suicide attempt should receive drugs with low potential for lethality in overdose situations (e.g., selective serotonin reuptake inhibitors) (337, 338). Poor compliance with medication regimens coupled with high overdose risk also suggests the dispensing of limited amounts of medication and random blood or urine toxicology screening to verify the use of both prescribed and nonprescribed medications by such patients.

In the majority of patients, however, signs and symptoms of depression and anxiety are related to alcohol intoxication or withdrawal and remit in the first few weeks of abstinence (339). Consequently, most psychiatrists feel that observation over a 3–4-week drug-free period should occur before diagnosis of a comorbid affective or anxiety disorder and prescription of a disorder-specific drug. Others suggest that in selected cases earlier initiation of treatment is warranted. For example, depressed patients with a prior history of major depression unrelated to periods of alcohol use and/or a strong family history of affective disorder are more likely to have a comorbid primary depression that should be treated as soon as detoxification is completed (45, 47, 267, 340). Tricyclic antidepressants should be used with caution for alcohol-dependent patients with comorbid depression. The risk of poor compliance, tricyclic-alcohol interactions, and the risk of overdose should be considered with such patients. In addition, tricyclic plasma levels may be lower than expected because of the alcohol-induced increase in liver microsomal oxidases (341, 342). Serotonin reuptake inhibitors may have less risk of morbidity and mortality in overdose situations and, therefore, are preferred (343). Lithium, valproate, or carbamazepine may be used with caution for patients with comorbid bipolar disorder.

The use of benzodiazepines for alcohol-dependent patients with comorbid anxiety or panic disorder is controversial. Benzodiazepines (and other CNS depressants) have high abuse potential in these patients. For patients with generalized or performance anxiety, β blockers (e.g., propranolol) and buspirone are preferable to benzodiazepines since they have no cross-tolerance with ethanol or other CNS depressants and minimal abuse potential. Buspirone has also been reported to reduce alcohol consumption in patients with high levels of comorbid anxiety (344, 345). In otherwise refractory cases of panic disorder, clonazepam or other long-acting benzodiazepines can be cautiously administered if the principles just outlined are observed.

Monoamine oxidase inhibitors have been used to treat patients with atypical depressions, but the risk of poor compliance with dietary and drug restrictions (including those for alcohol) and subsequent adverse reactions (e.g., hypertension) is high (346).

Chronic high-dose alcohol use can affect several different organ systems, including the gastrointestinal tract, the cardiovascular system, and the central and peripheral nervous systems. Alcohol-induced gastrointestinal problems include gastritis, ulcers of the stomach or duodenum, and, in approximately 15% of heavy users, cirrhosis of the liver and pancreatitis (347–349). Alcohol-dependent patients also experience higher than average rates of cancer of the esophagus, stomach, and other parts of the gastrointestinal tract (350).

Common comorbid cardiovascular conditions include low-grade hypertension and increased levels of triglycerides and low-density lipoprotein cholesterol, which increase the risk of heart disease. Cardiomyopathy occurs primarily among very heavy drinkers.

Endocrine consequences of chronic alcohol use for men include decreases in serum testosterone, loss of facial hair, breast enlargement, decreased libido, and impotence (351); endocrine consequences for women include amenorrhea, luteal phase dysfunction, anovulation, early menopause, and hyperprolactinemia (350). Blunting of the thyroid-stimulating hormone response to thyrotropin-releasing hormone, hypoglycemia, ketosis, and hyperuricemia have also been reported (352).

Alcohol-induced peripheral myopathy with muscle weakness, atrophy, tenderness, and pain is accompanied by elevations in creatine phosphokinase levels and the presence of myoglobin in the urine. Severe cases can involve rapidly progressive muscle wasting.

Many patients seeking treatment of alcohol dependence manifest cognitive abnormalities. In chronically heavy drinkers, dementia with characteristic cognitive deficits can occur. More commonly, however, one sees a subtle cognitive dysfunction that still may hamper patients' ability to comprehend or comply with a treatment plan (353). For such patients active involvement of family members or other responsible parties should take place at the beginning of and throughout treatment. Initial placement in a more structured (e.g., residential) treatment setting may also be indicated to assess the impact of cognitive problems on the patient's ability to comply with short- and long-term treatment. In patients who remain abstinent, reversal of alcohol-induced cognitive disturbance is often observed over time (354).

Nervous system sequelae of chronic alcohol use are related to vitamin deficiencies, particularly deficiencies in thiamin and other B vitamins; they include peripheral neuropathies, cognitive deficits, severe memory impairment, and degenerative changes in the cerebellum (355).

Wernicke's encephalopathy is characterized by ophthalmoplegia, ataxia, and confusion (204, 356). Ocular abnormalities include nystagmus, eye muscle palsies, and pupillary abnormalities. The mortality rate for acute untreated Wernicke's encephalopathy is 15%–20% (357, 358). Recovery is incomplete in 40% of the cases.

The vast majority (approximately 80%) of patients with Wernicke's disease also develop Korsakoff's syndrome (alcohol amnestic disorder), characterized by anterograde and retrograde amnesia, disorientation, poor recall, and impairment of recent memory, coupled with confabulation. Lesions in the mammillary bodies and thalamic nuclei may be the result of vitamin deficiencies or the direct toxic effects of alcohol. Recovery is variable. In more than one-half of the patients, elements of Korsakoff's syndrome are permanent.

Ataxia in alcohol-dependent patients is most often due to cerebellar dysfunction. Central demyelinization of the paraventricular gray matter of the diencephalon of the brain stem and glial proliferation are the major pathologic findings.

These neurological complications should be treated vigorously with B complex vitamins (e.g., thiamin, 50–100 mg/day i.m. or i.v.). Some patients may require treatment over a prolonged period, and improvement may occur up to 1 year after treatment is begun (359).

Alcoholic hallucinosis during or after cessation of prolonged alcohol use may respond to antipsychotic medication. Unlike the visual hallucinations that may occur during alcohol withdrawal, these are primarily auditory and occur in conjunction with a clear sensorium (360).

Alcohol dementia, characterized by impairment in short- and long-term memory, abstract thinking, judgment, and other higher cortical functions and by personality change, is seen in chronically heavy drinkers. Usually the memory deficits are less severe than in Korsakoff's syndrome or Alzheimer's disease (361). Neuropathological abnormalities in the frontal lobes, in the area surrounding the third ventricle, or diffusely through the cortex have been reported.

4. Pregnancy

Also refer to section III.H.3. Alcohol-related disorders may have adverse effects on the health of the pregnant woman, the course of the pregnancy, fetal development, early child development, and parenting behavior. The most well-established effect of in utero substance exposure is fetal alcohol syndrome. Reported effects of fetal alcohol syndrome in children exposed to high doses of alcohol in utero include low birth weight, poor coordination, hypotonia, neonatal irritability, retarded growth and development, craniofacial abnormalities (including microcephaly), cardiovascular defects, mild to moderate retardation, childhood hyperactivity, and impaired school performance (204, 362, 363).

Goals of treatment of pregnant women with alcohol use disorders include eliminating the use of alcohol, treating any comorbid psychiatric or general medical disorders, guiding the patient safely through the pregnancy, facilitating appropriate parenting behavior, and motivating the patient to remain in treatment after delivery to minimize the risk of relapse.

5. Age: the elderly

Two studies suggest that the treatment needs of older adults with alcohol use disorders may be different from those of younger patients. Liskow et al. (364) found that patients aged 58–77 required higher benzodiazepine doses during a 5-day detoxification and may need longer detoxification than patients under 33. Kofoed et al. (365) reported that VA patients aged 54 or older who received specialized services for the elderly in a VA program remained in treatment longer and were four times as likely to complete the program than elderly patients who received conventional services, although posttreatment relapse rates were comparable in the two groups.

V. COCAINE-RELATED DISORDERS: TREATMENT PRINCIPLES AND ALTERNATIVES

▶ A. OVERVIEW

The focus of this section is the treatment of patients with cocaine dependence or abuse. Treatment of these disorders may be complicated by episodes of intoxication and withdrawal, the treatment of which is discussed in sections V.E.1 and V.E.2, respectively.

Cocaine-related disorders are most commonly found in persons aged 18–30 and are almost equally distributed between males and females. In a 1991 study, 12% of the U.S. adult population reported using cocaine one or more times in their lifetimes. A community study conducted in the early 1980s indicated that about 0.2% of the adult population have had cocaine abuse at some time in their lives (2, p. 228). It is likely that the prevalence of abuse is now higher since the overall use of cocaine has increased since that time.

Cocaine smoking is associated with a more rapid progression from use to dependence or abuse than is intranasal use (366). Dependence is commonly associated with a progressive tolerance to the desirable effects of cocaine, leading to increasing doses. With continuing use there is a diminution of pleasurable effects due to tolerance and an increase in dysphoric effects. Few data are available on the long-term course of cocaine-related disorders (2).

The goals of treatment for patients with cocaine use disorders are identical to those for patients with other forms of substance use disorders; these are discussed in section III.A and include abstinence, relapse prevention, and rehabilitation.

Psychiatric management (section III.C) is an important component of a successful treatment plan.

▶ B. CHOICE OF TREATMENT SETTING

The range of available settings for substance-related disorders and the general criteria for choosing among them are described in section III.G. In general, the choice of a setting depends on the clinical characteristics of the patient, the preferences of the patient, the treatment needs, and the available alternatives. As in the treatment of all patients with substance-related disorders, the least restrictive setting that is likely to facilitate safe and effective treatment is preferred.

Several studies have indicated that most patients can be effectively treated for cocaine abuse in intensive outpatient programs (143, 367). Although in one nonrandomized study (368) a group of 149 inpatients fared better at 1-year follow-up than did patients treated in an outpatient setting, a randomized study (367) revealed no difference in outcome after 3 and 6 months between patients assigned to inpatient and partial hospital care.

C. PHARMACOLOGIC TREATMENTS FOR DEPENDENCE AND ABUSE

Although a number of studies have shown promising results with a variety of pharmacotherapeutic agents, no medication has been found to have clear-cut efficacy in the treatment of cocaine dependence (369–371). Consequently, pharmacologic treatment is not ordinarily indicated as an initial treatment for many patients with cocaine dependence. However, patients with more severe forms of cocaine dependence or individuals who do not respond to psychosocial treatment may be candidates for a trial of pharmacotherapy. Thus far, desipramine and amantadine appear to have had the most positive (although mixed) results, although other medications may prove to be more successful.

1. Drugs to reduce symptoms of cocaine abstinence or craving

Over 20 different medications have been studied in the search for an effective pharmacologic treatment for cocaine dependence. Most of these studies have been hampered by methodological problems, including lack of adequate controls and consistent outcome measures (e.g., urine tests rather than self-reports), failure to standardize the type and "dose" of the accompanying psychosocial interventions, lack of clarity about the importance of craving in the maintenance of cocaine dependence, the role of craving in the natural course of untreated cocaine abstinence syndrome, and lack of agreement as to the exact meaning of the term "craving" (372, 373).

Gawin et al. (374) found desipramine to be more effective than either lithium or placebo in reducing cocaine use by outpatients without coexisting mood disorders. More recent reports (375–377) have failed to confirm these positive findings, possibly because of differences in patient population and route of cocaine administration.

Initial studies of carbamazepine in the treatment of cocaine dependence yielded some favorable results (378), but subsequent double-blind, placebo-controlled studies failed to establish the efficacy of carbamazepine for these patients (379, 380).

Other agents used in the treatment of cocaine dependence have included pergolide (381), L-dopa/carbidopa (382), fluoxetine (383, 384), flupentixol (385), bupropion (386), amantadine (387), and maprotiline (388). All have shown some promise, but in relatively small, uncontrolled trials. An uncontrolled study of phenelzine (389) also yielded moderate success, but this treatment carries a high risk of hypertensive crisis in individuals who relapse to cocaine use, and it is therefore not recommended.

The mixed opioid agonist/antagonist buprenorphine has shown some promise in open trials in the treatment of patients dually dependent on cocaine and opioids (390, 391), although a large-scale double-blind clinical trial comparing patients maintained on buprenorphine with those receiving methadone showed no decrease in cocaine use among the former group (392). Work by Schottenfeld et al. (393) suggests that higher doses of buprenorphine (12–16 mg/day) may be effective. Larger-scale clinical trials funded by NIDA are currently examining the effectiveness of buprenorphine in this population.

2. Drugs to block the subjective effects of cocaine

Attempts to find a drug that blocks or attenuates the subjective (e.g., euphorigenic) effects of cocaine have included trials of imipramine (394), desipramine (375), bromocriptine (395, 396), trazodone, neuroleptics (397), and mazindol (398). However, there is no convincing evidence that, at doses that can be tolerated by patients, any of these medications is effective in this regard.

► D. PSYCHOSOCIAL TREATMENTS

Although a wide variety of treatment approaches have shown promise in preliminary studies, no therapeutic modality has been shown to be consistently superior to others in the treatment of cocaine-dependent patients. To date, several approaches show promise, but they need further study in larger-scale studies involving a broader range of patients. Both clinical and research experience suggest that intensive (i.e., more than once a week) outpatient psychosocial treatment focusing on abstinence is the preferred approach (399). Kang et al. (400) found that once-a-week psychosocial treatment (e.g., family therapy, psychotherapy, or group therapy) was generally ineffective, while Weddington et al. (373) reported a high degree of success among patients assigned to twice-a-week psychotherapy with or without medication.

1. Cognitive behavioral therapies

Studies demonstrating the efficacy of cognitive behavioral treatment strategies for cocaine-dependent patients are few in number. However, cognitive behavioral relapse prevention has been shown to be somewhat more effective than interpersonal therapy for patients with severe cocaine problems, but for patients whose cocaine problems were less severe the two treatments were equally effective (89). Recent 1-year follow-up showed a positive emerging effect of the psychotherapy (83).

2. Behavioral therapies

Studies of contingency contracting have shown positive outcomes during the period when the contract is in effect, promoting treatment compliance and abstinence (228). However, in a controlled trial, Higgins et al. (97) demonstrated the efficacy of contingency contracting (i.e., vouchers) in the outpatient treatment of cocaine dependence, with positive effects maintained during the 3 months after the contingency voucher program ended. Higgins et al. (95–97) studied the efficacy of a community reinforcement approach and found better outcomes from community reinforcement counseling plus incentives than from 12-step counseling. Cue exposure therapy has also been used in the treatment of cocaine use disorders, with equivocal results (104).

3. Psychodynamic psychotherapy

Well-controlled trials of psychodynamically oriented treatments for cocaine abuse or dependence are limited. A case series of patients successfully treated with individual psychodynamically oriented psychotherapy was reported by Schiffer (401), and there is a preliminary report revealing a high rate of retention with modified psychodynamically oriented group psychotherapy (116). Spitz has also described the use of group therapy for this population (402).

4. Comparisons of specific psychotherapeutic interventions

Carroll et al. (89) compared relapse prevention treatment using behavioral and cognitive approaches with interpersonal psychotherapy in a 12-week study of 42 outpatients with cocaine use disorders and found no significant differences in overall treatment outcome between the two groups, although patients with more severe cocaine abuse problems fared slightly better with relapse prevention. In a second study of outpatient treatment, Carroll et al. (403) randomly assigned 139 subjects to one of four conditions: a) relapse prevention plus desipramine, b) clinical management plus desipramine, c) relapse prevention plus placebo, or d) clinical management plus placebo. By the end of the 12- week trial, all groups showed significant improvement, but there were no main effects for psychotherapy or medication. Patients with greater baseline severity of cocaine use had better outcomes with relapse prevention than with clinical management, whereas those with less severity did better with desipramine than placebo. Depressed subjects had better cocaine use outcomes than nondepressed subjects, and they did better in relapse prevention than in clinical management (403). At 6- and 12-month follow-up, Carroll et al. (83) found evidence that subjects who received relapse prevention had better cocaine use outcomes than those who received clinical management, but there were no differences in cocaine use between the desipramine and placebo subjects.

Higgins et al. (96) compared behavioral treatment, consisting of contingency management procedures and community reinforcement, with traditional 12-step drug counseling in a random-assignment study. Although the sample size was relatively small, the results indicated better treatment retention at 24 weeks (58% versus 11%) and greater abstinence at 16 weeks (42% versus 5%) in patients treated with behavioral therapy. In the Higgins et al. trial (97), all patients received community reinforcement counseling, but only one group received contingent vouchers. The group with vouchers was more likely to complete 24 weeks of treatment (75% versus 40%), had a longer average duration of continuous cocaine abstinence (mean=11.7 weeks, SE=2.0, versus mean=6.0 weeks, SE=1.5), and showed significant improvement on the drug and psychiatric scales of the Addiction Severity Index.

A large-scale, multisite study is currently underway to compare the efficacy of outpatient supportive-expressive psychodynamic therapy (110), cognitive therapy (85), and addiction counseling. The various psychosocial approaches for patients with cocaine and opioid use disorders have recently been reviewed (404).

5. Self-help groups

See also section III.E.6. Twelve-step approaches, such as Narcotics Anonymous and Cocaine Anonymous, are commonly used in the management of cocaine dependence (405, 406). In more traditional settings, peer-led counseling groups have reportedly been useful in reducing recidivism (407). In a study of day hospital rehabilitation for patients with cocaine use disorders (247), greater participation in self-help programs at 3 months posttreatment predicted less cocaine use at 6 months posttreatment, even after pretreatment patient characteristics and degree of success in the day hospital program were controlled. These findings suggest that participation in self-help programs may improve outcome, independent of other treatment-related factors.

▶ E. CLINICAL FEATURES INFLUENCING TREATMENT

The treatment implications of various clinical features are summarized in section III.H. In addition to these considerations, specific patterns of comorbidities and sequelae need to be considered for patients with cocaine use disorders, including the management of intoxication and withdrawal states.

1. Management of intoxication

The treatment of acute cocaine intoxication has been the subject of relatively little systematic investigation. In general, since there is no specific cocaine antidote, treatment is typically symptomatic and supportive.

Cocaine intoxication can induce paranoid delusions. Although neuroleptic drugs have been reported to be effective, most individuals recover spontaneously within hours (372, 408) and thus require no treatment. Patients who become extremely agitated and/or potentially dangerous may require sedation (e.g., with a benzodiazepine). Acute cocaine use can also produce hypertension, tachycardia, and seizures. Animal data and some clinical experience suggest that all adrenergic blockers and dopaminergic antagonists should be avoided in treating acute cocaine intoxication. Labetalol has been cited in favorable case reports, but no clinical studies have been reported. Benzodiazepines are frequently used for acute cocaine intoxication, and favorable results have also been reported with ambient cooling (409). There is no evidence that anticonvulsants prevent cocaine-induced seizures, and they are not recommended for this purpose.

2. Management of withdrawal

Cessation of cocaine use does not always cause specific withdrawal symptoms, although anhedonia and drug craving are common (372). However, many people experience a characteristic withdrawal syndrome within a few hours to several days after the acute cessation of, or reduction in, heavy and prolonged cocaine use.

The clinical features and duration of the cocaine abstinence syndrome are still somewhat controversial and ill defined. An early uncontrolled outpatient study (372) characterized withdrawal as progressing through three phases: an acute "crash" phase, a period of more gradual withdrawal, and an extinction phase lasting 1 to 10 weeks. Acute withdrawal (crashing) is seen after periods of frequent high-dose use. Intense and unpleasant feelings of depression and fatigue, at times accompanied by suicidal ideation, have been described during this phase. More-recent inpatient studies (373, 410), however, have suggested that cessation of regular cocaine use is associated with relatively mild symptoms of depression, anxiety, anhedonia, sleep disturbance (i.e., insomnia or hypersomnia), increased appetite, and psychomotor retardation, which decrease steadily over several weeks.

Dopamine agonists, such as amantadine (200–400 mg/day), were initially thought to be effective in reducing symptoms of cocaine withdrawal, craving, and subsequent use (379, 411, 412), but two more-recent studies (373, 377) failed to confirm this finding. Similarly, initial studies of bromocriptine yielded promising results in the treatment of cocaine withdrawal (395, 413). Subsequently, Tennant and Sagherian (412) found a higher rate of cocaine-negative urine samples but a higher dropout rate among patients given bromocriptine than among patients given amantadine. Teller and Devenyi (414) found no reduction of cocaine craving in an inpatient study of bromocriptine, and Moscovitz et al. (415) found no significant difference between bromocriptine and placebo in reducing cocaine use in outpatients. There may be a subgroup of patients who will respond to some form of pharmacotherapy with reduced craving and, subsequently, reduced use (see section III.D). However, to date there are inadequate research data to help the psychiatrist identify such patients.

3. Comorbid psychiatric and general medical disorders

Several reports have addressed treatment of patients with comorbid psychiatric disorders who also have cocaine-related disorders (e.g., references 49, 55, 416–421). Specific treatments that have been reported effective in certain populations of patients with cocaine abuse include lithium for patients with comorbid bipolar disorder, desipramine for patients with comorbid depression, and bromocriptine for patients with comorbid ADHD (370, 416, 417, 422). In addition, Ziedonis and Kosten's double-blind trial (423) suggests that desipramine or amantadine treatment for depressed cocaine-abusing methadone maintenance patients may reduce cocaine use. Given the evidence to date, however, these treatments alone cannot be expected to reduce cocaine use in these patients and must therefore be accompanied by appropriate psychosocial treatment for cocaine use disorders (55, 416).

A range of general medical conditions are associated with the route of administration of cocaine. Intranasal use may cause sinusitis, irritation and bleeding of the nasal mucosa, a perforated nasal septum, or, when a Valsalva-like maneuver is performed to better absorb the drug, a pneumothorax. Smoking cocaine is associated with respiratory problems, such as coughing, bronchitis, and pneumonitis, resulting from irritation and inflammation of the tissues lining the respiratory tract. Puncture marks and "tracks," most commonly in the forearms, occur in persons who inject cocaine. HIV infection is associated with cocaine dependence as a result of frequent injections and increased promiscuous sexual behavior, while other sexually transmitted diseases, hepatitis, tuberculosis, and other lung infections are also seen (2).

General medical conditions independent of the route of administration of cocaine include a) weight loss and malnutrition due to appetite suppression, b) myocardial infarction, and c) stroke. Seizures, palpitations, and arrhythmias have also been observed. Among persons who sell cocaine, in particular, traumatic injuries due to violent behavior are common (2).

4. Pregnancy

Also refer to section III.H.3. Cocaine-related disorders may have adverse effects on the health of the pregnant woman, the course of the pregnancy, fetal development, early child development, and parenting behavior. Possible effects of cocaine use on the course of the pregnancy include irregularities in placental blood flow, abruptio placentae, and premature labor and delivery (2). Possible effects on fetal development include very low birth weight, congenital anomalies, malformations of the urogenital system, mild neurodysfunction, transient electroencephalogram abnormalities, cerebral infarction and seizures, vascular disruption syndrome, and smaller head circumference (2, 424–427). Cerebrovascular problems, including small brain hemorrhages, may be due to decreased placental blood flow and diminished fetal oxygen concentrations in cocaine-exposed fetuses (425).

Possible effects on early child development that have been reported in cocaine-exposed newborns include hypertonicity, spasticity and convulsions, hyperreflexia, irritability, and attention problems. However, the roles of exposure to cocaine or other substances, poor maternal nutrition, prematurity, low birth weight, and neonatal withdrawal in the development of these signs and symptoms remain unclear (428, 429). Signs of CNS irritability usually disappear within the first year of life, as do any differences in head circumference or retardation in brain growth. Studies in cocaine-exposed children reveal deficits in attention span at 7 months, and in utero exposure to amphetamines has been found to be associated with slightly lower IQs (albeit still in the normal range) in 4-year-olds (430). While no clear correlation between in utero drug exposure and subsequent intellectual or neurological development has been established, associated conditions, such as low birth weight, the complications of untreated (or undertreated) withdrawal, and congenital abnormalities, may have adverse effects on cognitive and psychosocial development.

For pregnant patients withdrawing from cocaine, consideration of the use of pharmacotherapies should take into account the risks and benefits to the mother and fetus. The possibility of concurrent heroin use should be considered.

VI. OPIOID-RELATED DISORDERS: TREATMENT PRINCIPLES AND ALTERNATIVES

▶ ## A. OVERVIEW

The focus of this section is on the treatment of patients with opioid dependence or abuse. Consistent with the DSM-IV criteria listed in section II.A, the ECA study indicated that 0.7% of the adult population have met DSM-III-R criteria for opioid dependence or abuse at some time in their lives and that the male-to-female ratio of those affected is 3:1 or 4:1 (431).

Treatment of opioid use disorders may be complicated by episodes of intoxication and withdrawal, the treatment of which is discussed in sections VI.E.1 and VI.E.2. Chronic opioid use typically leads to impairment in social, vocational, academic, and parental functioning. Comorbid general medical, psychiatric, and legal problems are also common. General medical conditions may be related to 1) the use of unsterile needles for intravenous drug self-administration (e.g., HIV infection, abscesses, "needle tracks"); 2) poor self-care and adverse living conditions (e.g., tuberculosis, malnutrition); and 3) the drug-using lifestyle (e.g., head trauma), as well as comorbid psychiatric disorders (see section VI.E.3). Finally, many opioid-dependent patients also abuse alcohol, cocaine, anxiolytics, sedatives, and/or other psychoactive substances and may become dependent on these as well.

Opioid dependence is associated with a high death rate—approximately 10 per 1,000 per year among untreated persons. Death most often results from overdose, accidents, injuries, or other general medical complications. Accidents and injuries due to violence associated with buying or selling drugs are also common and in some areas account for more opioid-related deaths than overdose or HIV infection.

The long-term course of opioid use is quite heterogeneous. Although many untreated individuals with an untreated opioid use disorder are able to maintain a pattern of abuse without ever meeting the DSM-IV diagnostic criteria for dependence, many do become dependent; among such patients, relapse following a long period of abstinence (e.g., after incarceration) is common. On the other hand, only about 10% of service personnel who became dependent on opioids in Vietnam continued use after their return home (although a substantial minority did become dependent on alcohol or amphetamines) (431). The latter finding suggests the importance of environmental and peer-related factors, along with drug availability, in the development and maintenance of this disorder.

The goals of treatment for patients with opioid use disorders are similar to those for patients with other substance use disorders (section III.A). Although some opioid-dependent patients are able to achieve abstinence from all opioid drugs, many require and benefit from opiate agonist maintenance (e.g., with methadone or LAAM).

Psychiatric management (section III.C) is an important component of a successful treatment plan. Denial and ambivalence about giving up opioid use often interfere with treatment compliance and should be addressed directly in both individual and group settings. Motivation for treatment is generally enhanced by the involvement of supportive family members, non-drug-using peers and appropriate role models. Periodic monitoring of patients for the presence of opioids and other drugs in breath, blood, or urine is a necessary component of any treatment program. Maintenance of a therapeutic alliance is often difficult with opioid-dependent patients, particularly those with comorbid antisocial personality disorder. Many such patients require an initial period of treatment in a structured drug-free setting in which there is a high level of staff experience and expertise in confronting denial and setting limits. The use of coercive pressure to encourage the patient to remain in treatment (e.g., through the legal system) can also be a useful external support for patients with poor impulse control and high levels of ambivalence about abstaining from nonprescribed substances.

▶ B. CHOICE OF TREATMENT SETTING

The range of available settings and the general criteria for choosing among them are described in section III.G. In general, the choice of a treatment setting depends on the clinical characteristics and preferences of the patient, the perceived treatment needs, and the available alternatives. As in the treatment of all patients, the least restrictive setting that is likely to facilitate safe and effective treatment is preferred.

Therapeutic communities have been shown to be effective in the treatment of patients with opioid dependence. Simpson and Sells (157) reported that in a large-scale study with a 12-year follow-up, individuals with opioid dependence treated in therapeutic communities had the most favorable outcomes, even after age and demographic variables were controlled for. However, these data are tempered by the fact that only 15%–25% of those admitted voluntarily completed the program (see section III.G.2.b).

Long-term treatment with methadone or LAAM is generally provided through specialized outpatient programs that are licensed to dispense these substances. Licensing requirements concerning these programs are discussed in section III.I.3.

▶ C. PHARMACOLOGIC TREATMENTS FOR DEPENDENCE AND ABUSE

1. Agonist substitution therapy

For many patients with chronic relapsing opioid dependence the treatment of choice is maintenance on long-acting opioids. Of these, methadone is the most thoroughly studied and widely used treatment for opioid dependence. LAAM is a longer-acting preparation that can be administered less frequently than methadone (discussed later in this section). Buprenorphine (section VI.E.2.d) is a partial opioid agonist that has shown promising results in the longer-term treatment of opioid dependence, but additional research is needed (392). The current formulation of buprenorphine for the treatment of opioid dependence is sublingual; an oral form remains to be developed. Experiments are being conducted on a combination of buprenorphine and low doses of naloxone to determine whether it reduces the chances for diversion and abuse.

The primary goals of methadone (or LAAM) maintenance are a) to achieve a stable maintenance dose that reduces opioid craving and illicit opioid use and b) to facilitate engagement of the patient in a comprehensive program designed to prevent dependence or abuse of other substances and promote rehabilitation.

Since maintenance on methadone leads to the development of physiologic dependence and perhaps other CNS adaptations, federal guidelines limit the use of this modality to patients with a prolonged (e.g., more than 1 year) history of opioid dependence including (with some carefully defined exceptions) demonstrated physiologic manifestations. For patients who meet these legal criteria, the choice of methadone maintenance treatment is a matter of patient preference, assessment of the patient's past response to treatment, the probability of achieving and maintaining abstinence with other treatment modalities, and the psychiatrist's assessment of the short- and long-term effects of continued use of illicit opioids on the patient's life adjustment and overall health status.

Methadone maintenance treatment has generally been shown to be effective in decreasing the psychosocial and general medical morbidity associated with opioid dependence, with overall improvements in health status, decreased mortality, decreased criminal activity, and improved social functioning. Several studies also support the usefulness of methadone maintenance in reducing the spread of HIV infection among patients who administer drugs by injection (191, 432).

No single dose of methadone is optimal for all patients. Some may benefit from maintenance on low doses (10–20 mg/day), while others require more than 100 mg/day to achieve maximum benefit. Although 40–60 mg/day of methadone is usually sufficient to block opioid withdrawal symptoms, higher doses (averaging 70–80 mg/day) are usually needed during maintenance treatment to block craving for opiates and associated drug use. In general, higher doses (i.e., >60 mg/day) are associated with better retention and outcome (146, 147). If higher doses are used, monitoring of plasma methadone concentrations may be helpful, with the aim of maintaining minimum levels of 150–200 ng/ml (433). Retention rates for patients in methadone maintenance programs exceed 60% at 6 months, with up to 90% reduction in illicit opioid use in the patients who remain in treatment (146, 434).

Key issues in methadone maintenance treatment include determining a dose sufficient to suppress opioid withdrawal and craving, deciding on the appropriate duration of treatment, and including this modality within a comprehensive rehabilitation program. Programs that stress rehabilitation and long-term methadone treatment have been associated with the availability of more general medical and psychiatric services (146–148) and higher overall program quality (146). A General Accounting Office study supported these findings and demonstrated that the majority of programs may fail to provide optimal treatment (435). In some studies, use of higher doses of methadone has been associated with better overall outcome (147); in others, high-dose methadone has been associated only with less heroin use (146). Behavioral monitoring, random urine testing to assess recent illicit drug use, and linking the results of urine tests to counseling and other contingencies also improve outcomes (148, 150).

LAAM is a long-acting preparation that also reduces craving for opioids. LAAM is usually prescribed in doses of 20–140 mg (average, 60 mg) (204). Some patients prefer LAAM to daily methadone since dosing can be as infrequent as three times per week (436), thus allowing for fewer clinic visits and expanded integration into work or other rehabilitative activities. While treatment with LAAM has been shown to be comparable to methadone treatment with respect to reduction of opioid use (436–438), retention rates are reportedly higher for patients treated with methadone at doses of 80–100 mg/day (204). In general, longer duration of LAAM treatment (i.e., >6 months) is associated with better outcome.

The criteria for withdrawing patients from long-term maintenance on methadone or LAAM include demonstrated progress toward a drug-free lifestyle, stability in personal and occupational adjustment, absence of other substance use disorders, and successful treatment and remission of any comorbid psychiatric disorder(s).

Precipitous discharge from maintenance programs and concurrent withdrawal of methadone are associated with a high rate of relapse to illicit opioid use (439, 440). Voluntary termination of methadone maintenance also carries a high risk of relapse, even for patients who have responded well to treatment. Patients who choose to voluntarily discontinue maintenance treatment should receive supportive treatment during detoxification and aftercare services to aid in maintaining abstinence (27). Patients who relapse repeatedly despite such support should be given the option of voluntary lifetime maintenance on methadone.

2. Opioid antagonist treatment

Maintenance on the opiate antagonist naltrexone is an alternative to methadone maintenance. The goal of treatment is to block the effects of the usual street doses of heroin or other opioids, thereby discouraging opioid use and facilitating extinction of classically conditioned drug craving (57, 77). Because of its long duration of action (24 to 72 hours, depending on the dose), naltrexone can be administered three times per week (100 mg p.o. on Monday and Wednesday, 150 mg on Friday). Because it has no abuse potential, naltrexone can be an important adjunct in the treatment of patients with opioid use disorders (441).

Adverse effects of naltrexone may include dysphoria, anxiety, and gastrointestinal distress. Like other opioid antagonists, naltrexone can precipitate severe withdrawal symptoms when administered to patients who are physiologically dependent on opioids. In general, naltrexone should be administered only to patients who have been withdrawn from opioids under medical supervision and have remained opioid free for at least 5 days after the use of heroin or other short-acting opioids, or 7 days after the last dose of methadone or other longer-acting opioids. Before naltrexone treatment is begun, a test dose of naloxone, 0.8 mg i.m., should be used to assess the degree of opioid dependence. The interval between completion of opioid detoxification and initiation of naltrexone treatment is a period of high risk for relapse. For this reason rapid opioid withdrawal, with use of clonidine and naltrexone (see section VI.E.2.c), has been used to shorten the interval between detoxification and initiation of naltrexone maintenance (74, 442). Repeated naloxone doses have also been used with clonidine to shorten opioid detoxification.

Although naltrexone is extremely effective when taken as prescribed, its utility is often limited by lack of patient compliance and/or low treatment retention. Compliance is improved when drug administration is directly observed and supervised by a designated health care professional, responsible family member, or work supervisor (75). Treatment retention is facilitated by family involvement in treatment planning and by the use of behavioral contingencies (i.e., reinforcement or punishment) (443, 444). Higher rates of success with naltrexone have also been reported for court-mandated treatment and for physicians or other professionals who are at risk of losing their professional licenses if they do not comply with treatment (445).

▶ D. PSYCHOSOCIAL TREATMENTS

Psychosocial interventions are a key component of a treatment plan that includes a strategy to facilitate abstinence from opioids (e.g., with the aid of an opioid antagonist) or that includes the use of an opiate agonist (e.g., methadone).

1. Cognitive behavioral therapies

Woody et al. (107, 109, 446, 447) randomly assigned methadone maintenance patients to one of three groups: a) drug counseling alone, b) drug counseling plus supportive-expressive psychotherapy, or c) drug counseling with cognitive behavioral therapy. Outcomes were determined at 7 and 12 months. In patients with moderate to high degrees of depression or other psychiatric symptoms, supportive-expressive or cognitive behavioral therapies were much more effective than drug counseling alone; for patients with low levels of psychiatric symptoms, all three treatment conditions were equally effective. These findings were essentially replicated in three community-based methadone maintenance clinics (448).

2. Behavioral therapies

A variety of behavioral techniques have been used in treating opioid-dependent patients. Cue exposure treatment has been demonstrated to be effective in reducing classically conditioned responses to drug-related cues in a small group of patients with opioid use disorders (104). The use of urine toxicology testing to monitor for illicit drug use and provision of rewards for abstinence or aversive consequences for illicit drug use have been shown to be effective in promoting treatment compliance and abstinence in both methadone maintenance and naltrexone programs during the period the contingencies are in effect (30, 75, 443, 449, 450). In one study (449), methadone take-home privileges contingent on two consecutive weeks of drug-free urine tests yielded a higher percentage of patients who were abstinent at 4 weeks than did control conditions.

McLellan et al. (148) evaluated whether the addition of contingency-based counseling, general medical care, and psychosocial services improved the efficacy of methadone maintenance treatment in a study of newly admitted opioid patients randomly assigned to three levels of care. Patients who received counseling and contingencies based on urine test results, in addition to methadone, had better drug use outcomes than those who received methadone only. Patients who, in addition, received on-site general medical and psychiatric care, employment services, and family therapy had the best outcomes of all three conditions. Methadone alone was effective treatment for only a small percentage of patients.

3. Psychodynamic psychotherapies

The utility of adding a psychodynamic therapy to a program of methadone maintenance has been investigated. Woody et al. (107, 448) found that supportive-expressive therapy was more effective than drug counseling alone for patients with high levels of other psychiatric symptoms (see section VI.D.1). Rounsaville et al. (113) attempted to compare the efficacy of a 6-month course of weekly individual interpersonal therapy with a low-contact comparison condition for individuals in a full-service methadone maintenance program (that included weekly group psychotherapy). Patients with opioid dependence who met the inclusion criteria (including the presence of an additional nonpsychotic psychiatric diagnosis) were randomly assigned to the two groups. However, only 5% of the eligible patients agreed to participate (compared to 60% in the Woody et al. study), and only about one-half completed the trial. The highly selective nature of the participants (i.e., 95% of eligible patients refused), the high attrition rate, and the lack of significant outcome differences between the two groups led to the conclusions that it is very difficult to engage opioid-dependent patients in individual interpersonal therapy and that the potential benefit of such treatment is unclear for those who participate.

4. Group and family therapy

Psychodynamically oriented group therapy, modified for substance-dependent patients, appears to be effective in promoting abstinence when combined with behavioral monitoring and individual supportive psychotherapy (116). McAuliffe (451) reported that group relapse prevention based on a conditioning model of addiction, when combined with self-help groups, was more effective than no treatment in reducing opioid use, unemployment, and criminal activities in recently detoxified patients.

Family therapy has been demonstrated to enhance treatment compliance and facilitate implementation and monitoring of contingency contracting with opioid-dependent patients (see section III.E.5).

5. Self-help groups

See also section III.E.6. Self-help groups, such as Narcotics Anonymous, are beneficial for some individuals in providing peer support for continued participation in treatment, avoiding drug-using peers and high-risk environments, confronting denial, and intervening early in patterns of thinking and behavior that often lead to relapse.

E. CLINICAL FEATURES INFLUENCING TREATMENT

The treatment implications of various clinical features are summarized in section III.H. In addition to these considerations, specific patterns of comorbidities and sequelae need to be considered for patients with opioid use disorders, including the management of intoxication and withdrawal states.

1. Management of intoxication

The care of patients with opioid use disorders is frequently complicated by episodes of relapse. Consequently, recognition and treatment of intoxication with opioids or other substances is an important aspect of ongoing treatment.

Acute opioid intoxication of mild to moderate degree usually does not require treatment. However, severe opioid overdose, marked by respiratory depression, may be fatal and requires treatment in a hospital emergency room or inpatient setting. The length of hospitalization depends on the severity of respiratory depression and associated general medical complications, the dose and half-life of the opioid used, the presence of other drugs of abuse, and the reason for the overdose. Uncomplicated overdose with an opioid that has a relatively short half-life (e.g., 3–4 hours for heroin) may be treated in an emergency room, with release after a few hours. Overdose with methadone or LAAM, however, requires closer observation for a minimum of 24–48 hours. Deliberate overdose as part of a suicide attempt requires thorough psychiatric evaluation in a hospital setting.

Patients with signs of respiratory depression, stupor, or coma need ventilatory assistance. An adequate airway should be established. Aspiration can be prevented by placing the patient on his or her side or by using a cuffed endotracheal tube. In cases where oral intake of opioids or other drugs within the previous 6 hours is suspected, gastric lavage should be carried out. In hypoglycemic patients, intravenous 50% glucose in water should be administered slowly. Pulmonary edema, where present, can be treated with positive-pressure ventilation.

Naloxone (Narcan), a pure narcotic antagonist, will reverse respiratory depression and other manifestations of opioid overdose. The usual dose is 0.4 mg (1 ml) i.v. A positive response, characterized by increases in respiratory rate and volume, a rise in systolic blood pressure, and pupillary dilation, should occur within 2 minutes. If there is no response, the same or a higher dose (e.g., 0.8 mg) of naloxone can be given twice more at 5-minute intervals. Failure to respond to naloxone suggests a concurrent, or completely different, etiology for the problem (e.g., barbiturate overdose, head injury). In patients who are physically dependent on opioids, naloxone may pre-

with opioid withdrawal. Some psychiatrists maintain that the abuse potential of CNS depressants for these patients is too great and may also precipitate craving for opioids and relapse. Others feel that for carefully selected patients and with appropriate monitoring, use of benzodiazepines over a relatively brief period (i.e., 1–2 weeks) may be helpful in ameliorating the often-debilitating insomnia that can accompany opioid withdrawal (458). Diphenhydramine, hydroxyzine, and sedating antidepressants (e.g., doxepin, amitriptyline, and trazodone) have also been used for this purpose. It should be noted that these medications may also be abused, although much less often than the benzodiazepines (74).

f) Acupuncture

Studies on the efficacy of acupuncture or electrostimulation in the treatment of opioid withdrawal have yielded conflicting findings (460–465). Wen and Cheung (466) reported favorable results with 40 patients who received acupuncture combined with electrical stimulation, although the study was subsequently thought to have inadequate controls (467). Experts remain divided on the effectiveness of acupuncture in the treatment of withdrawal (463).

3. Comorbid psychiatric disorders

a) Comorbid symptoms

The reduction of opioid use in patients with preexisting comorbid psychiatric disorders may precipitate the reemergence of previously controlled symptoms (e.g., depression, mania, psychosis), which may in turn increase the risk of relapse to substance use (433).

In prescribing medications for comorbid non-substance-related psychiatric disorders, psychiatrists should be alert to the dangers of medications with high abuse potential and to possible drug-drug interactions between opioids and other psychoactive substances (e.g., benzodiazepines) (444, 446, 468). For example, use of MAOIs should be avoided because of potential drug-drug interactions with cocaine, opioids, or alcohol. In general, benzodiazepines having a rapid onset, such as diazepam and alprazolam, should be avoided because of their abuse potential (469). However, benzodiazepines having a slow onset and substantially lower abuse potential (e.g., oxazepam or clorazepate) can probably be used safely for selected patients provided that appropriate controls are applied (470). All other psychotherapeutic drugs should be prescribed cautiously, with random blood or urine monitoring to ascertain compliance.

b) Other substance use disorders

Dependence on alcohol, cocaine, or other drugs of abuse is a frequent problem for opioid-dependent patients. Cocaine abuse was found to be a problem for about 60% of patients entering methadone programs (146). In studies of opioid-dependent patients in active treatment, rates of cocaine use as high as 40% or more have been reported (471–474). Similarly, heavy drinking is a problem for an estimated 15%–30% of methadone-maintained patients, and benzodiazepine abuse may be just as common in this population (475, 476). Comparable data regarding rates of comorbid substance use disorders in patients treated in naltrexone programs are not generally available.

Comorbid substance use disorders require special attention, since treatment directed at opioid dependence alone is unlikely to lead to cessation of other substance use. Treatment is generally similar to that described for individual substances elsewhere in this guideline. Increased frequency of behavioral monitoring (e.g., daily breath or twice-weekly urine toxicology testing), intensified counseling, contingency contracting, referral to specific self-help groups (e.g., AA), and specialized pharmacologic treatments (e.g., disulfiram) have all been used with varying degrees of success. Two studies suggest that higher methadone doses coupled with intensive outpatient treatment may decrease cocaine use by methadone-maintained patients (252).

Opioid-dependent patients who are also dependent on other substances, particularly CNS depressants, should be stabilized with methadone and then gradually withdrawn from other drugs. Efforts to abruptly eliminate all drugs of abuse will not be successful with all patients. In such cases, elimination of the drugs one at a time may be warranted.

Use of aversive contingencies, such as methadone dose reduction or even withdrawal, for continued abuse of cocaine (or sedatives or alcohol) by patients in methadone maintenance treatment is controversial. Some psychiatrists believe that requiring methadone withdrawal for persistent drug abuse causes many patients to cease or greatly limit use, while failure to enforce such limits implicitly gives patients license to continue use. Others believe that methadone withdrawal is never justified for patients abusing alcohol or other drugs because of the proven efficacy of methadone in reducing intravenous heroin use, improving social and occupational functioning, and providing the opportunity to continue to motivate patients to reduce other drug use.

4. Comorbid general medical disorders

The injection of opioids may result in the sclerosing of veins, cellulitis, abscesses, or, more rarely, tetanus infection. Other life-threatening infections associated with opioid use by injection include bacterial endocarditis, hepatitis, and HIV. HIV infection rates have been reported to be as high as 60% among persons dependent on heroin in some areas of the United States (2). Counseling on how to reduce HIV risk should be a routine part of treatment for intravenous opioid users (14).

Tuberculosis is a particularly serious problem among individuals who inject drugs, especially those dependent on heroin. Infection with the tubercle bacillus occurs in approximately 10% of these individuals. For non-HIV-infected patients who test positive for the purified protein derivative of tuberculin (PPD), the lifetime risk of developing active tuberculosis is approximately 10%, and the 1-year risk is 7%–10% (477). Guidelines regarding prophylactic treatment for patients with a positive skin test have been published (478).

In addition to the presence of life-threatening infections, opioid dependence is associated with a very high rate of death from overdose, accidents, injuries, or other general medical complications (2, p. 253).

5. Pregnancy

Also refer to section III.H.3. Opioid use disorders may have adverse effects on the health of the pregnant woman, the course of the pregnancy, fetal development, early child development, and parenting behavior. In pregnant women these effects include a) poor nourishment, with accompanying vitamin deficiencies or iron and folic acid deficiency anemias; b) general medical complications from frequent use of contaminated needles (abscesses, ulcers, thrombophlebitis, bacterial endocarditis, hepatitis, urinary tract infections, and HIV infection); c) sexually transmitted diseases (gonorrhea, chlamydia, syphilis, herpes); and d) hypertension.

Possible effects of opioid use and its resultant lifestyle on the course of the pregnancy include toxemia, miscarriage, premature rupture of membranes, and infections. Possible short- and long-term effects on the baby include low birth weight, prematurity, stillbirth, neonatal abstinence syndrome, and sudden infant death syndrome (426, 479, 480). Approximately one-half of the infants born to women with opioid dependence are physiologically dependent on opioids and may experience a moderate to severe withdrawal syndrome requiring pharmacologic intervention. However, when socioeconomic factors (e.g., family disruption, poverty) are controlled for, mild to moderate neonatal withdrawal does not appear to affect psychomotor or intellectual development (480).

The goals of treatment for the pregnant opioid-using patient include ensuring physiologic stabilization and avoidance of opioid withdrawal; preventing further abuse of illicit drugs or alcohol; improving maternal nutrition; encouraging participation in prenatal care and rehabilitation; reducing the risk of obstetrical complications, including low birth weight and neonatal withdrawal, which can be lethal if untreated; and arranging for appropriate postnatal care when necessary.

Pregnant patients who lack the motivation or psychosocial supports to remain drug free should be considered for methadone maintenance regardless of their previous history of treatment. Withdrawal from methadone is not recommended, except in cases where methadone treatment is logistically not possible. In cases where medical withdrawal is necessary, there are no data to suggest that withdrawal in one trimester is worse than in any other. On the other hand, a narcotic antagonist should never be given to a pregnant substance-using patient because of the risk of spontaneous abortion, premature labor, or stillbirth. Data on the safety of clonidine for pregnant patients are not available.

In a randomized comparison of enhanced and standard methadone maintenance for pregnant opioid-dependent women, Carroll et al. (481) found that enhanced treatment—consisting of standard treatment (daily methadone medication, weekly group counseling, and thrice-weekly urine screening) plus weekly prenatal care by a nurse-midwife, weekly relapse-prevention groups, positive contingency awards for abstinence, and provision of therapeutic child care during treatment visits—resulted in improved neonatal outcomes (longer gestations and higher birth weights) but did not affect maternal drug use.

6. Age: children and adolescents

Some psychiatrists prefer to avoid methadone maintenance as a first-line treatment for opioid dependence in adolescents since it may become a lifelong therapy. Although therapeutic communities are sometimes recommended, most adolescents have difficulty tolerating prolonged confinement in such programs unless the programs are specifically tailored to meet the clinical needs of this age group.

VII. RESEARCH DIRECTIONS

The treatment of patients with substance use disorders would be improved by research focusing on the following broad areas:

A. The factors that alter the development, clinical course, and prognosis of these disorders, including genetic, developmental, biological, cognitive, and socio-cultural factors, as well as comorbidity and the impact of early experience with abusable substances.
B. The effects of treatment modalities in current use, as well as those being de-veloped, on short-, intermediate-, and long-term outcomes in specific patient populations.
C. The differential efficacy of treatment programs, with specific attention to the site of treatment and the mix of specific treatment modalities used.
D. The intensity and staging of treatment (i.e., using different treatments in different settings at different phases of the disorder) and the interactive (i.e., additive, syn-ergistic, or antagonistic) effects of various treatment modalities when applied concurrently or in sequence.
E. The impact of sociodemographic, psychiatric, and general medical characteris-tics, as well as patient treatment preferences, on treatment, participation, com-pliance, and outcome.
F. Improved methods for the diagnosis and treatment of comorbid psychiatric and/or substance use disorders, including approaches for defining the precise temporal and etiologic relationships between substance use and other forms of psychopathology.
G. The biological, cognitive, and behavioral factors contributing to development of the prolonged abstinence syndrome in patients previously dependent on alco-hol, cocaine, or opioids.
H. The acute and chronic effects of abused substances on the morphology, bio-chemistry, and physiology of the brain, as revealed through brain imaging or other assessment techniques, and the time course of recovery from these effects once patients are drug free.
I. New pharmacotherapies that reduce craving in both active and abstinent sub-stance users.
J. New pharmacotherapies that may reverse the physiologic effects of chronic sub-stance use on the functioning of the brain and other affected organs.
K. Identification of both risk and protective factors that influence vulnerability to development of substance use disorders.
L. Organizational and managerial factors in the cost-effectiveness of treatment pro-grams.
M. Programmatic approaches aimed at prevention and early intervention for these disorders.

Selected examples of *specific* types of research that are needed are the following:

A. Studies to guide the identification of patient populations who will benefit from naltrexone for treatment of alcohol use disorders.
B. The development of more-effective pharmacotherapies for the treatment of co-caine dependence, including agents that reduce short- and long-term craving for cocaine.
C. The further development of pharmacotherapies with mixed agonist/antagonist properties that block the effects of opioids and reduce opioid craving. In ad-dition, the development of nonopioid medications for opioid withdrawal with better risk-benefit ratios than those of currently available agents.
D. Studies of the pathogenesis of substance-induced fetal abnormalities following in utero exposure to alcohol or cocaine.

E. The development of new pharmacotherapies for pregnant substance-abusing women that do not affect the fetus.

F. Studies of the efficacy of behavioral, psychosocial, and family-based interventions in the treatment of children and adolescents at risk for substance use disorders.

G. Studies to identify the gene or genes that influence the heritability of alcoholism and the development of techniques to alter the genetic makeup of individuals carrying this gene or genes.

VIII. DEVELOPMENT PROCESS

This practice guideline was developed under the auspices of the Steering Committee on Practice Guidelines. The process is detailed in the Appendix to this volume. Key features of the process included the following:

- initial drafting by a work group that included psychiatrists with clinical and research expertise in substance use disorders;
- a comprehensive literature review (see the following outline);
- the production of multiple drafts with widespread review by over 145 individuals and 36 organizations (see section IX);
- approval by the APA Assembly and Board of Trustees; and
- planned revisions at 3–5-year intervals.

Computerized searches of relevant literature were carried out for the period January 1980 to February 1993, and these were subsequently updated through March 1994. Databases accessed included MEDLINE and PsycLIT. In addition, specialized bibliographies were obtained from Ovid Technologies, from the Alcohol and Alcohol Problems Science Database of the National Institute on Alcohol Abuse and Alcoholism (NIAAA), and from the Office for Treatment Improvement of the Substance Abuse and Mental Health Services Administration (SAMHSA). The specific searches included the following:

A. MEDLINE (*Index Medicus*) searches were conducted for the following periods:

1. January 1980 to February 1993, with the following key words:
   a. "Substance abuse—treatment outcome," yielding 4,543 references.

2. January 1988 to February 1992, with the following key words:
   a. "Substance use disorders and substance dependence," yielding 2,427 references.
   b. "Alcoholism and substance abuse," yielding 8,515 references.

3. January 1992 to March 1994, with the following key words:
   a. "Substance abuse treatment outcome," yielding 83 references.

B. A PsycLIT search on CD-ROM (*Psychological Abstracts*) was conducted for the period January 1983 to December 1990, with the following key words:

1. "Drug abuse, substance abuse, alcoholism, aggressive behavior, violence," yielding 98 references.

2. "Alcohol abuse, alcoholism, aggressive behavior, violence," yielding 69 references.

C. A PsycLIT (Silver Platter 3.1) search was conducted for the following periods:
1. January 1987 to September 1992, with the following key words:
   a. "Alcohol and drug treatment outcome," yielding 14 references.
   b. "Drug abuse, relapse prevention, rehabilitation," yielding 25 references.
2. January 1980 to October 1993, with the following key words:
   a. "Drug abuse outcome," yielding 31 references.

D. Current Information Service (NIAAA) bibliographies from the Alcohol and Alcohol Problems Science Database (ETOH) for the period January 1992 to May 1993 were obtained for the following areas:
1. Evolution of DSM-III and DSM-IV, yielding 23 references.
2. Therapies for alcohol dependence, yielding 39 references.

E. An Ovid Technologies search was conducted in May 1990 for the period January 1983 to April 1990, with the following key words:
1. "Treatment of alcoholism," yielding 50 references.
2. "Clinical pharmacology of alcoholism," yielding 89 references.
3. "Dual diagnosis," yielding 62 references.

F. An Office for Treatment Improvement search was conducted for the period January 1987 to September 1990, with the following key words:
1. "Coexisting substance abuse and mental disorders," yielding 83 references.

Papers selected from the aforementioned databases for further review were those published in English-language, peer-reviewed journals. Preference was given to papers based on randomized, controlled clinical trials, or nonrandomized case-control studies, or cohort studies that used broadly accepted statistical techniques for analyzing data. Clinical reports involving descriptions of patients or groups of patients were also reviewed if the sample size was felt to be adequate for drawing conclusions about the efficacy of a given treatment or if an individual case report was thought to illustrate a particularly important clinical point. Epidemiologic studies and studies involving meta-analysis were also reviewed if the population sample or the number of studies was sufficiently large to constitute a representative sample of patients with substance use disorders or a specific patient subgroup.

Review articles and book chapters were also reviewed. Criteria for inclusion were publication in a well-regarded peer-reviewed psychiatric, substance abuse, or general medical journal or in a major psychiatric text published in the decade between 1983 and 1993.

IX. INDIVIDUALS AND ORGANIZATIONS THAT SUBMITTED COMMENTS

Allan J. Adler, M.D., F.R.C.P.(C)
John Ambre, M.D., Ph.D.
Lee H. Beecher, M.D.
Myron L. Belfer, M.D.
Thomas Beresford, M.D.
Mel Ira Blaustein, M.D.
Sheila B. Blume, M.D.
Peter A. Boxer, M.D., M.P.H.
Steve J. Brasington, M.D.
Peter Bridge, M.D.
William H. Bristow, Jr., M.D.
David W. Brook, M.D.
Mary D. Bublis, M.D.
Robert Byck, M.D.
Robert Paul Cabaj, M.D.
Jean Lud Cadet, M.D.
Kenneth Carter, M.D.
Domenic A. Ciraulo, M.D.
Wilson M. Compton, M.D.
Gerard J. Connors, Ph.D.
James R. Cooper, M.D.
Linda Cottler, Ph.D.
Francine Cournos, M.D.
Lino Covi, M.D.
Dorynne Czechowicz, M.D.
Amin N. Daghestani, M.D.
William C. Dalsey, M.D.
Dave M. Davis, M.D.
Prakash N. Desai, M.D.
O'Neil S. Dillon, M.D.
Stephen Dilts, M.D.
Edward F. Domino, M.D.
Mina K. Dulcan, M.D.
Robert L. DuPont, M.D.
Richard S. Epstein, M.D.
Juan B. Espinosa, M.D.
Cesar Fabiani, M.D.
Loretta Finnegan, M.D.
Phillip J. Flores, Ph.D.
Saul Forman, M.D.
Marshall Forstein, M.D.
Richard J. Frances, M.D.
Linda Fuller, D.O.
Marc Galanter, M.D.
Frank Henry Gawin, M.D.

William Goldman, M.D.
James Goodman, M.D.
Enoch Gordis, M.D.
David Gorelick, M.D.
Sheila Hafter Gray, M.D.
Michael K. Greenberg, M.D.
Shelly F. Greenfield, M.D., M.P.A.
Harry E. Gwirtsman, M.D.
Deborah Hasin, Ph.D.
Stephen T. Higgins, Ph.D.
Ken Hoffman, M.D., M.P.H.
Steven K. Hoge, M.D.
Kate Hudgins, Ph.D.
John R. Hughes, M.D.
Steven E. Hyman, M.D.
Christine L. Kasser, M.D.
Edward Kaufman, M.D.
Edward J. Khantzian, M.D.
Howard D. Kibel, M.D.
Lucy Jane King, M.D.
Donald F. Klein, M.D.
Thomas R. Kosten, M.D.
Mary Jeanne Kreek, M.D.
Barry J. Landau, M.D.
David C. Lanier, M.D.
Hyung Kon Lee, M.D.
Alan Leshner, Ph.D.
William L. Licamele, M.D.
Joyce H. Lowinson, M.D.
James F. Maddux, M.D.
Velandy Manohar, M.D.
Eric R. Marcus, M.D.
Sara Marriott, M.B.B.S., M.R.C.Psych.
Ronald L. Martin, M.D.
James R. McCartney, M.D.
James R. McKay, Ph.D.
Laura McNicholas, M.D.
Jack H. Mendelson, M.D.
Roger E. Meyer, M.D.
Norman S. Miller, M.D.
William R. Miller, Ph.D.
Kenneth Minkoff, M.D.
Peter M. Monti, Ph.D.
Jerome A. Motto, M.D.
Edgar P. Nace, M.D.

J.C. Negrete, M.D., F.R.C.P.(C)
Melvyn M. Nizny, M.D.
Edward V. Nunes, M.D.
Charles O'Brien, M.D., Ph.D.
Lisa Simon Onken, Ph.D.
John Peake, M.D.
Glen N. Peterson, M.D.
Herbert S. Peyser, M.D.
Ghulam Qadir, M.D.
Edward Reilly, M.D.
John A. Renner, Jr., M.D.
Vaughn I. Rickert, Psy.D.
E.B. Ritson, M.D.
Nicholas L. Rock, M.D.
Barbara R. Rosenfeld, M.D.
Richard Rothman, M.D.
A. John Rush, M.D.
Jane E. Sasaki, M.D.
Bernard Savariego, M.D.
Marc A. Schuckit, M.D.
Carlotta Schuster, M.D.
Edward J. Schwab, Ph.D.
Paul M. Schyve, M.D.
James H. Scully, M.D.
Linda Semlitz, M.D.
Edward C. Senay, M.D.
Cynthia M. Shappell, M.D.
Steven S. Sharfstein, M.D.

Dale Simpson, M.D.
Leslie Smith, M.D.
Mark B. Sobell, Ph.D.
Wesley E. Sowers, M.D.
Anderson Spickard, M.D.
Robert G. Stephens, M.D.
Robert S. Stephens, Ph.D.
Verner Stillner, M.D.
Richard T. Suchinsky, M.D.
William Tatomer, M.D.
Gene Tenelli, M.D.
Forest Tennant, M.D., Ph.D.
Jerome Tilles, M.D.
William G. Troyer, Jr., M.D.
Jalie A. Tucker, Ph.D.
George E. Vaillant, M.D.
Marsha L. Vannicelli, Ph.D.
John J. Verdon, Jr., M.D.
John G. Wagnitz, M.D., M.S.
Naimah Weinberg, M.D.
Sidney Weissman, M.D.
Joseph J. Westermeyer, M.D., Ph.D.
H.G. Wittington, M.D.
C. Roy Woodruff, Ph.D.
George E. Woody, M.D.
Henry H. Work, M.D.
Leon Wurmser, M.D.

Agency for Health Care Policy and Research
American Academy of Child and Adolescent Psychiatry
American Academy of Neurology
American Academy of Pediatrics
American Academy of Psychiatrists in Alcoholism and Addiction
American Association of Chairmen of Departments of Psychiatry
American Association of Community Psychiatrists
American Association of Pastoral Counselors
American Association of Psychiatric Administrators
American Association of Psychiatrists from India
American Association of Suicidology
American Board of Adolescent Psychiatry
American College of Emergency Physicians
American College of Neuropsychopharmacology
American Group Psychotherapy Association
American Medical Association
American Psychiatric Electrophysiology Association
American Psychoanalytic Association
American Psychological Association
American Psychosomatic Society
American Society of Group Psychotherapy and Psychodrama
Association for Academic Psychiatry

Association for Medical Education and Research in Substance Abuse
Association for the Advancement of Behavior Therapy
Baltimore-Washington Society for Psychoanalysis
Committee on Problems of Drug Dependence
Joint Commission on Accreditation of Health Care
National Association of Psychiatric Health Systems
National Association of Veterans Affairs Chiefs of Psychiatry
National Institute of Alcohol Abuse and Alcoholism
National Institute of Mental Health
National Institute on Drug Abuse
Pakistan Psychiatric Society of North America
Royal College of Psychiatrists
Society for Adolescent Medicine
Society of Biological Psychiatry

X. REFERENCES

The following coding system is used to indicate the nature of the supporting evidence in the summary recommendations and references:

[A] *Randomized clinical trial.* A study of an intervention in which subjects are prospectively followed over time; there are treatment and control groups; subjects are randomly assigned to the two groups; both the subjects and the investigators are blind to the assignments.

[B] *Clinical trial.* A prospective study in which an intervention is made and the results of that intervention are tracked longitudinally; study does not meet standards for a randomized clinical trial.

[C] *Cohort or longitudinal study.* A study in which subjects are prospectively followed over time without any specific intervention.

[D] *Case-control study.* A study in which a group of patients is identified in the present and information about them is pursued retrospectively or backward in time.

[E] *Review with secondary data analysis.* A structured analytic review of existing data, e.g., a meta-analysis or a decision analysis.

[F] *Review.* A qualitative review and discussion of previously published literature without a quantitative synthesis of the data.

[G] *Other.* Textbooks, expert opinion, case reports, and other reports not included above.

1. Institute of Medicine: A study of the evolution, effectiveness and financing of public and private drug treatment systems, in Treating Drug Problems, vol 1. Edited by Gerstein DR, Harwood HJ. Washington, DC, National Academy Press, 1990 [G]

2. American Psychiatric Association: Diagnostic and Statistical Manual of Mental Disorders, 4th ed. Washington, DC, APA, 1994 [G]

3. Elliot DS, Huizinga D, Menard S: Multiple Problem Youth: Delinquency, Substance Use and Mental Health. New York, Springer-Verlag, 1989 [F]

4. Milan R, Halikas JA, Meller JE, Morse C: Psychopathology among substance abusing juvenile offenders. J Am Acad Child Adolesc Psychiatry 1991; 30:569–574 [D]

5. Christie-Burke K, Burke JD, Regier JD, Rae DS: Age at onset of selected mental disorders in five community populations. Arch Gen Psychiatry 1990; 47:511–518 [D]

6. Bukstein OG, Brent DA, Kaminer Y: Comorbidity of substance abuse and other psychiatric disorders in adolescents. Am J Psychiatry 1989; 146:1131–1141 [F]

7. Mirin SM, Weiss RD, Michael J: Psychopathology in substance abusers: diagnosis and treatment. Am J Drug Alcohol Abuse 1988; 14:139–157 [D]

8. Deykin EY, Levy JC, Wells V: Adolescent depression, alcohol and drug abuse. Am J Public Health 1987; 7:178–182 [D]

9. Treffert DA: Marijuana use in schizophrenia: a clear hazard. Am J Psychiatry 1978; 135:1213–1215 [D]

10. Alterman AI, Erdlen DL, Laporte DJ, Erdlen FR: Effects of illicit drug use in an inpatient psychiatric population. Addict Behav 1982; 7:231–242 [D]

11. Inman DJ, Bascue LO, Skoloda T: Identification of borderline personality disorders among substance abuse inpatients. J Subst Abuse Treat 1985; 2:229–232 [D]

12. Hesselbrock MN, Meyer RE, Keener JJ: Psychopathology in hospitalized alcoholics. Arch Gen Psychiatry 1985; 42:1050–1055 [D]

13. Lesieur HR, Blume SB: Pathological gambling, eating disorders, and the psychoactive substance use disorders. J Addict Dis 1993; 12:89–102 [F]

14. Batki SL, Sorensen JL, Faltz B, Madover S: Psychiatric aspects of treatment of i.v. drug abusers with AIDS. Hosp Community Psychiatry 1988; 39:439–441 [G]

15. Trocki KT, Leigh BD: Alcohol consumption and unsafe sex: a comparison of heterosexuals and homosexual men. J Acquir Immune Defic Syndr 1991; 4:981–986 [D]

16. Ausubel DP: Methadone maintenance treatment: the other side of the coin. Int J Addict 1983; 18:851–862 [F]

17. Donovan JE, Jessor R: Structure of problem behavior in adolescence and young adulthood. J Consult Clin Psychol 1985; 53: 890–904 [C]

18. Dupont RL: Getting Tough on Gateway Drugs: A Guide for the Family. Washington, DC, American Psychiatric Press, 1984 [G]

19. Brook DW, Brook JS: The etiology and consequences of adolescent drug use, in Prevention and Treatment of Drug and Alcohol Abuse. Edited by Watson RR. Clifton, NJ, Humana Press, 1990 [G]

20. National Household Survey on Drug Abuse: Main Findings, 1992. Washington, DC, US Department of Health and Human Services, 1992 [D]

21. Allen CA, Cooke DJ: Stressful life events and alcohol misuse in women: a critical review. J Stud Alcohol 1985; 46:147–152 [F]

22. Cloninger CR, Bohman M, Sigvardsson S: Inheritance of alcohol abuse: cross-fostering analysis of adopted men. Arch Gen Psychiatry 1981; 38:861–868 [D]

23. Cloninger CR: Neurogenetic adaptive mechanisms in alcoholism. Science 1987; 236:410–416 [G]

24. Bohman M, Sigvardsson S, Cloninger CR: Maternal inheritance of alcohol abuse: cross-fostering analysis of adopted women. Arch Gen Psychiatry 1981; 38:965–969 [D]

25. Kendler KS, Heath AC, Neale MC, Kessler RC, Eaves LJ: Alcoholism and major depression in women: a twin study of the causes of comorbidity. Arch Gen Psychiatry 1993; 50:690–698 [D]

26. Khantzian EJ: The self-medication hypothesis of addictive disorders: focus on heroin and cocaine dependence. Am J Psychiatry 1985; 142:1259–1264 [F]

27. Nurco DN, Stephenson PE, Hanlon TE: Aftercare/relapse prevention and the self-help movement. Int J Addict 1991; 25: 1179–1200 [F]

28. Vaillant GE, Milofsky MS: Natural history of male alcoholism, IV: paths to recovery. Arch Gen Psychiatry 1982; 39:127–133 [E]

29. Vaillant GE: The Natural History of Alcoholism: Causes, Patterns, and Paths to Recovery. Cambridge, Mass, Harvard University Press, 1983 [E]

30. Vaillant GE: What can long-term follow-up teach us about relapse and prevention of relapse in addiction? Br J Addict 1988; 83:1147–1157 [C]

31. McLellan AT, Luborsky L, Woody GE, Druley KA, O'Brien CP: Predicting response to alcohol and drug abuse treatments: role of psychiatric severity. Arch Gen Psychiatry 1983; 40:620–625 [C]

32. Vaillant GE: A 20-year follow-up of New York addicts. Arch Gen Psychiatry 1973; 29:237–241 [C]

33. Brecht ML, Anglin MD, Woodward JA, Bonett DG: Conditional factors of maturing out: personal resources and preaddiction sociopathy. Int J Addict 1987; 22:55–69 [B]

34. Schuckit MA: Prediction of outcome among alcoholics. Drug Abuse and Alcoholism Newsletter 1988; 27(4) [F]

35. Institute of Medicine: Broadening the Base of Treatment for Alcohol Problems. Washington, DC, National Academy Press, 1990 [G]

36. Williams GD, Grant BF, Harford TC, Noble J: Population projections using DSM-III criteria: alcohol abuse and dependence, 1990–2000. Alcohol Health Res World 1989; 13:366–370 [D]

37. Annual Medical Examiner Data 1990: Data from the Drug Abuse Warning Network (DAWN) Statistical Series: Series 1, number 10-B, DHHS Publication (ADM) 91-1840. Rockville, Md, US Department of Health and Human Services, National Institute on Drug Abuse, 1991 [G]

38. US Centers for Disease Control: Alcohol-related mortality and years of potential life lost—United States, 1987. MMWR Morb Mortal Wkly Rep 1990; 39(11):173–177 [D]

39. US National Center for Health Statistics: Prevention Profile. Washington, DC, US Government Printing Office, 1992 [D]

40. Institute for Health Policy, Brandeis University: Substance Abuse: The Nation's Number One Health Problem: Key Indicators for Policy. Princeton, NJ, Robert Wood Johnson Foundation, October 1993 [G]

41. US Centers for Disease Control: Current trends: statewide prevalence of illegal drug use by pregnant women—Rhode Island. MMWR Morb Mortal Wkly Rep 1990; 39:225–227 [D]

42. Chasnoff IJ, Landress HJ, Barrett ME: The prevalence of illegal drug use or alcohol use during pregnancy and discrepancies in mandatory reporting in Pinellas County, Florida. N Engl J Med 1990; 322:1202–1206 [D]

43. Kessler RC, McGonagle KA, Zhao S, Nelson CB, Hughes M, Eshleman S, Wittchen H, Kendler KS: Lifetime and 12-month prevalence of DSM-III-R psychiatric disorders in the United States: results from the National Comorbidity Study. Arch Gen Psychiatry 1994; 51:8–19 [D]

44. Ross HE, Glaser FB, Germanson T: The prevalence of psychiatric disorders in patients with alcohol and other drug problems. Arch Gen Psychiatry 1988; 45:1023–1031 [D]

45. Mirin SM, Weiss RD: Substance abuse and mental illness, in Clinical Textbook of Addictive Disorders. Edited by Frances RJ, Miller SI. New York, Guilford Press, 1991 [G]

46. Mirin SM, Weiss RD: Psychiatric comorbidity in drug and alcohol addiction, in Comprehensive Handbook of Drug and Alcohol Addiction. Edited by Miller NS. New York, Guilford Press, 1991 [G]

47. Mirin SM, Weiss RD, Griffin ML, Michael JL: Psychopathology in drug abusers and their families. Compr Psychiatry 1991; 32: 36–51 [G]

48. Mirin SM, Weiss RD, Greenfield S: Psychoactive substance use disorders, in The Practitioner's Guide to Psychoactive Drugs, 3rd ed. Edited by Gelenberg A, Bassuk E, Schoonover S. New York, Plenum, 1991 [F]

49. Weiss RD, Mirin SM, Griffin ML, Michael JL: Psychopathology in cocaine abusers: changing trends. J Nerv Ment Dis 1988; 176:719–725 [C]

50. Weiss RD, Mirin SM, Griffin ML: Diagnosing major depression in cocaine abusers: the use of depression rating scales. Psychiatry Res 1989; 28:335–343 [E]

51. Crowley TJ, Chesluk D, Dilts S, Hart R: Drug and alcohol abuse among psychiatric admissions. Arch Gen Psychiatry 1974; 30: 13–20 [D]

52. Eisen SV, Grob MC, Dill DL: Substance Abuse in an Inpatient Population: A Comparison of Patients on Appleton and Generic Units: McLean Hospital Evaluative Service Unit Report 745. Belmont, Mass, McLean Hospital, 1988 [C]

53. Marlatt GA, Larimer ME, Baer JS, Quigley LA: Harm reduction for alcohol problems: moving beyond the controlled drinking controversy. Behav Ther 1993; 24:461–504 [F]

54. Rawson RA, Obert JL, McCann MJ, Mann AJ: Cocaine treatment outcome: cocaine use following inpatient, outpatient and no treatment. NIDA Res Monogr 1986; 67:271–277 [C]

55. Rounsaville BJ, Anton SF, Carroll K, Budde D, Prusoff BA, Gawin F: Psychiatric diagnoses of treatment-seeking cocaine abusers. Arch Gen Psychiatry 1991; 48:43–51 [C]

56. Marlatt GA, Gordon JR (eds): Relapse Prevention: Maintenance Strategies in the Treatment of Addictive Behaviors. New York, Guilford Press, 1985 [F]

57. Wikler A, Pescor FT: Classical conditioning of a morphine abstinence phenomenon, reinforcement of opioid-drinking behavior and "relapse" in morphine addicted rats. Psychopharmacologia 1967; 10:255–284 [A]

58. Childress AR, Ehrman R, Rohsenow DJ, Robbins SJ, O'Brien CP: Classically conditioned actors in drug dependence, in Substance Abuse: A Comprehensive Textbook. Edited by Lowinson JH, Ruiz P, Millman RB. Baltimore, Williams & Wilkins, 1992 [F]

59. Wise RA: The neurobiology of craving: implications for the understanding and treatment of addiction. J Abnorm Psychol 1988; 97:118–132 [F]

60. McLellan AT, Alterman AI, Cacciola J, Metzger D, O'Brien CP: A quantitative measure of substance abuse treatment programs: the Treatment Services Review. J Nerv Ment Dis 1992; 180:101–110 [G]

61. Khantzian EJ, Treece C: DSM-III psychiatric diagnosis of narcotic addicts: recent findings. Arch Gen Psychiatry 1985; 42:1067–1071 [D]

62. Fleisch B: Approaches in the Treatment of Adolescents With Emotional and Substance Abuse Problems. Rockville, Md, US Department of Health and Human Services, 1991 [G]

63. Friedman AS, Beschner GM: Treatment Services for Adolescent Substance Abusers: DHHS Publication ADM 85-1342. Rockville, Md, National Institute on Drug Abuse, 1985 [G]

64. Horvath AO, Luborsky L: The role of the therapeutic alliance in psychotherapy. J Consult Clin Psychol 1993; 61:561–573 [F]

65. Luborsky L, McLellan AT, Woody GE, O'Brien CP, Auerbach A: Therapist success and its determinants. Arch Gen Psychiatry 1985; 42:602–611 [A]

66. Miller WR, Rollnick S: Motivational Interviewing: Preparing People to Change Addictive Behavior. New York, Guilford Press, 1991 [G]

67. Khantzian EJ: The primary care therapist and patient needs in substance abuse treatment. Am J Drug Alcohol Abuse 1988; 14:159–167 [F]

68. Galanter M: Network therapy for addiction: a model for office practice. Am J Psychiatry 1993; 150:28–36 [F]

69. Daley DC, Marlatt GA: Relapse prevention: cognitive and behavioral interventions, in Substance Abuse: A Comprehensive Textbook. Edited by Lowinson JH, Ruiz P, Millman RB. Baltimore, Williams & Wilkins, 1992 [F]

70. Miller WR, Hester RK: The effectiveness of alcoholism treatment: what research reveals, in Treating Addictive Behaviors: Processes of Change. Edited by Miller WR, Heather NH. New York, Plenum, 1986 [F]

71. Jaffe JH: Drug addiction and drug abuse, in Goodman and Gilman's The Pharmacological Basis of Therapeutics, 7th ed. Edited by Gilman AG, Gilman LS, Rall TW, Murad F. New York, Macmillan, 1985 [F]

72. Liskow BI, Goodwin D: Pharmacological treatment of alcohol intoxication withdrawal and dependence: a critical review. J Stud Alcohol 1987; 48:356–370 [F]

73. Jaffe JH, Ciraulo DA: Drugs used in the treatment of alcoholism, in Diagnosis and Treatment of Alcoholism. Edited by Mendelson JH, Mello NK. New York, McGraw-Hill, 1985 [G]

74. Kleber HD: Opioids: detoxification, in Textbook of Substance Abuse Treatment. Edited by Galanter M, Kleber HD. Washington, DC, American Psychiatric Press, 1994 [G]

75. Meyer RE, Mirin SM, Zackon F: Community outcome on narcotic antagonists, in The Heroin Stimulus: Implications for a Theory of Addiction. Edited by Meyer RE, Mirin SM. New York, Plenum, 1979 [B]

76. Meyer RE, Mirin SM: A psychology of craving: implications of behavioral research, in Substance Abuse: Clinical Problems and Perspectives. Edited by Lowinson JH, Ruiz P. Baltimore, Williams & Wilkins, 1991 [F]

77. Wikler A: Dynamics of drug dependence: implications of a conditioning theory for research and treatment. Arch Gen Psychiatry 1973; 28:611–616 [F]

78. Gragg DM: Drugs to decrease alcohol consumption (letter). N Engl J Med 1982; 306:747 [G]

79. Banys P: The clinical use of disulfiram (Antabuse): a review. J Psychoactive Drugs 1988; 20:243–261 [F]

80. Fuller RK, Branchey L, Brightwell DR, Derman RM, Emrick CD, Iber FL, James KE, Lacoursiere RB, Lee KK, Lowenstam I, Maaney I, Neiderheiser D, Nocks JJ, Shaw S: Disulfiram treatment of alcoholism: a Veterans Administration cooperative study. JAMA 1986; 256:1449–1455 [A]

81. Howard MO, Elkins RL, Rimmele C, Smith JW: Chemical aversion treatment of alcohol dependence. Drug Alcohol Depend 1991; 29:107–143 [F]

82. Frawley PJ, Smith JW: Chemical aversion therapy in the treatment of cocaine dependence as part of a multimodal treatment program: treatment outcome. J Subst Abuse Treat 1990; 7:21–29 [C]

83. Carroll KM, Rounsaville BJ, Nich C, Gordon LT, Wirtz PW, Gawin FH: One year follow-up of psychotherapy and pharmacotherapy for cocaine dependence: delayed emergence of psychotherapy effects. Arch Gen Psychiatry 1994; 51:989–998 [C]

84. Beck AT, Emery GE, Greenberg RL: Anxiety Disorders and Phobias: A Cognitive Perspective. New York, Basic Books, 1985 [F]

85. Wright FD, Beck AT, Newman CF, Liese BS: Cognitive therapy of substance abuse: theoretical rationale. NIDA Res Monogr 1993; 137:123–146 [F]

86. Annis HM, Davis CS: Relapse prevention, in Handbook of Alcoholism Treatment Approaches. Edited by Hester RK, Miller WR. New York, Pergamon Press, 1989 [F]

87. Annis HM: A relapse prevention model for treatment of alcoholics, in Treating Addictive Behaviors: Process of Change. Edited by Miller WR, Heather NH. New York, Plenum, 1986 [F]

88. Annis HM, Davis CS: Self-efficacy and the prevention of alcoholic relapse: initial findings from a treatment trial, in Assessment and Treatment of Addictive Disorders. Edited by Baker TB, Cannon DS. New York, Praeger, 1988 [B]

89. Carroll KM, Rounsaville B, Gawin F: A comparative trial of psychotherapies for ambulatory cocaine abusers: relapse prevention and interpersonal psychotherapy. Am J Drug Alcohol Abuse 1991; 17:229–247 [B]

90. Cooney NL, Kadden RM, Litt MD, Getter H: Matching alcoholics to coping skills or interactional therapies: two-year follow-up results. J Consult Clin Psychol 1991; 59:598–601 [B]

91. Kadden RM, Cooney NL, Getter H, Litt MD: Matching alcoholics to coping skills or interactional therapies: posttreatment results. J Consult Clin Psychol 1989; 57:698–704 [B]

92. Miller W: Motivational interviewing with problem drinkers. Behav Psychother 1983; 11:147–172 [G]

93. Miller WR: Motivation for treatment: a review. Psychol Bull 1985; 98:84–107 [F]

94. Miller WR, Benefield RG, Tonigan JS: Enhancing motivation for change in problem drinking: a controlled study of two therapist styles. J Consult Clin Psychol 1993; 61:455–461 [B]

95. Higgins ST, Delaney DD, Budney AJ, Bickel WK, Hughes JR, Foerg F, Fenwick JW: A behavioral approach to achieving initial cocaine abstinence. Am J Psychiatry 1991; 148:1218–1224 [C]

96. Higgins ST, Budney AJ, Bickel WK, Hughes JR, Foerg F, Badger G: Achieving cocaine abstinence with a behavioral approach. Am J Psychiatry 1993; 150:763–769 [A]

97. Higgins ST, Budney AJ, Bickel WK, Foerg FE, Donham R, Badger GJ: Incentives improve outcome in outpatient behavioral treatment of cocaine dependence. Arch Gen Psychiatry 1994; 51:568–576 [B]

98. Azrin NH: Improvements in the community-reinforcement approach to alcoholism. Behav Res Ther 1976; 14:339–348 [B]

99. Crowley TJ: Contingency contracting treatment of drug-abusing physicians, nurses, and dentists. NIDA Res Monogr 1984; 46:68–83 [F]

100. Niaura RS, Rohsenow DJ, Binkoff JA, Monti PM, Pedraza M, Abrams DB: Relevance of cue reactivity to understanding alcohol and smoking relapse. J Abnorm Psychol 1988; 97:133–152 [F]

101. Klajner F, Hartman LM, Sobell MB: Treatment of substance abuse by relaxation training: a review of its rationale, efficacy and mechanisms. Addict Behav 1984; 9:41–55 [F]

102. Childress A, Ehrman R, McLellan A, O'Brien C: Update on behavioral treatments for substance abuse. NIDA Res Monogr 1988; 90:183–192 [F]

103. Monti PM, Rohsenow DJ, Rubonis AV, Niaura RS, Sirota AD, Colby SM, Goddard P, Abrams DB: Cue exposure with coping skills treatment for male alcoholics: a preliminary investigation. J Consult Clin Psychol 1993; 61:1011–1019 [B]

104. O'Brien CP, Childress AR, McLellan T, Ehrman R: Integrating systemic cue exposure with standard treatment in recovering drug dependent patients. Addict Behav 1990; 15:355–365 [C]

105. Cannon DS, Baker TB, Wehl CK: Emetic and electric shock alcohol aversion therapy: six and twelve month follow-up. J Consult Clinical Psychol 1981; 49:360–368 [A]

106. Holder HD, Longabaugh R, Miller WR, Rubonis AV: The cost effectiveness of treatment for alcoholism: a first approximation. J Stud Alcohol 1991; 52:517–540 [E]

107. Woody GE, Luborsky L, McLellan AT, O'Brien CP, Beck AT, Blaine J, Herman I, Hole A: Psychotherapy for opiate addicts: does it help? Arch Gen Psychiatry 1983; 40:639–645 [B]

108. Woody GE, McLellan AT, Luborsky L, O'Brien C: Psychotherapy for substance abusers. Psychiatr Clin North Am 1986; 9:547–562 [F]

109. Woody GE, McLellan AT, Luborsky L, O'Brien CP: Sociopathy and psychotherapy outcome. Arch Gen Psychiatry 1985; 42:1081–1086 [B]

110. Luborsky L: Principles of Psychoanalytic Psychotherapy: A Manual for Supportive-Expressive Therapy. New York, Basic Books, 1984 [F]

111. Ohehagen A, Berglund M, Appel CP, Andersson K, Nilsson B, Skjaerris A, Wedlin-Toftenow AM: A randomized study of long-term out-patient treatment in alcoholics. Alcohol Alcohol 1992; 27:649–658 [A]

112. Klerman G, Weissman M, Rounsaville B, Chevron E: Interpersonal Psychotherapy of Depression. New York, Basic Books, 1984 [F]

113. Rounsaville BJ, Glazer W, Wilber CH, Weissman MM, Kleber HD: Short-term interpersonal psychotherapy in methadone-maintained opiate addicts. Arch Gen Psychiatry 1983; 40:629–636 [B]

114. Zinberg S, Wallace J, Blume SB: Practical Approaches to Alcoholism Psychotherapy. New York, Plenum, 1978 [G]

115. Brandsma J, Pattison EM: The outcome of group psychotherapy in alcoholics: an empirical review. Am J Drug Alcohol Abuse 1985; 11:151–162 [F]

116. Khantzian EJ, Halliday KS, McAuliffe WE: Addiction and the Vulnerable Self: Modified Dynamic Group Therapy for Substance Abusers. New York, Guilford Press, 1990 [F]

117. Yalom ID, Bloch S, Bond G, Zimmerman E, Qualls B: Alcoholics in interactional group therapy: an outcome study. Arch Gen Psychiatry 1978; 35:419–425 [B]

118. Vannicelli M: Removing Roadblocks: Group Psychotherapy With Substance Abusers and Family Members. New York, Guilford Press, 1992 [G]

119. McKay JR, Longabaugh R, Beattie MC, Maisto SA: The relationship of pretreatment family functioning to drinking behavior during follow-up by alcoholic patients. Am J Drug Alcohol Abuse 1992; 18:445–460 [C]

120. Steinglass P, Bennett L, Wolin S, Reiss D: The Alcoholic Family. New York, Basic Books, 1987 [F]

121. Stanton MD: Family treatment approaches to drug abuse problems: a review. Fam Process 1979; 18:251–280 [F]

122. Heath A, Atkinson B: Systematic treatment of substance abuse: a graduate course. J Marital Family Therapy 1988; 14:411–418 [G]

123. Stanton MD: Course-work and self-study in the family treatment of alcohol and drug abuse: expanding health and Atkinson's curriculum. J Marital Family Therapy 1988; 14:419–427 [B]

124. Stanton MD, Thomas TC: Family Therapy of Drug Abuse and Addiction. New York, Guilford Press, 1982 [G]

125. Kaufman E, Kaufman P: Family Therapy of Drug and Alcohol Abuse. New York, Gardner Press, 1979, pp 147–186 [G]

126. Heath AW, Stanton MD: Family therapy, in Clinical Textbook of Addictive Disorders. Edited by Frances RJ, Miller SI. New York, Guilford Press, 1991 [F]

127. Getter H, Litt MD, Kadden RM, Cooney NL: Measuring treatment process in coping skills and interactional group therapies for alcoholism. Int J Group Psychother 1992; 42:419–430 [B]

128. Roehrich L, Goldman MS: Experience-dependent neuropsychological recovery and the treatment of alcoholism. J Consult Clin Psychol 1993; 61:812–821 [B]

129. Rohsenow DJ, Monti PM, Binkoff JA, Liepman MR, Nirenberg TD, Abrams DB: Patient-treatment matching for alcoholic men in communication skills vs cognitive-behavioral mood management training. Addict Behav 1991; 16:63–69 [B]

130. Annis HM, Chan D: The differential treatment model: empirical evidence from a personality typology of adult offenders. Criminal Justice and Behavior 1983; 10:159–173 [D]

131. Miller WR: Client/treatment matching in addictive behaviors. Behavior Therapist 1992; 15:7–8 [G]

132. McKay JR, Longabaugh R, Beattie MC, Maisto SA, Noel N: Changes in family functioning during treatment and drinking outcomes for high and low autonomy alcoholics. Addict Behav 1993; 18:355–363 [A]

133. McKay JR, Longabaugh R, Beattie MC, Maisto SA, Noel N: Does adding conjoint therapy to individually focused alcoholism treatment lead to better family functioning? J Subst Abuse 1993; 5:45–59 [B]

134. McKay JR, Maisto SA, O'Farrell TJ: End-of-treatment self-efficacy, aftercare, and drinking outcomes of alcoholic men. Alcohol Clin Exp Res 1993; 17:1078–1083 [A]

135. McKay JR, Maisto SA: An overview and critique of advances in the treatment of alcohol use disorders. Drugs and Society 1993; 8:1–29 [F]

136. Longabaugh R, Beattie MC, Noel N, Stout R, Malloy P: The effect of social investment on treatment outcome. J Stud Alcohol 1993; 54:465–478 [B]

137. McLellan AT, Woody GE, Luborsky L, O'Brien CP, Druley KA: Increased effectiveness of substance abuse treatment: a prospective study of patient-treatment matching. J Nerv Ment Dis 1983; 171:597–605 [C]

138. Miller WR, Hester RK: Inpatient treatment for alcoholism: who benefits? Am Psychol 1986; 41:794–805 [F]

139. Miller WR, Hester R: Matching problem drinkers with optimal treatments, in Treating Addictive Behaviors: Processes of Change. Edited by Miller WR, Heather NH. New York, Plenum, 1986 [F]

140. Nace EP, Davis CW, Gaspari JP: Axis II comorbidity in substance abusers. Am J Psychiatry 1991; 148:118–120 [D]

141. Hoffmann N, Halikas J, Mee-Lee D: The Cleveland Admission, Discharge, and Transfer Criteria: Model for Chemical Dependency Treatment Programs. Cleveland, Northern Ohio Chemical Dependency Treatment Directors Association, 1987 [G]

142. Hoffmann NG, Mee-Lee D: Patient Placement Criteria for the Treatment of Psychoactive Substance Use Disorders. Washington, DC, American Society of Addiction Medicine, 1991 [G]

143. McKay JR, McLellan AT, Alterman AI: An evaluation of the Cleveland criteria for inpatient treatment of substance abuse. Am J Psychiatry 1992; 149:1212–1218 [C]

144. Prochaska JO, DiClemente CC, Norcross JC: In search of how people change: applications to addictive behaviors. Am Psychol 1992; 47:1102–1114 [F]

145. Project MATCH (Matching Alcoholism Treatment to Client Heterogeneity): rationale and methods for a multisite clinical trial matching patients to alcoholism treatment. Alcohol Clin Exp Res 1993; 17:1130–1145 [A]

146. Ball J, Ross A: The Effectiveness of Methadone Maintenance Treatment. New York, Springer-Verlag, 1991 [C]

147. Joe GW, Simpson DD, Hubbard RL: Treatment predictors of tenure in methadone maintenance. J Subst Abuse 1991; 3:73–84 [C]

148. McLellan AT, Arndt IO, Metzger DS, Woody GE, O'Brien CP: The effects of psychological services in substance abuse treatment. JAMA 1993; 269:1953–1959 [B]

149. McLellan AT, Grissom GR, Brill P, Durell J, Metzger DS, O'Brien CP: Private substance abuse treatments: are some programs more effective than others? J Subst Abuse Treat 1993; 10:243–254 [C]

150. McLellan AT, Alterman AI, Metzger DS, Grissom GR, Woody GE, Luborsky L, O'Brien CP: Similarity of outcome predictors across opiate, cocaine, and alcohol treatments: role of treatment services. J Consult Clin Psychol 1994; 62:1141–1158 [D]

151. Apsler R, Harding WM: Cost-effectiveness analysis of drug abuse treatment: current status and recommendations for future research, in Background Papers on Drug Abuse Financing and Services Approach: Drug Abuse Services Research Series, number 1, DHHS Publication (ADM) 91-17777. Rockville, Md, National Institute on Drug Abuse, 1991 [E]

152. Dackis CA, Gold MS: Psychiatric hospitals for treatment of dual diagnosis, in Substance Abuse: A Comprehensive Textbook. Edited by Lowinson JH, Ruiz P, Millman RB. Baltimore, Williams & Wilkins, 1992 [F]

153. Hayashida M, Alterman AI, McLellan AT, O'Brien CP, Purtell JJ, Volpicelli JR, Raphaelson AH, Hall CP: Comparative effectiveness and costs of inpatient and outpatient detoxification of patients with mild-to-moderate alcohol withdrawal syndromes. N Engl J Med 1989; 320:358–365 [B]

154. Friedman AS, Glickman NW: Residential program characteristics for completion of treatment by adolescent drug abusers. J Nerv Ment Dis 1987; 165:418–424 [D]

155. McLellan AT: The psychiatrically severe drug abuse patients: methadone maintenance or therapeutic community? Am J Drug Alcohol Abuse 1984; 10:77–95 [A]

156. De Leon G, Rosenthal MS: Treatment in residential therapeutic communities, in Treatments of Psychiatric Disorders: A Task Force Report of the American Psychiatric Association, vol 2. Washington, DC, APA, 1989 [G]

157. Simpson DD, Sells SB (eds): Opioid Addiction and Treatment: A 12 Year Follow-Up. Melbourne, Fla, Robert E Krieger, 1990 [E]

158. De Leon GD, Wexler HK, Jainchill N: The therapeutic community: success and improvement rates 5 years after treatment. Int J Addict 1982; 17:703–747 [C]

159. De Leon G: The Therapeutic Community: Study of Effectiveness. NIDA Treatment Research Monograph Series, DHHS Publication (ADM) 85-1286. Rockville, Md, National Institute on Drug Abuse, 1984 [C]

160. Longabaugh R: Longitudinal outcome studies, in Alcoholism: Origins and Outcome. Edited by Rose RM, Barrett J. New York, Raven Press, 1988 [F]

161. Kleber HD, Slobetz F: Outpatient drug-free treatment, in Handbook on Drug Abuse. Edited by DuPont RL, Goldstein A, O'Donnell J. Rockville, Md, National Institute on Drug Abuse, 1979 [G]

162. McLellan AT, O'Brien CP, Metzger DS, Alterman AI, Cornish J, Urschel H: Is substance abuse treatment effective: compared to what? in Addictive States. Edited by O'Brien CP, Jaffe J. New York, Raven Press, 1992 [F]

163. Crumley FE: Substance abuse and adolescent suicidal behavior. JAMA 1990; 163:3051–3056 [F]

164. Schuckit MA: Primary male alcoholics with histories of suicide attempts. J Stud Alcohol 1986; 47:78–81 [D]

165. Rich CL, Young D, Fowler RC: San Diego suicide study, I: young vs old subjects. Arch Gen Psychiatry 1986; 43:577–582 [D]

166. Hawton K: Assessment of suicide risk. Br J Psychiatry 1987; 150:145–153 [F]

167. Murphy GE: Suicide and substance abuse. Arch Gen Psychiatry 1988; 45:593–594 [G]

168. Norstrom T: Alcohol and suicide in Scandinavia. Br J Addict 1988; 83:553–559 [E]

169. Dorpat TL: Drug automatism, barbiturate poisoning and suicide behavior. Arch Gen Psychiatry 1974; 31:216–220 [G]

170. Budde RD: Cocaine abuse and violent death. Am J Drug Alcohol Abuse 1989; 15:375–382 [D]

171. Langevin R, Paitich D, Orchard B, Handy L, Russon A: The role of alcohol, drugs, suicide attempts and situational strains in homicide committed by offenders seen for psychiatric assessment: a controlled study. Acta Psychiatr Scand 1982; 66:229–242 [D]

172. Luisada PV: The phencyclidine psychosis: phenomenology and treatment. NIDA Res Monogr 1978; 21:241–253 [C]

173. Brecher M, Wang BW, Wong H, Morgan JP: Phencyclidine and violence: clinical and legal issues. J Clin Psychopharmacol 1988; 8:398–401 [D]

174. Melges FT, Tinklenberg JR, Hollister LE, Gillespie HK: Temporal disintegration and depersonalization during marijuana intoxication. Arch Gen Psychiatry 1970; 23:204–210 [B]

175. Bowers MB Jr: Acute psychosis induced by psychotomimetic drug abuse, 1: clinical findings. Arch Gen Psychiatry 1972; 27: 437–439 [C]

176. Bowers MB Jr: Acute psychosis induced by psychotomimetic drug abuse, 2: neurochemical findings. Arch Gen Psychiatry 1972; 27:440–442 [C]

177. McLellan AT, Luborsky L, O'Brien CP: Alcohol and drug abuse treatment in three different populations: is there improvement and is it predictable? Am J Drug Alcohol Abuse 1986; 12:101–120 [C]

178. McLellan AT: "Psychiatric severity" as a predictor of outcome from substance abuse treatments, in Psychopathology and Addictive Disorders. Edited by Meyer RE. New York, Guilford Press, 1986 [G]

179. Penick EC, Powell BJ, Liskow BI, Jackson JO, Nickel EJ: The stability of coexisting psychiatric syndromes in alcoholic men after one year. J Stud Alcohol 1988; 49:395–405 [C]

180. Rounsaville BJ, Weissman MM, Wilber CH, Kleber HD: Pathways to opiate addiction: an evaluation of differing antecedents. Br J Psychiatry 1982; 141:437–446 [D]

181. Rounsaville BJ, Weissman MM, Kleber H, Wilber C: Heterogeneity of psychiatric diagnosis in treated opiate addicts. Arch Gen Psychiatry 1982; 39:161–166 [D]

182. Rounsaville BJ, Kosten TR, Weissman MM, Kleber HD: Prognostic significance of psychopathology in treated opioid addicts: a 2.5-year follow-up study. Arch Gen Psychiatry 1986; 43:739–745 [D]

183. Stone MH: The Fate of Borderline Patients: Successful Outcome and Psychiatric Practice. New York, Guilford Press, 1990 [G]

184. Tarter RE: Evaluation and treatment of adolescent substance abuse: a decision tree method. Am J Drug Alcohol Abuse 1990; 16:1–46 [G]

185. Rounsaville BJ, Dolinsky ZS, Babor TF, Meyer RE: Psychopathology as a predictor of treatment outcome in alcoholics. Arch Gen Psychiatry 1987; 44:505–513 [C]

186. Jaffe JH, Ciraulo DA: Alcoholism and depression, in Psychopathology and Addictive Disorders. Edited by Meyer RE. New York, Guilford Press, 1986 [F]

187. Hunt W, Barnet L, Branch L: Relapse rates in addiction programs. J Clin Psychol 1971; 27:455–456 [G]

188. Goodwin DW: Alcohol: clinical aspects, in Substance Abuse: A Comprehensive Textbook, 2nd ed. Edited by Lowinson JH, Ruiz P, Millman RB, Langrod JG. Baltimore, Williams & Wilkins, 1992 [G]

189. Bridge TP, Mirsky AF, Goodwin FK (eds): Psychological, Neuropsychiatric, and Substance Abuse Aspects of AIDS: Advances in Biochemical Psychopharmacology, vol 44. New York, Raven Press, 1988 [G]

190. Sorensen JL, Costantini MF, London JA: Coping with AIDS: strategies for patients and staff in drug abuse treatment programs. J Psychoactive Drugs 1989; 21:435–440 [F]

191. Ball JC, Lange WR, Myers CP, Friedman SR: Reducing the risk of AIDS through methadone maintenance treatment. J Health Soc Behav 1988; 29:214–226 [C]

192. Novick DM: The medically ill substance abuser, in Substance Abuse: A Comprehensive Textbook, 2nd ed. Edited by Lowinson JH, Ruiz P, Millman RB, Langrod JG. Baltimore, Williams & Wilkins, 1992 [G]

193. Tuberculosis and human immunodeficiency virus infection: recommendations of the Advisory Committee for the Elimination of Tuberculosis (ACET). MMWR Morb Mortal Wkly Rep 1989; 38:236–238, 243–250 [G]

194. Woods JR, Plessinger MA, Clark KA: Effect of cocaine on uterine blood flow and fetal oxygenation. JAMA 1987; 257:957–961 [G]

195. Szeto HH: Maternal-fetal pharmacokinetics and fetal dose-response relationships. Ann NY Acad Sci 1989; 562:42–55 [F]

196. Dattel BJ: Substance abuse in pregnancy. Semin Perinatol 1990; 14:179–187 [F]

197. Fulroth RF, Durand DJ, Nicherson BG, Espinoza AM: Prenatal cocaine exposure is not associated with a large increase in the incidence of SIDS (abstract). Pediatr Res 1989; 25:215A [C]

198. Fried PA: Postnatal consequences of maternal marijuana use. NIDA Res Monogr 1985; 59:61–72 [C]

199. Little RE, Asker RL, Sampson PD, Renwick JH: Fetal growth and moderate drinking in early pregnancy. Am J Epidemiol 1986; 123:270–278 [C]

200. Meeker JE, Reynolds PC: Fetal and newborn death associated with maternal cocaine use. J Anal Toxicol 1990; 14:378–382 [D]

201. Handler A, Kistin N, Davis F, Ferre C: Cocaine use during pregnancy: perinatal outcomes. Am J Epidemiol 1991; 133:818–824 [D]

202. Tabor BL, Smith-Wallace T, Yonekura ML: Perinatal outcome associated with PCP versus cocaine use. Am J Alcohol Abuse 1990; 16:337–348 [D]

203. Vinci R, Parker S, Bauchner H, Zuckerman B, Cabral H: Maternal cocaine use and impaired fetal oxygenation (abstract). Pediatr Res 1989; 25:231A [C]

204. Ciraulo DA, Shader RI: Clinical Manual of Chemical Dependence. Washington, DC, American Psychiatric Press, 1991 [F]

205. Finnegan LP, Kendall SR: Maternal and neonatal effects of alcohol and drugs, in Substance Abuse: A Comprehensive Textbook, 2nd ed. Baltimore, Williams & Wilkins, 1992 [G]

206. Blume SB: Is social drinking during pregnancy harmless? there is reason to think not. Adv Alcohol Subst Abuse 1985; 5:209–219 [F]

207. Griffin ML, Weiss RD, Mirin SM, Lange U: A comparison of male and female cocaine abusers. Arch Gen Psychiatry 1989; 46:122–126 [D]

208. Winfield I, George LK, Swartz M, Blazer DG: Sexual assault and psychiatric disorders among a community sample of women. Am J Psychiatry 1990; 147:335–341 [D]

209. Ladwig GB, Andersen MD: Substance abuse in women: relationship between chemical dependency of women and past reports of physical and/or sexual abuse. Int J Addict 1989; 24:739–754 [D]

210. Stevens S, Arbiter N, Glider P: Women residents: expanding their role to increase treatment effectiveness in substance abuse programs. Int J Addict 1989; 24:425–434 [G]

211. Reilly D: Family factors in the etiology and treatment of youthful drug abuse. Family Therapy 1976; 2:149–171 [G]

212. Stanton MD, Landau-Stanton J: Therapy with families of adolescent substance abusers, in Treatment Choices for Alcohol and Drug Abuse. Edited by Milkman HB, Sederer LI. Lexington, Mass, Lexington Books, 1990 [G]

213. Catalano RF, Hawkins JD, Wells EA, Miller J, Brewer D: Evaluation of the effectiveness of adolescent drug abuse treatment, assessment of risks for relapse, and promising approaches for relapse prevention. Int J Addict 1991; 25:1085–1140 [F]

214. Barnes GM: Alcohol use among older persons: findings from a western New York State general population survey. J Am Geriatr Soc 1979; 27:244–250 [D]

215. McCourt WF, Williams AF, Schneider L: Incidence of alcoholism in a state mental hospital population. Q J Stud Alcohol 1971; 32:1085–1088 [D]

216. Atkinson JH, Schuckit MA: Geriatric alcohol and drug misuse and abuse. Advances in Substance Abuse 1983; 3:195–237 [G]

217. Atkinson RM (ed): Alcohol and Drug Abuse in Old Age. Washington, DC, American Psychiatric Press, 1984 [G]

218. Abrams RC, Alexopoulos G: Geriatric addictions, in Clinical Textbook of Addictive Disorders. Edited by Frances RJ, Miller SI. New York, Guilford Press, 1991 [G]

219. National Institute on Alcohol Abuse and Alcoholism: Alcohol and minorities. Alcohol Alert, issue 23 (PH 347), January 1994, pp 1–4 [G]

220. Institute of Medicine: The treatment of special populations: overview and definitions, in Broadening the Base of Treatment for Alcohol Problems. Washington, DC, National Academy Press, 1990 [G]

221. Dolan MP, Roberts WR, Penk WE, Robinowitz R, Atkins HG: Personality differences among black, white and Hispanic-American male heroin addicts on MMPI content scales. J Clin Psychol 1983; 39:807–813 [D]

222. Cabaj RP: Substance abuse in the gay and lesbian community, in Substance Abuse: A Comprehensive Textbook, 2nd ed. Edited by Lowinson JH, Ruiz P, Millman RB. Baltimore, Williams & Wilkins, 1992 [G]

223. Liles RE, Childs D: Similarities in family dynamics of incest and alcohol abuse. Alcohol Health and Res World 1986; Fall:66–69 [G]

224. Kosten TR, Rounsaville BJ, Kleber HD: Parental alcoholism in opioid addicts. J Nerv Ment Dis 1985; 173:461–469 [D]

225. O'Farrell T: Marital and family therapy in alcoholism treatment. J Subst Abuse Treat 1989; 6:23–29 [F]

226. Leukefeld CG, Tims FM: Compulsory treatment for drug abuse. Int J Addict 1990; 25:621–640 [F]

227. Beane EA, Beck JC: Court based civil commitment of alcoholics and substance abusers. Bull Am Acad Psychiatry Law 1991; 19:359–366 [D]

228. Anker AL, Crowley TJ: Use of contingency contracts in specialty clinics for cocaine abuse. NIDA Res Monogr 1981; 41:452–459 [B]

229. Conditions for the use of narcotic drugs, Code of Federal Regulations (CFR), 21 CFR Part 291.505, April 1994 [G]

230. Helzer JE, Burnam A, McEvoy LT: Alcohol abuse and dependence, in Psychiatric Disorders in America. Edited by Robins LN, Regier DA. New York, Free Press, 1991 [E]

231. Hasin DS, Grant B, Endicott J: The natural history of alcohol abuse: implications for definitions of alcohol use disorders. Am J Psychiatry 1990; 147:1537–1541 [C]

232. Rosenberg H: Prediction of controlled drinking by alcoholics and problem drinkers. Psychol Bull 1993; 113:129–139 [F]

233. Baer JS, Marlatt GA, Kivlahan DR, Fromme K, Larimer ME, Williams E: An experimental test of three methods of alcohol risk reduction with young adults. J Consult Clin Psychol 1992; 60:974–979 [A]

234. Kivlahan DR, Marlatt GA, Fromme K, Coppel DB, Williams E: Secondary prevention with college drinkers: evaluation of an alcohol skills training program. J Consult Clin Psychol 1990; 58:805–810 [A]

235. Apsler R: Evaluating the cost-effectiveness of drug abuse treatment services. NIDA Res Monogr 1991; 113:57–66 [E]

236. McLellan AT: Patient-Treatment Matching and Outcome Improvement in Alcohol Rehabilitation: Institute of Medicine Report on Future Directions in Research and Treatment of Alcohol Dependence. Washington, DC, National Academy of Sciences, 1989 [G]

237. McKay JR, Murphy R, Longabaugh R: The effectiveness of alcoholism treatment: evidence from outcome studies, in Psychiatric Treatment: Advances in Outcome Research. Edited by Mirin ST, Gossett J, Grob MC. Washington, DC, American Psychiatric Press, 1991 [F]

238. Moos RH, Finney JW, Cronkite RC. Alcoholism Treatment. Context, Process, and Outcome. New York, Oxford University Press, 1990 [F]

239. McCrady BS, Noel NE, Abrams DB, Stout RL, Nelson HF, Hay WM: Effectiveness of three types of spouse-involved behavioral alcoholism treatment. J Stud Alcohol 1986; 47:459–467 [A]

240. O'Farrell TJ, Cutter HS, Floyd FJ: Evaluating behavioral marital therapy for male alcoholics: effects on marital adjustment and communication from before to after treatment. Behav Ther 1985; 16:147–167 [A]

241. Bunn JY, Booth BM, Loveland Cook CA, Blow FC, Fortney JC: The relationship between mortality and intensity of inpatient alcoholism treatment. Am J Public Health 1984; 84:211–214 [C]

242. Walsh DC, Hingson RW, Merrigan DM, Morelock Levenson S, Cupples A, Heeren T, Coffman GA, Becker CA, Barker TA, Hamilton SK, McGuire TG, Kelly CA: A randomized trial of treatment options for alcohol-abusing workers. N Engl J Med 1991; 325:775–782 [A]

243. Annis HM: Is inpatient rehabilitation of the alcoholic cost-effective? in Controversies in Alcoholism and Substance Abuse. New York, Haworth Press, 1986 [F]

244. McCrady B, Longabaugh R, Fink E, Stout R, Beattie M, Ruggieri-Authelet A: Cost-effectiveness of alcoholism treatment in partial hospital versus inpatient settings after brief inpatient treatments: 12-month outcomes. J Consult Clin Psychol 1986; 54:708–713 [B]

245. Fink EB, Longabaugh R, McCrady BM, Stout RL, Beattie M, Ruggieri-Authelet A, McNiel D: Effectiveness of alcoholism treatment in partial versus inpatient settings: twenty-four-month outcomes. Addict Behav 1985; 10:235–248 [C]

246. McLachlan JFC, Stein RI: Evaluation of a day clinic for alcoholics. J Stud Alcohol 1982; 43:261–272 [G]

247. McKay JR, Alterman AI, McLellan AT, Snider EC: Treatment goals, continuity of care, and outcome in a day hospital substance abuse rehabilitation program. Am J Psychiatry 1994; 151: 254–259 [C]

248. Volpicelli JR, Alterman AI, Hagashida M, O'Brien CP: Naltrexone in the treatment of alcohol dependence. Arch Gen Psychiatry 1992; 49:876–880 [A]

249. O'Malley SS, Jaffe A, Chang G, Schottenfeld MD, Meyer RE, Rounsaville BJ: Naltrexone and coping skills therapy for alcohol dependence: a controlled study. Arch Gen Psychiatry 1992; 49:881–887 [A]

250. Eskelson CD, Hameroff SR, Kanel JS: Ethanol increases serum β-endorphin levels in rats. Anesth Analg 1980; 59(7) [G]

251. Wilkinson CW, Crabbe JC, Keith LD, Kendall JW, Dorsa DM: Influence of ethanol dependence on regional brain content of β-endorphin in the mouse. Brain Res 1986; 378:107–114 [G]

252. Stine SM, Freeman M, Burns B, Charney DS, Kosten TR: Effects of methadone dose on cocaine abuse in a methadone program. Am J Addictions 1992; 1:294–303 [B]

253. Marchner J: The pharmacology of alcohol-sensitizing drugs, in Pharmacological Treatments for Alcoholism. Edited by Edwards G, Littleton J. New York, Methuen, 1984 [F]

254. Peachey JE: A review of the clinical use of disulfiram and calcium carbamide in alcoholism treatment. Clin Psychopharmacol 1981; 1:368–375 [F]

255. Fox R: Disulfiram—alcohol side effects. JAMA 1968; 204:271–272 [B]

256. Fuller RF, Roth HP: Disulfiram for the treatment of alcoholism: an evaluation in 128 men. Ann Intern Med 1979; 90:901–904 [A]

257. Arana GW, Hyman SE: Handbook of Psychiatric Drug Therapy, 2nd ed. Boston, Little, Brown, 1991 [G]

258. Peachey JE, Brien JF, Loomis CW: A study of the calcium carbamide-ethanol interaction in man: symptom response. Alcohol Clin Exp Res 1980; 4:322–329 [A]

259. Peachey JE: Clinical uses of the alcohol-sensitizing drugs, in Pharmacological Treatments for Alcoholism. Edited by Little EG. New York, Croom Helm, 1984 [G]

260. Lister RG, Nutt DJ: Alcohol antagonists—the continuing quest. Alcohol Clin Exp Res 1988; 12:566–569 [G]

261. Keso L, Salaspuro M: Inpatient treatment of employed alcoholics: a randomized clinical trial of Hazelden-type and traditional treatment. Alcohol Clin Exp Res 1990; 14:584–589 [A]

262. Gerrein JR, Rosenberg CM, Manohar V: Disulfiram maintenance in outpatient treatment of alcoholism. Arch Gen Psychiatry 1973; 28:798–802 [A]

263. Ciraulo DA, Barnhill J, Boxenbaum H: Pharmacokinetic interaction of disulfiram and antidepressants. Am J Psychiatry 1985; 142:1373–1374 [B]

264. Fawcett J, Clark DC, Aagesen CA, Pisani VD, Tilkin JM, Sellers D, McGuire M, Gibbons RD: A double-blind, placebo-controlled trial of lithium carbonate therapy for alcoholism. Arch Gen Psychiatry 1987; 44:248–256 [A]

265. Dorus W, Ostrow D, Anton R, Cushman P, Collins JF, Schaefer M, Charles HL, Desai P, Hayashida M, Malkerneker U, Willengring M, Fiscella R, Sather MR: Lithium treatment of depressed and nondepressed alcoholics. JAMA 1989; 262:1646–1652 [A]

266. Mason BT, Kocsis JH: Desipramine treatment of alcoholism. Psychopharmacol Bull 1991; 27:155–161 [A]

267. Nunes EV, McGrath PJ, Quitkin FM, Stewart JP, Harrison W, Tricamo E, Ocepek-Welikson K: Imipramine treatment of alcoholism with comorbid depression. Am J Psychiatry 1993; 150: 963–965 [A]

268. Naranjo CA, Kadlec KE, Sanheuza P, Woodley-Remus D, Sellars EM: Fluoxetine differentially alters alcohol intake and other consummatory behavior in problem drinkers. Clin Pharmacol Ther 1990; 47:490–498 [B]

269. Lawrin MO, Naranjo CA, Sellars EM: Identification and testing of new drugs for modulating alcohol consumption. Psychopharmacol Bull 1986; 22:1020–1025 [G]

270. Cornelius JR, Salloum IM, Cornelius MD, Ehler JB, Perel JM: Fluoxetine vs placebo in depressed alcoholics. Presented at New Clinical Drug Evaluation Unit (NCDEU) Meeting, Marco Island, Fla, June 1994 [A]

271. Silber A: Rationales for the technique of psychotherapy with alcoholics. Int J Psychoanal Psychother 1974; 2:328–347 [G]

272. Chaney EF: Social skills training, in Handbook of Alcoholism Treatment Approaches. Edited by Hester RK, Miller WR. New York, Pergamon Press, 1989 [F]

273. Monti PM, Abrams DB, Binkoff JA, Zwick WR, Liepman MR, Nirenberg TD, Rohsenow DJ: Communication skills training, communication skills training with family and cognitive behavioral mood management training for alcoholics. J Stud Alcohol 1990; 51:263–270 [A]

274. Longabaugh R, Rubin A, Malloy P, Beattie M, Clifford PR, Noel N: Drinking outcomes of alcohol abusers diagnosed as antisocial personality disorder. Alcohol Clin Exp Res 1994; 18:778–785 [B]

275. Miller WR, Munoz RF: How to Control Your Drinking, revised ed. Albuquerque, University of New Mexico Press, 1982 [F]

276. Sanchez-Craig M: Therapist's Manual for Secondary Prevention of Alcohol Problems: Procedures for Teaching Moderate Drinking and Abstinence. Toronto, Addiction Research Foundation, 1984 [F]

277. Bandura A: Self-efficacy: toward a unifying theory of behavioral change. Psychol Rev 1977; 84:191–215 [F]

278. Burling TA, Reilly PM, Moltzen JO, Ziff DC: Self-efficacy and relapse among inpatient drug and alcohol abusers: a predictor of outcome. J Stud Alcohol 1989; 50:354–360 [C]

279. Edwards G, Brown D, Duckitt A, Oppenheimer E, Sheehan M, Taylor C: Outcome of alcoholism: the structure of patient attributions as to what causes change. Br J Addict 1987; 82:533–545 [C]

280. Hunt GM, Azrin NH: A community reinforcement approach to alcoholism. Behav Res Ther 1973; 11:91–104 [A]

281. Chick J, Ritson B, Connaughton J, Stewart A, Chick J: Advice vs extended treatment for alcoholism: a controlled study. Br J Addict 1988; 83:159–170 [A]

282. Babor TF: Avoiding the Horrible and Beastly Sin of Drunkenness: Does Dissuasion Make a Difference? Storrs, University of Connecticut School of Medicine, 1992 [G]

283. Bien TH, Miller WR, Tonigan JS: Brief interventions for alcohol problems: a review. Addiction 1993; 88:315–336 [F]

284. Anderson P, Scott E: The effect of general practitioners' advice to heavy drinking men. Br J Addict 1992; 87:891–900 [A]

285. Moos RH, Moos B: The process of recovery from alcoholism, III: comparing functioning in families of alcoholics and matched control families. J Stud Alcohol 1984; 45:111–118 [F]

286. McCrady BS, Stout R, Noel N, Abrams D, Nelson HF: Effectiveness of three types of spouse-involved behavioral alcoholism treatment. Br J Addict 1991; 86:1415–1424 [F]

287. Bowers T, Al-Redha MR: A comparison of outcome with group/marital and standard/individual therapies with alcoholics. J Stud Alcohol 1990; 51:301–309 [A]

288. Noel NE, McCrady BS, Stout RL, Fisher-Nelson H: Predictors of attrition from an outpatient alcoholism treatment program for couples. J Stud Alcohol 1987; 48:229–235 [B]

289. Litt MD, Babor TF, DelBoca FK, Kadden RM, Cooney NL: Types of alcoholics, II: application of an empirically derived typology to treatment matching. Arch Gen Psychiatry 1992; 49:609–614 [A]

290. Maisto SA, O'Farrell TJ, McKay JR, Connors GJ, Pelcovits M: Factors in maintaining sobriety following alcohol treatment. Alcohol Treatment Q 1989; 6:143–150 [C]

291. Walker RD, Donovan DM, Kivlahan DR, O'Leary MR: Length of stay, neuropsychological performance and aftercare: influences on alcoholism treatment outcome. J Clin Consult Psychol 1983; 51:900–911 [B]

292. McLatchie BH, Lomp KG: An experimental investigation of the influence of aftercare on alcohol relapse. Br J Addict 1988; 83:1045–1054 [B]

293. Gilbert FS: The effect of type of aftercare follow-up on treatment outcome among alcoholics. J Stud Alcohol 1988; 49:149–159 [A]

294. Ito J, Donovan D: Aftercare in alcoholism treatment: a review, in Treating Addictive Behaviors: Processes of Change. Edited by Miller WR, Heather NH. New York, Plenum, 1986 [F]

295. O'Farrell TJ, Choquette KA, Cutter HS, Brown ED, McCourt WF: Behavioral marital therapy with and without additional couples relapse prevention sessions for alcoholics and their wives. J Stud Alcohol 1993; 54:652–666 [B]

296. Alcoholics Anonymous: The Big Book. New York, Alcoholics Anonymous World Services, 1973 [G]

297. Nowinski J, Baker S, Carroll K: 12 Step Facilitation Therapy Manual: DHHS Publication (ADM) 92–1893. Rockville, Md, US Department of Health and Human Services, 1992 [G]

298. Cross GM, Morgan CW, Mooney AJ, Martin CA, Rafter JA: Alcoholism treatment: a ten year follow-up study. Alcohol Clin Exp Res 1990; 14:169–173 [C]

299. Gilbert FS: Development of a "steps questionnaire." J Stud Alcohol 1991; 52:353–360 [C]

300. Emrick C: Alcoholics Anonymous: affiliation processes and effectiveness as treatment. Alcohol Clin Exp Res 1987; 11:416–423 [G]

301. McCrady BS, Irvine S: Self-help groups, in Handbook of Alcoholism Treatment Approaches. Edited by Hester RK, Miller WR. Elmsford, NY, Pergamon Press, 1989 [G]

302. Tallaksen CM, Bohmer T, Bell H: Blood and serum thiamin and thiamin phosphate esters concentrations in patients with alcohol dependence syndrome before and after thiamin treatment. Alcohol Clin Exp Res 1992; 16:320–325 [B]

303. Bond NW, Homewook J: Wernicke's encephalopathy and Korsakoff's psychosis: to fortify or not to fortify? Neurotoxicology 1991; 13:353–355 [F]

304. Blass JP, Gibson GE: Abnormality of a thiamine-requiring enzyme in patients with Wernicke-Korsakoff syndrome. N Engl J Med 1977; 297:1367–1370 [G]

305. Shaw JM, Kolesar GS, Sellers EM, Kaplan HL, Sandor P: Development of optimal treatment tactics for alcohol withdrawal. J Clin Psychopharmacol 1981; 1:382–389 [B]

306. Naranjo CA, Sellers EM, Chater K, Iversen P, Roach C, Sykora K: Nonpharmacologic intervention in acute alcohol withdrawal. Clin Pharmacol Ther 1983; 34:214–219 [A]

307. Whitfield CL, Thompson G, Lamb A, Spencer V, Pfeifer M, Browning-Ferrando M: Detoxification of 1,024 alcoholic patients without psychoactive drugs. JAMA 1978; 239:1409–1410 [B]

308. Femino J, Lewis DC: Clinical Pharmacology and Therapeutics of the Alcohol Withdrawal Syndrome: Monograph 272. Rockville, Md, National Institute on Alcohol Abuse and Alcoholism, 1982 [F]

309. Rosenbloom A: Emerging treatment options in the alcohol withdrawal syndrome. J Clin Psychiatry 1988; 49(Dec suppl):28–32 [G]

310. Victor M: Treatment of alcohol intoxication and the withdrawal syndrome: a critical analysis of the use of drugs and other forms of therapy. Psychosom Med 1966; 28:636–650 [G]

311. Saitz R, Mayo-Smith MF, Roberts MS, Redmond HA, Bernard DR, Calkins DR: Individualized treatment for alcohol withdrawal. JAMA 1994; 272:519–523 [A]

312. Bradley KA: Management of alcoholism in the primary care setting. West J Med 1992; 156:273–277 [F]

313. Woo E, Greenblatt DJ: Massive benzodiazepine requirements during acute alcohol withdrawal. Am J Psychiatry 1979; 136:821–823 [G]

314. Sellers EM, Naranjo CA: New strategies for the treatment of alcohol withdrawal. Psychopharmacol Bull 1983; 22:88–91 [F]

315. Seppala T, Aranko K, Mattila MJ, Shrotriay RC: Effects of alcohol on buspirone and lorazepam actions. Clin Pharmacol Ther 1982; 32:201–207 [A]

316. Gessner PK: Treatment of the alcohol withdrawal syndrome. Substance Abuse 1979; 1:2–5 [G]

317. Gessner PK: Drug withdrawal therapy of the alcohol withdrawal syndrome, in Biochemistry and Pharmacology of Ethanol, vol 2. Edited by Majchowicz E, Moble E. New York, Plenum, 1979 [G]

318. Gross GA: The use of propranolol as a method to manage acute alcohol detoxification. J Am Osteopathic Assoc 1982; 82:206–207 [B]

319. Zilm DH, Sellers EM, MacLeod SM: Propranolol effect on tremor in alcohol withdrawal. Ann Intern Med 1975; 83:234–236 [G]

320. Sellers EM, Zilm DH, Macleod SM: Chlordiazepoxide and propranolol treatment of alcoholic withdrawal (abstract). Clin Res 1975; 23:610A [A]

321. Kraus MI, Gottlieb LD, Horwitz RI, Anscher M: Randomized clinical trial of atenolol in patients with alcohol withdrawal. N Engl J Med 1985; 313:905–909 [A]

322. Wilkins AJ, Jenkins WJ, Steiner JA: Efficacy of clonidine in treatment of alcohol withdrawal state. Psychopharmacology (Berl) 1983; 81:78–80 [A]

323. Robinson BJ, Robinson GM, Maling TJ, Johnson RH: Is clonidine useful in the treatment of alcohol withdrawal? Alcohol Clin Exp Res 1989; 13:95–98 [A]

324. Smith DE: Use of psychotropic drugs in alcoholism treatment: a summary. Addictions Alert 1989; 2:47–48 [F]

325. Gorelick DA, Wilkins JN: Special aspects of human alcohol withdrawal. Rec Dev Alcohol 1986; 4:283–305 [G]

326. Greenblatt DJ, Shader RI: Treatment of the alcohol withdrawal syndrome, in Manual of Psychiatric Therapeutics. Edited by Shader RI. Boston, Little, Brown, 1975 [G]

327. Sandor P, Sellers EM, Dumbrell M, Khouw V: Effect of short- and long-term alcohol use on phenytoin kinetics in chronic alcoholics. Clin Pharmacol Ther 1981; 30:390–397 [G]

328. Shaw GK: Alcohol dependence and withdrawal. Br Med Bull 1982; 38:99–102 [F]

329. Rothstein E: Prevention of alcohol withdrawal seizure: the roles of diphenylhydantoin and chlordiazepoxide. Am J Psychiatry 1973; 130:1381–1382 [B]

330. Sampliner R, Iber FL: Diphenylhydantoin control of alcohol withdrawal seizures: results of a controlled study. JAMA 1974; 230:1430–1432 [A]

331. Wilbur R, Kulik FA: Anticonvulsant drugs in alcohol withdrawal: use of phenytoin, primidone, carbamazepine, valproic acid and the sedative anticonvulsants. Am J Hosp Pharm 1981; 38:1138–1148 [F]

332. Poutanen P: Experience with carbamazepine in the treatment of withdrawal symptoms in alcohol abusers. Br J Addict 1979; 74:201–204 [B]

333. Malcolm R, Ballenger JC, Sturgis ET, Anton R: Double-blind controlled trial comparing carbamazepine to oxazepam treatment of alcohol withdrawal. Am J Psychiatry 1989; 146:617–621 [A]

334. Chu NS: Carbamazepine: prevention of alcohol withdrawal seizures. Neurology 1979; 29:1397–1401 [G]

335. Post RM, Ballenger JC, Putnam F, Bunney WE: Carbamazepine in alcohol withdrawal syndromes: relationship to the kindling model (letter). J Clin Psychopharmacol 1983; 3:204 [G]

336. Wilson A, Vulcano B: A double-blind, placebo-controlled trial of magnesium sulfate in the ethanol withdrawal syndrome. Alcohol Clin Exp Res 1984; 8:542–545 [A]

337. Robins E: The Final Months: A Study of the Lives of 134 Persons Who Committed Suicide. New York, Oxford University Press, 1981 [D]

338. Berglund M: Suicide in alcoholism: a prospective study of 88 suicides, I: the multidimensional diagnosis at first admission. Arch Gen Psychiatry 1984; 41:888–891 [C]

339. Linnoila MI: Anxiety and alcoholism. J Clin Psychiatry 1989; 50:26–29 [G]

340. Nunes EV, Quitkin FM, Brady R, Stewart JW: Imipramine treatment of methadone maintenance patients with affective disorder and illicit drug use. Am J Psychiatry 1991; 148:667–669 [B]

341. Ciraulo DA, Jaffe JH: Tricyclic antidepressants in the treatment of depression associated with alcoholism. J Clin Psychopharmacol 1981; 1:146–150 [F]

342. Ciraulo DA, Barnhill JG, Jaffe JH: Clinical pharmacokinetics of imipramine and desipramine in alcoholics and normal volunteers. Clin Pharmacol Ther 1988; 43:509–518 [B]

343. Cornelius JR, Salloum IM, Cornelius MD, Perel JM, Thase ME, Ehler JG, Mann JJ: Fluoxetine trial in suicidal depressed alcoholics. Psychopharmacol Bull 1993; 29:195–199 [B]

344. Bruno F: Buspirone in the treatment of alcoholic patients. Psychopathology 1989; 22(suppl 1):49–59 [A]

345. Kranzler HR, Burleson JA, Del Boca FK, Babor TF, Korner P, Brown J, Bohn MJ: Buspirone treatment of anxious alcoholics: a placebo-controlled trial. Arch Gen Psychiatry 1994; 51:720–731 [A]

346. Schottenfeld RS, O'Malley SS, Smith L, Rounsaville BJ, Jaffe JH: Limitation and potential hazards of MAOI's for the treatment of depressive symptoms in abstinent alcoholics. Am J Drug Alcohol Abuse 1989; 15:339–344 [G]

347. Galamos JT: Alcoholic liver disease: fatty liver, hepatitis, and cirrhosis, in Gastroenterology. Edited by Berk JE. Philadelphia, WB Saunders, 1985 [G]

348. Lieber CS: Pathogenesis of alcoholic liver disease: an overview, in Alcohol and the Liver. Edited by Fisher MM, Rankin JG. New York, Plenum, 1977 [G]

349. Lieber CS, Leo MA: Alcohol and the liver, in Medical Disorders of Alcoholism: Pathogenesis and Treatment. Edited by Lieber CS. Philadelphia, WB Saunders, 1982 [G]

350. Mendelson JH, Babor TF, Mello NK, Pratt H: Alcoholism and prevalence of medical and psychiatric disorders. J Stud Alcohol 1986; 47:361–366 [D]

351. Van Thiel DH, Gavaler JS: Endocrine effects of chronic alcohol abuse: hypothalamic-pituitary-gonadal axis, in Alcohol and the Brain: Chronic Effects. Edited by Tarter RE, Van Thiel DH. New York, Plenum, 1985 [B]

352. Korsten MA, Lieber CS: Medical complications of alcoholism, in The Diagnosis and Treatment of Alcoholism. Edited by Mendelson JH, Mello NK. New York, McGraw-Hill, 1985 [G]

353. Gorenstein EE: Cognitive-perceptual deficit in an alcoholism spectrum disorder. J Stud Alcohol 1987; 48:310–318 [D]

354. Bowden SC: Separating cognitive impairment in neurologically asymptomatic alcoholism from Wernicke-Korsakoff syndrome: is the neuropsychological distinction justified? Psychol Bull 1990; 107:355–366 [F]

355. Rindi G: Alcohol and thiamine of the brain. Alcohol 1989; 24:493–495 [G]

356. Turner S, Daniels L, Greer S: Wernicke's encephalopathy in an 18-year-old woman. Br J Psychiatry 1989; 154:261–262 [G]

357. Naidoo DP, Bramdev A, Cooper K: Wernicke's encephalopathy and alcohol-related disease. Postgrad Med J 1991; 67:978–981 [C]

358. McNamara ME, Campbell JJ, Recupero PR: Wernicke-Korsakoff syndrome (letter). J Neuropsychiatry Clin Neurosci 1991; 3:232 [G]

359. Martin PR, Eckardt MJ, Linnoila M: Treatment of chronic organic mental disorders associated with alcoholism. Recent Dev Alcohol 1989; 7:329–350 [G]

360. Saravay S, Pardes H: Auditory elementary hallucinations in alcohol withdrawal psychosis. Arch Gen Psychiatry 1967; 16: 652–658 [D]

361. Williams CM, Skiller AE: The cognitive effects of alcohol abuse: a controlled study. Br J Addict 1990; 85:911–917 [B]

362. Lemoine P, Harroussea H, Borteyru JP: Les enfants de parents alcooliques: anomalies observées à propos de 127 cas. Ouest Medical 1968; 25:477–482 [C]

363. Clarren SK, Smith DW: The fetal alcohol syndrome. N Engl J Med 1978; 298:1063–1067 [G]

364. Liskow BI, Rinck C, Campbell J: Alcohol withdrawal in the elderly. J Stud Alcohol 1989; 50:414–421 [D]

365. Kofoed LL, Tolson RL, Atkinson RM, Toth RL, Turner JA: Treatment compliance of older alcoholics: an elder-specific approach is superior to "mainstreaming." J Stud Alcohol 1987; 48:47–51 [B]

366. Gorelick DA: Progression of dependence in male cocaine addicts. Am J Drug Alcohol Abuse 1992; 18:13–19 [C]

367. Alterman AI, O'Brien CP, August DS, Snider EC, Droba M, Cornish JW, McLellan AT, Hall CP, Raphaelson AH, Schrade FX: Effectiveness and costs of inpatient versus day hospital cocaine rehabilitation. J Nerv Ment Dis 1994; 182:157–163 [A]

368. Budde D, Rounsaville B, Bryant K: Inpatient and outpatient cocaine abusers: clinical comparisons at intake and one-year follow-up. J Subst Abuse Treat 1992; 9:337–342 [C]

369. Kosten TR: Pharmacotherapeutic interventions for cocaine abuse: matching patients to treatments. J Nerv Ment Dis 1989; 177:379–389 [F]

370. Gorelick DA: Overview of pharmacologic treatment approaches for alcohol and other drug addiction. Psychiatr Clin North Am 1993; 16:141–156 [F]

371. Kosten TR, McCance-Katz E: New pharmacotherapies, in American Psychiatric Press Review of Psychiatry, vol 14. Edited by Oldham J, Riba MB. Washington, DC, American Psychiatric Press, 1995 [G]

372. Gawin FH, Kleber HD: Abstinence symptomatology and psychiatric diagnosis in chronic cocaine abusers. Arch Gen Psychiatry 1986; 43:107–113 [B]

373. Weddington WW, Brown BS, Haertzen CA, Cone EJ, Dax EM, Herning RI, Michaelson BS: Changes in mood, craving and sleep during short-term abstinence reported by male cocaine addicts. Arch Gen Psychiatry 1990; 47:861–868 [C]

374. Gawin FH, Kleber HD, Byck R, Rounsaville BJ, Kosten TR, Jatlow PI, Morgan C: Desipramine facilitation of initial cocaine abstinence. Arch Gen Psychiatry 1989; 46:117–121 [A]

375. Arndt I, Dorozynsky L, Woody G, McLellan AT, O'Brien CP: Desipramine treatment of cocaine abuse in methadone maintenance patients. NIDA Res Monogr 1989; 95:322–323 [A]

376. Weddington WW Jr, Brown BS, Haertzen CA, Hess JM, Mahaffey JR, Kolar AF, Jaffee JH: Comparison of amantadine and desipramine combined with psychotherapy for treatment of cocaine dependence. Am J Drug Alcohol Abuse 1991; 17:137–152 [A]

377. Kosten TP, Morgan CM, Falcione J, Schottenfeld RS: Pharmacotherapy for cocaine-abusing methadone-maintained patients using amantadine or desipramine. Arch Gen Psychiatry 1992; 49:894–898 [A]

378. Halikas JA, Crosby RD, Carlson GA, Crea F, Graves NM, Bowers LD: Cocaine reduction in unmotivated crack users using carbamazepine versus placebo in a short-term, double-blind crossover design. Clin Pharmacol Ther 1991; 50:81–95 [A]

379. Cornish JW, Alterman AA, Maany I, Droba M, O'Brien CP: Amantadine and carbamazepine treatment for cocaine abuse, in CME Syllabus and Scientific Proceedings in Summary Form, 145th Annual Meeting of the American Psychiatric Association. Washington, DC, APA, 1992 [G]

380. Montoya ID, Levin FR, Fudala P, Gorelick DA: A double-blind comparison of carbamazepine and placebo treatment of cocaine dependence. NIDA Res Monogr 1994; 141:435 [A]

381. Malcolm R, Hutto BR, Phillips JD, Ballenger JC: Pergolide mesylate treatment of cocaine withdrawal. J Clin Psychiatry 1991; 52:39–40 [C]

382. Wolfsohn R, Angrist B: A pilot trial of levodopa/carbidopa in early cocaine abstinence (letter). J Clin Psychopharmacol 1990; 10:440–442 [C]

383. Pollack MH, Rosenbaum JF: Fluoxetine treatment of cocaine abuse in heroin addicts. J Clin Psychiatry 1991; 52:31–33 [E]

384. Batki SL, Manfredi LB, Jacob P III, Jones RT: Fluoxetine for cocaine dependence in methadone maintenance: quantitative plasma and urine cocaine/benzoylecgonine concentrations. J Clin Psychopharmacol 1993; 13:243–250 [B]

385. Gawin FH, Allen D, Humblestone B: Outpatient treatment of "crack" cocaine smoking with flupenthixol decanoate: a preliminary report. Arch Gen Psychiatry 1989; 46:322–325 [B]

386. Margolin A, Kosten T, Petrakis I, Avants SK, Kosten T: An open pilot study of bupropion and psychotherapy for the treatment of cocaine abuse in methadone-maintained patients. NIDA Res Monogr 1991; 105:367–368 [B]

387. Kosten TR, Morgan CH, Schottenfeld RS: Amantadine and desipramine in the treatment of cocaine abusing methadone maintained patients. NIDA Res Monogr 1991; 105:510–511 [A]

388. Brotman AW, Witkie SM, Gelenberg AJ, Falk WE, Wojcik J, Leahy L: An open trial of maprotiline for the treatment of cocaine abuse: a pilot study. J Clin Psychopharmacol 1988; 8:125–127 [C]

389. Golwyn DH: Cocaine abuse treated with phenelzine. Int J Addict 1988; 23:897–905 [B]

390. Kosten TR, Kleber HD, Morgan C: Treatment of cocaine abuse with buprenorphine. Biol Psychiatry 1989; 26:170–172 [C]

391. Gastfriend DR, Mendelson JH, Mello NK, Teoh SK: Preliminary results of an open trial of buprenorphine in the outpatient treatment of combined heroin and cocaine dependence. NIDA Res Monogr (in press) [B]

392. Johnson RE, Jaffe JH, Fudala PJ: A controlled trial of buprenorphine treatment for opioid dependence. JAMA 1992; 267:2750–2755 [A]

393. Schottenfeld RS, Pakes J, Ziedonis D, Kosten TR: Buprenorphine: dose-related effects on cocaine and opioid use on cocaine-abusing opioid-dependent humans. Biol Psychiatry 1993; 34:66–74 [B]

394. Rosecan JS: The treatment of cocaine addiction with imipramine, L-tyrosine, and L-tryptophan. Presented at the VII World Congress of Psychiatry, Vienna, July 11–16, 1983 [G]

395. Dackis CA, Gold MS: Bromocriptine as treatment of cocaine abuse. Lancet 1985; 1:1151–1152 [E]

396. Gutierrez-Esteinou R, Baldessarini RJ, Cremens MC, Campbell A, Teicher MH: Interactions of bromocriptine with cocaine (letter). Am J Psychiatry 1988; 145:1173 [E]

397. Gawin FH: Neuroleptic reduction of cocaine-induced paranoia but not euphoria? Psychopharmacology (Berl) 1986; 90:142–143 [G]

398. Margolin A, Azants SK, Kosten TR, Nichou C: A double-blind study of mazindol for the treatment of cocaine abuse in newly abstinent cocaine abusing methadone-maintained patients: a preliminary report. NIDA Res Monogr 1994; 141:446 [A]

399. Washton AM: Treatment of cocaine abuse. NIDA Res Monogr 1986; 67:263–270 [B]

400. Kang S-Y, Kleinman PH, Woody GE, Millman RB, Todd TC, Kemp J, Lipton DS: Outcomes for cocaine abusers after once-a-week psychosocial therapy. Am J Psychiatry 1991; 148:630–635 [A]

401. Schiffer F: Psychotherapy of nine successfully treated cocaine abusers: techniques and dynamics. J Subst Abuse Treat 1988; 5:131–137 [E]

402. Spitz HI: Cocaine abuse: therapeutic group approaches, in Cocaine Abuse: New Directions in Treatment and Research. Edited by Spitz HI, Rosecan JS. New York, Brunner/Mazel, 1987 [G]

403. Carroll KM, Rounsaville BJ, Gordon LT, Nich C, Jatlow P, Bisighini RM, Gawin FH: Psychotherapy and pharmacotherapy for ambulatory cocaine abusers. Arch Gen Psychiatry 1994; 51: 177–187 [B]

404. Carroll KM, Rounsaville BJ: Psychosocial treatments, in American Psychiatric Press Review of Psychiatry, vol 14. Edited by Oldham JM, Riba MB. Washington, DC, American Psychiatric Press, 1995 [G]

405. Wesson DR, Smith DE: Cocaine: treatment perspectives. NIDA Res Monogr 1985; 61:193–203 [F]

406. Washton AM: Cocaine Addiction. New York, WW Norton, 1989 [F]

407. Galanter M, Egelko S, DeLeon G, Rohrs C: A general hospital day program combining peer-led and professional treatment of cocaine abusers. Hosp Community Psychiatry 1993; 44:644–649 [C]

408. Satel SL, Price LH, Palumbo JM, McDougle CJ, Krystal JH, Gawin F, Charney DS, Heninger GR, Kleber HD: Clinical phenomenology and neurobiology of cocaine dependence: a prospective inpatient study. Am J Psychiatry 1991; 148:1712–1716 [C]

409. Goldfrank LR, Hoffman RS: The cardiovascular effects of cocaine. Ann Emerg Med 1991; 20:165–175 [F]

410. Satel SL, Southwick SM, Gawin FH: Clinical features of cocaine-induced paranoia. Am J Psychiatry 1991; 148:495–498 [C]

411. Handelsman L, Chordia PL, Escovar IL, Marion IJ, Lowinson JH: Amantadine for treatment of cocaine dependence in methadone-maintained patients (letter). Am J Psychiatry 1988; 145: 533 [C]

412. Tennant FS, Sagherian AA: Double-blind comparison of amantadine hydrochloride and bromocriptine mesylate for ambulatory withdrawal from cocaine dependence. Arch Intern Med 1987; 147:109–112 [A]

413. Giannini AJ: Bromocriptine therapy in cocaine withdrawal. J Clin Pharmacol 1987; 27:267–270 [A]

414. Teller DW, Devenyi P: Bromocriptine in cocaine withdrawal—does it work? Int J Addict 1988; 23:1197–1205 [C]

415. Moscovitz H, Brookoff D, Nelson L: A randomized trial of bromocriptine for cocaine users presenting to the emergency department. J Gen Intern Med 1993; 8:1–4 [A]

416. Nunes EV, McGrath PJ, Wager S, Quitkin FM: Lithium treatment for cocaine abusers with bipolar spectrum disorders. Am J Psychiatry 1990; 147:655–657 [B]

417. Cocores JA, Patel MD, Gold MS, Pottash AC: Cocaine abuse, attention deficit disorder, and bipolar disorder. J Nerv Ment Dis 1987; 175:431–432 [G]

418. Gawin FH, Kleber HD: Cocaine abuse treatment: open trial with desipramine and lithium carbonate. Arch Gen Psychiatry 1984; 41:903–909 [B]

419. Weiss RD, Pope HG Jr, Mirin SM: Treatment of chronic cocaine abuse and attention deficit disorder, residual type, with magnesium pemoline. Drug Alcohol Depend 1985; 15:69–72 [E]

420. Khantzian EJ: An extreme case of cocaine dependence and marked improvement with methylphenidate treatment. Am J Psychiatry 1983; 140:784–785 [G]

421. Giannini AJ, Malone DA, Giannini MC, Price WA, Loiselle RH: Treatment of depression in chronic cocaine and phencyclidine abuse with desipramine. J Clin Pharmacol 1986; 26:211–214 [C]

422. Arndt IO, McLellan AT, Dorozynsky L, Woody G, O'Brien CP: Desipramine treatment for cocaine dependence: role of antisocial personality disorder. J Nerv Ment Dis 1994; 182:151–156 [A]

423. Ziedonis DM, Kosten TR: Depression as a prognostic factor for pharmacological treatment of cocaine dependence. Psychopharmacol Bull 1991; 27:337–343 [A]

424. Urogenital anomalies in the offspring of women using cocaine during early pregnancy—Atlanta, 1968–1980. MMWR Morb Mortal Wkly Rep 1989; 38:536, 541–542 [D]

425. Chasnoff IJ, Burns WJ, Schnoll SH: Cocaine use in pregnancy. N Engl J Med 1985; 313:666–669 [F]

426. Ward SLD, Bautista DB, Derry MK, Mills KSC, Durfee M, Lisbin A, Keens TG: Incidence of SIDS in infants of substance abusing mothers (abstract). Pediatr Res 1989; 25:106A [D]

427. Fulroth RF, Phillips B, Durand DJ: Perinatal outcome of infants exposed to cocaine and/or heroin in utero. Am J Dis Child 1989; 143:905–910 [C]

428. Schneider JW, Chasnoff IJ: Cocaine abuse during pregnancy: its effects on infant motor development—a clinical perspective. Topics in Acute Care and Trauma Rehabilitation 1987; 2:59–69 [F]

429. Neuspiel DR, Hamel SC, Hochberg E, Greene J, Campbell D: Maternal cocaine use and infant behavior. Neurotoxicol Teratol 1991; 13:229–233 [C]

430. Delaney-Black V, Roumell N, Shankaran S, Bedard M: Maternal cocaine use and infant outcomes (abstract). Pediatr Res 1990; 25:242A [G]

431. Robins LN, Regier DA (eds): Psychiatric Disorders in America. New York, Free Press, 1991 [G]

432. Metzger DS, Woody GE, McLellan AT, O'Brien CP, Druley P, Navaline H, DePhillippis D, Stolley P, Abrutyn E: Human immunodeficiency virus seroconversion among intravenous drug users in- and out-of-treatment: an 18-month prospective follow-up. J Acquir Immune Defic Syndr 1993; 6:1049–1056 [C]

433. Schottenfeld RS, Kleber HD: Methadone maintenance, in Comprehensive Textbook of Psychiatry, 6th ed. Edited by Kaplan HI, Sadock BJ. Baltimore, Williams & Wilkins, 1995 [F]

434. Hubbard RL, Marsden ME, Rachal JV: Drug Abuse Treatment: A National Study of Effectiveness. Chapel Hill, University of North Carolina Press, 1989 [C]

435. General Accounting Office: Methadone Maintenance: Some Treatment Programs Are Not Effective; Greater Federal Oversight Needed: Publication GAO/HRD90-104. Washington, DC, US Government Printing Office, 1990 [G]

436. Tennant FS Jr, Rawson RA, Pumphrey E, Seecof R: Clinical experiences with 959 opioid-dependent patients treated with levo-alpha-acetylmethadol (LAAM). J Subst Abuse Treat 1986; 3:195–202 [B]

437. Ling W, Klett CJ, Gillis RD: A cooperative clinical study of methadyl acetate. Arch Gen Psychiatry 1978; 35:345–353 [B]

438. Zangwell BC, McGahan P, Dorozynsky L, McLellan AT: How effective is LAAM treatment? clinical comparison with methadone. NIDA Res Monogr 1986; 67:249–255 [B]

439. Des Jarlais DC, Joseph H, Dole VP: Long-term outcomes after termination from methadone maintenance treatment. Ann NY Acad Sci 1981; 362:231–238 [C]

440. McGlothlin WH, Anglin DM: Shutting off methadone: costs and benefits. Arch Gen Psychiatry 1981; 38:885–892 [B]

441. Gonzalez JP, Brogden RD: Naltrexone: a review of its pharmacodynamic and pharmacokinetic properties and therapeutic efficacy in the management of opioid dependence. Drugs 1988; 35:192–213 [F]

442. Brewer C, Rezae H, Bailey C: Opioid withdrawal and naltrexone induction in 48–72 hours with minimal drop-out, using a modification of the naltrexone-clonidine technique. Br J Psychiatry 1988; 153:340–343 [B]

443. Anton RF, Hogan I, Jalali B, Riordan CE, Kleber HD: Multiple family therapy and naltrexone in the treatment of opiate dependence. Drug Alcohol Depend 1981: 8:157–168 [A]

444. Kleber HD: Treatment of drug dependence: what works. Int Rev Psychiatry 1989; 1:81–100 [F]

445. Washton AM, Pottash AC, Gold MS: Naltrexone in addicted business executives and physicians. J Clin Psychiatry 1984; 45:39–41 [B]

446. Woody GE, McLellan AT, O'Brien CP: Treatment of behavioral and psychiatric problems associated with opiate dependence. NIDA Res Monogr 1984; 46:23–35 [G]

447. Woody GE, McLellan AT, Luborsky L, O'Brien CP: Twelve-month follow-up of psychotherapy for opiate dependence. Am J Psychiatry 1987; 144:590–596; correction, 1989; 146:1651 [B]

448. Woody GE, McLellan AT, Luborsky L, O'Brien CP: Psychotherapy in community methadone programs: a validation study. Am J Psychiatry 1995; 152:1302–1308 [B]

449. Stitzer ML, Iguchi MY, Felch LJ: Contingent take-home incentive: effects on drug use of methadone maintenance patients. J Consult Clin Psychol 1992; 60:927–934 [B]

450. Brahen LS, Henderson RK, Capone T, Kordal N: Naltrexone treatment in a jail work-release program. J Clin Psychiatry 1984; 45:49–52 [A]

451. McAuliffe WE: A randomized controlled trial of recovery training and self-help for opioid addicts in New England and Hong Kong. J Psychoactive Drugs 1990; 22:197–209 [B]

452. Kleber HD: Detoxification from narcotics, in Substance Abuse: Clinical Problems and Perspectives. Edited by Lowinson J, Ruiz P. Baltimore, Williams & Wilkins, 1981 [F]

453. Jasinski DR, Johnson RE, Kuchel TR: Clonidine in morphine withdrawal: differential effects on signs and symptoms. Arch Gen Psychiatry 1985; 42:1063–1076 [B]

454. Kleber HD, Topazian M, Gaspari J, Riordan CE, Kosten T: Clonidine and naltrexone in the outpatient treatment of heroin withdrawal. Am J Drug Alcohol Abuse 1987; 13:1–17 [B]

455. Gold MS, Pottash AC, Sweeny DR, Kleber HD: Opiate withdrawal using clonidine. JAMA 1980; 243:343–346 [B]

456. Vining E, Kosten TR, Kleber HD: Clinical utility of rapid clonidine-naltrexone detoxification or opioid abuse. Br J Addict 1988; 83:567–575 [B]

457. Charney DS, Heninger GR, Kleber HD: The combined use of clonidine and naltrexone as a rapid, safe, and effective treatment of abrupt withdrawal from methadone. Am J Psychiatry 1986; 143:831–837 [B]

458. O'Connor PG, Waugh ME, Schottenfeld RS, Diakogiannis IA, Rounsaville BJ: Ambulatory opiate detoxification and primary care: a role for the primary care physician. J Gen Intern Med 1992; 7:532–534 [B]

459. Mello NK, Mendelson JH: Buprenorphine suppresses heroin use by heroin addicts. Science 1980; 207:657–659 [A]

460. Ellison F, Ellison W, Daulouede JP, Daubech JF, Pautrizel B, Bourgeois M, Tignol J: Opiate withdrawal and electro-stimulation: double-blind experiments. Encephale 1987; 13:225–229 [A]

461. Alling A, Johnson BD, Elmoghazy E: Cranial electro stimulation (CES) use in the detoxification of opiate dependent patients. J Subst Abuse Treatment 1990; 7:173–180 [F]

462. Ter Riet G, Kleijnen J, Knipschild P: A meta-analysis of studies into the effect of acupuncture on addiction. Br J Gen Pract 1990; 40:379–382 [E]

463. National Council Against Health Fraud: Acupuncture: the position paper of the National Council Against Health Fraud. Am J Acupuncture 1991; 19:273–279 [F]

464. Brewington V, Smith M, Lipton D: Acupuncture as a detoxification treatment: an analysis of controlled research. J Subst Abuse Treat 1994; 11:289–307 [G]

465. Ulett GA: Beyond Yin and Yang: How Acupuncture Really Works. St Louis, Warren H Green, 1992, pp 1–170 [G]

466. Wen HL, Cheung SYC: Treatment of drug addiction by acupuncture and electrical stimulation. Am J Acupuncture 1973; 1:71–75 [B]

467. Whitehead PC: Acupuncture in the treatment of addiction: a review and analysis. Int J Addict 1978; 13:1–16 [F]

468. Kleber HD, Weissman MM, Rounsaville BJ: Imipramine as treatment for depression in addicts. Arch Gen Psychiatry 1983; 40:649–653 [A]

469. Sellers EM, Ciraulo DA, DuPont RL, Griffiths RR, Kosten TR, Romach MK, Woody GE: Alprazolam and benzodiazepine dependence. J Clin Psychiatry 1993; 54(suppl 10):64–75 [F]

470. Griffiths RR, McLeod DR, Bigelow GE, Liebson IA, Roache JD, Nowowieski P: Comparison of diazepam and oxazepam: preference, liking and extent of abuse. J Pharmacol Exp Ther 1984; 229:501–508 [A]

471. Kosten TR, Schumann B, Wright D, Carney MK, Gawin FH: A preliminary study of desipramine in the treatment of cocaine abuse in methadone maintenance patients. J Clin Psychiatry 1987; 48:442–444 [B]

472. Kosten TR, Gawin FH, Rounsaville BJ, Kleber HD: Cocaine abuse among opioid addicts: demographic and diagnostic factors in treatment. Am J Drug Alcohol Abuse 1986; 12:1–16 [C]

473. Kosten TR, Rounsaville BJ, Kleber HD: A 2.5-year follow-up of cocaine use among treated opioid addicts: have our treatments helped? Arch Gen Psychiatry 1987; 44:281–284 [C]

474. Condelli WS, Fairbank JA, Dennis ML, Rachal JV: Cocaine use by clients in methadone programs: significance, scope and behavioral interventions. J Subst Abuse Treat 1991; 8:203–212 [F]

475. Anglin MD, Almog IJ, Fisher DG, Peters KR: Alcohol use by heroin addicts: evidence for an inverse relationship: a study of methadone maintenance and drug-free treatment samples. Am J Drug Alcohol Abuse 1989; 15:191–207 [D]

476. Stimmel B, Cohen M, Sturiano V, Hanbury R, Korts D, Jackson G: Is treatment for alcoholism effective in persons on methadone maintenance? Am J Psychiatry 1983; 140:862–866 [B]

477. American Thoracic Society: Diagnostic standards and classification of tuberculosis. Am Rev Respir Dis 1990; 142:725–735; correction, 1990; 142:1470 [G]

478. Dooley SW Jr, Castro KG, Hutton MD, Mullan RJ, Polder JA, Snider DE Jr: Guidelines for preventing the transmission of tuberculosis in health-care settings, with special focus on HIV-related issues. MMWR Morb Mortal Wkly Rep 1990; 39:1–29 [G]

479. Kaltenbach KK, Nathanson L, Finnegan LP: Temperament characteristics of infants born to drug dependent women (abstract). Pediatr Res 1989; 25:15A [D]

480. Suffet F, Brotman R: A comprehensive care program for pregnant addicts: obstetrical, neonatal and child development outcomes. Int J Addict 1984; 19:199–219 [C]

481. Carroll KM, Chang G, Behr H, Clinton B, Kosten TR: Improving treatment outcome in pregnant, methadone-maintained women. Am J Addiction 1995; 4:56–59 [B]

PRACTICE GUIDELINE FOR THE
Treatment of Patients With Nicotine Dependence

WORK GROUP ON NICOTINE DEPENDENCE

John R. Hughes, M.D., Chair

Susan Fiester, M.D.
Michael Goldstein, M.D.
Michael Resnick, M.D.
Nicholas Rock, M.D.
Douglas Ziedonis, M.D.

NOTE TO THE READER

In this practice guideline, treatment recommendations are discussed in sections IV and V and are summarized in Section I. Data regarding the safety and efficacy of available treatments are reviewed in section III.

This practice guideline was approved in July 1996 and was published in *The American Journal of Psychiatry* in October 1996.

CONTENTS

INTRODUCTION

This practice guideline provides guidance on the care of patients with nicotine dependence. Cigarette use is the most common cause of nicotine dependence, and almost all of the data available are derived from studies of cigarette users; thus, this document will focus on cigarette smoking. The recommendations in the guideline generally apply to all smokers even though not all smokers meet DSM-IV criteria for nicotine dependence (1). This is because most of the principles for treating nicotine dependence apply to non-nicotine-dependent smokers as well. Many smokers have comorbid psychiatric conditions (2), which are not described in this guideline; thus, the psychiatrist caring for a patient who smokes should consider, but not be limited to, the treatments recommended in this practice guideline.

This guideline is intended for psychiatrists. However, the data summarized in this guideline should be useful to all clinicians caring for nicotine-dependent patients.

This guideline focuses on three groups of smokers likely to be seen by psychiatrists (table 1).

Concurrent with the development of the present guideline, the Agency for Health Care Policy Research (AHCPR) developed its *Clinical Practice Guideline on Smoking Cessation* (3). The AHCPR guideline focuses on primary care providers but also includes recommendations for smoking cessation specialists and health care administrators. The present guideline builds upon the AHCPR guideline by focusing on specific populations (table 1) not covered in the AHCPR guidelines. In addition, the APA guideline complements the AHCPR guideline in providing detail on the more intensive therapies. Psychiatrists interested in providing smoking cessation treatments should be familiar with the AHCPR guidelines (3).

This practice guideline is limited to recommendations for treatment. Actions to change public policy toward tobacco are very important to decreasing the prevalence of smoking and psychiatrists are strongly urged to support such actions. APA's *Position Statement on Nicotine Dependence* (4) lists the more important actions needed. These include: a) encouraging appropriate diagnosis and treatment of nicotine dependence as a comorbid condition with other psychiatric disorders; b) increasing state and federal taxes on tobacco products and applying the proceeds of such taxes to the prevention, treatment, and research of nicotine dependence; c) changing the warning labels on tobacco products to include the high likelihood of developing dependence on nicotine; and d) advocating for health insurance coverage of treatment of nicotine dependence by qualified health professionals.

Prevention and treatment of smoking in young persons are also very important. This guideline focuses on adults. Modifications for treating adolescents are briefly discussed in section V.C.2. Psychiatrists are referred to *Preventing Tobacco Use Among Young People: A Report of the Surgeon General* (5) for more information on preventing and treating adolescent smoking.

TABLE 1. Target Populations

1. Patients who smoke and are being seen by a psychiatrist for a psychiatric disorder other than nicotine dependence or withdrawal
2. Smokers who have failed initial treatments for smoking cessation and need more intensive treatment that could be provided by a psychiatrist
3. Psychiatric patients who smoke and are temporarily confined to smoke-free inpatient wards, residential facilities, etc.

DEVELOPMENT PROCESS

This practice guideline was developed under the auspices of the Steering Committee on Practice Guidelines. The process is detailed in the Appendix to this volume. Key features of the process included:

- initial drafting by a work group that included psychiatrists with clinical and research expertise in nicotine dependence;
- a comprehensive literature review (description follows);
- the production of multiple drafts with widespread review, in which 23 organizations and over 76 individuals submitted comments (see section VII);
- approval by the APA Assembly and Board of Trustees;
- planned revisions at 3- to 5-year intervals.

A computerized search of the relevant literature from MEDLINE and PsycLIT databases for all years available (i.e., 1966–1995 and 1974–1995, respectively) was conducted using the terms "cigarettes," "nicotine," "smoking," and "tobacco." No exclusion criteria were used. This search produced 675 relevant treatment articles. Other databases searched were the Center for Disease Control and Prevention's *Bibliography on Smoking and Health* (6), the Oxford Collaborative Trials Registry (7), and the bibliography of the AHCPR *Clinical Practice Guideline on Smoking Cessation* (3). In addition, references in empirical articles and narrative and meta-analytic reviews were used to locate articles.

For brevity, meta-analyses and reviews of treatments for smoking are usually cited in the guideline instead of original studies. However, the conclusions of the work group are based on knowledge of the individual studies included in these meta-analyses and reviews and on other pertinent studies.

EVIDENCE RATINGS

Each recommendation in the guideline receives one of three categories of endorsement using a bracketed Roman numeral following the statement. The three categories are based on the scientific literature and on clinical expertise and represent varying levels of clinical confidence in the recommendation. Three varying degrees of clinical confidence are noted:

[I] Recommended with substantial clinical confidence. These recommendations are usually based on several well-controlled clinical trials that reported similar findings or represent key principles of clinical psychiatric care with broad expert consensus.

[II] Recommended with moderate clinical confidence. These recommendations are usually based on a few positive studies or on less-consistent data from many sources.

[III] Recommended with lower clinical confidence or recommended on the basis of individual circumstances. These recommendations usually have not been adequately tested or have conflicting reports about efficacy but are consistent with expert opinion and with accepted principles of treatment of smoking.

I. EXECUTIVE SUMMARY

The following executive summary is not intended to stand by itself. The treatment of smoking cessation requires the consideration of many factors and cannot be adequately reviewed in a brief summary. The reader is encouraged to consult the relevant portions of the guideline when specific treatment recommendations are sought.

Recommended psychiatric management strategies that all smokers should receive are listed in table 7 (see page 255).

Table 8 lists the recommended treatments and their ratings (see page 255).

There are a number of promising treatments for nicotine dependence that may be recommended based on individual circumstances. These include intensive behavior therapy [III], educational/supportive groups [III], exercise [III], hypnosis [III], anorectics [III], antidepressants [III], buspirone [III], higher-than-normal dose transdermal nicotine [III], mecamylamine [III], nicotine inhaler [III], and sensory replacement [III].

Treatments that *cannot be* recommended at this time for the treatment of nicotine dependence (either because of data indicating lack of efficacy or lack of sufficient evidence supporting efficacy) include: contingency contracting, cue exposure, hospitalization, nicotine fading, physiological feedback, relaxation, 12-step therapy, ACTH, acupuncture, anticholinergics, benzodiazepines, β blockers, glucose, homeopathics, lobeline, naltrexone, nutritional aids, reduction devices, silver nitrate, sodium bicarbonate, and stimulants.

Psychiatrists should assess the smoking status of all their patients on a regular basis. If the patient is a smoker, the psychiatrist discusses interest in quitting and gives explicit advice to motivate the patient to stop smoking, including a personalized reason the patient should stop [I]. When possible, advice may come from multiple sources in addition to the psychiatrist; e.g., from other physicians, nurses, social workers, etc. [I]. Written materials may be used as well as face-to-face interventions [II]. Since many psychiatric patients are not ready to quit, the goal of advice will often be to motivate patients to contemplate cessation by reviewing the benefits of quitting, discussing barriers to quitting, and offering support and treatment [III]. If the patient is interested in stopping smoking, a quit date should be elicited, treatment prescribed, and follow-up arranged [II]. The minimal initial treatment for those who wish to quit includes written materials, brief counseling, and a follow-up visit or call 1–3 days after the quit date [II].

If the patient has failed serious attempts without formal treatment, failed with nonpharmacological therapies, had serious withdrawal symptoms, or appears highly nicotine dependent, transdermal nicotine is recommended [I]. If the patient prefers or if ad-lib dosing is needed, nicotine gum can be used instead of transdermal nicotine [I]. If used alone, nicotine gum is to be taken on an every-hour basis [I]. If the patient is a highly nicotine-dependent or heavy smoker, higher-dose nicotine gum should be used [I]. Nicotine gum can also be used on an ad-lib basis to supplement transdermal nicotine therapy [II].

If the patient has had trouble stopping smoking for nonwithdrawal reasons (e.g., due to skills deficits), he or she is a candidate for multicomponent behavior therapy [I]. The more effective components of behavior therapy appear to be skills training/relapse prevention; rapid smoking, in which patients inhale cigarette smoke every few seconds; and stimulus control strategies [III]. Some smokers also appear to benefit from group support [III].

Combined behavior therapy and nicotine replacement improves outcome over either treatment alone and is recommended when available and acceptable to the patient [I]; however, attending behavior therapy should not be a prerequisite to receiving nicotine replacement therapy [I].

For the smoker who has failed adequate treatment, as described previously, and who is interested in making another attempt to stop smoking, the psychiatrist should assess the adequacy of prior treatments and evaluate the patient for ongoing or residual alcohol, drug, or psychiatric problems that need treatment [II]. If the patient has previously failed an adequate trial of transdermal nicotine and relapse appeared to be withdrawal related, three options are reasonable: a) ad-lib nicotine gum added to transdermal nicotine [II], b) oral or transdermal clonidine [II], or c) nicotine nasal spray [II]. If relapse was due to reasons other than withdrawal (e.g., stress), multicomponent behavior therapy should be considered [I]. If the patient has previously attended such therapy, more intensive individual behavior therapy (e.g., 1–2 times/week for 2–3 weeks) should be considered [III].

Psychiatric and general medical patients who smoke and are on smoke-free wards should receive clear instructions about the no smoking policy, advice to stop smoking, and education about the symptoms and time course of nicotine withdrawal [III]. Those patients who wish to use the smoke-free ward to initiate a stop smoking attempt may receive the therapies outlined previously [I]. Patients who do not wish to stop smoking permanently and who evidence nicotine withdrawal may be instructed in behavioral strategies to decrease withdrawal symptoms [III] and provided nicotine replacement (patch or gum) [II].

There is a possibility that smoking cessation might modify psychiatric symptoms (see table 6, page 252) such that it interferes with the diagnosis and treatment of psychiatric disorders (8). Cessation can also dramatically alter blood levels of some psychiatric medications (see table 5, page 251) (8) [II].

II. DISEASE DEFINITION, EPIDEMIOLOGY, AND NATURAL HISTORY

A. DSM-IV NICOTINE USE DISORDERS

DSM-IV includes nicotine dependence and nicotine withdrawal as disorders. Nicotine abuse is not included because clinically significant psychosocial problems from tobacco use are rare (9). Nicotine intoxication is also not included as it is very rare.

B. SPECIFIC FEATURES OF DIAGNOSIS

1. Nicotine dependence

Examples of how the generic DSM-IV criteria for substance dependence apply to nicotine dependence are illustrated in table 2. The applicability and reliability of the DSM diagnosis of nicotine dependence appears high (10); however, its validity has not been well tested.

TABLE 2. DSM-IV Diagnostic Criteria for Substance Dependence and Examples of Their Application to Nicotine Dependence (10)

A maladaptive pattern of substance use, leading to clinically significant impairment or distress, as manifested by three (or more) of the following, occurring at any time in the same 12-month period:

Criteria	Examples
Tolerance, as defined by either	
A need for markedly increased amounts of the substance to achieve intoxication or desired effect	Most smokers escalate use to 1 pack/day or more by age 25
Markedly diminished effect with continued use of the same amount of the substance	Absence of nausea, dizziness, etc.
Withdrawal, as manifested by either	
The characteristic withdrawal syndrome for the substance	See table 4
The substance is taken to relieve or avoid withdrawal symptoms	Many smokers light up immediately after being in a smoke-free area
The substance is often taken in larger amounts or over a longer period than was intended	Most smokers do not intend to smoke 5 years later, but in fact, over 70% continue to use
There is persistent desire or unsuccessful effort to cut down substance use	77% of smokers have tried to stop, 55% of these have not been able to stop despite repeated attempts and only 5%–10% of self-quitters are successful
A great deal of time is spent in activities necessary to obtain the substance, use the substance or recover from its effects	Leaving worksite to smoke
Important social, occupational or recreational activities are given up or reduced because of substance use	Not taking a job due to on-job smoking restrictions
The substance use is continued despite knowledge of having a persistent or recurrent physical or psychological problem that is likely to have been caused or exacerbated by the substance	Many smokers have heart disease, chronic obstructive pulmonary disease or ulcers and continue to smoke

Another widely used measure of nicotine dependence is the Fagerstrom Tolerance Questionnaire or the more recent version—the Fagerstrom Test for Nicotine Dependence (table 3) (11, 12). Scores of greater than seven on these scales indicate nicotine dependence.

The severity of nicotine dependence can be illustrated by the fact that only 33% of self-quitters remain abstinent for 2 days and fewer than 5% are ultimately successful on a given quit attempt (13, 14). The strength of nicotine dependence via cigarette smoking is due to several factors: a) nicotine produces a multiplicity of positive reinforcing effects (e.g., improved concentration and mood, decreased anger and weight), b) a bolus of nicotine reaches the brain within 10 seconds after inhalation, producing an almost instantaneous effect, c) nicotine dose can be precisely controlled by the way a cigarette is smoked, d) smoking occurs frequently (e.g., a pack-a-day smoker self-administers nicotine about 200 times a day), and e) there are many cues for smoking (15).

Nicotine dependence and withdrawal can develop with all forms of tobacco use (i.e., cigarettes, chewing tobacco, snuff, pipes, and cigars) and can be maintained with nicotine replacement (i.e., nicotine gum, patch, and nasal spray) (16, 17). The ability of these products to induce or maintain dependence and withdrawal increases with the rapidity of absorption of nicotine, nicotine dose, and availability of the product (15).

TABLE 3. Items and Scoring for Fagerstrom Test for Nicotine Dependence (11)

Questions	Answers	Points
1. How soon after you wake up do you smoke your first cigarette?	Within 5 minutes	3
	6–30 minutes	2
	31–60 minutes	1
	After 60 minutes	0
2. Do you find it difficult to refrain from smoking in places where it is forbidden; e.g., in church, at the library, in the cinema, etc.?	Yes	1
	No	0
3. Which cigarette would you hate most to give up?	The first one in the morning	1
	All others	0
4. How many cigarettes/day do you smoke?	10 or less	0
	11–20	1
	21–30	2
	31 or more	3
5. Do you smoke more frequently during the first hours of waking than during the rest of the day?	Yes	1
	No	2
6. Do you smoke if you are so ill that you are in bed most of the day?	Yes	1
	No	0

Smoking has been labeled the most important preventable cause of death and disease (18, 19). Smoking is responsible for 20% of all deaths in the U.S., and 45% of smokers will die of a tobacco-induced disorder (20). Cigarette smoking causes lung, oral, and other cancers, cardiovascular disease, chronic obstructive pulmonary disease, peptic ulcers, gastrointestinal disorders, maternal/fetal complications, and other disorders (20, 21). Secondhand smoke causes the deaths of thousands of nonsmokers and morbidity in children and other relatives of smokers (22, 23). Smokeless tobacco, pipes, and cigars also cause oral cancers and other problems (20). Although nicotine itself might cause health problems, most of the tobacco-induced disorders appear to be due to the carcinogens and carbon monoxide in tobacco smoke rather than nicotine itself (24, 25). Smoking cessation dramatically reduces the risk of heart disease and cancer and prevents continuation of the decline in lung function in those with chronic obstructive lung disease (18).

2. Nicotine withdrawal

The DSM-IV criteria for nicotine withdrawal are listed in table 4. In addition to these symptoms, craving for tobacco, a desire for sweets, increased coughing, and impaired performance on vigilance tasks may occur (16, 17). Withdrawal symptoms begin within a few hours and peak 24–48 hours after cessation (17). Most symptoms last an average of 4 weeks, but hunger and craving can last 6 months or more (17). Nicotine withdrawal symptoms are due, in large part, to nicotine deprivation (16, 17). Cessation of smoking can cause slowing on EEG, decreases in cortisol and catecholamine levels, sleep EEG changes, and a decline in metabolic rate (16). The mean heart rate decline is about 8 beats per minute, and the mean weight gain is 2–3 kg (16). Withdrawal is usually most severe from cigarette abstinence compared to other forms of tobacco and nicotine medications (16, 17). As with all withdrawal syndromes, the severity varies among patients (16).

Cessation of smoking can produce clinically significant changes in the blood levels of several psychiatric medications (table 5) (8). For example, smoking decreases clo-

TABLE 4. DSM-IV Diagnostic Criteria for Nicotine Withdrawal

A. Daily use of nicotine for at least several weeks

B. Abrupt cessation of nicotine use, or reduction in the amount of nicotine used, followed within 24 hours by four (or more) of the following signs:

    1. dysphoric or depressed mood
    2. insomnia
    3. irritability, frustration or anger
    4. anxiety
    5. difficulty concentrating
    6. restlessness
    7. decreased heart rate
    8. increased appetite or weight gain

C. The symptoms in Criterion B cause clinically significant distress or impairment in social, occupational, or other important areas of functioning

D. The symptoms are not due to a general medical condition and are not better accounted for by another mental disorder

---

TABLE 5. Effect of Abstinence From Smoking on Blood Levels of Psychiatric Medications (8)

Abstinence Increases Blood Levels

Clomipramine	Doxepin	Oxazepam
Clozapine	Fluphenazine	Nortriptyline
Desipramine	Haloperidol	Propranolol
Desmethyldiazepam	Imipramine	

Abstinence Does Not Increase Blood Levels

Amitriptyline	Ethanol	Midazolam
Chlordiazepoxide	Lorazepam	Triazolam

Effect of Abstinence on Blood Levels Is Unclear

Alprazolam	Chlorpromazine	Diazepam

---

zapine and haloperidol levels by 30% (8). This effect appears to be due, not to nicotine, but rather to the effects of benzopyrenes and related compounds on the P450 system.

Withdrawal symptoms can also mimic, disguise, or aggravate the symptoms of other psychiatric disorders or side effects of medications (table 6) (8). For example, when an alcoholic smoker who is also nicotine dependent is admitted to a smoke-free ward for alcohol detoxification, his or her anxiety, depression, difficulty concentrating, insomnia, irritability, and restlessness could be due to or aggravated by nicotine withdrawal. Also, although uncommon, cessation appears to be able to precipitate a relapse of major depression, bipolar disorder, and alcohol/drug problems (2, 26).

C. EPIDEMIOLOGY AND NATURAL HISTORY

At present, approximately 50% of the U.S. adult population have never smoked, 25% are current smokers (48 million), and 25% are ex-smokers (11). Among current smokers, most are cigarette smokers, with fewer than 5% using cigars, pipes, or smokeless tobacco (11). The mean number of cigarettes smoked per day is about 20. Between 8% and 15% of smokers are occasional or light smokers (<5 cigarettes/day) (11). The prevalence of smoking has declined dramatically in the U.S.; however, this decline has not been uniform and has abated recently (27). The prevalence of smoking has declined less in those who are younger, female, non-Caucasian, less educated, or poor and those with psychiatric or alcohol/drug problems (27).

TABLE 6. Some Examples of Nicotine Withdrawal Symptoms That Can Be Confused With Other Psychiatric Conditions (8)

Anxiety	Irritability
Depression	Restlessness
Increased REM sleep	Weight gain
Insomnia	

The median age of initiation of smoking is 15 (5). Psychiatric predictors of initiation of smoking include use and abuse of alcohol and other drugs, attention deficit disorders, and depressive symptoms; however, smoking precedes the normal age at onset for most psychiatric disorders (2). Twin studies have found that the heritability of smoking is as great as, if not greater than, that for alcoholism (28, 29). Some of the heritability of smoking is shared with and some is independent of that for alcoholism (30).

Within a few years of daily smoking, most smokers begin to develop dependence (5). For example, 50% of smokers in their twenties meet DSM criteria for dependence (31). Also, within a few years of daily smoking, smokers note withdrawal symptoms upon cessation (5). Among older adult daily smokers, 87% (40 million) are estimated to meet DSM-IV criteria for nicotine dependence (32).

About one-third of adults who smoke make a serious attempt to stop smoking each year (27). Over 90% of these attempts to quit are made without formal treatment (27). With self-quitting, 33% of smokers are abstinent for 2 days and 3%–5% are abstinent for 1 year, after which little relapse occurs (13, 14). Most smokers make several quit attempts, so that 50% of smokers eventually quit (27). Smokers with a past or present history of anxiety, depression, or schizophrenia are less likely to stop smoking (2, 8, 33, 34). This could be due to several factors, including increased nicotine withdrawal or nicotine dependence, less social support, or fewer coping skills (2). Smokers who have current alcohol abuse/dependence problems are unlikely to stop smoking unless their alcohol problem resolves (34). Whether alcohol/drug abusers in recovery are less likely to stop smoking is unclear (34).

About 50% of adults who attempt to stop smoking will meet DSM-IV criteria for nicotine withdrawal (17). Smokers who have withdrawal-induced depression or severe craving are less likely to successfully stop smoking (2, 17). In addition, fear of weight gain appears to be a major deterrent to cessation attempts, especially among women (35). The presence of cues for smoking is thought to be crucial in producing withdrawal; thus, withdrawal during inpatient stays on smoke-free units is often not as severe as expected (16).

III. TREATMENT PRINCIPLES AND ALTERNATIVES

▶ A. INTRODUCTION

There are many similarities between nicotine and other drug dependencies (36, 37). There are also significant differences. For example, although nicotine dependence produces dramatic health problems, it usually does not produce significant interpersonal, financial, legal, or psychological problems. Thus, the present guidelines will in some respects be similar to and in others different than the *American Psychiatric As-*

sociation Practice Guideline for the Treatment of Patients with Substance Use Disorders: Alcohol, Cocaine, Opioids (38; included in this volume).

The following sections contain data regarding the likely impact of a variety of treatments for patients who smoke. It is important to note that the bulk of these data are derived from studies of patient groups who are not under psychiatric care. (Exceptions to this are noted.) Expert judgment has been used to determine the applicability of these data to the populations under consideration in this guideline.

► B. GOALS OF TREATMENT

Long-term abstinence is the ultimate goal of the treatment of nicotine dependence. Initial goals include moving smokers from not contemplating smoking cessation, to contemplating cessation, to initiating a quit attempt, to quitting for a short period [II] (39). Whether harm reduction (e.g., switching to low nicotine cigarettes or cutting down on the number of cigarettes smoked) is an acceptable goal is debatable because the health benefits from these actions are not well demonstrated, compensatory behaviors occur, and patients may consider harm reduction as a "safe haven," which will undermine later cessation attempts (40). Whether long-term use of nicotine medication is necessary in some smokers is also debatable (41). Management of withdrawal is an important goal in and of itself, especially for those on smoke-free wards (8). Nicotine intoxication is rare; its treatment is not covered here, and the reader is referred to other sources (42).

► C. ASSESSMENT

The patient's current smoking status (e.g., current smoker, ex-smoker, never smoked, number of cigarettes/day) needs to be routinely determined. The comprehensiveness of subsequent assessment is determined by the goals and characteristics of potential interventions; i.e., different assessments are necessary to guide the application of brief advice, the intensive treatment of prior treatment failures, or the relief of nicotine withdrawal in an inpatient setting.

1. Readiness to change and motivation to quit

About 40% of current smokers are not considering stopping smoking in the foreseeable future (43). These patients may be uninformed, demoralized about their ability to change, or defensive and resistant to change. Many psychiatric patients are probably in this phase (33, 44). Another 40% of current smokers are ambivalent about quitting (43). These smokers have given serious thought to giving up smoking but are not yet ready to commit to quitting. About 20% of current smokers are intending to quit smoking in the next few months (43). Many of these patients have made a quit attempt in the past year or have taken small steps toward quitting, such as cutting down on the number of cigarettes that they smoke. Making distinctions based on readiness to change is important because, as outlined in section III.D.3., smokers who are not considering quitting appear to need different treatments than those who are ambivalent about stopping or those presently interested in stopping.

2. Diagnosing nicotine dependence

Quantifying a smoker's degree of nicotine dependence is important because highly nicotine-dependent smokers are more likely to need more intensive therapy, especially pharmacotherapy (see section III.F.). Table 2 illustrates the DSM-IV criteria for substance dependence, with examples of how they apply to nicotine dependence

(10). Although the DSM system has not been formally tested as a measure to guide therapy, it does appear to be reliable and to have prospective validity (45–47).

The Fagerstrom scale assessments (table 3), widely used in treatment studies, have proven reliability and validity (12, 48). They have been shown to predict success at stopping smoking and, more importantly, to predict which smokers especially benefit from nicotine gum or nasal spray (see section III.F.2.e.).

Several other markers of nicotine dependence have been proposed; e.g., number of cigarettes/day, time to first cigarette (an item on the Fagerstrom scale), cotinine levels, amount of withdrawal on last attempt, and number of unsuccessful quit attempts. However, with the possible exception of time to first cigarette (48), these have yet to be shown to have significant treatment utility.

In summary, both the DSM-IV and Fagerstrom scale assessments are recommended [II].

3. Motivators for and barriers to quitting

The most common reasons for trying to stop smoking are to improve health and in response to social pressure (49). The most common barriers are fear of weight gain, fear of withdrawal, and fear of failure (49). Assessment of motivators and barriers appears helpful in motivating patients and is recommended [III] (50). Exacerbation of psychiatric symptoms is likely an additional barrier for psychiatric patients (39).

4. Smoking history

Seventy percent of smokers have tried to stop in the past (27); thus, the lessons learned and patient perceptions about these prior attempts need to be assessed [III]. The more important areas to be assessed include the smoker's reasons for quitting, any change in psychiatric functioning when he or she tried to stop, cause of relapse (e.g., whether the relapse was related to withdrawal symptoms or exacerbation of a psychiatric disorder), how long he or she remained abstinent, whether he or she sought treatment before, adequacy of prior treatment in terms of dose and duration, compliance with treatment, whether he or she believed treatment helped, and his or her expectations about future treatments [III].

5. Psychosocial factors

Since social support is a major predictor of cessation (51), the smoking status (e.g., never smoked, ex-smoker, current smoker) of others in the household and close friends should be assessed [III]. If others in the household are current smokers, their willingness to quit at the same time as the patient or not to smoke in front of the patient should be determined. Whether and how others in the household and friends have supported or undermined prior quit attempts should be assessed.

6. Patient preferences

Smokers vary in their treatment preferences. Many patients have strong likes or dislikes about pharmacotherapy, group therapy, and individual therapy. Patients sometimes prefer to stop smoking on a certain date. These preferences and their basis should be elicited and should be considered when developing a treatment plan [III].

7. Nicotine/cotinine and carbon monoxide levels

Nicotine and cotinine levels can be measured in blood, saliva, and urine (52). Nicotine level can reflect smoking over the last few hours; whereas the level of cotinine, a metabolite of nicotine, is sensitive to smoking in the last 7 days and offers a better measure of total daily nicotine exposure (52). Measurement of cotinine level has been proposed to help guide nicotine replacement, but the utility of this strategy has not been well tested (53). Carbon monoxide level is usually measured by breath and reflects smoking only over the last few hours (52). The major asset of carbon monoxide level is that it is easily measured and can be used to verify cessation when patients are using nicotine replacement (52). Carbon monoxide measurement can be used to motivate cessation or reinforce abstinence, but its efficacy is unclear (54).

Patients usually are truthful about their smoking status and the number of cigarettes smoked per day (55). Thus, although the described measures show promise as helpful assessments, at present they are not necessary for evaluation of smoking cessation.

8. Overall psychiatric/general medical evaluation

Psychiatric assessment in smokers places special emphasis on screening for affective and substance use disorders because these disorders are prevalent among smokers and have been shown to interfere with smoking cessation [I] (2, 34). Smokers should also be briefly screened for the signs and symptoms of most common causes of morbidity and mortality among smokers; i.e., cardiovascular disease, lung cancer, and chronic obstructive pulmonary disease (20, 21). Among smokeless tobacco, cigar, and pipe users, mouth and upper airway cancers are the most common causes of tobacco-induced mortality, and patients should be screened for their presence (20, 21).

▶ D. PSYCHIATRIC MANAGEMENT

In this guideline, psychiatric management refers to the skills and techniques that are critical to the care of all patients with nicotine dependence (table 7), regardless of what specific techniques are used (table 8). These techniques are common to all smoking interventions and should be used with all smokers. Meta-analyses have found such techniques to increase quit rates by a factor of 1.5 to 2.0 (3, 56–58). In addition to the present guideline, several other descriptive reviews of the skills and techniques critical to smoking interventions have been published (59–67).

TABLE 7. Strategies of Psychiatric Management for Patients Who Smoke

- Assess smoking behavior, motivation to quit, motivators for and barriers to quitting
- Establish a therapeutic alliance
- Advise patient to stop
- Assist in cessation
- Arrange follow-up

TABLE 8. Recommended Treatments for Nicotine Dependence

Psychosocial Therapies	Somatic Therapies
Multicomponent behavior therapy [I]	Nicotine gum [I]
Skills training/relapse prevention [II]	Transdermal nicotine [I]
Stimulus control [II]	Nicotine gum or transdermal nicotine + behavior therapy [I]
Rapid smoking [II]	Nicotine gum + transdermal nicotine [II]
Self-help materials [II]	Clonidine [II]
	Nicotine nasal spray [II]

1. Establishing a therapeutic alliance

Nicotine dependence is a chronic relapsing disorder; e.g., most smokers require 5–7 attempts before they finally quit for good (27). Many patients don't realize it usually takes several attempts to stop smoking, and they will need to be remotivated to attempt to quit after a failure [II] (61). Because of this, it is important to establish a therapeutic relationship such that the patient will return to the psychiatrist for subsequent quit attempts, if necessary (61).

Advice is best given in a nonjudgmental, empathic, supportive manner [III] (39, 61). No studies have been conducted to test whether confrontational styles of interventions used in treating other drug dependencies are useful with smoking. In patients with a present or past psychiatric disorder, it is important to convey the message that simply having a psychiatric disorder is not a reason not to make a quit attempt [II] (63, 68).

2. The treatment setting

Treatment best occurs in a system that encourages cessation (61). The psychiatrist should consider making his or her worksite smoke-free (61, 69). Achieving this on psychiatric inpatient units may be especially important, as discussed later in section IV.C.3.a.

3. Initial interventions

a) Increasing motivation and readiness to change

Smokers who are not ready to stop or are ambivalent about stopping smoking are given motivational interventions such as personalized information and feedback on the risks of smoking that are particular to the individual patient [III] (39). If feelings of demoralization are uncovered, they can be addressed by informing the patient that even the most committed smokers make several quit attempts before they are finally successful [III]. Revisiting smoking cessation at periodic intervals, especially when smoking-related illnesses (e.g., bronchitis) or other special situations (e.g., pregnancy, child with asthma) occur, can sometimes motivate smokers to consider quitting [II]. Documenting smoking status in the medical record may help to facilitate such follow-up.

Smokers may express negative feelings or fears about quitting. Problem solving around these fears appears helpful [III]. Clarification and legitimation of their feelings and expressions of support and respect also may be helpful [III]. It is useful to explore the smoker's reasons for smoking as well [III]. Smokers who become chronically ambivalent may benefit from encouragement to take small steps toward action, such as reducing the number of cigarettes they smoke or trying to quit for just 24 hours [III]. The psychiatrist supports self-efficacy by identifying and praising past behavioral change and encouraging the use of strategies effective in the past. Finally, and most importantly, no matter what the smoker's level of motivation, direct advice to stop smoking should be given [I].

Strategies such as those mentioned have been formalized in the stages of change and motivational enhancement models. There are only a few studies verifying the efficacy of providing advice for smoking cessation based on stages of change (70). Although motivational enhancement therapy appears to be effective for alcohol dependence, its effectiveness with nicotine dependence has not been tested. On the other hand, clinical experience indicates that these approaches may be useful [III].

b) Initial intervention for patients who wish to stop

The most widely used initial interventions are the National Cancer Institute's 4 *As* strategies based on smokers seen in general medical settings. The program consists of four steps, or four *As* (61):

- *Ask* and record smoking status (covered in section III.C.).
- *Advise* to stop: Clear direct advice to stop smoking is essential. It is best to elicit a personal reason to stop smoking from the patient. One of the best ways to elicit such reasons is to ask if the patient has thought about stopping before and why he or she was interested in stopping on the most recent occasion.
- *Assist* the patient in addressing cessation: The psychiatrist should elicit a commitment to quit. If a specific quit date is agreed upon, the psychiatrist should offer treatments at that time or immediately before the quit date. If the patient is not ready to make a commitment to a quit date, the psychiatrist should plan to readdress smoking at a later date, encourage the patient to reconsider, and offer to help if the patient changes his or her mind. In addition, the psychiatrist should give written materials focused on either motivating the patient to make a quit attempt or suggesting tips on how to make the cessation attempt successful.
- *Arrange* follow-up: If the patient is attempting smoking cessation, the psychiatrist or the psychiatrist's staff should call or see the patient 1–3 days after the quit date. Waiting 7–10 days after the quit date is usually too long, as many patients relapse in the first few days after the quit date (13).

Brief advice by the physician based on protocols similar to the National Cancer Institute approach typically doubles quit rates from approximately 5% to 10% [I] (3, 56–58, 71, 72). Advice from nonphysicians is also effective (3, 58), and advice from multiple sources is more effective (3, 58). Although not tested, brief advice is probably less successful in those psychiatric patients who have poor self-esteem and a more chaotic social, environmental, and psychologic status. Nevertheless, such brief advice from the psychiatrist and other psychiatric personnel (e.g., nurses, social workers) is a recommended treatment because it is a base therapy upon which other therapies can be added as needed [I].

4. Educating about nicotine dependence and its treatment

Many smokers don't realize their smoking may be a form of nicotine dependence (11). Key points to convey to patients include: a) the large majority of smokers try multiple times before they finally quit, but with persistence half of all smokers quit; b) the nature (see table 4) and duration (4 weeks or longer) of true withdrawal symptoms; c) nicotine withdrawal can be relieved with nicotine replacement; and d) most smokers fail early on, but if the smoker is able to remain abstinent for 3 months, relapse is unlikely [III] (61).

5. Timing of cessation attempt

The timing of the cessation attempt is based on the patient's readiness to change (see section III.D.3.b.) and the psychiatrist's evaluation of whether the patient's psychiatric status is sufficiently stable [III] (68). Thus, cessation of smoking would likely not be recommended when the patient is exhibiting psychiatric symptoms but could be recommended when symptoms have abated and maintenance psychotherapy or pharmacotherapy is underway [II] (68).

Since smoking cessation can induce withdrawal symptoms that could interfere with psychiatric diagnosis and treatment and since cessation can change the blood levels of several psychiatric medications (tables 4 and 5) (8), it may be best to recommend cessation when no major changes in the treatment of a psychiatric disorder are underway [III] (68). If cessation has to be delayed, the psychiatrist should be sure to keep cessation on the treatment goal list to address at a later time [I].

On the other hand, sometimes smoking cessation may be integrated into the lifestyle changes that are a part of certain psychiatric treatment (e.g., during cessation of alcohol use) (see section V.A.1.). Also, admission to a smoke-free inpatient unit can be used to motivate a cessation attempt. Finally, intervention is indicated if the patient has recently been diagnosed with a smoking-related illness, as smokers with such illnesses generally have higher success rates (49, 73) (see section V.B.1.).

6. Abrupt versus gradual cessation

Most patients use and most clinicians recommend abrupt cessation of smoking rather than gradual reduction (74). Gradual reduction has been thought to be less successful because patients appear to have difficulty achieving further reductions once smoking 5–10 cigarettes per day (53). On the other hand, most of the scientific data available suggest no difference in the outcomes of abrupt versus gradual cessation (3, 53, 56, 75); thus, patient preferences to use gradual reduction should be respected [III]. However, with a gradual approach, patients should be advised to set a date by which they will completely stop [III] and not to use nicotine replacement therapy until they have stopped using cigarettes [II].

7. Dealing with weight gain concerns

One of the most common fears around smoking cessation is weight gain (76). On average, smokers weigh 2–3 kg less than persons who have never smoked and when they stop smoking they gain weight until they are similar in weight to those who have never smoked (35). The large majority of smokers gain weight over the first few months postcessation, but many later lose much or all of this weight. Women who are already trying to keep weight off gain the most (77).

Even though the health benefits of stopping smoking clearly outweigh the health risks of weight gain (35), fear of weight gain is a major deterrent to smoking cessation, especially among women (77). However, weight gain after stopping smoking does not cause relapse to smoking (17). In fact, concentrated efforts to control weight gain by dieting during abstinence increase, not decrease, relapse back to smoking (78, 79). This may be because trying to stop smoking and trying to diet at the same time is just too difficult. Rather than dieting, increasing physical activity upon cessation, learning healthy eating strategies, or convincing the smoker to tolerate a moderate amount of weight gain over the first 3 months and to work on losing weight later on can be recommended [III] (80). Nicotine gum, but not the nicotine patch, appears to delay weight gain and could be used to delay attempts to control weight until relapse to smoking is less likely [III] (81).

8. Advising about alcohol and caffeine use

Alcohol use is a risk factor in most studies of smoking relapse (82); thus, either diminishing alcohol intake or abstaining from alcohol is recommended [III]. Caffeine use typically does not change with cessation (17), and whether caffeine use is a risk factor for relapse is unclear (83). Smoking increases the metabolism of caffeine, and smoking cessation increases caffeine levels by 50%–60% (84). Since many of the symptoms of caffeine intoxication and nicotine withdrawal overlap (e.g., anxiety, insomnia, restlessness), reducing caffeine intake postcessation might be helpful; however, the one study to test this hypothesis was negative (84). In addition, abruptly stopping caffeine could induce a withdrawal syndrome of its own (85). In summary, with this contradictory evidence, patient preferences on whether to change caffeine intake should be respected [III].

9. Follow-up visits

The first follow-up should occur within 1–3 days after the quit date, as the majority of smokers relapse in the first few days [I] (13). The scheduling of further follow-ups should be determined by the patient's perceived need, past history of cessation, past psychiatric history, whether he or she is taking a medication whose blood level might increase with cessation (table 5), and whether he or she is taking antismoking medications that require visits to monitor side effects or plan tapering [III].

At follow-up, the psychiatrist assesses whether the patient has smoked and, if so, the number of cigarettes smoked per day [II] (61). The psychiatrist also assesses the severity of withdrawal symptoms, the onset of any psychiatric symptoms or alcohol/drug use, how the patient dealt with high-urge situations, any medication side effects, etc., and tailors the treatment accordingly [II] (61). Most, but not all, studies suggest that brief follow-ups (including telephone calls) increase quit rates [II] (57, 58).

10. Dealing with slips and relapses

Since smoking even one cigarette during a cessation attempt very often portends a full-blown relapse (86), reports of slips should prompt immediate planning around either changes in behavior therapy (e.g., discuss ways to avoid or cope with situation that led to slip) or pharmacotherapy (e.g., increase dose, change medications) [III]. If the patient has fully relapsed, the psychiatrist should praise the patient for even limited success [III]. The patient and the psychiatrist should then discuss what was learned with this quit attempt and when the patient would like to think about trying again [III]. Most patients who relapse continue to be interested in stopping smoking; thus, the psychiatrist should discuss setting a time to reconsider another cessation attempt [III].

E. SPECIFIC PSYCHOSOCIAL TREATMENTS

1. Behavior therapies

a) Introduction

Behavioral therapy is based on the theory that learning processes operate in the development, maintenance, and cessation of smoking. Many of the recommendations described under psychiatric management (see section IV.A.3.) are actually based on the principles of behavioral therapy. The following sections briefly describe formal behavioral techniques for cessation. For more information, the reader is referred to several recent descriptive (51, 62, 65, 67, 71, 72, 74, 87–91) and meta-analytic (3, 57) reviews of behavior therapy.

b) Goals

Major goals of behavior therapy are to change the antecedents (including cognitions) to smoking, to reinforce nonsmoking, and to teach skills to avoid smoking in high-risk situations.

c) Efficacy

There are over 100 controlled prospective studies verifying the efficacy of behavior therapy (57, 71, 72, 92). Typically, behavioral therapies are a multimodal package of several of the specific treatments described later in this guideline. In most reviews/meta-analyses, 6-month quit rates with behavior therapy packages are 20%–25%, and behavior therapy typically increases quit rates twofold over control groups (3, 56, 57, 71, 72, 90, 92). Given this large database of efficacy, multimodal behavior therapy is a recommmended first-line therapy [I].

d) Specific techniques

Although multimodal behavior therapies have been validated, much less research is available on the efficacy of the individual techniques in the behavioral therapy package. The following sections review each technique and indicate those that are recommmended treatments.

(1) Skills training/relapse prevention

Skills training, relapse prevention, and their variants (problem solving, coping skills, and training in stress management) have patients anticipate a large number of situations or processes that are likely to lead to urges to smoke or to prompt a slip (e.g., a party, an argument, a thought). Early on in cessation, it is often best to avoid high-risk situations (91). Later, patients plan strategies to cope with these situations. Behavioral coping includes removing oneself from the situation, substituting other behaviors (e.g., exercising, taking a walk), or utilizing skills to manage the triggers (e.g., refusal skills, assertiveness, time management). Cognitive coping includes identifying maladaptive thoughts, challenging them, and substituting more effective thought patterns (e.g., reminding oneself of why it is important to stop smoking or that the urge will pass). Another target is to prevent the abstinence violation effect that transforms a slip to a relapse (e.g., not viewing a slip as a catastrophe).

The results of individual trials specifically testing relapse prevention have been mixed (91, 93). However, two recent meta-analyses concluded problem solving/skills training/relapse prevention significantly increases cessation rates (3, 56); thus, skills training/relapse prevention is a recommended component treatment [II].

(2) Stimulus control

Stimulus control usually includes self-monitoring prior to a quit attempt to facilitate identification of stimuli associated with smoking (74). Stimulus control also includes initially removing or avoiding cues associated with smoking to reduce urges to smoke. Patients are encouraged to discard all cigarettes, remove lighters, ashtrays, and matches, and avoid other smokers and situations associated with smoking.

Studies of whether stimulus control is effective on its own have produced mixed results (3). However, stimulus control appears to be a very helpful procedure in multicomponent treatment in that it serves as the base for many behavioral techniques (e.g., relapse prevention); thus, stimulus control is a recommended treatment component of behavior therapy [II].

(3) Aversive therapy

The rationale of aversive therapy is to make smoking more aversive and less reinforcing by inducing mild nicotine intoxication symptoms of nausea, dizziness, etc., when the patient smokes. The original version of this type of treatment was rapid smoking, in which patients inhale cigarette smoke every few seconds (71, 72). Many well-controlled studies of rapid smoking have been conducted, and most reviews and meta-analyses have concluded rapid smoking is efficacious (3, 51, 56, 71, 72, 74, 92). Compliance with rapid smoking, as with all aversive therapies, is difficult, and a strong therapeutic alliance or a priori contracts may be used to improve compliance [III]. Other, less-aversive versions of therapy include focused smoking, in which smokers smoke at a regulated rate, and smoke holding and rapid puffing, in which patients smoke rapidly but do not inhale. Whether these less-aversive techniques are as effective as rapid smoking is debatable (51, 71, 72, 74, 92).

Although most therapists no longer use rapid smoking because of health and compliance concerns, rapid smoking appears to be safe in healthy patients (51, 71, 72, 74) and those with medical disorders may be able to participate with medical supervision [II]. In summary, rapid smoking is a recommended component of behavior therapy for those smokers willing to comply [II].

(4) Social support
Although many studies indicate social support for stopping smoking is a predictor of cessation, attempts to harness social support as an intervention have been mostly unsuccessful (51, 72, 74). Buddy systems, increasing cohesion in group therapy, and teaching spouses to reinforce not smoking have not consistently increased quit rates (3, 51, 72, 74). The lack of success of such interventions is likely related to their failure to influence the level of support. A recent study that was successful in enhancing levels of social support did enhance smoking cessation outcome (94). Most clinicians and programs address social support because lack of social support appears to undermine cessation attempts (95). In summary, social support lacks sufficient evidence to be recommended but is a promising treatment.

(5) Contingency management
In this procedure, smokers are either reinforced for not smoking with the presentation of some reward or punished for smoking by the loss of some reward. For example, patients place a deposit that is either refunded contingent on not smoking or forfeited for smoking, using carbon monoxide level as an objective measure of smoking. Contingency contracting is effective while the contingency is in place, but whether this effect persists after the contingency is removed is unclear (51, 72, 74). Thus far, procedures to wean smokers from such contingency procedures have not been developed. Meta-analysis of long-term studies does not support the efficacy of contingency contracting with smoking (3). In summary, contingency contracting lacks sufficient evidence to be recommended.

(6) Cue exposure
Cue exposure involves repeatedly exposing patients to real or imagined situations that evoke potent urges to smoke in an attempt to extinguish the ability of these situations to evoke urges to smoke. Four randomized, controlled trials of cue exposure have been published (96–99), and meta-analysis does not support the efficacy of cue exposure (3). In summary, cue exposure lacks sufficient evidence to be recommended.

(7) Nicotine fading
In this procedure, patients gradually reduce the nicotine yield of their cigarette. This technique should not be confused with reducing the number of cigarettes per day, which was covered in section III.D.6. With nicotine fading, some smokers increase the number of cigarettes or smoke each cigarette more intensely, but overall nicotine consumption is significantly reduced (51, 71, 72, 74, 90). The evidence that this treatment increases quit rates is mixed (51, 71, 72, 90), and meta-analyses do not support its ef-

ficacy (3, 56). In summary, nicotine fading lacks sufficient evidence to be recommended.

(8) Relaxation

Relaxation is often taught to manage relapse situations associated with anxiety. Although often used in multicomponent programs, relaxation itself usually has not been shown to increase smoking cessation (51, 71, 72, 74, 90), and meta-analysis does not support its efficacy (3). In summary, relaxation lacks sufficient evidence to be recommended.

(9) Physiological feedback

The rationale for this procedure is that giving patients immediate and concrete positive feedback of the benefits of not smoking by showing them that their carbon monoxide level declines with cessation will reinforce not smoking. Controlled trials of the efficacy of such feedback have produced mixed results (55, 56), and the one meta-analysis did not support its efficacy (3). Thus, physiological feedback lacks sufficient evidence to be recommended.

e) Implementation

Both group and individual formats have been used for behavioral therapies for smoking cessation (57, 58, 74). Groups are often used to increase social support for stopping smoking, and individual therapy is used to tailor treatment to the specific problems of the individual smoker. Meta-analyses suggest little difference in outcomes across group versus individual therapy (3, 57, 58). Thus, patient preferences and availability of specific treatments should be considered when recommending group versus individual therapy [III].

Since two-thirds of patients relapse in the first week (13, 86), most treatment is optimally timed before or very soon after cessation [I]. In most cessation programs, several sessions occur over the few weeks immediately prior to and immediately after the quit date (74).

The most common providers of behavior therapy are voluntary organizations (e.g., the American Lung Association), wellness programs, or health educators/psychologists in health care organizations (100). A major problem is that, although clearly effective, behavior therapy is often not available to patients or available only intermittently, is costly, and is not integrated into the health care system (60, 100, 101). As a result, many of those motivated to quit forego behavior therapy (60, 101).

Although recent studies of matching particular behavior therapies to particular types of smokers have been published (102, 103), at present there are insufficient data to recommend specific matching strategies. Psychiatric patients, including those with substance abuse/dependence, are more likely to benefit from behavior therapy because of their high incidence of psychosocial problems, poor coping skills and, often, past history of benefit from such therapy (68).

2. Self-help materials

The major goals of self-help materials are to increase motivation and impart cessation skills. Written manuals are the most common form of self-help material, although recently computer and video versions have been developed (87, 104). Most self-help materials are behaviorally oriented. Whether self-help interventions used without additional contact or support increase smoking cessation is debatable (14, 57, 71, 72, 74, 87, 92). Reactive telephone counseling via a hot-line appears to increase cessation when added to other self-help interventions (104–106), and meta-analyses suggest a small positive effect (3, 57). Self-help materials appear to be more effective in patients who are less nicotine-dependent (107, 108) and more motivated (87). Use of multiple modes of therapy (e.g., written materials plus phone contact) appears to enhance the effectiveness of self-help (58, 87, 104). Tailoring materials to the specific needs and concerns of each patient also appears helpful (70, 108). In summary, self-help materials are recommended as part of a behavioral therapy package [II].

3. Educational and supportive groups

The goals of educational and supportive groups are to teach patients the harms of smoking and benefits of cessation and to provide group reinforcement for not smoking. The efficacy of education and group support in themselves (i.e., without the behavioral techniques listed above) is debatable (3, 71, 72, 109). On the other hand, the clinical experience of the Work Group on Nicotine Dependence and other clinicians is that group support is important for some patients; thus, educational and supportive groups are considered a promising therapy [III].

4. Hypnosis

The usual goal of hypnotherapy for smoking cessation is to implant nonconscious suggestions that will deter smoking; e.g., smoking will be unpleasant. Three meta-analyses reported hypnosis was efficacious (56, 57, 92); however, the most recent meta-analysis did not (3). In addition, several quantitative reviews concluded the efficacy of hypnosis was unproven (51, 62, 74). Much of this discordance is because most hypnosis trials have poor methodologies and were excluded from consideration in some meta-analyses or reviews. Given the conflicting evidence, hypnosis is rated as a promising treatment [III].

5. Other therapies

The goal of 12-step programs for smoking cessation (as modified from Alcoholics Anonymous) is to have the smoker accept that he or she is powerless over smoking and work through 12 goals (or steps) that help break down denial. Several organizations have outlined how to apply the 12-step model to smoking, and a national self-help organization—Nicotine Anonymous—exists (110). However, there are no scientific tests of 12-step programs for smoking cessation.

Exercise might be helpful as it is thought to increase self-esteem, relieve stress, emphasize the new role of an abstinent smoker as a healthy person, and help manage weight gain. Controlled evaluations of exercise for smoking cessation have produced mixed results, but more recent studies have been positive (111, 112). The major difficulty has been poor compliance with high-intensity exercise regimens. Although recent research indicates psychological benefit occurs with low-intensity activity, whether increasing low-level activity might be helpful in smoking cessation has not been tested. In summary, exercise/activity is a promising therapy.

Biofeedback, family therapy, interpersonal therapy, and psychodynamic therapy have been used with other drug dependencies (38) and might be applicable to smoking cessation; however, there are either no or only a few descriptions of adapting these to treat smoking. In summary, none of these treatments have sufficient evidence to be recommended. (Acupuncture is covered with somatic therapies in the next section.)

F. SOMATIC TREATMENTS

1. Introduction

Pharmacotherapies can be divided into replacement therapy, antagonist therapy, therapies to make drug intake aversive, and nonnicotine medications that mimic nicotine effects (113, 114). Nonmedication somatic therapies include acupuncture and devices. The following are brief descriptions of these therapies. For more information, the reader is referred to recent descriptive (51, 56, 62, 67, 71, 72, 101, 113–123) and meta-analytic (3, 57, 92, 115, 124–129) reviews.

2. Nicotine replacement therapy

a) Goals

The goal of nicotine replacement therapy is to relieve withdrawal, which will allow the patient to focus on habit and conditioning factors when attempting to stop smoking. After the acute withdrawal period, nicotine replacement therapy is gradually reduced so that little withdrawal should occur.

b) Description of products

(1) Nicotine gum

Nicotine ingested through the gastrointestinal tract is extensively metabolized on first pass through the liver (42). Nicotine gum (nicotine polacrilex) avoids this problem via buccal absorption (42). The gum contains 2 or 4 mg of nicotine that can be released from a resin by chewing (113). The original recommendation was to use one piece of 2-mg gum every 15–30 minutes as needed for craving. More recent work suggests scheduled dosing (e.g., 1 piece of 2-mg gum/hour), and 4-mg gum for highly nicotine-dependent smokers is more effective (62, 113). The original recommended duration of treatment was 3 months. Many experts believe longer treatment is more effective; however, the two trials of longer duration produced contradictory results (41).

Nicotine absorption from the gum peaks 30 minutes after beginning to use the gum (42). Venous nicotine levels from 2- and 4-mg gum are about one-third and two-thirds, respectively, of the steady-state (i.e., between cigarettes) levels of nicotine achieved with cigarette smoking (42). Nicotine via cigarettes is absorbed directly into the arterial circulation; thus, arterial levels from smoking are 5–10 times higher than those from the 2- and 4-mg gums (130). Absorption of nicotine in the buccal mucosa is decreased by an acidic environment; thus, patients should not use beverages (e.g., coffee, soda, juice) immediately before, during, or after nicotine gum use (130). Nicotine gum (2- and 4-mg doses) has recently been approved as an over-the-counter medication.

(2) Nicotine patch

The four transdermal formulations take advantage of ready absorption of nicotine across the skin (115, 131, 132). Three of the patches are for 24-hour use and one is for 16-hour (waking) use. Starting doses are 21–22 mg/24-hour patch and 15 mg/16-hour patch. Patches are applied daily each morning beginning upon cessation of smoking. Nicotine via patches is slowly absorbed so that on the first day venous nicotine levels peak 6–10 hours after administration. Thereafter, nicotine levels remain fairly steady with a decline from peak to trough of 25% to 40% with 24-hour patches (131). Nicotine levels obtained with the use of patches are typically half those obtained by smoking (131).

After 4–6 weeks patients are usually tapered to a middle dose (e.g., 14 mg/24 hours or 10 mg/16 hours) and then again in 2–4 weeks to the lowest dose (7 mg/24 hours or 5 mg/16 hours). Most, but not all, studies indicate abrupt cessation of the use of patches often causes no significant withdrawal; thus, tapering may not be necessary (133). The recommended total duration of treatment is usually 6–12 weeks (115, 133). Two nicotine patches are now available over the counter. The treatment schedule for one of these patches is now 6 weeks only with no tapering.

(3) Nicotine nasal spray

Nicotine nasal spray is a nicotine solution in a nasal spray bottle similar to those used with antihistamines (133–135). This treatment is likely to be marketed in the United States in 1996. Nasal sprays produce droplets that average about 1 mg per administration. This formulation produces a more rapid rise in nicotine levels than does nicotine gum; the rise in nicotine levels produced by nicotine spray falls between those produced by nicotine gum and cigarettes. Peak nicotine levels occur within 10 minutes, and venous nicotine levels are about two-thirds those of between-cigarette levels (136). Smokers are to use the product ad-lib up to 30 times/day for 12 weeks, including a tapering period.

(4) Nicotine inhalers

These are plugs of nicotine placed inside hollow cigarette-like rods. The plugs produce a nicotine vapor when warm air is passed through them (137–139). Absorption from nicotine inhaler is primarily buccal rather than respiratory (140). More recent versions of inhalers produce venous nicotine levels that rise more quickly than with nicotine gum but less quickly than with nicotine nasal spray, with nicotine blood levels of about one-third that of between-cigarette levels (141). The inhaler is to be used ad-lib for about 12 weeks.

(5) Other nicotine delivery devices

Nicotine lozenges for buccal absorption are available in some countries, but not in the United States.

(6) Lobeline

Lobeline is a nontobacco drug that shares tolerance with nicotine on several measures (142). It has been included in several over-the-counter antismoking medications. The pharmacokinetics of lobeline in humans has not been reported.

c) Efficacy

(1) Nicotine withdrawal

Nicotine replacement therapy is often used solely for the purpose of relieving withdrawal symptoms in outpatient or inpatient settings. Many studies have shown nicotine replacement therapy decreases withdrawal symptoms in outpatient settings (16, 17). Anxiety, anger/irritability, depression, difficulty concentrating, and impatience are usually relieved by nicotine replacement; whereas insomnia and weight gain are not consistently decreased (16, 17). This is true for nicotine gum, patch, spray, and inhaler. Nicotine gum appears to be more likely to delay weight gain than nicotine patch (101). Nicotine gum at 2-mg ad-lib appears less likely to reduce craving than nicotine patch or nasal spray; however, this may be a dose-related issue, as the 4-mg dose appears to better reduce craving (143). Whether nicotine gum, patch, nasal spray, or inhaler is better at relieving withdrawal is unknown. Higher doses of nicotine replacement therapy only marginally decrease withdrawal symptoms (101). Whether nicotine inhaler or lobeline decreases withdrawal symptoms is unclear (138, 144).

(2) Long-term abstinence with adjunctive psychosocial therapy

Eleven meta-analyses of over 50 studies that included a psychosocial therapy (usually behavior therapy) along with nicotine replacement all conclude that nicotine gum and nicotine patch increase long-term quit rates by a factor of 1.6–2.4 (3, 56–58, 101, 115, 124, 126, 127, 133, 145, 146). The three studies of nicotine nasal spray reported increases in abstinence in the same range (135, 147, 148). The one study of nicotine inhaler found a tripling of the quit rate (138). Lobeline has not been shown to be effective (113, 123, 149). Higher doses of nicotine gum are more effective in more nicotine-dependent patients (115, 127). Whether higher doses of nicotine patch are more efficacious is debatable (53).

(3) Long-term abstinence with minimal adjunctive therapy

Often, interventions for smoking cessation consist of brief advice (10 minutes) plus a prescription for nicotine replacement. Although early reviews indicated nicotine gum was not more effective than placebo in this setting, more recent meta-analyses indicate nicotine gum increases quit rates by a factor of around 1.5 (3, 57, 58, 92, 101, 115, 124, 126, 127). In addition, controlled studies have found that nicotine gum doubles quit rates even when given with no adjunctive therapy; i.e., in an over-the-counter setting (FDA Advisory Panel Hearings, Sept. 29, 1995). The nicotine patch is clearly effective when given with minimal therapy and doubles quit rates (3, 34, 56, 101, 115, 127, 133, 146). Both the 24- and 16-hour patch double quit rates even in an over-the-counter setting (FDA Advisory Panel Hearing, March 17, 1996). Finally, although nicotine gum and patch are efficacious in these settings, overall quit rates are low (e.g., 10%–20%). Nicotine nasal spray, nicotine inhaler, and lobeline have not been tested in this setting.

(4) Patch plus gum

Three controlled trials indicate using nicotine gum (2 mg) ad-lib in addition to a nicotine patch increases quit rates over either therapy used alone (119). Such combined therapy does not appear to significantly increase side effects; thus, this is a recommended treatment [II].

(5) Summary of recommendations

Nicotine patches and nicotine gum are recommended initial pharmacotherapies for smoking cessation [I]. Nicotine nasal spray is also recommended but because it has a smaller empirical base and appears to have significant side effects (see section III.F.2.d.3), it is recommended as a treatment for those who have failed to stop smoking using the nicotine patch or gum [II]. Because of a limited database, the nicotine inhaler is classified as a promising treatment. Lobeline lacks sufficient evidence of efficacy to be recommended.

d) Side effects

(1) Nicotine gum

Major side effects from nicotine gum are very rare and side effects rarely deter use (24). Minor side effects are of mechanical origin (e.g., difficulty chewing, sore jaw) or of local pharmacological origin (e.g., burning in mouth, throat irritation). Tolerance develops to most side effects over the first week (24). Education about proper use of the gum (e.g., do not chew too vigorously) decreases side effects (24). Originally, some disorders were listed as contraindications to use of nicotine gum (e.g., cardio-vascular disease, pregnancy, hypertension), but given that nicotine blood levels are much lower with nicotine gum than with cigarettes, these contraindications have been dropped (24, 25).

The only psychiatric/psychological side effect of nicotine gum is the continuance of nicotine dependence (15). Abrupt cessation of nicotine gum can produce withdrawal symptoms similar to, but less intensive than, that from cigarettes (15). Gradual reduction in the use of nicotine gum usually produces no or very minor symptoms (15). About 10%–20% of those who stop smoking with the help of nicotine gum continue to use nicotine gum for 9 months or more, but few use the gum longer than 2 years (41). There are several lines of evidence that most long-term use is not dependence. For example, all but 1%–2% of smokers eventually stop gum use, the amount of gum use at long-term follow-up is minimal (usually 12 mg/day), the amount of gum use decreases over time, and weaning off the gum usually requires only education and reassurance even in long-term users (15, 41, 150). Instead, long-term use appears to most often represent the patient's desire to extend the duration of therapy for fear of returning to smoking if nicotine gum use is stopped. Harmful effects of long-term use of nicotine gum have not been studied but are unlikely given the absence of exposure to carcinogens or carbon monoxide and the much lower levels of nicotine from nicotine gum than from cigarettes (24, 25).

(2) Nicotine patch

Significant medical problems with nicotine patches have not been found (24, 25, 115, 151). The most common minor side effects are skin reactions (50%), insomnia and increased or vivid dreams (15% with 24-hour patches), and nausea (5%–10%) (24, 115, 151). Tolerance to these side effects usually develops within a week. Rotation of patch sites decreases skin irritation. Although debatable, insomnia reported in the first week postcessation appears to be mostly due to nicotine withdrawal rather than the nicotine patch itself (152). A 24-hour patch can be removed before bedtime to determine if the insomnia is due to the nicotine patch. Insomnia usually abates without treatment after 4–7 days. Although one series of case reports suggested concomitant use of cigarettes and nicotine patches caused myocardial infarction, later analyses and prospective empirical studies in smokers with active heart disease indicated this prior report was incorrect (23). Abrupt cessation of the nicotine patch does not appear to produce significant withdrawal symptoms, and long-term use has not been a problem (151).

(3) Nicotine nasal spray

The major side effects from nicotine nasal spray are nasal and throat irritation, rhinitis, sneezing, coughing, and watering eyes (135, 147, 148). One or more of these occur in over three-quarters of the patients. Long-term nasal problems from use of nicotine nasal spray is usually not a problem (147). Whether abrupt cessation of nasal spray produces withdrawal has not been studied. Nicotine nasal spray does appear to have some dependence liability, as indicated by the fact that in some studies, several patients who quit smoking with nicotine nasal spray continued to use it for long periods (147).

(4) Nicotine inhaler

No serious medical side effects have been reported with nicotine inhalers (137). About half of subjects report throat irritation or coughing (138). Whether some patients use nicotine inhalers for long periods or have withdrawal upon cessation of inhaler use has not been tested.

(5) Lobeline

Major side effects, including abuse/dependence, from lobeline have not been reported (149).

e) Implementation

(1) Indications

How to decide to whom to give nicotine replacement therapy is debatable (48, 60, 88, 101, 115, 153, 154). Nicotine gum (especially the 4-mg dose) and nicotine nasal spray are more helpful in highly nicotine-dependent patients (as measured by the Fagerstrom scale); however, even patients who are less dependent appear to obtain some benefit from nicotine gum (12). The package insert for nicotine patches states they are to be used only by those who smoke 15 cigarettes per day or more. No such minimum is given for nicotine gum. On the other hand, nicotine patches are beneficial to both highly and less nicotine-dependent smokers (12, 115, 127, 151). Whether highly nicotine-dependent smokers would most benefit from nicotine gum, patch, or nasal spray has not been tested (113).

Number of cigarettes per day, presence of significant withdrawal during prior quit attempts, and time to first cigarette have also been proposed as indicators for the use of nicotine replacement therapy, but there are no data on the utility of these indicators. Some have suggested that nicotine replacement therapy be used only if the patient is enrolled in behavior therapy; however, the data clearly show that nicotine replacement therapy is effective in the absence of behavior therapy (see section III.F.2.c.3).

In summary, nicotine replacement should be considered in all smokers who have seriously tried to quit on their own and failed [III]. Use of nicotine replacement in smokers with cardiovascular disease or who are pregnant is discussed in sections V.B.2. and V.C.3., respectively. Although nicotine gum and patches are available over the counter, psychiatrists still need to be involved in their use by encouraging use when appropriate, supplementing package instructions, and providing adjunctive psychiatric management and, when appropriate, psychosocial and other pharmacological therapies.

(2) Pretreatment evaluation

Some have suggested precessation cotinine level is a useful benchmark to examine the percent of nicotine replaced by nicotine medication therapy and thus make decisions on whether higher doses should be used. Whether this improves treatment is controversial (53).

(3) Length of treatment

Most treatment optimally lasts 4–6 weeks before tapering [III]. Some have advocated longer-term use of nicotine replacement therapy and even a nicotine maintenance program. Two prospective trials differed in whether longer treatment with nicotine gum produced higher abstinence rates (155, 156). A recent meta-analysis of nicotine patches did not find that longer treatment was associated with higher quit rates (133).

3. Antagonists

a) Goals

The goal of antagonist therapy is to prevent cigarettes from producing positive reinforcing and subjective effects.

b) Mecamylamine

Mecamylamine is a noncompetitive blocker of both central nervous system and peripheral nicotinic receptors (124, 157, 158) that decreases the positive subjective effects from cigarettes (157, 158). When mecamylamine is given to smokers who are not trying to stop smoking, they initially increase their smoking in an attempt to overcome the blockade produced by mecamylamine (157, 158). Mecamylamine does not precipitate withdrawal in humans, perhaps because it is an indirect blocker (157, 158).

Early studies suggested some short-term efficacy with mecamylamine, but the high doses used produced significant dropout rates because of side effects (157, 158). Side effects included abdominal cramps, constipation, dry mouth, and headaches. Based on a theory that combined blockade and agonist therapy might be beneficial (159), a recent study combined low doses of mecamylamine and nicotine patch and produced a significant increase in long-term efficacy with few side effects (160).

Antagonists have not been effective in opioid drug dependence because of compliance problems (161). Smokers tend to be more compliant than opioid abusers; thus, nicotine antagonists might be effective. Behavioral programs to insure compliance similar to those used with alcohol and cocaine dependence might also be helpful (161). In summary, mecamylamine lacks sufficient evidence to be recommended but is considered promising.

c) Naltrexone

Naltrexone is a long-acting form of the opioid antagonist naloxone. The rationale for using naltrexone for smoking cessation is that the performance-enhancing and other positive effects of nicotine may be opioid mediated (162). Most, but not all, studies have found that naltrexone increases smoking (interpreted again as an attempt to overcome blockade) (123, 163). There are no data on naltrexone as a cessation treatment nor on what happens to cigarette use in alcoholics treated with naltrexone. The few side effects from naltrexone include elevated liver enzymes, nausea, and blockade of analgesia from narcotic pain relievers (123). In summary, at this time, naltrexone lacks sufficient evidence to be recommended.

4. Medications that make intake aversive

a) Goals

Medications in this class produce unpleasant events when the patient ingests the medication. Disulfiram treatment for alcoholism (164) is the most widely known example of this class.

b) Silver acetate

This medication combines with sulfides in tobacco smoke to produce a bad taste. Silver acetate has been tested as a gum and as a pill; neither form has consistently been shown to be effective (3, 56, 123, 149). In fact, the FDA recently pulled silver acetate from over-the-counter sales because of lack of efficacy (149). As with disulfiram, compliance appears to be quite poor; thus this treatment might be effective if used in conjunction with a behavioral compliance program. The major side effect of concern is argyrism (silver poisoning), which produces discoloration of skin. This appears to be very rare at the doses used for smoking cessation (149). In summary, silver acetate lacks sufficient evidence to be recommended.

5. Medications that mimic nicotinic effects

a) Clonidine

Clonidine is a postsynaptic α_2 agonist that dampens sympathetic activity originating at the locus ceruleus (123, 125, 165). It appears to have some efficacy for alcohol and opioid withdrawal and thus was tried with nicotine withdrawal as well (123, 125). Several clinical trials used oral or transdermal clonidine in doses of 0.1–0.4 mg/day for 2–6 weeks with and without behavior therapy. Three meta-analytic reviews reported clonidine doubles quit rates (56, 125, 165), but a fourth disagreed (3).

The most common side effects of clonidine are dry mouth, sedation, and constipation (165). Postural hypotension, rebound hypertension, and depression are rare with smoking cessation treatment (165). Several studies have suggested clonidine is more effective in women than in men; however, many studies have failed to find this association (165).

Although clonidine appears to increase quit rates similar to that of nicotine replacement therapy, the quantity and quality of the scientific studies on clonidine are less than that for nicotine replacement therapy. Nevertheless, clonidine may be an alternative for smokers who prefer not to receive nicotine and for smokers who have failed nicotine replacement therapy [II].

b) Anxiolytics

Anxiety is a prominent symptom of nicotine withdrawal (16). In addition, smoking decreases some measures of anxiety and may reduce stress-induced anxiety (166); thus, temporarily replacing the anxiolytic effects of nicotine with another medication during the first weeks of cessation might make cessation easier. Diazepam appears to decrease tobacco withdrawal, but in a well-conducted long-term clinical trial, diazepam did not increase abstinence (123). β Blockers can act as anxiolytics. Placebo-controlled trials of metoprolol, oxprenolol, and propranolol have not found that they decrease craving or increase abstinence rates (123). Older trials found that the non-benzodiazepine anxiolytics meprobamate and hydroxyzine were not effective for smoking cessation (123). In summary, the above anxiolytics do not have sufficient evidence to be recommended.

Buspirone is a serotonergic agonist, which acts as an anxiolytic but produces minimal, if any, sedation, abuse potential, or physical dependence. Major side effects to buspirone are rare. Some short-term trials have reported that buspirone appeared to reduce nicotine withdrawal, but others have failed to find this (123). Buspirone improved short-term smoking cessation rates in unselected smokers and improved abstinence in high-anxiety smokers (123). Because of its favorable side effect profile and some evidence of efficacy, buspirone is classed as a promising therapy.

c) Antidepressants

A past history of depression and dysphoria prior to, at the onset of, or during smoking cessation predicts failure to stop smoking; thus, antidepressants might be useful in helping smokers with these problems stop smoking (2, 167). In the only published long-term clinical trials, imipramine had no effect on smoking cessation (123), but a more recent trial of nortriptyline was positive (168). Two trials with fluoxetine were completed some time ago but the results were never published or presented (123). Short-term, trials with doxepin, tryptophan, and bupropion in unselected groups of smokers have also reported promising results (123).

Many antidepressants have substantial side effects and a long delay in efficacy; thus, these treatments may not be acceptable to the general population of smokers. A more focused approach might be treatment with antidepressants prior to cessation in the 30%–40% of smokers with a past history of depression or in smokers who are dysphoric at the time of smoking cessation. In summary, antidepressants are considered a promising treatment.

d) Stimulants

The goal here is to replace the stimulant effects of nicotine (e.g., improved energy and concentration) with a medication in the first weeks of cessation. The one long-term study of a stimulant found that amphetamines did not increase abstinence (123). A recent uncontrolled trial suggests methylphenidate decreases tobacco withdrawal (169). Finally, if stimulants were found to be effective, whether dependence on the stimulant occurs would need to be examined. In summary, stimulants lack sufficient evidence to be recommended.

e) Anorectics

Anorectics were used initially to combat postcessation hunger and weight gain because these are two of the most widely cited reasons for difficulty in stopping smoking (77). Short-term trials of women with weight concerns reported that both fenfluramine and phenylpropanolamine reduced postcessation weight gain and some withdrawal symptoms and increased abstinence (123). The results are intriguing, given the data that controlling weight by adding a dieting component to a multicomponent program worsens rather than improves abstinence rates (78, 79). Fenfluramine and phenylpropanolamine have few side effects. In summary, both of these medications lack sufficient evidence to be recommended but are considered promising.

6. Sensory replacement

Black pepper extracts (170), capsaicin (171), denicotinized tobacco (172), flavorings (173), and regenerated (denicotinized) smoke (174) all decrease cigarette craving or withdrawal or substitute for the satisfaction from cigarettes in laboratory tests. A citric acid inhaler has been developed and showed some promise in two clinical trials (175, 176). As expected, this treatment has very few side effects. Since sensory treatments could be used not only as a stand-alone therapy but also as an adjunct to traditional pharmacotherapies, this appears to be a promising treatment.

7. Other medications

Sodium bicarbonate has been used to decrease the rate of urinary elimination of nicotine and thereby decrease withdrawal symptoms (123). ACTH has been used to decrease postcessation hypoglycemia (123). Anticholinergics have been used to reduce a hypothesized cholinergic rebound upon smoking cessation (123). Dextrose has been used to prevent smokers from mislabeling hunger as nicotine craving (123). Homeopathic remedies and nutritional supplements have also been proposed. For all of these treatments, the basic rationale and mechanism of action is suspect and controlled trials of long-term abstinence are lacking (123); thus, all lack sufficient evidence to be recommended.

8. Acupuncture

One common rationale for the use of acupuncture for smoking cessation is that acupuncture can release endorphins that assist in cessation. Controlled studies comparing advice versus sham acupuncture sites do not consistently show efficacy (3, 57, 177, 178); thus, this treatment lacks sufficient evidence to be recommended.

9. Devices

Filters have been used to help smokers gradually reduce the amount of smoking. Short-term studies show smokers compensate for such changes to some extent (90, 179). The few studies of the efficacy of filters are inconclusive (90, 179). A small computer has been developed that uses self-monitoring data to then program a set of times to smoke. The computer gradually eliminates cigarettes by increasing the inter-cigarette interval. There are no published controlled studies with the device. In summary, there is not sufficient evidence to recommend devices as a treatment.

▶ G. COMBINED PSYCHOSOCIAL AND SOMATIC THERAPY

The goal of combined therapy is to provide treatment for withdrawal and to concurrently develop antismoking skills. Most meta-analyses and most experimental trials indicate that, unlike other dependencies, formal psychosocial treatment is not essential to obtain benefits from somatic therapies. In other words, nicotine replacement therapy (34, 56–58, 92, 115, 124, 126, 127, 129, 133, 146) and clonidine (125, 165) increase quit rates by a factor of 1.5 to 2.0, both when given with brief advice plus follow-up (i.e., similar to psychiatric management) and when given with formal psychosocial therapy.

Although nicotine replacement is effective without formal psychosocial therapy, it is important to note that in most studies, combining nicotine replacement with a behavior therapy gives substantially higher quit rates than either behavior therapy or nicotine replacement alone (34, 53, 129). Thus, combined therapy is a recommended treatment [I].

IV. FORMULATION AND IMPLEMENTATION OF A TREATMENT PLAN

▶ A. ADULT PATIENTS WHO ARE BEING SEEN BY PSYCHIATRISTS AND WHO CURRENTLY USE TOBACCO

1. Introduction

There are only a handful of controlled studies of treating smoking among psychiatric patients (2, 34, 180); thus, much of what is recommended in this section is based on treating smokers who do not have a current psychiatric disorder plus the general principles of treating psychiatric patients. The guidelines that follow are similar to those offered by others for psychiatric patients who smoke (63, 68, 69, 181).

2. Assessment

Assessment of psychiatric patients focuses on five points [II]. First, is the patient presently motivated to quit smoking? If not, then motivational strategies should be used.

If the smoker is ready to quit, then a concrete discussion of cessation procedures should occur. Second, are there any psychiatric reasons for concern about whether this is the best time for cessation; e.g., is the patient about to undergo a new therapy, is the patient presently in crisis, or is there a problem that is so pressing that time is better spent on this problem than on cessation [II]? Third, what is the likelihood that cessation would worsen the nonnicotine psychiatric disorder [II] (2) and can that possibility be diminished with frequent monitoring, use of nicotine replacement therapy, or other therapies? Fourth, what is the patient's ability to mobilize coping skills to deal with cessation [II]? If coping skills are low, would the patient benefit from individual or group behavior therapy? Fifth, is the patient highly nicotine-dependent or does the patient have a history of relapse due to withdrawal symptoms or increased psychiatric symptoms [I]? If so, which medication might be of help?

3. Psychiatric management

a) Increasing readiness/motivation
Since it appears that most psychiatric patients are not ready to make a quit attempt (44), most often treatment will consist of enhancing motivation and dealing with anticipated barriers to cessation (61). Fears of withdrawal symptoms or of worsening psychiatric problems may be dealt with by problem solving, increased monitoring by the therapist, and behavior therapy or nicotine replacement [III].

b) Stepped care approaches
Since the large majority of smokers quit on their own or with minimal treatment (27, 182), most existing algorithms/guidelines rely on a stepped care approach with minimal interventions early on and more intensive interventions for those who are not able to stop with minimal interventions (48, 88, 153, 154). There are three issues to consider with this approach: 1) Most smokers who quit on their own require several attempts before they succeed (27); thus, any success later in the algorithm cannot be attributed to the specific treatment being given at that point. 2) Early cessation of smoking can prevent much of the devastating consequences of smoking (18); thus, delaying delivering a treatment known to be effective could allow a serious, irreversible consequence of smoking (e.g., an acute myocardial infarction) to occur. 3) The notion that most smokers can quit on their own or will need only minimal treatment is based on research on smokers without a history of psychiatric problems (27). Smokers with psychiatric problems appear to be 2–3 times less likely to successfully stop smoking than smokers without psychiatric problems (2, 8, 33); thus, psychiatric patients require more intensive interventions earlier on [II].

c) Timing
It may be helpful to have smoking cessation listed as a goal on the master treatment plan for smokers [I]. When and how cessation advice is best delivered must be determined by the patient's status; e.g., smoking cessation is not likely to be successful when the patient is in crisis [III]. The best time for cessation would appear to be when the patient is psychiatrically stable, there are no recent or planned changes in medications, and no urgent problems take precedence [III].

d) Monitoring
Cessation appears to exacerbate psychiatric symptoms, and these symptoms undermine smoking cessation in a small subset of patients (2); thus, patients with a present

or past psychiatric history are contacted optimally 2–3 days postcessation and often thereafter to assess mood, problems, etc. [II]. The blood levels of many psychiatric medications increase substantially when patients taking such medications stop smoking, and these increases could worsen side effects or cause toxicity (table 5) (8); thus, blood levels and medication side effects should be monitored [II].

4. Use of psychosocial treatments

Although brief interventions, self-help, and supportive therapy have been shown to be effective with general medical patients, such minimal therapies may not be sufficient in patients with psychiatric problems. In addition, psychiatric patients often have fewer social supports, coping skills, etc. These two considerations suggest behavioral therapy should be considered even in the early quit attempts for these patients [II]. Since many psychiatric patients have experience with individual or group therapy, patient preferences should be considered in choosing between the two [III]. If the patient has specific problems that undermine cessation (e.g., problems with assertiveness), the therapist might work on this issue in individual therapy while the patient continues a group therapy [III].

5. Use of pharmacotherapy

Since psychiatric patients appear to have more withdrawal symptomatology when they stop smoking (2), use of nicotine replacement therapy even in early cessation attempts is recommended [II]. Given that compliance with nicotine gum is difficult (183), nicotine nasal spray has abuse potential (15), and clonidine has frequent side effects (165), the nicotine patch is recommended as the usual initial pharmacotherapy [I]. Although many psychiatric patients smoke large numbers of cigarettes and inhale cigarette smoke deeply (8), using higher-than-normal doses of nicotine for heavier smokers has not consistently been shown more effective (53). However, supplementation of nicotine patch with ad-lib use of nicotine gum appears to help patients over the rough times and should be considered [II] (119).

Those patients who smoke fewer than 15 cigarettes per day are candidates for starting with an intermediate rather than high-dose patch or for using nicotine gum instead [II] (151). Whether the 24- or 16-hour patch is better is debatable (133, 151). Twenty-four-hour patches may better relieve morning craving but appear to cause insomnia (131, 132). Longer durations of patch therapy have not been found more effective (133); thus, a 6- to 12-week duration of therapy is recommended [II].

If the patient has a preference for nicotine gum, then the gum is best used with scheduled dosing (e.g., 1 piece of gum/hour) rather than ad-lib dosing, and the 4-mg dose is recommended for heavy smokers (more than 25 cigarettes/day) or more nicotine-dependent smokers [II] (143, 184, 185). In any of the situations in which nicotine gum is used, strong encouragement to comply with use recommendations is necessary [II]. The optimal duration of nicotine gum therapy is debatable (113). Clinically, some patients appear to require long durations of treatment; i.e., 6 months or longer. Given the lack of medical harm from nicotine gum and that almost all smokers eventually stop using the gum (41), patient preference for duration of gum use should be the major determinant for duration of treatment [III]. Some clinicians have suggested that some smokers will need nicotine maintenance for life. Given the absence of empirical data on this, proactive encouragement of maintenance is not recommended.

If the patient has a strong objection to nicotine replacement therapy, clonidine may be used [II]. Clonidine delivered via patch therapy may improve compliance. Usually 0.1–0.4 mg of clonidine per day is needed [II] (125, 165). If this therapy is used, interactions of clonidine side effects (e.g., sedation) with psychiatric status should be monitored [II] (165).

Among patients with a past history of a psychiatric disorder but who are no longer taking psychiatric medications or in active psychotherapy, restarting psychiatric medications or psychotherapy prior to cessation may dampen withdrawal problems and prevent remission of the psychiatric illness (2, 167). Although the efficacy of this strategy has not been tested, if the patient or physician believes psychiatric symptomatology has precipitated relapses in prior cessation attempts, reinstitution of psychiatric treatment should be considered (2).

B. SMOKERS WHO HAVE FAILED INITIAL TREATMENT

1. Definition of group

This group is composed of smokers who have failed a trial of a known effective formal therapy (e.g., behavior therapy or nicotine replacement).

2. Assessment

a) Adequacy of prior therapy

As with treatment failures with other psychiatric disorders, a first consideration is the adequacy of prior treatment [III]. How many sessions of behavior therapy were attended? What was the quality of the behavior treatment in the last quit attempt? What were the doses of gum or patch used? What was the duration of therapy? What was the level of compliance with the psychosocial or somatic therapy? How long did the patient remain abstinent?

b) Cause of relapse

Another important consideration is to determine the perceived cause of the relapse [III]. Was the relapse due to uncontrolled withdrawal symptoms, environmental stressors, alcohol use, negative or positive mood, or being around other smokers? Were there factors (e.g., fatigue, life disappointments, family/social stressors) that undermined cessation?

c) Motivation to stop

The clinician should encourage the patient to try to quit again, and if the patient agrees, a new quit date should be set [II]. What was the patient's satisfaction with prior treatments? What did he or she learn from prior failures? If the patient is not ready to try again, what are his or her fears and what are the barriers to attempting again? What changes does the patient think need to be made before another attempt is made?

d) Search for comorbidity

Most smokers have not been assessed for psychiatric or alcohol/drug abuse problems initially and such problems interfere with cessation (2, 167); thus, screening for such disorders is indicated [II]. In prior studies, 15%–20% of heavy smokers have current and up to 35% have past alcohol problems (186) Similarly, 40% of smokers seeking treatment have a past history of depression (2, 167).

3. Psychiatric management/use of psychosocial and pharmacological treatments

a) Prior treatment inadequate

If the prior treatment appeared appropriate but was inadequately implemented, the therapy may be repeated with changes to insure the fidelity of therapy, compliance, adequate dose and duration, etc. [III].

b) Prior treatment adequate

If the prior treatment was appropriate and adequate, the psychiatrist should attempt to determine whether the relapse was due to withdrawal symptoms versus nonwithdrawal causes.

(1) Relapse due to withdrawal

If the prior relapse appeared to be caused by withdrawal symptomatology and the patient has not previously been treated with nicotine replacement, nicotine patch therapy is appropriate [I]. If the patient has been adequately treated with nicotine patch therapy, then clonidine [II], nicotine patch plus nicotine gum [II], nicotine nasal spray [II], or higher-dose nicotine patch [III] may be considered. Simply re-treating with nicotine patch therapy is not very effective (135, 148, 187, 188). Use of nicotine nasal spray is recommended because this delivery mode produces a more bolus-like effect that might better relieve withdrawal and craving [III] (136).

Use of nicotine nasal spray initially and then switching to nicotine patch or the concomitant use of nicotine nasal spray and nicotine patch have also been proposed (119) but have not been tested. The rationale for the use of clonidine is simply to try a medication from a different class. A final possibility is symptomatic treatment based on the type of withdrawal symptoms (e.g., antidepressants for withdrawal-induced depression). Although logical, this strategy has not been adequately tested.

(2) Relapse due to nonwithdrawal stressor

If the smoker has relapsed due to a stressful life event and has not previously been treated with behavior therapy, it should be considered. If the patient has already had behavior therapy, two choices are available: 1) more intensive behavior therapy [III] or 2) behavior therapy with a different content or format; i.e., group therapy, individual therapy, combined individual and group therapy, or involvement of family members [III]. Whether these treatments would be effective for those who have failed prior behavior therapy has not been tested. Switching to nonbehavioral psychosocial treatments (e.g., hypnosis or 12-step therapy) is not recommended because there is no empirical support for their efficacy.

(3) Combined therapy

Sometimes it is difficult to distinguish withdrawal versus nonwithdrawal causes of relapse. In this case, the patient may be a candidate for combined pharmacological and behavior therapy (128, 129) [II].

(4) Referral

When the treating psychiatrist does not have the knowledge necessary to implement the treatments outlined here or if the strategies are administered and the smoker is not able to quit, referral to someone who specializes in treating nicotine dependence should be considered [III].

(5) Inpatient programs

An inpatient model for smoking cessation has been described (189) and appears to produce high quit rates, especially given the highly nicotine-dependent smokers enrolled. There are no controlled trials that substantiate this at the current time.

C. TREATMENT OF SMOKERS ON SMOKE-FREE WARDS

1. Introduction

This section focuses on psychiatric patients on smoke-free wards, but the same principles apply to smokers on general medical wards seen in consultation and to smokers in smoke-free nonmedical settings; e.g., residential care settings. Controlled studies of treating nicotine withdrawal symptoms on medical or psychiatric inpatient wards have not been published; thus, the recommendations below are based on treating withdrawal in outpatient settings (16, 17).

2. Assessment

a) Withdrawal

Assessment focuses on reports of a history of withdrawal symptoms in prior hospitalizations, withdrawal during prior voluntary quit attempts, or significant fear of withdrawal [III].

b) Smoking cessation

An inpatient stay may be an opportune time for initiating treatment for nicotine dependence (e.g., because of intensity of exposure to medical staff, diagnosis of medical condition, removal from usual smoking cues). It may therefore be helpful to include smoking cessation on the master treatment plan whenever relevant. Smokers should be assessed for their readiness and motivation for change as described in section III.C.1. [I] (39). Those considering quitting should be asked about their interest in using the temporary abstinence of the smoke-free unit as the beginning of an attempt to stop smoking permanently [III].

3. Psychiatric management

a) System issues

It is very difficult to motivate inpatients to stop smoking unless the unit is smoke-free (69, 190); thus, a smoke-free psychiatric unit is recommended [I]. Although many inpatient units have been concerned about going smoke-free, the large majority have found it less difficult than anticipated (69, 190). Studies before and after institution of smoke-free units indicate no increases in aggression, disruption, discharges against medical advice, use of medications or restraints, or admission refusals (190). One of the most important issues is to prevent psychiatric staff who smoke from either purposefully or inadvertently undermining smoke-free restrictions. Permitting staff to smoke while on the inpatient unit or in contact with patients may increase the difficulty for patients who are trying to quit.

Giving special off-ward privileges to allow patients to smoke or labeling off-ward passes as "smoking breaks" implicitly condones smoking (69, 190). In addition, there are risks in allowing the patient smoking breaks; e.g., if the patient has suicidal ideation or a history of eloping or acting out on passes [III]. Policies that provide breaks for both smokers and nonsmokers (on the same schedule) may be preferable to policies that provide smokers with extra passes. Other recommendations for implementing a smoke-free unit are discussed in recent reviews (69, 190).

b) Patient education

Patients need to be educated about the rationale for a smoke-free unit; i.e., it is not to force patients to stop smoking but to prevent secondhand smoke exposure to other patients and to be consistent with the institution's goal to encourage healthy behaviors [II] (69, 190). Patients should also be educated about the goal of treatment; i.e., to reduce withdrawal symptoms and, if patients are interested, to help them begin a cessation attempt [II]. Many patients are unaware of the valid symptoms of nicotine withdrawal and their time course; thus, education about these can be helpful [II] (69, 190).

c) Monitoring

Patients need to be monitored for changes in psychiatric symptoms, as withdrawal can worsen anxiety, insomnia, concentration, and weight gain and can cause clinically significant increases in the levels of several psychiatric medications [III] (tables 4 and 5) (2, 8). For example, many alcoholics smoke. Thus, during alcohol detoxification on a smoke-free ward, how much of the irritability, anxiety, insomnia, restlessness, difficulty concentrating, and depression is due to alcohol versus nicotine withdrawal is unclear. Although nicotine withdrawal is thought to be milder, there is substantial between-person variability such that some alcoholic smokers have nicotine withdrawal symptoms that are more severe than their alcohol withdrawal symptoms (191). Similarly, when patients with schizophrenia are hospitalized and given higher doses of medications, any increases in restlessness could be due to nicotine withdrawal rather than neuroleptic-induced akathisia. Finally, cessation of smoking can cause dramatic increases in blood levels of some medications; e.g., clozapine levels can increase 40% when smokers are deprived of nicotine (192).

4. Use of psychosocial treatments

The efficacy of psychosocial treatments for withdrawal symptoms has not been tested (16); however, the clinical experience of the Work Group on Nicotine Dependence suggests several strategies [III]. Relaxation tapes can be used to alleviate anxiety. Anger can be averted by temporarily avoiding interactions. Insomnia can be decreased by improving sleep hygiene. Weight gain can be combated by increasing activity. Distraction and activities aimed at keeping busy can be used to get through craving episodes. Support groups for those going smoke-free and support from family and significant others for going smoke-free can be helpful as well.

5. Use of pharmacological therapies

Nicotine withdrawal during hospitalization is often not as severe as anticipated because of the absence of smoking cues, the distraction of the primary problem, the effects of medications, etc. Thus, prophylactic pharmacotherapy should be considered only when patients complain of withdrawal symptoms or if withdrawal signs are observed [I]. Exceptions to this rule would be those patients who are so concerned about nicotine withdrawal that they will not accept hospitalization without treatment for withdrawal. In this scenario, given the low risk of nicotine replacement, prophylactic treatment with nicotine replacement may have advantages over giving extra passes for smoking breaks [III]. The advantages of nicotine gum include the patient's ability to self-titrate nicotine dose and to stop using it immediately before intermittent smoking (e.g., during passes) [III]. In addition, many patients find that only a few pieces of gum per day are sufficient to prevent withdrawal symptoms (69, 190). The nicotine patch has the advantage of improved compliance and stable nicotine replacement. This may be especially advantageous in differentiating nicotine withdrawal from other psychiatric symptoms (8). One disadvantage of nicotine gum and patch is that patients may smoke while using them [III]. Although not desirable, this appears to be unlikely to produce significant adverse effects (193).

V. CLINICAL FEATURES INFLUENCING TREATMENT

▶ ## A. PSYCHIATRIC DISORDERS

1. Alcohol/drug use/abuse

Some 15%–20% of heavy smokers have current alcohol dependence or abuse (34). Smokers who have current alcohol/drug problems are unlikely to stop smoking permanently without overcoming the alcohol/drug problems (34); thus, in most cases, alcohol/drug abuse problems should be treated prior to or concurrent with the treatment of nicotine dependence [II]. About 80% of alcohol/drug abusers who are in treatment are smokers (1, 34). About half of such smokers are not presently interested in stopping smoking (34) and thus would benefit from treatments to increase motivation and readiness to change [II]. For the other half interested in stopping, whether it is best for them to stop smoking at the same time as they stop alcohol/drug use or to stop smoking immediately after or long after stopping alcohol/drug use is unclear (34). One rationale for stopping smoking at the same time as stopping alcohol/drug use is that use of each substance serves as a cue for use of the other substance; thus, by stopping both substances, such cues are eliminated. The major rationale for stopping smoking after stopping drinking/drug use is that often stopping drinking is a more urgent concern and that stopping two drug dependencies at the same time is just too difficult. Given the absence of empirical data, patient preferences for when to stop smoking in relation to alcohol/drug abuse treatment should be respected [III].

A common concern is that smoking cessation will cause relapse to alcohol/drug use. Most of the available data do not support this (34). In two studies, 80%–85% of recovering alcoholics reported no increased craving for alcohol nor did they relapse to alcohol use when they stopped smoking (2, 34). In fact, correlational studies suggest smoking cessation may decrease the probability of relapse to alcohol (34). However, frequent monitoring during smoking abstinence is recommended in this group to help prevent the other 15%–20% from relapsing to drinking during smoking cessation [III]. Although not empirically tested, smokers who have a history of increased desire for alcohol during abstinence from smoking could either reenter or intensify ongoing therapy for alcoholism or could be prescribed a course of disulfiram [III]. There are very little data on how to tailor a smoking cessation program to the specific needs of recovering alcoholics; e.g., whether such patients need a more intensive program, would do better in a 12-step or behavior therapy program, or would need higher-than-normal dose nicotine replacement because they are more nicotine dependent

(34). However, recent studies suggest treatment of smoking may be effective either during or after treatment for alcoholism [III] (34, 194).

2. Depression

Among patients seeking smoking cessation treatment, 25%–40% have a past history of major depression and many have minor dysthymic symptoms (2, 167). Since both have been shown to predict poor smoking cessation rates and since one study reported that 33% of those with a history of bipolar disorder and 18% of those with a history of unipolar depression relapsed to depression during smoking cessation (26), the psychiatrist should consider starting or restarting psychotherapy or pharmacotherapy for depression in patients who state that depression intensified with cessation or that cessation caused depression [III]. This recommendation is based on the results of recent trials that found that cognitive behavioral therapy for depression and antidepressants improved smoking cessation rates in those with a past history of depression or who had symptoms of depression (168, 180, 195). Finally, for a smoker with a past history of depression currently taking antidepressant medication, it is important to note that some antidepressant levels will increase with smoking cessation [II] (8).

3. Schizophrenia

Patients with schizophrenia who smoke are often not interested in stopping (33, 44, 196). Thus, strategies to motivate these patients to commit to quit are especially important [III]. When patients with schizophrenia do try to stop, many are unsuccessful (33); thus, intensive treatments are appropriate even with early attempts [III]. The high prevalence of alcohol and illicit drug abuse in patients with schizophrenia (33) can interfere with smoking cessation [II]. The blood levels of some antipsychotics can increase dramatically with cessation and nicotine withdrawal can mimic the akathisia, depression, difficulty concentrating, and insomnia seen in patients with schizophrenia (see section IV.C.3.c.).

4. Other psychiatric disorders

There is insufficient information to make specific recommendations about tailoring treatment of smoking cessation to the needs of smokers with other psychiatric disorders. In general, when psychiatric patients make an attempt at smoking cessation, they should be followed closely to monitor for more severe nicotine withdrawal, exacerbation of their psychiatric disorder, and possible side effects due to cessation-induced increases in medication levels [III] (8).

B. CONCURRENT GENERAL MEDICAL DISORDERS

1. General management

Often, psychiatrists are asked to see general medical patients in consultation. In addition, many psychiatric patients who smoke have smoking-induced medical illnesses. In fact, the onset or diagnosis of a smoking-related medical illness provides an opportunity for motivating the patient to make a quit attempt (73). Smokers who have recently been diagnosed with a tobacco-related illness (e.g., a heart attack) have a substantially greater success rate at smoking cessation (73). Since many of these patients will quit on their own without treatment (73), a stepped-care approach is appropriate with these patients [III] (48). In this approach, patients are given minimal therapies initially unless there are particular reasons to use more intense interventions (e.g., current active alcohol dependence). With this approach, the clinician needs to follow these high-risk patients closely to initiate treatment promptly because many patients will relapse after minimal treatment [I] (48, 73). If minimal treatment fails, a more intensive treatment should be tried.

If the patient is hospitalized for a medical problem when he or she decides to stop smoking, withdrawal may not be a problem while the patient is in the hospital; thus, nicotine replacement therapy may not be necessary [III] (48, 73). However, many patients find that withdrawal symptoms occur upon return to their natural environs (16); thus, these patients should be followed very closely after discharge to determine whether nicotine replacement therapy is indicated [I].

In patients with general medical problems, it is important to remember that smoking interferes with administration of many treatment medications, increases risks of anesthesia and surgery, and impairs healing (42). That smokers are at very high risk for lung cancer, chronic obstructive lung disease, heart disease, ulcers, etc., needs to be considered in all medical evaluations (61).

Finally, several childhood illnesses are associated with secondhand smoking (e.g., upper respiratory illnesses) (22, 23). Pointing out this relationship is often a motivator for patients to stop smoking.

2. Cardiovascular disease

Patients either at risk for or who already have cardiovascular disease should be made aware of three facts to increase their motivation to stop smoking [II]: 1) The risks of cardiovascular disease decrease markedly in the first year after smoking cessation and are near normal by 5 years postcessation (197). 2) Stopping smoking also substantially increases post-myocardial-infarction survival (197). 3) Stopping smoking is much more important than changing diet, weight, or exercise (197). The one anecdotal observation of heart attacks occurring while using nicotine patches has been refuted by empirical studies that show that the nicotine patch is safe in patients with stable cardiac disease (193).

3. Pulmonary disease

Smoking cessation improves many respiratory symptoms (sometimes cough is transiently worse in the first few weeks) (16) but causes no or little reversal in pulmonary function (197, 198). In most cases, cessation does stop the accelerated decline in lung function with chronic obstructive pulmonary disease (197). Smokers who persist in smoking despite pulmonary disease appear to be highly nicotine dependent with a high incidence of alcohol problems (64, 199); thus, treatment with nicotine replacement therapy and screening for alcoholism are especially important in this group [III]. Also, smoking cessation increases theophylline levels up to 40% (42). Some have suggested pulmonary function changes due to smoking can be used as motivators in such patients, but this has not been well tested (50, 55).

4. Cancer

The risk for cancer declines with increasing duration of abstinence from smoking (197). In those who already have cancer, cessation improves the quality of life (73, 197); thus, cancer patients should still be advised to stop smoking [I].

C. DEMOGRAPHIC AND PSYCHOSOCIAL VARIABLES

1. Elderly

The rates of smoking in those over 65 are lower than in younger persons (15%–20%) (200). Cessation in this age group is still beneficial both in terms of the length and quality of life (197, 200). There are programs tailored to the elderly, but these have not been well tested to see if they are better than nontailored programs (200, 201). Behaviorally based programs appear to be effective and are recommended with the qualification that cognitive deficits and depression are common in this group [II]. The elderly do not appear to have greater side effects with nicotine replacement therapy (202), and this treatment should be considered [II].

2. Youth

Despite a large public health effort, the prevalence of smoking in teens has actually increased in the last 3 years (Monitoring the Future, 1995, unpublished data). This increase appears to be associated with tobacco advertising (5). Although policy initiatives focused on illegal sales, taxation, and vending machines are essential to combating smoking among youth, providing treatment for smoking cessation also could be helpful. Young smokers appear to develop nicotine dependence fairly quickly, in that many have withdrawal when they try to quit, and most find it difficult to stop (5). Smoking is highly correlated with alcohol/drug problems in youth (37); thus, screening for comorbidity in this group appears important. There are few studies of smoking cessation treatments for adolescents, and none that show high long-term quit rates (5); however, the Work Group on Nicotine Dependence found no reason to believe that the psychiatric management strategies (table 7) and the psychosocial treatments (table 8) effective in adults would not be effective in youth; thus, these are recommended [III]. Whether nicotine replacement therapy would be of help in this group has not been tested (5); however, based on the results from adults, youth who are nicotine dependent (e.g., have withdrawal symptoms upon cessation) should be considered for nicotine replacement therapy [III].

3. Gender

Although earlier studies suggested women were less likely to succeed in stopping smoking, more recent data suggest women are quitting at same rate as men (203). The factors that undermine cessation in women appear to be depression, social support, and weight gain (203). Some data have suggested men do better with nicotine replacement therapy (203) and women do better with clonidine (165); however, these findings have not been consistently replicated. Whether women have more withdrawal symptoms and are more influenced by social support than are men is also unclear (204). There are no replicable empirical data on how to tailor smoking treatments to the needs of women (203).

Smoking during pregnancy is associated with increased perinatal complications and low-birth-weight babies (205). How much of the low birth weight is due to nicotine-induced vasoconstriction of the placental artery or carbon-monoxide-induced hypoxemia is unclear (205, 206). If a woman stops smoking within the first two trimesters, her risk of having a low-birth-weight child is near normal (205). Female smokers who do not stop early on in pregnancy appear to be highly nicotine dependent (24). Behavior therapy tailored to this group appears to be effective and is recommended [II] (73, 205). Weight gain concerns and depression may undermine resistance to cessation in this group and need to be addressed [III] (73, 205). Many pregnant smokers relapse immediately postpartum (73, 205); thus, special emphasis on maintaining abstinence postpartum is indicated [II].

The use of nicotine replacement therapy in pregnancy is debatable (23, 206). Recent preclinical data suggest nicotine itself could adversely affect the developing central nervous system (207); however, the level of nicotine to which the fetus is exposed is much lower from nicotine gum and patch than from cigarettes. Nicotine replacement therapy should still be considered in pregnant women who have tried to stop during their pregnancy but have not been able to do so because of withdrawal symptoms [III]. If nicotine replacement is used, the woman should understand the benefits and risks of nicotine replacement therapy, and the clinician should consider a lower dose and a shorter duration of treatment to reduce fetal exposure to nicotine [III].

4. Race/ethnicity

In examining the association of race, culture, or ethnicity with nicotine and other drug dependence, it is important to differentiate sociodemographic factors (e.g., income, education) from race/ethnicity factors (208). Blacks are less likely to initiate smoking, smoke fewer cigarettes per day (11), and appear to be less likely to become nicotine dependent (31), but have higher cotinine levels and are less likely to stop smoking than whites (208). There are no replicable empirical data on how to change the form or content of cessation therapies for blacks versus for whites (208).

5. Socioeconomic status

Smokers who are nonprofessionals, less educated, or poorer are more likely to start smoking and, once they start, are less likely to stop (11, 209). Although not well studied, smokers of low socioeconomic status probably have less social support for cessation and may have less knowledge of the harm from smoking and the benefits of cessation (209). Finally, these smokers have less access to formal therapies for smoking cessation (209). One study of providing free smoking cessation therapy (i.e., nicotine replacement therapy) to low-income smokers found quit rates similar to those of higher socioeconomic groups (210). There are no replicable results to indicate how to modify treatment for smokers of low socioeconomic status.

▶ D. TYPE OF TOBACCO

1. Cigarettes

The data and conclusions cited in the previous sections are for treatment of cigarette smoking. Cigarettes comprise over 95% of tobacco consumption in the United States (11). Cigarettes are very dependence producing because the inhalation route produces high arterial concentrations of nicotine that very quickly reach the brain (15, 42). In addition, the cigarette is a delivery device that allows easy titration of the dose to achieve different effects (15, 42). Finally, the high availability of cigarettes and multiple cues for their use make cessation difficult (15, 42).

2. Smokeless tobacco

The prevalence of smokeless tobacco use has increased dramatically in the last decade (211). Most users are young men (212). Smokeless tobacco provides nicotine via buccal absorption (211, 212), with a slower rate of nicotine absorption but resultant nicotine blood levels similar in magnitude to those produced by cigarettes (42, 213). Smokeless tobacco use can induce nicotine dependence, including a withdrawal syndrome (42, 213). Smokeless tobacco use produces medical harm including gingivitis, oral cancers, etc. (211–213). Often, smokeless tobacco users have detectable and readily observable oral lesions that can be used as motivators (211).

Although the cessation rates with behavior therapy are somewhat low in smokeless tobacco users, behavioral therapy appears effective and is recommended [II] (5, 211, 213). The single study of nicotine gum showed no efficacy (214). The efficacy of the nicotine patch, nonnicotine mint snuff, or other pharmacotherapies for cessation of smokeless tobacco have not been tested. Nevertheless, given that smokeless tobacco users appear nicotine dependent, a trial of nicotine patch therapy is indicated in those who have failed because of withdrawal symptoms [III].

3. Patients who smoke pipes/cigars

The major distinction among pipe and cigar smokers is whether they are primary or secondary (i.e., previously used cigarettes) users, as secondary pipe/cigar users smoke more intensely (213) and thus may be more nicotine dependent. Although nicotine dependence is likely to occur in some pipe and cigar users, there is no empirical data on nicotine dependence or its treatment in this group. However, based on the data from adults, pipe and cigar smokers who are nicotine dependent should benefit from the same treatments recommended for cigarette smokers [III].

VI. RESEARCH DIRECTIONS

Several reviews have outlined research directions for developing treatments for smokers without concomitant psychiatric disorders (60, 66, 101, 213, 215–217); thus, the following section will focus only on research directions for the psychiatric aspects of smoking.

A. EPIDEMIOLOGY AND NATURAL HISTORY OF NICOTINE DEPENDENCE

Nicotine dependence per se has been studied much less than has alcohol or other drug dependencies. To our knowledge there are only two population-based studies of the prevalence and correlates of nicotine dependence using the DSM-IV criteria (32, 218) and only one using the Fagerstrom scale (219). Serial cross-sectional and longitudinal epidemiological studies of nicotine dependence are needed to determine a) whether the prevalence of nicotine dependence among smokers is increasing over time, b) whether certain groups (e.g., the poor, those with nonnicotine drug dependencies, those with a history of depression) are especially vulnerable to developing nicotine dependence if they take up smoking, and c) the natural history of nicotine dependence (e.g., how soon does it develop, whether some smokers are immune to developing dependence).

B. EPIDEMIOLOGY AND NATURAL HISTORY OF SMOKING IN PSYCHIATRIC PATIENTS

Although the natural history of smoking initiation and cessation is quite well described, similar studies in psychiatric patients are almost completely absent. Studies of the prevalence and incidence of initiation and cessation of smoking, movement through the stages of change, rates of quit attempts, relapse rates, etc., are needed for smokers with major psychiatric disorders.

▶ C. MORBIDITY FROM SMOKING IN PSYCHIATRIC PATIENTS

How often psychiatric patients die from smoking-related diseases is not known. Demonstration that many psychiatric patients die from smoking-related illnesses might help motivate psychiatrists to be more aggressive in their treatment of nicotine dependence. Prior case-control mortality studies of psychiatric disorders have often not factored in the much higher rates of smoking in psychiatric patients; e.g., the high rates of cancer in depressed patients may be more related to their smoking habits than the competence of their immune system.

▶ D. PATIENT-TREATMENT MATCHING

As indicated previously, there are a few empirically based studies of treatment-matching strategies for smokers with different levels of motivation to quit (39, 70), for different types of behavior therapy (102, 103), and for the use of nicotine gum (12) or nasal spray (147) in highly versus less-nicotine-dependent patients. At present there are contradictory data on how to determine which patients need nicotine replacement (101). We are unaware of any data on how to select patients that especially need behavior therapy. Most importantly for this guideline, there are no data on how smokers with alcohol/drug abuse, anxiety, depression, or other psychiatric disorders should be matched to specific treatments.

▶ E. TREATMENT OF SMOKING IN PATIENTS WITH A CURRENT PSYCHIATRIC DISORDER

One study has shown that behavioral/cognitive therapy for depression is especially helpful with smokers with mild depressive symptoms (180, 195). Other studies have tested treatments for smoking among those with alcohol and other drug dependencies, but none have had much success (34). As described earlier, smokers with non-nicotine psychiatric/drug disorders appear to have more difficulty stopping smoking (2, 167); thus, studies of efficacy of treatments of different content and duration in smokers with past or present histories of specific psychiatric disorders, especially depression and schizophrenia, are needed.

▶ F. TREATMENT OF WITHDRAWAL ON SMOKE-FREE UNITS

As described earlier, several studies have found that smoke-free units are not as difficult to manage as predicted (190). However, because smoking cessation causes nicotine withdrawal symptoms that overlap with many psychiatric symptoms (e.g., irritability, insomnia), cessation has been hypothesized to interfere with psychiatric diagnosis, to worsen several psychiatric disorders, to cause relapse in some patients in remission, to mimic or worsen side effects from several medications, and to substantially increase blood levels of several medications (2, 8). Whether these effects are clinically significant needs to be studied.

VII. INDIVIDUALS AND ORGANIZATIONS THAT SUBMITTED COMMENTS

We thank Barbara Lascelles for her excellent secretarial help with the multiple drafts of this document.

Dave Abrams, M.D.
Andrew Baillie, Ph.D.
Tim Baker, M.D.
Richard Balon, M.D.
Thomas Bittker, M.D.
C.H. Blackton, M.D.
John Blamphin
Sheila Blume, M.D.
Ralph Bohm, M.D.
David W. Brook, M.D.
Sara Charles, M.D.
George J. Cohen, M.D.
Sheldon Cohen, M.D.
Dave M. Davis, M.D.
Praksash N. Desai, M.D.
Leah Dickstein, M.D.
Karl Olov Fagerstrom, M.D.
Michael Fiore, M.D., M.P.H.
Saul Forman, M.D.
Tom Glynn, Ph.D.
Larry S. Goldman, M.D.
Marion Goldstein, M.D.
John Grabowski, Ph.D.
Sheila Hafter Gray, M.D.
Donna Grossman, J.D., M.P.H.
Harry A. Guess, M.D., Ph.D.
Frederick G. Guggenheim, M.D.
Joseph Hagan, M.D.
Dorothy Hatsukami, M.D.
Al Herzog, M.D.
Richard B. Heyman, M.D.
Richard Hurt, M.D.
Corinne G. Husten, M.D., M.P.H.
Martin Jarvis, M.D.
Elaine M. Johnson, Ph.D.
Nalini V. Juthani, M.D.
Lori Karan, M.D.
Robert Kimmich, M.D.
Martha Kirkpatrick, M.D.

Thomas Kittke, M.D.
Harry Lando, Ph.D.
Alan I. Leshner, Ph.D.
Edward Lichtenstein, Ph.D.
Velandy Manohar, M.D.
Ronald Martin, M.D.
Tom McClcllan, M.D.
Roy Menninger, M.D.
Michael Meyers, M.D.
Jane Moore
Jerome Motto, M.D.
Rodrigo Munoz, M.D.
Jim Nininger, M.D.
Claire Palmer
Christi Patten, Ph.D.
Roger Peele, M.D.
Herbert S. Peyser, M.D.
Paul Pilkonis, Ph.D.
Robert F. Prien, Ph.D.
Ghulam Qadir, M.D.
Vaughn I. Rickert, Psy.D.
Jed E. Rose, Ph.D.
Pedro Ruiz, M.D.
Mitchell L. Schare, Ph.D.
Charles Schuster, Ph.D.
Paul M. Schyve, M.D.
Saul Shiffman, Ph.D.
Chris Silagy, M.D.
John Slade, M.D.
Nada Stotland, M.D.
William R. Tatomer, M.D.
Robert Trachtenberg, J.D.
Carol Martinez Weber, M.D.
Joseph Westermeyer, M.D., Ph.D.
Douglas M.C. Wilson, M.D.
Steven H. Woolf, M.D., M.P.H.
Valery W. Yandow, M.D.

Agency for Health Care Policy Research
American Academy of Clinical Psychiatrists

American Academy of Pediatrics
American Association of Suicidology
American College of Cardiology
American College of Preventive Medicine
American Medical Association
American Psychoanalytic Association
American Society of Addiction Medicine
Association for Advancement of Behavior Therapy
Center for Substance Abuse Prevention
Center for Tobacco Research and Intervention
The Cochrane Collaboration
The Menninger Foundation
National Association of VA Chiefs of Psychiatry
National Cancer Institute
National Institute on Drug Abuse
National Institutes of Health
National Institute of Mental Health
Pakistan Psychiatric Society of North America
Royal College of Psychiatrists
Society for Adolescent Medicine
Western Psychiatric Institute and Clinic

VIII. REFERENCES

The following coding system is used to indicate the nature of the supporting evidence in the summary recommendations and references:

[A]   *Randomized clinical trial.* A study of an intervention in which subjects are prospectively followed over time; subjects are randomly assigned to treatment and control groups; both the subjects and the investigators are blind to the assignments, except psychosocial treatments may not be double-blind.

[B]   *Clinical trial.* A prospective study in which an intervention is made and the results of that intervention are tracked longitudinally; study does not meet standards for a randomized clinical trial.

[C]   *Cohort or longitudinal study.* A study in which subjects are prospectively followed over time without any specific intervention.

[D]   *Case-control study.* A study in which a group of patients is identified in the present and information about them is pursued retrospectively or backward in time and compared to matched control subjects.

[E]   *Review with secondary data analysis.* A structured analytic review of existing data; e.g., a meta-analysis or a decision analysis.

[F]   *Review.* A qualitative review and discussion of previously published literature without a quantitative synthesis of the data.

[G]   *Other.* Textbooks, expert opinion, case reports, and other reports not included above.

1. American Psychiatric Association: Diagnostic and Statistical Manual of Mental Disorders, 4th ed. Washington, DC, APA 1994 [G]

2. Glassman AH: Cigarette smoking: implications for psychiatric illness. Am J Psychiatry 1993; 150:546–553 [F]

3. US Department of Health and Human Services: Clinical Practice Guideline #18 Smoking Cessation. Washington, DC, US Government Printing Office, 1996 [E]

4. American Psychiatric Association Council on Research: Position statement on nicotine dependence. Am J Psychiatry 1995; 152:481–482 [G]

5. US Department of Health and Human Services: Preventing Tobacco Use Among Young People: A Report of the Surgeon General. Washington, DC, US Government Printing Office, 1994 [F]

6. US Department of Health and Human Services: Bibliography on Smoking and Health: Selected Annotations. Washington, DC, US Government Printing Office, 1994 [G]

7. Silagy C, Gray S, Fowler G, Lancaster T: Development of a prospective register of smoking cessation trials. Control Clin Trials (in press) [E]

8. Hughes JR: Possible effects of smoke-free inpatient units on psychiatric diagnosis and treatment. J Clin Psychiatry 1993; 54:109–114 [F]

9. Hughes JR: Nicotine withdrawal, dependence, and abuse, in DSM-IV Sourcebook, vol 1. Edited by Widiger TA, Frances AJ, Pincus HA, First MB, Ross R, Davis W. Washington, DC, American Psychiatric Association, 1994, pp 109–116 [F]

10. Hughes JR: Smoking as a drug dependence: a reply to Robinson and Pritchard. Psychopharmacology (Berl) 1993; 113:282–283 [G]

11. Giovino GA, Henningfield JE, Tomar SL, Escobedo LG, Slade J: Epidemiology of tobacco use and dependence. Epidemiol Rev 1995; 17:48–65 [F]

12. Fagerstrom K, Schneider NG: Measuring nicotine dependence: a review of the Fagerstrom Tolerance Questionnaire. J Behav Med 1989; 12:159–182 [F]

13. Hughes JR, Gulliver SB, Fenwick JW, Cruser K, Valliere WA, Pepper SL, Shea PJ, Solomon LJ: Smoking cessation among self-quitters. Health Psychol 1992; 11:331–334 [C]

14. Cohen S, Lichtenstein E, Prochaska JO, Rossi JS, Gritz ER, Carr CR, Orleans CT, Schoenbach VJ, Biener L, Abrams D, DiClemente CC, Curry S, Marlatt GA, Cumming KM, Emont SL, Giovino G, Ossip-Klein D: Debunking myths about self-quitting. Am Psychol 1989; 44:1355–1365 [A]

15. Hughes JR: Dependence potential and abuse liability of nicotine replacement therapies. Biomed Pharmacother 1989; 43:11–17 [F]

16. Hughes JR, Higgins ST, Hatsukami D: Effects of abstinence from tobacco: a critical review, in Research Advances in Alcohol and Drug Problems, vol 10. Edited by Kozlowski LT, Annis HM, Cappell HD, Glaser FB, Goodstadt MS, Israel Y, Kalant H, Sellers EM, Vingilis ER. New York, Plenum, 1990, pp 317–398 [F]

17. Hughes JR, Hatsukami DK: The nicotine withdrawal syndrome: a brief review and update. Int J Smoking Cessation 1992; 1:21–26 [F]

18. US Department of Health and Human Services: Health Consequences of Smoking Cessation: A Report of the US Surgeon General. Washington, DC, US Government Printing Office, 1990 [F]

19. US Department of Health and Welfare: Smoking and Health: A Report of the Surgeon General. Washington, DC, US Government Printing Office, 1979 [F]

20. Peto R, Lopez AD, Boreham J, Thun M, Heath C Jr: Mortality from tobacco in developed countries: indirect estimation from national vital statistics. Lancet 1992; 339:1268–1278 [G]

21. Bartecchi CE, MacKenzie TD, Schrier RW: The human costs of tobacco use, part II. N Engl J Med 1994; 330:975–980 [F]

22. US Department of Health and Human Services: The Health Consequences of Involuntary Smoking: A Report of the Surgeon General. Washington, DC, US Government Printing Office, 1986 [F]

23. Office of Health and Environmental Assessment: Respiratory Health Effects of Passive Smoking: Lung Cancer and Other Disorders. Washington, DC, US Government Printing Office, 1992 [F]

24. Hughes JR: Risk/benefit of nicotine replacement in smoking cessation. Drug Saf 1993; 8:49–56 [F]

25. Benowitz NL: Toxicity of nicotine: implications with regard to nicotine replacement therapy, in Nicotine Replacement: A Critical Evaluation. Edited by Pomerleau OF, Pomerleau CS, Fagerstrom KO, Henningfield JE, Hughes JR. New York, Alan R Liss, 1988, pp 187–217 [F]

26. Glassman AH, Covey LS, Dalack GW, Stetner F, Rivelli SK, Fleiss J, Cooper TB: Smoking cessation, clonidine, and vulnerability to nicotine among dependent smokers. Clin Pharmacol Ther 1993; 54:670–679 [A]

27. US Department of Health and Human Services: National trends in smoking cessation, in The Health Benefits of Smoking Cessation: A Report of the Surgeon General. Washington, DC, US Government Printing Office, 1990, pp 580–616 [F]

28. Hughes JR: Genetics of smoking: a brief review. Behavior Therapy 1986; 17:335–345 [F]

29. Heath AC, Madden PAF: Genetic influences on smoking behavior, in Behavior Genetic Approaches in Behavioral Medicine: Perspectives on Individual Differences. Edited by Turner JR, Cardon LR, Hewitt JK. New York, Plenum, 1995, pp 45–66 [F]

30. Swan GE, Carmelli D, Rosenman RH, Fabstig RR, Christian JC: Smoking and alcohol consumption in adult male twins: genetic heritability and shared environmental influences. J Subst Abuse 1990; 2:39–50 [B]

31. Breslau N, Kilbey MM, Andreski P: DSM-III-R nicotine dependence in young adults: prevalence, correlates and associated psychiatric disorders. Addiction 1994; 89:743–754 [G]

32. Hale KL, Hughes JR, Olivcto AH, Helzer JE, Higgins ST, Bickel WK, Cottler LB: Nicotine dependence in a population-based sample, in Problems of Drug Dependence, 1992: NIDA Research Monograph 132. Edited by Harris LS. Rockville, Md, National Institute on Drug Abuse, 1993, pp 181 [G]

33. Ziedonis DM, Kosten TR, Glazer WM, Frances RJ: Nicotine dependence and schizophrenia. Hosp Comm Psychiatry 1994; 45:204–206 [F]

34. Hughes JR: Clinical implications of the association between smoking and alcoholism, in Alcohol and Tobacco: From Basic Science to Policy: NIAAA Research Monograph 30. Edited by Fertig J, Fuller R. Washington, DC, US Government Printing Office, 1995, pp 171–181 [F]

35. Klesges RC, Meyers AW, LaVasque ME: Smoking, body weight and their effects on smoking behavior: a comprehensive review of the literature. Psychol Bull 1989; 106:204–230 [F]

36. US Department of Health and Human Services: Tobacco use compared to other drug dependencies, in The Health Consequences of Smoking: Nicotine Addiction: A Report of the US Surgeon General. Washington, DC, US Government Printing Office, 1988, pp 241–376 [F]

37. Henningfield JE, Clayton R, Pollin W: Involvement of tobacco in alcoholism and illicit drug use. Br J Addict 1990; 85:279–292 [G]

38. American Psychiatric Association: Practice guideline for the treatment of patients with substance use disorders: alcohol, cocaine, opioids. Am J Psychiatry 1995; 152(Nov suppl):1–59 [G]

39. Prochaska JO, Goldstein MG: Process of smoking cessation: implications for clinicians. Clin Chest Med 1991; 12:727–735 [F]

40. Hughes JR: Applying harm reduction to smoking. Tobacco Control 1995; 4:S33–S38 [F]

41. Hughes JR: Long-term use of nicotine-replacement therapy, in New Developments in Nicotine-Delivery Systems. Edited by Henningfield JE, Stitzer ML. New York, Carlton, 1991, pp 64–71 [F]

42. Benowitz NL: Pharmacologic aspects of cigarette smoking and nicotine addiction. N Engl J Med 1988; 319:1318–1330 [F]

43. Velicer WF, Fava JL, Prochaska JO, Abrams DB, Emmons KM, Pierce JP: Distribution of smokers by stage in three representative samples. Prev Med 1995; 24:401–411 [G]

44. Hall RG, Duhamel M, McClanahan R, Miles G, Nason C, Rosen S, Schiller P, Tao-Yonenaga L, Hall SM: Level of functioning, severity of illness, and smoking status among chronic psychiatric patients. J Nerv Ment Dis 1995; 183:468–471 [G]

45. Breslau N, Kilbey MM, Andreski P: Nicotine dependence and major depression: new evidence from a prospective investigation. Arch Gen Psychiatry 1993; 50:31–35 [C]

46. Breslau N: Psychiatric comorbidity of smoking and nicotine dependence. Behav Genet 1995; 25:95–101 [G]

47. Woody GE, Cottler LB, Cacciola J: Severity of dependence: data from the DSM-IV field trials. Addiction 1993; 88:1573–1579 [G]

48. Pomerleau CS, Majchrzak MJ, Pomerleau OF: Nicotine dependence and the Fagerstrom Tolerance Questionnaire: a brief review. J Subst Abuse 1989; 1:471–477 [F]

49. Orleans CT: Treating nicotine dependence in medical settings: a stepped-care model, in Nicotine Addiction: Principles and Management. Edited by Orleans CT, Slade JD. New York, Oxford University Press, 1993, pp 145–161 [G]

50. Orleans CT, Glynn TJ, Manley MW, Slade JD: Minimal-contact quit smoking strategies for medical settings. Ibid, pp 181–220 [F]

51. US Department of Health and Human Services: Treatment of tobacco dependence, in The Health Consequences of Smoking: Nicotine Addiction. Washington, DC, US Government Printing Office, 1988, pp 459–560 [F]

52. Benowitz NL: The use of biologic fluid samples in assessing tobacco smoke consumption. NIDA Res Monogr 1983; 48:6–26 [F]

53. Hughes JR: Treatment of nicotine dependence: is more better? JAMA 1995; 274:1390–1391 [F]

54. Lerman C, Orleans CT, Engstrom PF: Biological markers in smoking cessation treatment. Semin Oncology 1993; 20:359–367 [F]

55. Velicer WF, Prochaska JO, Rossi JS, Snow MG: Assessing outcome in smoking cessation studies. Psychol Bull 1992; 111:23–41 [F]

56. Law M, Tang JL: An analysis of the effectiveness of interventions intended to help people stop smoking. Arch Intern Med 1995; 155:1933–1941 [E]

57. Baillie A, Mattick RP, Hall W, Webster P: Meta-analytic review of the efficacy of smoking cessation interventions. Drug and Alcohol Rev 1994; 13:157–170 [E]

58. Kottke TE, Battista RN, DeFriese GH, Brekke ML: Attributes of successful smoking cessation interventions in medical practice: a meta-analysis of 39 controlled trials. JAMA 1988; 259:2882–2889 [E]

59. Fiore MC: Cigarette smoking. Med Clin North Am 1992; 76:289–547 [F]

60. Abrams DB: Treatment issues: towards a stepped-care model. Tobacco Control 1993; 2:S17–S37 [F]

61. Glynn TJ, Manley MW: How To Help Your Patients Stop Smoking. Washington, DC, US Government Printing Office, 1989 [G]

62. Sachs DPL: Advances in smoking cessation treatment. Current Pulmonology 1991; 12:139–198 [F]

63. Goldstein MG, Niaura R, Abrams DB: Pharmacological and behavioral treatment of nicotine dependence: nicotine as a drug of abuse, in Medical Psychiatric Practice, vol 1. Edited by Stoudemire A, Fogel BS. Washington, DC, American Psychiatric Press, 1991, pp 541–596 [F]

64. Sachs DPL, Leischow SJ: Pharmacological approaches to smoking cessation. Clin Chest Med 1991; 12:9–10 [F]

65. Hughes JR: Behavioral support programs for smoking cessation. Modern Medicine 1994; 62:22–26 [F]

66. Orleans CT, Slade JD (eds): Nicotine Addiction: Principles and Management. New York, Oxford University Press, 1993 [F]

67. Mattick RP, Baillie A, An Outline for Approaches to Smoking Cessation: Quality Assurance Project. Canberra, Australian Government Publishing Service, 1992 [F]

68. Hughes JR, Francis RJ: How to help psychiatric patients stop smoking. Psychiatr Serv 1995; 46:435–445 [G]

69. Hurt RD, Eberman KM, Slade JD, Karan L: Treating nicotine addiction in patients with other addictive disorders, in Nicotine Addiction: Principles and Management. Edited by Orleans CT, Slade JD. New York, Oxford University Press, 1993, pp 310–326 [F]

70. Prochaska JO, DiClemente CC, Velicer WF, Rossi JS: Standardized, individualized, interactive and personalized self-help programs for smoking cessation. Health Psychol 1993; 12:399–405 [A]

71. Schwartz JL: Methods of smoking cessation. Med Clin North Am 1992; 76:451–476 [E]

72. Schwartz JL: Review and Evaluation of Smoking Cessation Methods: The United States and Canada. Washington, DC, US Department of Health and Human Services, 1987 [E]

73. Gritz ER, Kristeller JL, Burns DM: Treating nicotine addiction in high-risk groups and patients with medical co-morbidity, in Nicotine Addiction: Principles and Management. Edited by Orleans CT, Slade JD. New York, Oxford University Press, 1993, pp 279–309 [F]

74. Lando HA: Formal quit smoking treatments. Ibid, pp 221–244 [F]

75. Cinciripini PM, Lapitsky L, Seay S, Wallfisch A, Kitchens K: The effects of smoking schedules on cessation outcome: can we improve on common methods of gradual and abrupt nicotine withdrawal? J Consult Clin Psychol 1995; 63:388–399 [A]

76. French SA, Jeffery RW: Weight concerns and smoking: a literature review. Ann Behav Med 1995; 17:234–244 [F]

77. Gritz ER, Klesges RC, Meyers AW: The smoking and body weight relationship: implications for intervention and post-cessation weight control. Ann Behav Med 1989; 11:144–153 [F]

78. Hall SM, Tunstall CD, Vila KL, Duffy J: Weight gain prevention and smoking cessation: cautionary findings. Am J Public Health 1992; 82:799–803 [A]

79. Pirie PL, McBride CM, Hellerstedt W, Jeffery RW, Hatsukami DK, Allen S, Lando H: Smoking cessation in women concerned about weight. Am J Public Health 1992; 82:1238–1243 [A]

80. McBride CM, French SA, Pirie PL, Jeffrey RW. Changes over time in weight concerns among women smokers engaged in the cessation process. Ann Behav Med (in press) [A]

81. Perkins KA: Issues in the prevention of weight gain after smoking cessation. Ann Behav Med 1994; 16:46–52 [F]

82. Shiffman SM: Relapse following smoking cessation: a situational analysis. J Consult Clin Psychol 1982; 50:71–86 [C]

83. Hughes JR, Oliveto AH: Caffeine and alcohol intake as predictors of smoking cessation and tobacco withdrawal. J Subst Abuse 1993; 5:305–310 [C]

84. Oliveto AH, Hughes JR, Terry SY, Bickel WK, Higgins ST, Pepper SL, Fenwick JW: Effects of caffeine on tobacco withdrawal. Clin Pharmacol Ther 1991; 50:157–164 [A]

85. Hughes JR: Caffeine withdrawal, dependence, and abuse, in DSM-IV Sourcebook, vol 1. Edited by Widiger TA, Frances AJ, Pincus HA, First MB, Ross R, Davis W. Washington, DC, American Psychiatric Association, 1994, pp 129–134 [F]

86. Kenford SL, Fiore MC, Jorenby DE, Smith SS, Wetter D, Baker TB: Predicting smoking cessation: who will quit with and without the nicotine patch. JAMA 1994; 271:589–594 [C]

87. Curry SJ: Self-help interventions for smoking cessation. J Consult Clin Psychol 1993; 61:790–803 [F]

88. Brown RA, Goldstein MG, Niaura R, Emmons KM, Abrams DB: Nicotine dependence: assessment and management, in Psychiatric Care of the Medical Patient. Edited by Stoudemire A, Fogel BS. New York, Oxford University Press, 1993, pp 877–901 [F]

89. Fisher EB Jr, Lichtenstein E, Haire-Joshu D, Morgan GD, Rehberg HR: Methods, successes, and failures of smoking cessation programs. Annu Rev Med 1993; 44:481–513 [F]

90. Glasgow RE, Lichtenstein E: Long-term effects of behavioral smoking cessation interventions. Behavior Therapy 1987; 18:297–324 [F]

91. Mermelstein RJ, Karnatz T, Reichmann S: Smoking, in Principles and Practice of Relapse Prevention. Edited by Wilson PH. New York, Guilford Press, 1992, pp 43–68 [F]

92. Viswesvaran C, Schmidt FL: A meta-analytic comparison of the effectiveness of smoking cessation methods. J Appl Psychol 1992; 77:554–561 [E]

93. Curry S, McBride C: Relapse prevention for smoking cessation: review and evaluation of concepts and interventions. Annu Rev Public Health 1994; 15:345–366 [F]

94. Gruder CL, Mermelstein RJ, Kirkendol S, Hedeker D, Wong SC, Schreckengost J, Warnecke RB, Burzette R, Miller TQ: Effects of social support and relapse prevention training as adjuncts to a televised smoking-cessation intervention. J Consult Clin Psychol 1993; 61:113–120 [A]

95. Havassy B, Hall S, Wasserman D: Social support and relapse: commonalities among alcoholics, opiate users and cigarette smokers. Addict Behav 1991; 16:235–246 [C]

96. Corty E, McFall R: Response prevention in the treatment of cigarette smoking. Addict Behav 1984; 9:405–408 [A]

97. Lowe M, Green L, Kurtz S, Ashenberg Z, Fisher EJ: Self-initiated, cue extinction, and covert sensitization procedures in smoking cessation. J Behav Med 1980; 3:357–372 [A]

98. Raw M, Jarvis M, Feyerabend C, Russell MAH: Comparison of nicotine chewing gum and psychological treatments for dependent smokers. Br Med J 1980; 281:481–482 [B]

99. Raw M, Russell MAH: Rapid smoking, cue exposure and support in the modification of smoking. Behav Res Ther 1980; 18:363–372 [A]

100. Davis RM: The delivery of smoking cessation services: current status and future needs. Tobacco Control 1993; 2:S63–S78 [F]

101. Hughes JR: Pharmacotherapy for smoking cessation: unvalidated assumptions, anomalies and suggestions for further research. J Consult Clin Psychol 1993; 61:751–760 [E]

102. Digiusto E, Bird KD: Matching smokers to treatment: self-control versus social support. J Consult Clin Psychol 1995; 63:290–295 [A]

103. Zelman DC, Brandon TH, Jorenby DE, Baker TB: Measures of affect and nicotine dependence predict differential response to smoking cessation treatments. J Consult Clin Psychol 1992; 60:943–952 [A]

104. Gould RA, Clum GA: A meta-analysis of self-help treatment approaches. Clin Psychol Rev 1993; 13:169–186 [E]

105. Lichtenstein E, Glasgow RE, Lando HA, Ossip-Klein DJ: Telephone counseling for smoking cessation: rationale and review of evidence. Health Education Res 1996; 11:243–257 [F]

106. Orleans CT, Schoenbach VJ, Wagner EH, Quade D, Salmon MA, Pearson DC, Fiedler J, Porter CQ, Kaplan BH: Self-help quit smoking interventions: effects of self-help materials, social support instructions and telephone counseling. J Consult Clin Psychol 1991; 59:439–448 [A]

107. COMMIT Research Group: Community intervention trial for smoking cessation (COMMIT), II: changes in adult cigarette smoking prevalence. Am J Public Health 1995; 85:193–200 [A]

108. Strecher VJ, Kreuter M, Den Boer DJ, Kobrin S, Hospers HJ, Skinner CS: The effects of computer-tailored smoking cessation messages in family practice settings. J Fam Pract 1994; 39:262–270 [A]

109. Hajek P, Belcher M, Stapleton J: Enhancing the impact of groups: an evaluation of two group formats for smokers. Br J Clin Psychol 1985; 24:289–294 [A]

110. Casey K: If Only I Could Quit: Recovering From Nicotine Addiction. Center City, Minn, Hazelden Foundation, 1987 [G]

111. Marcus BH, Albrecht AE, Niaura RS, Abrams DB, Thompson PD: Usefulness of physical exercise for maintaining smoking cessation in women. Am J Cardiol 1991; 68:406–407 [A]

112. Marcus BH, Albrecht AE, Niaura RS, Taylor ER, Simkin LR, Feder SI, Abrams DB, Thompson PD: Exercise enhances the maintenance of smoking cessation in women. Addict Behav 1995; 20:87–92 [A]

113. Hughes JR: Treatment of nicotine dependence, in Pharmacological Aspects of Drug Dependence: Toward an Integrative Neurobehavioral Approach: Handbook of Experimental Psychology Series, vol. 11. Edited by Schuster CR, Gust SW, Kuhar MJ. New York, Springer-Verlag, 1996, pp 599–618 [F]

114. Jarvik ME, Henningfield JE: Pharmacological adjuncts for the treatment of tobacco dependence, in Nicotine Addiction: Principles and Management. Edited by Orleans CT, Slade JD. New York, Oxford University Press, 1993, pp 245–261 [F]

115. Silagy C, Mant D, Fowler G, Lodge M: Meta-analysis on efficacy of nicotine replacement therapies in smoking cessation. Lancet 1994; 343:139–142 [E]

116. Lee EW, D'Alonzo GE: Cigarette smoking, nicotine addiction and its pharmacologic treatment. Arch Intern Med 1993; 153:34–48 [F]

117. Nunn-Thompson CL, Simon PA: Pharmacotherapy for smoking cessation. Clin Pharm 1989; 8:710–720 [F]

118. Pomerleau O, Pomerleau C, Fagerstrom K, Henningfield JE, Hughes JR: Nicotine Replacement: A Critical Evaluation. New York, Haworth Press, 1988 [F]

119. Fagerstrom K: Combined use of nicotine replacement products. Health Values 1994; 18:15–20 [F]

120. Rose JE: Transdermal nicotine and nasal nicotine administration as smoking cessation treatments, in The Clinical Management of Nicotine Dependence. Edited by Cocores JA. New York, Springer-Verlag, 1991, pp 196–207 [F]

121. Prignot J: Pharmacological approach to smoking cessation. Eur Respir J 1989; 2:550–560 [F]

122. Jackson PH, Stapleton JA, Russell MAH, Merriman RJ: Predictors of outcome in a general practitioner intervention against smoking. Prev Med 1986; 15:244–253 [A]

123. Hughes JR: Non-nicotine pharmacotherapies for smoking cessation. J Drug Dev 1994; 6:197–203 [F]

124. Cepeda-Benito A: Meta-analytical review of the efficacy of nicotine chewing gum in smoking treatment programs. J Consult Clin Psychol 1993; 61:822–830 [E]

125. Covey LS, Glassman AH: A meta-analysis of double-blind placebo-controlled trials of clonidine for smoking cessation. Br J Addict 1991; 86:991–998 [E]

126. Gourlay SG, McNeil JJ: Antismoking products. Med J Aust 1990; 153:699–707 [C]

127. Tang JL, Law M, Wald N: How effective is nicotine replacement therapy in helping people to stop smoking? Br Med J 1994; 308:21–25 [E]

128. Hughes JR: Combining behavioral therapy and pharmacotherapy for smoking cessation: an update, in Integrating Behavior Therapies With Medication in the Treatment of Drug Dependence: NIDA Research Monograph 150. Edited by Onken LS, Blaine JD, Boren JJ. Rockville, Md, National Institute on Drug Abuse, 1995, pp 92–109 [E]

129. Hughes JR: Combined psychological and nicotine gum treatment for smoking: a critical review. J Subst Abuse 1991; 3:337–350 [E]

130. Henningfield JE, Stapleton JM, Benowitz NL, Grayson RF, London ED: Higher levels of nicotine in arterial than in venous blood after cigarette smoking. Drug Alcohol Depend 1993; 33:23–29 [G]

131. Palmer KJ, Faulds D: Transdermal nicotine: a review of its pharmacodynamic and pharmacokinetic properties, and therapeutic use as an aid to smoking cessation. Drugs 1992; 44:498–529 [F]

132. Hughes JR, Glaser M: Transdermal nicotine for smoking cessation. Health Values 1993; 17:24–31 [F]

133. Fiore MC, Smith SS, Jorenby DE, Baker TB: The effectiveness of the nicotine patch for smoking cessation: a meta-analysis. JAMA 1994; 271:1940–1946 [E]

134. Perkins KA, Grobe JE, Stiller RL, Fonte C, Goettler JE: Nasal spray nicotine replacement suppresses cigarette smoking desire and behavior. Clin Pharmacol Ther 1992; 52:627–634 [A]

135. Schneider NG, Olmstead R, Mody FV, Doan K, Franzon M, Jarvik ME, Steinberg C: Efficacy of a nicotine nasal spray in smoking cessation: a placebo-controlled, double-blind trial. Addiction 1995; 90:1671–1682 [A]

136. Sutherland G, Russell MAH, Stapleton J, Feyerabend C, Ferno O: Nasal nicotine spray: a rapid nicotine delivery system. Psychopharmacology (Berl) 1992; 108:512–518 [G]

137. Leischow SJ: Nicotine vaporiser: review of results, in Future Directions in Nicotine Replacement Therapy. Chester, England, Adis, 1994, pp 99–103 [F]

138. Tonnesen P, Norregaard J, Mikkelsen K, Jorgensen S, Nilsson F: A double-blind trial of a nicotine inhaler for smoking cessation. JAMA 1993; 269:1268–1271 [A]

139. Rose JE, Behm FM: Refined cigarette smoke as a method for reducing nicotine intake. Pharmacol Biochem Behav 1987; 28:305–310 [A]

140. Russell MAH, Jarvis MJ, Sutherland G, Feyerabend C: Nicotine replacement in smoking cessation. JAMA 1987; 257:3262–3265 [G]

141. Sutherland G, Russell MAH, Stapleton JA, Feyerabend C: Glycerol particle cigarettes: a less harmful option for chronic smokers. Thorax 1993; 48:385–387 [A]

142. Davison GC, Rosen RC: Lobeline and reduction of cigarette smoking. Psychol Rep 1972; 31:443–456 [A]

143. Sachs DPL: Effectiveness of 4 mg nicotine polacrilex for the initial treatment of high-dependent smokers. Arch Intern Med 1995; 155:1973–1980 [A]

144. Rose JE, Behm FM: Lobeline aerosol reduces craving for cigarettes, in Proceedings of the 1st Meeting of the Society for Research on Nicotine and Tobacco. Bethesda, Md, Society for Research on Nicotine and Tobacco, 1995, p 65 [A]

145. Lam WL, Sze PC, Sacks HS, Chalmer TC: Meta-analysis of randomized controlled trials of nicotine chewing gum. Lancet 1987; 2:27–29 [E]

146. Po ALW: Transdermal nicotine in smoking cessation. Eur J Clin Pharmacol 1993; 45:519–528 [E]

147. Sutherland G, Stapleton JA, Russell MAH, Jarvis MJ, Hajek P, Belcher M, Feyerabend C: Randomised controlled trial of nasal nicotine spray in smoking cessation. Lancet 1992; 340:324–329 [A]

148. Hjalmarson A, Franzon M, Westin A, Wiklund O: Effect of nicotine nasal spray on smoking cessation. Arch Intern Med 1994; 154:2567–2572 [A]

149. US Department of Health and Human Services: Smoking deterrent drug products for over-the-counter human use: establishment of a monograph. Federal Register 1982; 47:490–500 [G]

150. Hurt RD, Offord KP, Lauger GG, Marusic Z, Fagerstrom K, Enright PL, Scanlon PD: Cessation of long-term nicotine gum use: a prospective, randomized trial. Addiction 1995; 90:407–413 [A]

151. Fiore MC, Jorenby DE, Baker TB, Kenford SL: Tobacco dependence and the nicotine patch: clinical guidelines for effective use. JAMA 1992; 268:2687–2694 [F]

152. Wetter DW, Fiore MC, Baker TB, Young TB: Tobacco withdrawal and nicotine replacement influence objective measures of sleep. J Consult Clin Psychol 1995; 63:658–667 [A]

153. Cox JL: Algorithms for nicotine withdrawal therapy. Health Values 1993; 17:41–50 [G]

154. Hughes JR: An algorithm for smoking cessation. Arch Fam Med 1994; 3:280–285 [G]

155. Fagerstrom KO, Melin B: Nicotine chewing gum in smoking cessation: efficacy, nicotine dependence, therapy duration, and clinical recommendations, NIDA Res Monogr 1985; 53:102–109 [F]

156. Hatsukami DK, Huber M, Callies A, Skoog K: Physical dependence on nicotine gum: effect of duration of use. Psychopharmacology (Berl) 1993; 111:449–456 [A]

157. Clarke PBS: Nicotinic receptor blockade therapy and smoking cessation. Br J Addict 1991; 86:501–505 [F]

158. Stolerman IP, Goldfarb T, Fink R, Jarvik ME: Influencing cigarette smoking with nicotine antagonists. Psychopharmacologia 1973; 28:247–259 [F]

159. Rose JE, Levin ED: Concurrent agonist-antagonist administration for the analysis and treatment of drug dependence. Pharmacol Biochem Behav 1991; 41:219–226 [A]

160. Rose JE, Behm FM, Westman EC, Levin ED, Stein RM, Ripka GV: Mecamylamine combined with nicotine skin patch facilitates smoking cessation beyond nicotine patch treatment alone. Clin Pharmacol Ther 1994; 56:86–99 [G]

161. Rounsaville BJ: Can psychotherapy rescue naltrexone treatment of opioid addiction?, in Integrating Behavior Therapies With Medication in the Treatment of Drug Dependence: NIDA Research Monograph 150. Edited by Onken LS, Blaine JD, Boren JJ. Rockville, Md, National Institute on Drug Abuse, 1995, pp 37–52 [F]

162. Pomerleau OF, Pomerleau CS: Neuroregulators and the reinforcement of smoking: towards a biobehavioral explanation. Neurosci Biobehav Rev 1984; 8:503–513 [F]

163. Sutherland G, Stapleton JA, Russell MAH, Feyerabend C: Naltrexone, smoking behaviour and cigarette withdrawal. Psychopharmacology (Berl) 1995; 120:418–425 [A]

164. Fuller RK: Antidipsotropic medications, in Handbook of Alcoholism Treatment Approaches: Effective Alternatives. Edited by Hester RK, Miller WR. New York, Pergamon Press, 1989, pp 117–127 [F]

165. Gourlay SG, Benowitz NL: Is clonidine an effective smoking cessation therapy? Drugs 1995; 50:197–207 [E]

166. Parrott AC: Stress modulation over the day in cigarette smokers. Addiction 1995; 90:233–244 [G]

167. Hall SM, Munoz RF, Reus VI, Sees KL: Nicotine, negative affect, and depression. J Consult Clin Psychol 1993; 61:761–767 [F]

168. Humfleet G, Hall S, Reus V, Sees K, Mufloz R, Triffleman E: The efficacy of nortriptyline as an adjunct to psychological treatment for smokers with and without depressive histories, in Problems of Drug Dependence, 1995: NIDA Research Monograph, vol. 162. Edited by Adler M. Rockville, Md, National Institute on Drug Abuse, 1996, p 334 [A]

169. Robinson MD, Anastasio GD, Little JM, Sigmon JL, Menscer D, Pettice YJ, Norton HJ: Ritalin for nicotine withdrawal: Nesbitt's paradox revisited. Addict Behav 1995; 20:481–490 [B]

170. Rose JE, Behm FM: Inhalation of vapor from black pepper extract reduces smoking withdrawal symptoms. Drug Alcohol Depend 1994; 34:225–229 [A]

171. Behm FM, Rose JE: Reducing craving for cigarettes while decreasing smoking intake using capsaicin-enhanced low tar cigarettes. Exp Clin Psychopharmacol 1994; 2:143–153 [A]

172. Butschky MF, Bailey D, Henningfield JE, Pickworth WB: Smoking without nicotine delivery decreases withdrawal in 12-hour abstinent smokers. Pharmacol Biochem Behav 1995; 50:91–96 [A]

173. Levin ED, Behm FM, Rose JE: The use of flavor in cigarette substitutes. Drug Alcohol Depend 1990; 26:155–160 [A]

174. Behm FM, Levin ED, Lee YK, Rose JE: Low-nicotine regenerated smoke aerosol reduces desire for cigarettes. J Subst Abuse 1990; 2:237–247 [A]

175. Westman EC, Behm FM, Rose JE: Airway sensory replacement combined with nicotine replacement for smoking cessation. Chest 1995; 107:1358–1364 [A]

176. Behm FM, Schur C, Levin ED, Tashkin DP, Rose JE: Clinical evaluation of a citric acid inhaler for smoking cessation. Drug Alcohol Depend 1993; 31:131–138 [A]

177. Schwartz JL: Evaluation of acupuncture as a treatment for smoking. Am J Acupuncture 1988; 16:135–142 [E]

178. Ter-Riet G, Kleinjnen J, Knipschild P: A meta-analysis of studies into the effect of acupuncture on addiction. Br J Gen Pract 1990; 40:379–382 [E]

179. Glasgow RE, Klesges RC, Klesges LM, Vasey MW, Gunnarson DF: Long-term effects of a controlled smoking program: a 2/2 year follow-up. Behavior Therapy 1985; 16:303–307 [F]

180. Hall SM, Munoz RF, Reus VI: Cognitive-behavioral intervention increases abstinence rates for depressive history smokers. J Consult Clin Psychol 1994; 62:141–146 [A]

181. Dalack GW, Glassman AH: A clinical approach to help psychiatric patients with smoking cessation. Psychiatr Q 1992; 63:27–38 [G]

182. Fiore MC, Novotny TE, Pierce JP, Giovino GA, Hatziandreu EJ, Newcomb PA, Surawicz TS, Davis RM: Methods used to quit smoking in the United States. JAMA 1990; 263:2760–2765 [G]

183. Hughes JR: Problems of nicotine gum, in Pharmacologic Treatment of Tobacco Dependence: Proceedings of the World Congress, November 3–5, 1985. Edited by Ockene JK. Cambridge, Mass, Institute for the Study of Smoking Behavior and Policy, 1986, pp 141–147 [F]

184. Tonnesen P, Fryd V, Hansen M, Helsted J, Gunnersen A, Forchammer H, Stockner M: Effect of nicotine chewing gum in combination with group counseling in the cessation of smoking. N Engl J Med 1988; 318:15–27 [A]

185. Killen JD, Fortmann SP, Newman B, Varady A: Evaluation of a treatment approach combining nicotine gum with self-guided behavioral treatments for smoking relapse prevention. J Consult Clin Psychol 1990; 58:85–92 [A]

186. Hughes JR: Smoking and alcoholism, in Behavioral Approaches to Addiction. Edited by Hatsukami DK, Cox J. New York, Cahners, 1994, pp 1–3 [G]

187. Gourlay SG, Forbes A, Marriner T, Pethica D, McNeil JJ: Double blind trial of repeated treatment with transdermal nicotine for relapsed smokers. Br Med J 1995; 311:363–366 [A]

188. Tonnesen P, Norregaard J, Sawe U, Simonsen K: Recycling with nicotine patches in smoking cessation. Addiction 1993; 88:533–539 [A]

189. Hurt RD, Dale LC, Offord KP, Bruce BK, McClain FL, Eberman KM: Inpatient treatment of severe nicotine dependence. Mayo Clin Proc 1992; 67:823–828 [B]

190. Resnick MP: Treating nicotine addiction in patients with psychiatric co-morbidity, in Nicotine Addiction: Principles and Management. Edited by Orleans CT, Slade JD. New York, Oxford University Press, 1993, pp 327–336 [F]

191. Hughes JR, Higgins ST, Bickel WK: Nicotine withdrawal versus other drug withdrawal syndromes: similarities and dissimilarities. Addictions 1994; 89:1461–1470 [F]

192. Haring C, Barnas C, Saria A, Humpel C, Fleischhacker WW: Dose-related plasma levels of clozapine. J Clin Psychopharmacol 1989; 9:71–72 [G]

193. Working Group for the Study of Transdermal Nicotine in Patients With Coronary Artery Disease: Nicotine replacement therapy for patients with coronary artery disease. Arch Intern Med 1994; 154:989–995 [A]

194. Hurt RD, Eberman KM, Croghan IT, Offord KP, Davis LJ Jr, Morse RM, Palmen MA, Bruce BK: Nicotine dependence treatment during inpatient treatment for other addictions: a prospective intervention trial. Alcohol Clin Exp Res 1994; 18:867–872 [B]

195. Hall SM, Munoz RF, Reus VI, Sees KL: Mood management and nicotine gum in smoking treatment: a therapeutic contact and placebo controlled study. J Consult Clin Psychol (in press) [A]

196. Lohr JB, Flynn K: Smoking and schizophrenia. Schizophr Res 1992; 8:93–102 [F]

197. US Department of Health and Human Services: Psychological and behavioral consequences and correlates of smoking cessation, in Health Benefits of Smoking Cessation: A Report of the US Surgeon General. Washington, DC, US Government Printing Office, 1990, pp 517–578 [F]

198. Anthonisen NR, Connett JE, Kiley JP, Altose MD, Bailey WC, Buist AS, Conway WA Jr, Enright PL, Kanner RE, O'Hara P, Owens GR, Scanlon PD, Tashkin DP, Wise RA: Effects of smoking intervention and the use of an inhaled anticholinergic bronchodilator on the rate of decline of FEV1: the Lung Health Study. JAMA 1994; 272:1497–1505 [A]

199. Kennedy JA, Crowley TJ, Cottler LB, Mager DE: Substance use diagnoses in smokers with lung disease. Am J Addiction 1993; 2:126–130 [G]

200. Rimer BK, Orleans CT: Older smokers, in Nicotine Addiction: Principles and Management. Edited by Orleans CT, Slade JD. New York, Oxford University Press, 1993, pp 385–395 [F]

201. Rimer BK, Orleans CT, Fleisher L, Cristinzio S, Resch N, Telepchak J, Keintz MK: Does tailoring matter? the impact of a tailored guide on ratings and short-term smoking-related outcomes for older smokers. Health Education Res 1994; 9:69–84 [A]

202. Repsher LH, Transdermal Nicotine Study Group: Smoking cessation by women and older persons: results from the Transdermal Nicotine Study Group. Modern Medicine 1994; 62:34–38 [A]

203. Solomon LJ, Flynn BS: Women who smoke, in Nicotine Addiction: Principles and Management. New York, Oxford University Press, 1993, pp 339–349 [F]

204. Grunberg NE, Winders SE, Wewers ME: Gender differences in tobacco use. Health Psychol 1991; 10:143–153 [F]

205. US Department of Health and Human Services: The Health Consequences of Smoking For Women: A Report of the Surgeon General. Washington, DC, US Government Printing Office, 1980 [F]

206. Benowitz NL: Nicotine replacement therapy during pregnancy. JAMA 1991; 266:3174–3177 [F]

207. Naeye RL: Cognitive and behavioral abnormalities in children whose mothers smoked cigarettes during pregnancy. J Dev Behav Pediatr 1992; 13:425–428 [G]

208. Ramirez AG, Gallion KJ: Nicotine dependence among blacks and Hispanics, in Nicotine Addiction: Principles and Management. Edited by Orleans CT, Slade JD. New York, Oxford University Press, 1993, pp 350–364 [F]

209. Marsh A, McKay S: Poor Smokers. London, Policy Studies Institute, 1994 [F]

210. Howard TS, Hughes JR: Smoking cessation and the nicotine patch (letter). JAMA 1995; 274:214 [B]

211. US Department of Health and Human Services: The Health Consequences of Using Smokeless Tobacco: A Report of the Advisory Committee to the Surgeon General. Washington, DC, US Government Printing Office, 1986 [F]

212. US Department of Health and Human Services: Smokeless Tobacco or Health: Smoking and Tobacco Control Monograph 2. Washington, DC, US Government Printing Office, 1992 [F]

213. US Department of Health and Human Services: The Health Consequences of Smoking: Nicotine Addiction: A Report of the US Surgeon General. Washington, DC, US Government Printing Office, 1988 [F]

214. Hatsukami D, Jensen J, Allen S, Grillo M, Bliss R: The effects of behavioral and pharmacological treatment on smokeless tobacco users. J Consult Clin Psychol 1996; 64:153–161 [A]

215. Ockene JK, Kristeller JL: Tobacco, in The American Psychiatric Press Textbook of Substance Abuse Treatment. Edited by Galanter M, Kleber HD. Washington, DC, American Psychiatric Press, 1994, pp 157–177 [F]

216. Benowitz NL: Nicotine replacement therapy: what has been accomplished. Can we do better? Drugs 1993; 45:157–170 [F]

217. Jarvik ME, Schneider NG: Nicotine, in Substance Abuse: A Comprehensive Textbook. Edited by Lowinson JH, Ruiz P, Millman RB, Langrod JG. Baltimore, Williams & Wilkins, 1992, pp 334–356 [F]

218. Anthony JC, Warner LA, Kessler RC: Comparative epidemiology of dependence on tobacco, alcohol, controlled substances, and inhalants: basic findings from the National Comorbidity Survey. Exp Clin Psychopharmacol 1994; 2:244–268 [G]

219. Fagerstrom K, Kunze M, Schoberberger JC, Breslau N, Hughes JR, Hurt RD, Puska P, Ramstrom L, Zatonski W: Nicotine dependence versus prevalence of smoking: comparisons between countries and categories of smokers. Tobacco Control 1996; 5:52–56 [G]

PRACTICE GUIDELINE FOR THE
Treatment of Patients With Schizophrenia

WORK GROUP ON SCHIZOPHRENIA

Marvin I. Herz, M.D., Chair

Robert P. Liberman, M.D.
Jeffrey A. Lieberman, M.D.
Stephen R. Marder, M.D.
Thomas H. McGlashan, M.D.
Richard J. Wyatt, M.D.
Philip Wang, M.D. (Consultant)

In this practice guideline, treatment recommendations are discussed in sections IV and V and are summarized in section I. Data regarding the safety and efficacy of available treatments are reviewed in section III.

This practice guideline was approved in December 1996 and was published in *The American Journal of Psychiatry* in April 1997.

CONTENTS

INTRODUCTION

This guideline seeks to summarize data to inform the care of patients with schizophrenia. It begins at the point where the psychiatrist has diagnosed an adult patient as suffering from schizophrenia according to the criteria for this disorder defined in DSM-IV (1) and has evaluated the patient to ascertain the presence of other mental disorders (including alcohol- or substance-related disorders) and other general medical factors that may affect the diagnosis or treatment of the patient. The purpose of this guideline is to assist the psychiatrist in caring for a patient with schizophrenia. It should be noted that many patients have comorbid conditions that cannot be described completely with one DSM diagnostic category. The psychiatrist caring for a patient with schizophrenia should consider, but not be limited to, the treatments recommended in this practice guideline. Psychiatrists care for patients with schizophrenia in many different settings and serve a variety of functions; the recommendations in this guideline are primarily intended for psychiatrists who provide, or coordinate, the overall care of the patient with schizophrenia.

This document concerns patients 18 years of age and older. While many of the issues are similar, the assessment and treatment of children and younger adolescents are sufficiently different to warrant a separate guideline; the reader is referred to the guideline on this topic of the American Academy of Child and Adolescent Psychiatry (2).

DEVELOPMENT PROCESS

This practice guideline was developed under the auspices of the Steering Committee on Practice Guidelines. The process is detailed in the Appendix to this volume. Key features of the process include the following:

- initial drafting by a work group that included psychiatrists with clinical and research expertise in schizophrenia;
- a comprehensive literature review (description follows);
- the production of multiple drafts with widespread review, in which 15 organizations and over 90 individuals submitted comments (see section VII);
- approval by the APA Assembly and Board of Trustees;
- planned revisions at 3- to 5-year intervals.

The following computerized searches of relevant literature were conducted:

1. In MEDLINE and PsycLIT, for the period 1966–1993 the following key words were used: "conventional antipsychotic medications and tranquilizing agents, neuroleptic drugs, effective drug therapy"; "adjunctive treatments"; "ECT"; "individual psychotherapy"; "group psychotherapy"; "family interventions"; "vocational rehabilitation"; and "psychosocial skills."
2. In MEDLINE, PsycLIT, and MEDLARS, for the period 1966–1993 the following key words were used: "clozapine and efficacy and side effect profile."
3. In MEDLINE, for the period 1991–1995 the following key words were used: "schizophrenia treatment and group therapy, group homes, psychiatric department hospitals, day care, ambulatory care, outpatients"; "substance abuse and dependence"; and "patient readmission."
4. In MEDLINE, for the period 1985–1995 the following key words were used: "schizophrenia and vocational rehabilitation and social skills training, assertive community treatment, training in community living, family psychoeducation, behavioral family therapy, behavioral family management, token economy."

I. SUMMARY OF RECOMMENDATIONS

The following executive summary is intended to provide an overview of the organization and scope of recommendations in this practice guideline. The treatment of patients with schizophrenia requires the consideration of many factors and cannot adequately be reviewed in a brief summary. The reader is encouraged to consult the relevant portions of the guideline when specific treatment recommendations are sought. This summary is not intended to stand by itself.

▶ A. CODING SYSTEM

Each recommendation is identified as falling into one of three categories of endorsement, indicated by a bracketed Roman numeral following the statement. The three categories represent varying levels of clinical confidence regarding the efficacy of the treatment for the disorder and conditions described.

[I]   Recommended with substantial clinical confidence.
[II] Recommended with moderate clinical confidence.
[III] May be recommended on the basis of individual circumstances.

▶ B. GENERAL CONSIDERATIONS

Schizophrenia is a chronic condition that frequently has devastating effects on many aspects of the patient's life and carries a high risk of suicide and other life-threatening conditions. The care of most patients involves multiple efforts to reduce the frequency and severity of episodes and to reduce the overall morbidity and mortality of the disorder. Many patients require comprehensive and continuous care over the course of their lives with no limits as to duration of treatment [I].

Goals and strategies of treatment vary according to the phase and severity of illness. Specific guidelines for choosing among the various treatment options within each illness phase are presented.

1. Acute phase

During the acute phase, the aim is to facilitate the alleviation or reduction of acute symptoms with concomitant improvement in role functioning [I].

a) Assessment

Each patient should have a thorough initial workup that includes a complete psychiatric and general medical history, a mental status examination, and a physical examination that includes a neurological evaluation [I]. Basic laboratory tests should be conducted to rule out conditions that can mimic schizophrenia, to determine the presence of comorbid conditions, to establish a baseline for the administration of antipsychotic medications, and to guide routine medical care when necessary (e.g., for chronically ill individuals who have not been receiving routine medical care) [I]. Patients who are abusing alcohol or drugs or who have alcohol- or drug-induced psychosis should receive appropriate short-term treatment (e.g., detoxification) and long-term treatment [I]. The risk of self-harm, the risk of harm to others, and the presence of command hallucinations should be evaluated and appropriate precautions should be taken whenever there are questions about the safety of the patient or others [I].

b) Choice of treatment setting

Patients should be cared for in the least restrictive setting that is likely to be safe and to allow for effective treatment [I]. The psychiatrist should weigh the relative risks and the benefits of different settings on the basis of an evaluation of the condition of the patient, the need for particular treatments, family functioning, social supports, the preferences of the patient and family, and treatment resources that are available in the community. Hospitalization is indicated for patients who are felt to pose a serious threat of harm to themselves or others, who are unable to care for themselves, or who have general medical or psychiatric problems that are not safely or effectively treated in a less intensive setting [I]. Although efforts should be made to hospitalize patients voluntarily, involuntary hospitalization may be indicated if patients refuse and requirements of the local jurisdiction are met.

Alternative treatment settings, such as partial hospitalization, home care, family crisis therapy, crisis residential care, and assertive community treatment, should be considered for patients who do not need formal hospitalization for their acute episodes but who require more intensive services than can be expected in a typical outpatient setting [I].

c) Psychiatric management

In the acute phase, the specific treatment goals are to prevent harm, control disturbed behavior, suppress symptoms, effect a rapid return to the best level of functioning, develop an alliance with the patient and family, formulate short- and long-term treatment plans, and connect the patient with appropriate maintenance and follow-up care in the community [I].

Psychosocial interventions are aimed at reducing overstimulating or stressful life events in a structured and predictable environment [I]. The psychiatrist should provide information to the patient on the nature and management of his or her illness, in a manner that is appropriate to the patient's ability to assimilate the information [I].

If the patient has contact with his or her family and if the patient agrees, the psychiatrist should initiate a relationship with the family [I]. Educational meetings, "survival workshops" that teach the family how to cope with schizophrenia, and referrals to local and national support groups are often helpful [III].

d) Antipsychotic medications

Antipsychotic medications are indicated for nearly all acute psychotic episodes in patients with schizophrenia [I]. Although under some circumstances it may be reasonable to delay treatment for several days, psychiatrists should avoid withholding medications for longer periods as this may delay the patient's recovery and place the patient at risk of suicide and other dangerous behaviors [I].

It is important for the psychiatrist to assess the ability of the patient to participate in the decision about medication treatment. When an acutely psychotic patient refuses medication and is dangerous, the physician may consider administering it despite the patient's objection [I]. In less emergent circumstances, the physician should assess the patient's competency to refuse medication [I], while continuing to attempt to enlist the patient's cooperation with treatment.

Because of their efficacy and safety, conventional antipsychotic medications and risperidone are all reasonable first-line medications for patients in acute phases of schizophrenia [I]. The newer antipsychotics—olanzapine, sertindole (not yet approved by the Food and Drug Administration), and quetiapine (not yet approved)—may also be appropriate first choices for some patients, although there are fewer published data supporting their efficacy and safety [III]. In choosing among these medications, the psychiatrist should consider past treatment responses, side effect profile, patient preferences for a particular medication, and intended route of administration. Side effects include extrapyramidal side effects of high-potency antipsychotic medications and drowsiness, dizziness, dry mouth, and constipation from low-potency medications [I]. Mid-potency conventional medications may be preferable for patients who find both low- and high-potency medications difficult to tolerate [I]. Risperidone, olanzapine, sertindole, and quetiapine may cause fewer extrapyramidal side effects at clinically effective doses [II].

The clinician should also consider the preferred route of medication administration. If a patient is a candidate for a long-acting depot antipsychotic, the oral form of the depot medication is a logical choice [I]. Long-acting depot medications are not usually prescribed for acute psychotic episodes, although they may be indicated for the patient receiving involuntary antipsychotic medication or the sporadically compliant patient [II]. Risperidone and the newer antipsychotic medications (olanzapine, sertindole, and quetiapine) are not currently available in long-acting depot forms.

It is important to select a dose that is both effective and not likely to cause serious side effects. If a high-potency conventional antipsychotic medication is selected, the effective daily dose is likely to be in the range of 5 to 20 mg of haloperidol or 300 to 1000 mg of chlorpromazine equivalents [I]. For risperidone the daily dose should be in the range of 4 to 6 mg, for olanzapine it should be 10 to 20 mg, and for sertindole it should be 12 to 24 mg; for quetiapine the optimal dose range has not been established yet. Unless there is evidence that the patient is having uncomfortable side effects, the patient should be monitored in this range for at least 3 weeks [II]. During this phase, it may be important for clinicians to be patient and to avoid the temptation to prematurely escalate the dose for patients who are responding slowly [I]. The use of high doses during the first days of treatment ("rapid neuroleptization") should be avoided because of lack of effectiveness and risk of adverse effects [I].

If the patient is not improving, it may be useful to measure the plasma level to help establish whether 1) the dose is too low for an adequate response; 2) the dose is too high and may be causing side effects, such as akathisia, agitation, or akinesia; 3) other medications given concurrently, young or old age, or medical illness affects the pharmacodynamics of the medication; or 4) noncompliance is a problem [II]. The clinical correlates of plasma levels are the best established for haloperidol [I].

If noncompliance is a problem, discussion with the patient about the rationale for medication treatment can be helpful, as can administering the medication orally in liquid form or intramuscularly [III]. If the patient is complying and has an adequate plasma concentration but is not responding, then alternative treatment methods should be considered. These can include raising the dose for a finite period of time, such as 2 weeks, or trying an antipsychotic from a different class [I]. Risperidone [II] or one of the newer antipsychotics [III]—olanzapine, sertindole, or quetiapine—may have advantages at this stage.

When patients fail to respond to adequate trials (4 to 6 weeks at an adequate dose) of at least one antipsychotic medication, a trial of clozapine should be considered except for patients who have specific contraindications to it (e.g., history of blood dyscrasias, inability to comply with monitoring requirements) [I]. Clozapine should also be considered for patients with violent behavior who have not responded to an adequate trial of at least one antipsychotic medication [I]. Patients who experience intolerable side effects, including tardive dyskinesia, in trials of two antipsychotic agents from different classes may also be candidates for clozapine [I]. A clozapine trial should last for at least 3 months at a dose of 200–600 mg/day [I].

e) Other medications

Lithium, carbamazepine, valproic acid, or a benzodiazepine is commonly added to an antipsychotic medication when the patient continues to demonstrate active psychotic symptoms despite an adequate antipsychotic medication trial [III]. However, none of these adjuncts has demonstrated the effectiveness of clozapine, and these adjunctive medications should be reserved for treatment-resistant patients for whom clozapine is not appropriate [II].

Adjunctive medications are also commonly prescribed for comorbid conditions in schizophrenia. Benzodiazepines may be helpful for managing both anxiety and agitation during the acute phase of treatment [I]. Antidepressants should be considered for persistent depressive symptoms [I].

Medications are used to treat extrapyramidal side effects and other side effects of antipsychotic medications. Decisions regarding the use of medications for side effects depend on the severity and degree of distress associated with the side effect and on consideration of other potential strategies, including lowering the dose of the antipsychotic medication or switching to a different antipsychotic medication. Prophylactic antiparkinsonian medications may be considered, especially for patients taking high-potency antipsychotics who have a prior history of acute extrapyramidal side effects, those who prefer prophylactic medications, or those for whom the occurrence of side effects would contribute to noncompliance or negative attitudes toward treatment [II]. The benefit of using prophylactic antiparkinsonian medications should be weighed against the potential for side effects [I].

Catatonic and treatment-resistant schizophrenic patients may be candidates for ECT when pharmacologic treatments are not effective or are contraindicated [III].

2. Stabilization phase

During the stabilization phase, the aims of treatment are to minimize stress on the patient and provide support to minimize the likelihood of relapse, enhance the patient's adaptation to life in the community, and facilitate continued reduction in symptoms and consolidation of remission [I].

If a patient has improved with a particular medication regimen, he or she should, when possible, continue taking the same medication at the same dose for the next 6 months before a lower maintenance dose is considered for continued treatment [I]. Premature lowering of the dose or discontinuation of the medication during this phase may lead to relatively rapid relapse [I].

Psychotherapeutic interventions remain supportive and may include education for patient and family about the course and outcome of the illness, as well as factors that influence the course and outcome, including treatment compliance [III]. Patients should be helped with the transition to life in the community and helped to adjust to their lives outside the hospital through realistic goal setting [III]. Undue pressure to perform at high levels vocationally and/or socially, as well as an overly stimulating treatment environment, can be overly stressful to patients during this phase and increase the risk of relapse [I].

3. Stable phase

The goals of treatment during the stable phase are to ensure that the patient is maintaining or improving his or her level of functioning and quality of life, that prodromal symptoms and/or increases in schizophrenic symptoms are effectively treated, and that monitoring for adverse treatment effects continues [I].

a) Assessment

Ongoing monitoring and assessment during the stable phase are necessary to determine whether patients might benefit from alteration of treatment [I]. In addition to encouraging patients and those who interact with them to describe any changes, questions about specific symptoms and side effects should be raised [I].

The frequency of psychiatric assessments depends on the specific nature of the treatment and expected fluctuations of the illness. For example, patients given depot antipsychotic medications must be evaluated at least monthly, patients receiving clozapine must be evaluated (hematologically) weekly, and those who are going through potentially stressful changes in their lives must sometimes be assessed daily [III]. The use of formal or standardized instruments for some assessments (e.g., for monitoring tardive dyskinesia) is convenient and provides documentation which others can easily follow [I].

b) Psychiatric management and specific psychosocial treatments

As the patient becomes relatively asymptomatic and more motivated, supportive but increasingly specific psychosocial treatment strategies can be introduced [II]. Where indicated, these include reeducation in basic living skills, social skills training, cognitive rehabilitation, and beginning vocational rehabilitation [II]. For patients who do not have severe positive symptoms, psychosocial interventions, such as individual or group therapy, are often beneficial [II]. Patients with marked deficit states, however, may require a continuation of more structured, supportive, and nonstressful strategies [III]. Involvement with family members should be ongoing [I]. Patients should be monitored for prodromal symptoms and behaviors, and appropriate interventions should be made when prodromal symptoms appear.

c) Antipsychotic medications

In the stable phase, conventional antipsychotic medications are effective for reducing the risk of relapse [I]. The long-term efficacy of risperidone [II] and the newer agents [III]—olanzapine, sertindole, and quetiapine—has not been adequately studied; however, on the basis of their efficacy in treating acute episodes of schizophrenia, it may be reasonable to expect that they possess efficacy in the stable phase.

The long-term management plan in the stable phase should balance side effects with the risk of relapse [I]. There are likely to be benefits associated with the use of lower doses (300–600 mg of chlorpromazine equivalents per day), such as improved compliance, better subjective state, and perhaps better community adjustment [II]. However, these advantages should be weighed against a somewhat greater risk of relapse and more frequent exacerbations of schizophrenic symptoms [I]. Long-acting depot antipsychotic medications may be preferable to oral antipsychotic medications for many patients who are in the stable phase of treatment [I]. Risperidone [II] and the newer antipsychotic agents [III] (olanzapine, sertindole, and quetiapine) are not currently available in long-acting depot form; however, they may be useful during the stable phase for patients who experience extrapyramidal side effects with conventional antipsychotics and who are compliant with daily oral doses.

Stable patients who do not have positive symptoms may be candidates for dose reduction [II]. It is prudent to reduce the medication dose gradually, to a level of at least one-fifth the usual maintenance dose, as long as the patient remains stable.

Review of the need for maintenance antipsychotic medication and the required dose should be done at least annually [II]. Patients with only one episode of positive symptoms who have had no symptoms during the following year of maintenance therapy may be considered for a trial period without medication [III]. For patients who have experienced multiple episodes, maintenance antipsychotic medication treatment should be continued in most cases for at least 5 years and possibly indefinitely [III]. Continuing antipsychotic medications indefinitely should also be considered for patients with a history of serious suicide attempts or violent, aggressive behavior [III].

When a decision is made to discontinue antipsychotic medication, additional precautions should include slow, gradual dose reduction over many months, more frequent visits, and the use of early intervention strategies [II]. In this context, the psychiatrist should educate the patient and the family about early signs of relapse and should collaborate with them to develop plans for action should these signs appear.

d) Early intervention

The treatment program should be organized to respond quickly when a patient, family member, or friend reports prodromal symptoms or behaviors or exacerbations of schizophrenic symptoms in the patient [I]. Early use of supportive therapeutic techniques and a higher medication dose as indicated can be very helpful in reducing the likelihood of relapse and hospitalization [I]. During prodromal episodes, patients and family members should be seen more frequently for treatment, monitoring, and support, and assertive outreach including home visits should be used when indicated [III].

II. DISEASE DEFINITION, NATURAL HISTORY, AND EPIDEMIOLOGY

▶ A. CLINICAL FEATURES

Schizophrenia is a major psychotic disorder. Its essential features consist of a mixture of characteristic signs and symptoms that have been present for a significant length of time during a 1-month period (or for a shorter time if successfully treated), with some signs of the disorder persisting for at least 6 months (1). The symptoms involve multiple psychological processes, such as perception (hallucinations), ideation, reality testing (delusions), thought processes (loose associations), feeling (flatness, inappropriate affect), behavior (catatonia, disorganization), attention, concentration, motivation (avolition, impaired intention and planning), and judgment. No single symptom is pathognomonic of schizophrenia. These psychological and behavioral characteristics are associated with a variety of impairments in occupational or social functioning. Although there can be marked deterioration with impairments in multiple domains of functioning (e.g., learning, self-care, working, interpersonal relationships, and living skills), the disorder is noted for great heterogeneity across individuals and variability within individuals over time. It is also associated with an increased incidence of general medical illness (3) and mortality (4–9), especially from suicide, which occurs in up to 10% of patients (10–12).

The characteristic symptoms of schizophrenia have often been conceptualized as falling into two broad categories—positive and negative (or deficit) symptoms—with a third category, disorganized, recently added because statistical analyses have revealed that it is a dimension independent of the positive symptom category, where it was previously included. The positive symptoms include delusions and hallucinations. Disorganized symptoms include disorganized speech (13) (thought disorder) and disorganized behavior and poor attention. Negative symptoms include restricted range and intensity of emotional expression (affective flattening), reduced thought and speech productivity (alogia), anhedonia, and decreased initiation of goal-directed behavior (avolition) (14).

According to DSM-IV, subtypes of schizophrenia are defined by the predominant symptoms at the time of the most recent evaluation and therefore may change over time. These subtypes include paranoid type, in which preoccupation with delusions or auditory hallucinations is prominent; disorganized type, in which disorganized speech and behavior and flat or inappropriate affect are prominent; catatonic type, in which characteristic motor symptoms are prominent; undifferentiated type, which is a nonspecific category used when none of the other subtype features are predominant; and residual type, where there is an absence of prominent positive symptoms but continuing evidence of disturbance (e.g., negative symptoms or positive symptoms in an attenuated form) (15). Although the prognostic and treatment implications of these subtypes are variable, the disorganized type tends to be the most severe and the paranoid type to be the least severe (16).

Other mental disorders and general medical conditions may be comorbid with schizophrenia. Along with general medical conditions, the most common comorbid disorder appears to be substance use disorder, especially abuse of alcohol (17) and stimulants, such as cocaine and amphetamines (18); other commonly abused substances are nicotine, cannabis, phencyclidine (PCP), and LSD (19, 20). Such comorbidities can worsen the course and complicate treatment (21, 22). Symptoms of other mental disorders, especially depression but also obsessive and compulsive symptoms, somatic concerns, dissociative symptoms, and other mood or anxiety symptoms, may also be seen with schizophrenia. Whether they represent symptom or disorder levels of comorbidity, these features can significantly worsen prognosis (23) and often require specific attention and treatment planning. General medical conditions are often present, and individuals may be at special risk for those associated with poor self-care or institutionalization (e.g., tuberculosis), substance use (e.g., emphysema and other cigarette-related pathology, HIV-related disease), and antipsychotic-induced movement disorders. Some individuals with schizophrenia develop psychosis-induced polydipsia, which can lead to water intoxication and hyponatremia.

▶ B. NATURAL HISTORY AND COURSE

The onset of schizophrenia typically occurs during adolescence or early adulthood. It affects men and women with equal frequency. The peak age at onset for males, however, is the early 20s, and for women it is the late 20s and early 30s (12). The majority of patients alternate between acute psychotic episodes and stable phases with full or partial remission. Interepisode residual symptoms are common. This often-chronic illness can be characterized by three phases that merge into one another without absolute, clear boundaries between them. These phases form the structure for integrating treatment approaches described in this guideline.

- *Acute phase.* During this florid psychotic phase, patients exhibit severe psychotic symptoms, such as delusions and/or hallucinations and severely disorganized thinking, and are usually unable to care for themselves appropriately. Negative symptoms often become more severe as well.

- *Stabilization phase.* During this phase, acute psychotic symptoms decrease in severity. This phase may last for 6 or more months after the onset of an acute episode.
- *Stable phase.* Symptoms are relatively stable and, if present at all, are almost always less severe than in the acute phase. Patients can be asymptomatic; others may manifest nonpsychotic symptoms, such as tension, anxiety, depression, or insomnia. When negative (deficit) symptoms and/or positive symptoms, such as delusions, hallucinations, or thought disorder, persist, they are often present in attenuated, nonpsychotic forms (e.g., circumstantiality rather than looseness, illusions rather than hallucinations, overvalued ideas rather than delusions).

The onset of the first psychotic episode may be abrupt or insidious, but the majority of individuals display some type of prodromal phase manifested by the slow and gradual development of a variety of signs and symptoms (e.g., social withdrawal, loss of interest in school or work, deterioration of hygiene and grooming, unusual behavior, outbursts of anger). Eventually a symptom characteristic of the active phase appears, marking the disturbance as schizophrenia. Before a patient in the stable phase relapses, there is usually a prodromal period in which there may be nonpsychotic dysphoric symptoms, attenuated forms of positive symptoms, or idiosyncratic behaviors. This prodromal period usually lasts for several days to a few weeks but may last for several months (see section III.E.4).

Most longitudinal studies of schizophrenia suggest that its course is variable, with some individuals free of further episodes, the majority displaying exacerbations and remissions, and a small proportion remaining chronically severely psychotic (24–29). Because of the differences in diagnostic criteria used in studies, an accurate and comprehensive summary of the long-term outcome of schizophrenia is not possible. Complete remission (i.e., a return to full premorbid functioning) is not common in this disorder. Of the patients who remain ill, some appear to have a relatively stable course, whereas others show a progressive worsening associated with severe disability. Early in the illness, negative symptoms may be prominent and apparent primarily as prodromal features. Subsequently, positive symptoms appear. Because these positive symptoms are particularly responsive to treatment, they typically diminish, but in many individuals negative symptoms persist between episodes of positive symptoms. There is some suggestion that negative symptoms may become steadily more prominent in some individuals during the course of the illness (30).

There are some prognostic variables that are of value in predicting long-term outcome. For example, better outcomes are associated, on average, with female gender, family history of affective disorder, absent family history of schizophrenia, good premorbid functioning, higher IQ, married marital status, acute onset with precipitating stress, fewer prior episodes (both number and length), a phasic pattern of episodes and remissions, advancing age, minimal comorbidity, paranoid subtype, and symptoms that are predominantly positive (delusions, hallucinations) and not disorganized (thought disorder, disorganized behavior) or negative (flat affect, alogia, avolition) (15, 16, 27, 30–51). It appears that the course is influenced by culture and societal complexity, with better outcomes in developing countries (50).

C. EPIDEMIOLOGY

Lifetime prevalence of schizophrenia varies, but the results of most studies collectively average out to a rate of slightly less than one case per 100 persons in the population (9, 52–55). In the Epidemiologic Catchment Area Study using DSM-III criteria for schizophrenia, for example, the lifetime prevalence rates across four U.S. sites (Los Angeles, St. Louis, Baltimore, and New Haven, Conn.) ranged from 0.6% to 1.9% of the population (56, 57). The disorder appears to be uniformly distributed worldwide, although pockets of high or low prevalence may exist (55). The risk of developing schizophrenia is enhanced if one's relatives have the disorder, especially if they are first-degree relatives or if more than one is affected (9, 55, 58–62).

Risk is also increased if a person is single, is from an industrialized nation, is in a lower socioeconomic class, lives in an urban center, experienced problems in utero (e.g., Rh incompatibility, starvation, influenza) or perinatal complications, was born during the winter, or recently experienced some stressful life event (9, 55, 58–62).

Because schizophrenia usually appears early in life and can often be chronic, the costs of the disorder are substantial. Schizophrenia accounted for 2.5% of total direct health care expenditures, or about $16–$19 billion, in 1990 (63). Indirect costs from such factors as loss of productivity and family burden are estimated at $46 billion (63, 64). Unemployment rates can reach 70%–80% in severe cases (65), and it is estimated that schizophrenic patients constitute 10% of the totally and permanently disabled (63). Homelessness and schizophrenia have been linked; it has been estimated that about one-third of homeless single adults suffer from severe mental illness, largely schizophrenia (65, 66).

III. TREATMENT PRINCIPLES AND ALTERNATIVES

▶ A. GENERAL ISSUES

The development of a treatment plan for an individual with schizophrenia requires the consideration of many issues, including cross-sectional issues (e.g., current clinical status) and longitudinal issues (e.g., frequency, severity, treatments, and consequences of past episodes). Whenever feasible, treatment planning should attempt to involve the patient and family in an active collaboration using an integrated approach with appropriate pharmacologic, psychotherapeutic, psychosocial, and rehabilitative interventions that are empirically titrated to the patient's response and progress. Many patients require comprehensive and continuous care over the course of their lives, with no limits as to duration of treatment. In addition to treating patients directly, the psychiatrist frequently functions as a collaborator, consultant, and/or supervisor with other mental health professionals in a team approach.

At present, there is no cure for schizophrenia. However, treatment can decrease morbidity and mortality associated with the disorder. The general goals of treatment are to decrease the frequency, severity, and psychosocial consequences of episodes and to maximize psychosocial functioning between episodes. The specific goals of treatment depend on the phase of the illness and other specific characteristics of the patient. In addition, many patients with schizophrenia need specific community, supportive, and rehabilitative services to address the impairments in role function associated with their disorder.

▶ B. PSYCHIATRIC MANAGEMENT

Psychiatric management includes a set of interventions, from those described in this section. Some of these interventions have been included in the concept of "supportive psychotherapy," and others are included in the concept of "clinical management." Treatment of a patient with schizophrenia is facilitated by a comprehensive understanding of the patient, including his or her needs and goals, intrapsychic conflicts and defenses, coping styles, and strengths. The psychiatrist should attempt to understand the biological, interpersonal, social, and cultural factors that affect the patient's adjustment. The psychiatrist should provide education about schizophrenia, facilitate adherence to a medication regimen that is satisfactory to both the patient and psychiatrist, and attempt to help the patient solve practical problems, giving practical advice and guidance when needed.

Specific components of psychiatric management include the following: establishing and maintaining a therapeutic alliance; monitoring the patient's psychiatric status; providing education regarding schizophrenia and its treatments; determining the need for medication and other specific treatments and developing an overall treatment plan; enhancing adherence to the treatment plan; increasing understanding of and adaptation to the psychosocial effects of the illness; identifying and initiating treatment for new episodes as early as possible and addressing factors that precipitate and/or perpetuate episodes; initiating efforts to relieve family distress and improve family functioning; and facilitating access to services and coordinating resources among the mental health and other systems of care.

1. Establishing and maintaining a therapeutic alliance

It is important for the psychiatrist who is treating the patient to establish and maintain a supportive therapeutic alliance, which forms the foundation on which treatment is conducted (67). This allows the psychiatrist to gain essential information about the patient and allows the patient to develop trust in the psychiatrist and a desire to cooperate with treatment. As much as possible, there should be continuity of care with the same psychiatrist over time, thereby facilitating this process. Such a relationship allows the psychiatrist to learn more about the patient as a person and the vicissitudes of the disorder over time for that person.

2. Monitoring the patient's psychiatric status

The psychiatrist should remain vigilant for changes in psychiatric status. Collaboration with family members and significant others is especially important because individuals with schizophrenia often lack insight into the nature of their illness (68) and because moderate changes in mood, behavior, or thought processes may herald the onset of an acute episode with potentially serious consequences. Monitoring can be enhanced by knowledge gained over time about a patient's particular prodromal symptoms and behaviors that preceded prior episodes (67, 69–71). At times it may be necessary to reevaluate the diagnosis as new information becomes available.

3. Providing education regarding schizophrenia and its treatments

Patients with schizophrenia and their families often benefit from education and feedback with regard to the illness, prognosis, and treatment. Frequently, the patient's ability to understand and retain this information varies over time, and it may be impeded by periods of active psychosis or the presence of cognitive deficits. Therefore, this process should be an ongoing one in which the psychiatrist introduces facts about the illness, with adequate therapeutic attention to the psychological factors that may impede the patient's ability to use the information. Patient education over an extended period may help the patient to become a collaborator in the treatment of this persistent illness. In this capacity, the patient will know when to report prodromal symptoms, which could help the psychiatrist to intervene before the onset of a full-blown exacerbation. In addition, an understanding of the importance of various treatments, and the likely consequences of discontinuation, may eventually reduce the likelihood that the patient will abruptly stop a treatment (e.g., medication) without first discussing the options with his or her psychiatrist. Printed material on the disorder and its treatments is frequently quite helpful. Family members frequently play an important role in the care of patients with schizophrenia and therefore also benefit from ongoing education. Further, family members may be more likely than patients to recognize and report the appearance of prodromal symptoms (72).

4. Determining the need for medication and other specific treatments and developing an overall treatment plan

Patients with schizophrenia benefit from a variety of treatments, including medication and psychosocial interventions. Schizophrenia is a long-term illness, and the needs of an individual patient may vary over time. The psychiatrist works with the patient (and family, when appropriate) to develop a treatment plan. Frequently, the plan involves several health care providers, in which case a plan for coordinating the care is necessary. The psychiatrist should monitor the patient for changes in clinical status, including beneficial or adverse responses to a particular treatment, and modify the treatment plan accordingly. Treatment planning for patients with schizophrenia is an iterative process, in which treatments are implemented and modified over time, depending on patient response and preferences.

5. Enhancing adherence to the treatment plan

Schizophrenia is a long-term disorder, and adherence to carefully designed treatment plans can significantly improve the patient's health status. However, not uncommonly, patients with this disorder stop taking medications, miss clinic appointments, and fail to report essential information to their psychiatrists. Frequent causes of noncompliance are denial of illness (73), stigma associated with the illness, cultural beliefs, the need to take daily medication even in the stable phase, and the patient's experience of unpleasant medication side effects, especially akathisia (74, 75). All of the principal antipsychotic medications can be associated with unpleasant, and rarely, dangerous side effects. Encouraging the patient to report side effects and attempting to diminish or eliminate them can significantly improve medication compliance. Also, it is important for patients to understand that in the stable phase medication may only be prophylactic in preventing relapse (76, 77). If a patient stops taking medication during the stable phase, he or she may feel better, with less sedation or other side effects. As a result, the patient may come to the false conclusion that the medication is not helping. Other types of treatment (e.g., psychotherapy groups) may at times be experienced as unpleasant by patients. The psychiatrist should create an atmosphere in which the patient can feel free to discuss what he or she experiences as negative in the treatment process so that dropouts are minimized. It is helpful to reassess the treatment plan in collaboration with the patient and attempt to modify it in accord with the patient's preferences and needs.

When a patient does not appear for appointments or is noncompliant in other ways, assertive outreach including telephone calls and home visits may be very helpful in reengaging the patient in treatment. This outreach can be carried out by the psychiatrist and/or other designated team members in consultation with the psychiatrist.

6. Increasing understanding of and adaptation to the psychosocial effects of the disorder

Frequently, the psychosocial effects of schizophrenia leave many patients with emotional, social, familial, academic, occupational, and financial issues that require therapeutic assistance.

The psychiatrist should assist the patient in coping with his or her environment, including interpersonal relationships, work and living conditions, and other medical or health-related needs. Examples of such assistance include helping the patient avoid embarrassment by not telling others about delusions or hallucinations, assisting the patient in managing current life stresses, and encouraging the patient to develop a sense of increased control over and responsibility for his or her life. Working in collaboration with patients to set realistic and achievable short- and long-term goals can be useful because patients can increase their sense of self-worth through achieving these goals, thereby reducing the demoralization that many patients experience.

Patients who have children may need help assessing and meeting their children's needs, both during and in the wake of acute episodes. Patients may need help making appropriate plans to meet their children's needs. At times, it may be important to help the parent with schizophrenia to obtain a psychiatric evaluation for his or her child. Individuals with schizophrenia who are considering having children may benefit from genetic counseling (78).

7. Promoting early recognition of episodes and initiation of treatment and assisting in identification of factors that precipitate or perpetuate episodes

The psychiatrist should help the patient and family members to identify early signs and symptoms of acute episodes. Such identification can help the patient to gain a feeling of mastery over the illness and can help to ensure that adequate treatment is instituted as early as possible in the course of an episode, thus reducing the likelihood of relapse (72). Assertive outreach efforts may be necessary at these times (see section III.E.4).

8. Initiating efforts to relieve family distress and improve family functioning

Often family members experience considerable distress in dealing with the family member who has a diagnosis of schizophrenia. They benefit from education about symptoms and behaviors associated with that diagnosis, about the schizophrenic patient's vulnerability to stress, and about how to deal with disturbed and disturbing behaviors. Family members also benefit from support and guidance. In addition, their role as potential allies in the treatment process can be very helpful for the patient. Many families will achieve a higher level of functioning and satisfaction with the introduction of specific educational and problem-solving approaches, which are discussed in section III.E.2.

9. Facilitating access to services and coordinating resources among mental health, general medical, and other service systems

Patients with schizophrenia often require an array of psychiatric, general medical, rehabilitative, and social services. The psychiatrist managing the care of a patient with this disorder often works in collaboration with other mental health professionals, other general health providers (including primary care physicians), and staff from a variety of social service agencies. The psychiatrist should work with team members, the patient, and the family to ensure that such services are coordinated and that referrals for additional services are made when appropriate. It is important that disability income support is secured when indicated.

C. PHARMACOLOGIC TREATMENTS

Pharmacologic treatments are a critical component of the treatment for patients with schizophrenia. Medications are used for the treatment of acute episodes, the prevention of future episodes, and improvement of symptoms between episodes. Antipsychotic medications (including conventional antipsychotic medications, clozapine, risperidone, and other new medications) are the principal pharmacologic treatment for patients with schizophrenia. In addition, mood stabilizers and other adjunctive agents are frequently beneficial for subgroups of patients.

The following section is organized by medication. For each medication (or class of medication) the available data regarding efficacy are reviewed. Short-term efficacy has generally been measured by reductions in positive or negative symptoms among treated patients during 6- to 12-week medication trials. An advantage of studies that measure changes in positive or negative symptoms is that they clearly demonstrate how well a medication can achieve a reduction in the target symptoms. What is sometimes less clear is how such reductions in symptoms relate to improvements in patient functioning.

Long-term efficacy has usually been measured by reductions in either relapse or rehospitalization rates among treated patients over the course of several years. The utility of relapse rates depends on the measure that is used. Relapse rates based on symptom reemergence have varied markedly from study to study, in part because different criteria for types and severity of symptoms have been used to define relapse. Commonly, a predefined change in score on a symptom scale is used to determine the presence of a relapse. Typically, the symptom scales assign greater weight to positive, as opposed to negative, symptoms. Rehospitalization rates, on the other hand, offer the advantage of reflecting both symptoms and functioning, but they are also affected by other clinical and nonclinical determinants of hospitalization. Rehospitalization rates tend to be more conservative estimates of relapse (occurring at a rate of 1%–10% per month after discontinuation of therapy) than are rates of reemergence of psychotic symptoms (5%–20% per month) (79).

Side effects associated with medications and other issues in implementing treatment with medications, including the need for laboratory or other monitoring, are also discussed. Issues to be considered in determining when and how to use each possible medication in the overall treatment of an individual patient are addressed in section IV in the context of the various phases of treatment.

1. Antipsychotic medications

In this guideline the term "antipsychotic" refers to several classes of medications (see table 1), which include the conventional antipsychotic medications (often referred to as "neuroleptics") and clozapine and risperidone (often referred to as "atypical antipsychotics"). Olanzapine and two other new (but as yet unmarketed) medications are evaluated to the extent possible on the basis of the limited data available at this time.

a) Conventional antipsychotic medications

Conventional antipsychotics include all antipsychotic medications except clozapine, risperidone, and three newer medications. The conventional antipsychotic medica-

TABLE 1. Commonly Used Antipsychotic Medications

Medication	Therapeutically Equivalent Oral Dose (mg/day)	Degree of Extrapyramidal Side Effects
Conventional antipsychotics		
Phenothiazines		
Fluphenazine	2	+++
Trifluoperazine	5	+++
Perphenazine	10	++/+++
Mesoridazine	50	+
Chlorpromazine	100	++
Thioridazine	100	+
Butyrophenone		
Haloperidol	2	+++
Others		
Thiothixene	5	+++
Molindone	10	+
Loxapine	15	++/+++
New antipsychotics		
Clozapine	50	0?
Risperidone	1–2	+
Olanzapine	2–3?	0 – +?
Sertindole	2–3?	0 – +?
Quetiapine	50–100?	0 – +?

tions are equally effective in the treatment of psychotic symptoms of schizophrenia (with the exception of mepazine and promazine), although they vary in potency and their propensity to induce side effects. The conventional antipsychotics are usually classified into three groups according to their antipsychotic potency. The high-potency agents include haloperidol and fluphenazine; the intermediate-potency medications include loxapine and perphenazine; and the low-potency agents include chlorpromazine and thioridazine.

(1) Goals and efficacy

(a) Acute phase

The evidence supporting the effectiveness of these agents in reducing psychotic symptoms in acute schizophrenia comes from studies carried out in the 1960s (80, 81) as well as numerous clinical trials that have taken place since then (79, 82). Each of these studies compared one or more antipsychotic medications with either a placebo or a sedative agent, such as diazepam, morphine, or phenobarbital (83), that served as a control. Nearly all of these studies found that the antipsychotic medication was superior for treating schizophrenia. These studies demonstrated the efficacy of antipsychotic medications for every subtype and subgroup of schizophrenic patients. Moreover, Klein and Davis (84) and Davis et al. (82) reviewed studies that compared more than one antipsychotic medication and found that, with the exception of mepazine and promazine, all of these agents were equally effective.

Conventional antipsychotic medications are effective in diminishing most symptoms of schizophrenia. In a review of five large studies comparing an antipsychotic to a placebo, Klein and Davis (84) found that patients who received an antipsychotic demonstrated decreases in positive symptoms, such as hallucinations, uncooperativeness, hostility, and paranoid ideation. The patients also improved in thought disorder, blunted affect, withdrawal-retardation, and autistic behavior.

These findings—along with decades of clinical experience with these agents—indicate that antipsychotic treatment can reduce the positive symptoms (hallucinations, delusions, bizarre behaviors) and negative symptoms (apathy, affective blunting, alogia, avolition) associated with schizophrenic psychosis. Approximately 60% of patients treated with antipsychotic medication for 6 weeks improve to the extent that they achieve a complete remission or experience only mild symptoms, compared to only 20% of patients treated with placebo. Forty percent of medication-treated patients continue to show moderate to severe psychotic symptoms, compared to 80% of placebo-treated patients. Eight percent of medication-treated patients show no improvement or worsening, compared to nearly one-half of placebo-treated patients (79, 81). A patient's prior history of a medication response is a fairly reliable predictor of how the patient will respond to a subsequent trial (85, 86).

(b) Stabilization phase

Empirical research provides relatively little guidance for psychiatrists who are making decisions about medication and dose during this phase. The use of antipsychotic medications during this phase is based on the clinical observation that patients relapse abruptly when medications are discontinued during this phase of treatment.

(c) Stable phase

A large number of studies (87, 88) have compared relapse rates for stabilized patients who were kept on their medication regimens and those who were changed to placebo. During the first year only about 30% of those continuing to take medications relapsed, whereas about 65% of those taking placebo relapsed. Even when compliance with medication treatment was assured by the use of depot medications, as many as 24% of patients relapsed in a year (89). Hogarty et al. (90) found that among outpatients maintained with antipsychotic medications for 2 to 3 years who had been stable and judged to be at low risk of relapse, 66% relapsed in the year after medication withdrawal. Kane (88) reviewed studies in which the medications of well-stabilized patients were discontinued and found that 75% of patients relapsed within 6–24 months.

A number of studies have focused on the use of antipsychotic medications after recovery from a first episode of schizophrenia. Carefully designed double blind studies indicate that 40% to 60% of patients relapse if they are untreated during the year following recovery from a first episode (91, 92).

(2) Side effects

Antipsychotic medications can cause a broad spectrum of side effects. Many are the result of pharmacologic effects on neurotransmitter systems in regions other than the target site for the intended therapeutic effects of the medication (e.g., extrapyramidal side effects). Other side effects are of unclear pathophysiology (e.g., leukopenia).

Side effects can interfere with antipsychotic treatment in various ways. The manifestations of these effects can obscure the therapeutic effects of antipsychotic medications and prevent patients and psychiatrists from determining the benefits of treatment at a specific dose range (93). In addition, they can affect patients' compliance with treatment (74).

(a) Common side effects

i) Sedation.   Sedation is the most common single side effect of antipsychotic medications (82). Most patients experience some sedation, particularly with the low-potency agents, such as chlorpromazine, but it occurs to some extent with all antipsychotic medications.

Sedation is most pronounced in the initial phases of treatment. Most patients develop some tolerance to the sedating effects with continued administration. For agitated patients, the sedating effects of these medications in the initial phase of treatment can have therapeutic benefits. However, when sedation persists into maintenance treatment, causing daytime drowsiness, it becomes a problem. Lowering of the daily dose, consolidation of divided doses into one evening dose, or changing to a less sedating antipsychotic medication can be helpful.

ii) Anticholinergic and antiadrenergic effects.   The anticholinergic effects of antipsychotic medications (along with the effects of anticholinergic antiparkinsonian medications when concurrently administered) can produce a variety of adverse effects, including dryness of mouth, blurring of vision, constipation, tachycardia, and urinary retention. These can occur in one form or another in 10% to 50% of treated patients (94, 95). These side effects can be particularly troublesome for older patients (e.g., older men with benign prostatic hypertrophy) (94).

Although most of these effects are mild and tolerable, serious consequences can occur. For example, death can result from ileus of the bowel if not detected in time. In addition, some patients experience problems with thermoregulation and can develop hyperthermia, particularly in warm weather.

Central anticholinergic toxicity can lead to impaired memory and cognition, confusion, delirium, somnolence, and hallucinations (96, 97). These symptoms can affect the patient's response to psychosocial or rehabilitation programs and may impair the individual's efforts to become reintegrated into the community. Such symptoms are more likely to occur with medications that have more potent anticholinergic effects and in elderly or medically debilitated patients. Cessation of treatment usually results in reversal of symptoms. In cases where it is clear that anticholinergic effects are responsible, parenteral physostigmine (0.5–2.0 mg i.m. or i.v.) may be used to reverse the symptoms, although this should be done only under close medical monitoring.

Tachycardia can result from the anticholinergic effects of antipsychotic medications but may also occur as a result of postural hypotension. Hypotension is caused by the antiadrenergic effects of antipsychotic medications. When this is severe it can lead to syncopal episodes. Patients who experience severe postural hypotension must be cautioned against getting up quickly and without assistance. The elderly are particularly prone to this adverse effect, and syncopal episodes may contribute to an increased incidence of hip fractures in elderly women. Other management strategies include the use of support stockings, increased dietary salt, and administration of the salt/fluid-retaining corticosteroid fludrocortisone, to increase intravascular volume. Tachycardia due to anticholinergic effects without hypotension can be managed with low doses of a peripherally acting β blocker (e.g., atenolol) (98).

iii) Neurologic effects.   EXTRAPYRAMIDAL SIDE EFFECTS.   Of the spectrum of adverse effects of antipsychotic medications, the neurologic side effects are the most troublesome (99, 100). Although the various types of antipsychotic agents differ in their propensity for causing these side effects, they are all capable of producing them, although such effects are less likely with clozapine and risperidone (at least at low doses) (101–103). Extrapyramidal side effects can broadly be divided into acute and chronic categories. Acute extrapyramidal side effects are signs and symptoms that occur in the first days and weeks of antipsychotic medication administration, are dose dependent, and are reversible upon medication dose reduction or discontinuation.

Chronic extrapyramidal side effects are signs and symptoms that occur after months and years of antipsychotic medication administration, are not clearly dose dependent, and may persist after medication discontinuation.

There are four types of acute extrapyramidal side effects: parkinsonism, dystonia, and akathisia, which are quite common, and neuroleptic malignant syndrome, which occurs infrequently but is potentially life threatening (104–107). Detailed descriptions and differential diagnoses of the extrapyramidal side effect syndromes are provided in the "Medication-Induced Movement Disorders" section of DSM-IV. Approximately 60% of patients who receive acute treatment with antipsychotic medication develop clinically significant extrapyramidal side effects in one form or another (99, 100, 108). Some patients may develop more than one form at the same time.

- *Medication-induced parkinsonism.* Medication-induced parkinsonism, characterized by the symptoms of idiopathic Parkinson's disease (rigidity, tremor, akinesia, and bradykinesia), has been found in 20% of patients treated with antipsychotics (104, 109). These symptoms arise in the first days and weeks of antipsychotic medication administration and are dose dependent. Curiously, some patients who develop parkinsonian symptoms may, upon substantial dose increases, experience a lessening, rather than worsening, of symptoms. This unexpected result has been hypothesized to be due to an increase in the intrinsic anticholinergic activity provided by antipsychotic medications at higher doses (110). Medication-induced parkinsonism resolves after discontinuation of antipsychotic medication, although some cases of persisting symptoms have been reported.

  Akinesia or bradykinesia is a feature of medication-induced parkinsonism; a patient with this condition appears to be slow moving, indifferent to stimuli, and emotionally constricted. It has been noted alone or with other extrapyramidal side effects in almost one-half of patients treated with antipsychotics. In very severe cases, it may mimic catatonia. Depressive symptoms can also be present in over 50% of patients with akinesia, in which case the syndrome is termed "akinetic depression" (111, 112).

  Symptoms of medication-induced parkinsonism need to be carefully distinguished from negative symptoms of schizophrenia. Parkinsonian side effects usually respond to a reduction in antipsychotic medication dose (if this can be done while preserving the antipsychotic effects of treatment) or treatment with antiparkinsonian medication. Because of concern about exacerbating psychotic symptoms, the traditional dopamimetic medication for parkinsonian symptoms (L-dopa) is generally not used to treat medication-induced parkinsonism. Instead, anticholinergic antiparkinsonian medications are the treatment of choice (113). In addition to anticholinergic antiparkinsonian medications, weak dopamimetic medications, such as amantadine, can be used as second-line or additional treatments. The efficacy of these medications is good, but some patients who improve with antiparkinsonian medication continue to have residual parkinsonian symptoms.

- *Dystonia.* Acute dystonia is characterized by the spastic contraction of discrete muscle groups. Dystonic reactions occur in 10% of patients initiating therapy. Risk factors include young age, male gender, use of high-potency medications, high doses, and intramuscular administration. Dystonic reactions frequently arise after the first few doses of medication (90% occur within the first 3 days) (114). They can occur in various body regions but most commonly affect the neck, eyes, and torso (107). The specific name of the reaction is derived from the specific anatomic region that is affected. Hence, the terms "torticollis," "laryngospasm," "oculogyric crisis," and "opisthotonos" are used to describe dystonic reactions in specific body regions (115). These reactions are sudden in onset, are dramatic in appearance, and can cause patients great distress. For some patients these conditions, e.g., laryngospasm, can be dangerous and even life threatening.

Acute dystonic reactions respond dramatically to the administration of anticholinergic or antihistaminic medication, usually given parenterally (intramuscularly or intravenously). Afterwards, these patients are usually maintained with an oral regimen of anticholinergic antiparkinsonian medication to prevent the recurrence of acute dystonic reactions.

- *Akathisia.* Akathisia is characterized by somatic restlessness that is manifest subjectively and objectively in 20%–25% of patients treated with antipsychotics (105, 112). Patients characteristically complain of an inner sensation of restlessness and an irresistible urge to move various parts of their bodies. Objectively, this appears as increased motor activity. The most common form involves pacing and an inability to sit still. This side effect is often extremely distressing to patients, is a frequent cause of noncompliance with antipsychotic treatment, and, if allowed to persist, can produce dysphoria and possibly aggressive or suicidal behavior (116).

  Akathisia is less responsive to treatment than are parkinsonism and dystonia. A first step that may improve akathisia symptoms is a small, slow reduction in antipsychotic dose. Anticholinergic antiparkinsonian medications have limited efficacy but are usually the first line of treatment, particularly if the patient also has another extrapyramidal side effect, e.g., medication-induced parkinsonism or dystonia, that warrants their use. Centrally acting β blockers, such as propranolol, have been suggested by some to be the most effective form of treatment for akathisia (117), although the need remains for further double-blind, controlled comparisons of treatments. Propranolol is usually administered at doses between 30 to 90 mg/day, which is titrated to produce clinical response while blood pressure and pulse rate are monitored. Benzodiazepines can also be used to treat akathisia. Lorazepam and clonazepam are the most commonly used, but most benzodiazepines may be beneficial. A common problem that arises in assessing patients with akathisia is distinguishing this side effect from psychomotor agitation associated with the psychosis. This may be a difficult clinical distinction to make. Mistaking akathisia for psychotic agitation and raising the dose of antipsychotic medication usually leads to worsening of the akathisia, while treating psychotic agitation as akathisia (by adding either an anticholinergic agent or a β blocker) will have little benefit. In such cases the nonspecific effects of benzodiazepines on akathisia and agitation can be useful, although the dose necessary for therapeutic effects on psychotic agitation usually is higher than that required for akathisia (118).

- *Prophylactic treatment.* Given the high rate of acute extrapyramidal side effects among patients receiving antipsychotic medications, the prophylactic use of antiparkinsonian medications may be considered. The benefit of this approach has been demonstrated in several studies. For example, Hanlon et al. (119) found that only 10% of patients taking perphenazine with an antiparkinsonian medication developed an extrapyramidal side effect, in contrast to 27% of patients without an antiparkinsonian medication. The risk is that some patients may be treated unnecessarily with these medications (118). In addition, the presence of acute extrapyramidal side effects can provide useful clinical information (e.g., as a risk factor for subsequent development of tardive dyskinesia). Prophylactic antiparkinsonian medication may be considered for patients with a prior history of susceptibility to acute extrapyramidal side effects and for patients whose anticipated negative attitudes and noncompliance with treatment may be reinforced by the occurrence of adverse reactions.

The various medications used to treat acute extrapyramidal side effects are listed in table 2. The major differences among the anticholinergic medications are in their potencies and durations of action. Patients who are very sensitive to anticholinergic side effects (e.g., dry mouth, blurred vision, constipation) may require lower doses or less potent preparations (e.g., trihexyphenidyl, procyclidine hydrochloride). The need for anticholinergic medications should be reevaluated after the acute phase of treatment is over and whenever the dose of antipsychotic medication is changed. If the dose of antipsychotic medication is lowered, anticholinergic medication may no longer be necessary or may be given at a lower dose.

- *Neuroleptic malignant syndrome.* Neuroleptic malignant syndrome is characterized by the triad of rigidity, hyperthermia, and autonomic instability, including hypertension and tachycardia (106), and it is often associated with elevated serum creatine kinase activity. This condition can be sudden and unpredictable in its onset, is frequently misdiagnosed, and can be fatal in 5%–20% of cases if untreated (121). The prevalence is uncertain, but neuroleptic malignant syndrome may occur in as many as 1%–2% of patients treated with antipsychotic medications (121). Neuroleptic malignant syndrome usually occurs early in the course of treatment, often within the first week after treatment is begun or the dose is increased. Risk factors include young age, male gender, preexisting neurological disability, physical illness, dehydration, rapid escalation of dose, use of high-potency medications, and use of intramuscular preparations.

The first step in treatment is to discontinue the antipsychotic medication; then supportive treatment for the fever or cardiovascular symptoms should be provided. Treatments that have been used to accelerate the reversal of the condition include dopamine agonists, such as bromocriptine, pergolide, and lisuride, and antispasticity agents, such as dantrolene sodium (122). Recently, another antispasticity compound, azumolene, was suggested as a potential treatment for neuroleptic malignant syndrome (123). After several weeks of recovery, patients may be retreated with antipsychotic medication cautiously (124). Generally, treatment is resumed with a lower-potency antipsychotic medication than the precipitating agent, with gradually increased doses.

TABLE 2. Selected Medications for Treating Acute Extrapyramidal Side Effects[a]

Generic name	Trade Name	Dose (mg/day)	Duration of Action (hours)
Benztropine mesylate	Cogentin	0.5–6.0	24
Trihexyphenidyl hydrochloride	Artane	1–15	6–12
Amantadine	Symmetrel	100–300	12

[a]Adapted from *Drug Information for the Health Care Professional* (120, p. 290).

TARDIVE DYSKINESIA. Tardive dyskinesia is a hyperkinetic abnormal involuntary movement disorder caused by sustained exposure to antipsychotic medication that can affect neuromuscular function in any body region but is most commonly seen in the oral-facial region (95, 125). (For a description of tardive dyskinesia and its differential diagnosis see DSM-IV.)

Tardive dyskinesia may arise after exposure to any antipsychotic medication except clozapine. (While there is substantial evidence that patients treated with clozapine do not develop tardive dyskinesia, for risperidone there have been insufficient numbers of patients treated on a long-term basis to draw firm conclusions about its tardive dyskinesia risk; a case report of such an association has been published [126].) Tardive dyskinesia occurs at a rate of approximately 4% per year of antipsychotic medication treatment in adult psychiatric populations (95, 125). Various factors are associated with greater vulnerability to tardive dyskinesia. Schizophrenia itself may be associated with a risk of spontaneous dyskinesia indistinguishable from medication-induced tardive dyskinesia (127). Other risk factors include older age, female gender combined with postmenopausal status, diagnosis of affective disorder (particularly major depressive disorder), concurrent general medical disease such as diabetes, and use of high doses of antipsychotic medications (128–130). Although the majority of patients who develop tardive dyskinesia have mild symptoms, a proportion (approximately 10%) develop symptoms of moderate or severe degrees.

Patients receiving antipsychotic medication treatment on a sustained basis (for more than 4 weeks) should be evaluated regularly (approximately every 3 months or more often, depending on the frequency of visits) for side effects, including extrapyramidal side effects and signs of tardive dyskinesia. Once symptoms are identified, a workup to rule out potential idiopathic causes of tardive dyskinesia should be performed (95). This includes a standard neurologic examination, a family history check for neurologic disease (e.g., Huntington's disease), and laboratory tests (SMA-18, CBC, and T_4 measurement).

If idiopathic causes are ruled out, the patient may be considered to have tardive dyskinesia and treatment options should be considered. Discontinuation of medication should be considered only if the patient is in full remission or very stable with few residual positive symptoms or if the patient insists on stopping medication. The options include dose reduction and switching to a newer antipsychotic medication. The dose can gradually (over 12 weeks) be reduced by 50%. Frequently, this will lead to a decrease or remission of tardive dyskinesia. An initial increase in symptoms after withdrawal or dose reduction (withdrawal dyskinesia) may also occur in some patients. With sustained medication exposure without dose reduction after the development of tardive dyskinesia, the likelihood of reversibility diminishes. In some cases symptoms can persist despite long periods of time without medication. Despite the fact that continued treatment with antipsychotic medication increases the chances for persistence of tardive dyskinesia symptoms, the severity of tardive dyskinesia does not seem to increase over time at steady, moderate doses.

If medication discontinuation or dose reduction does not produce substantial improvement in tardive dyskinesia symptoms within 6 to 12 months, then the severity and degree of distress the symptoms cause the patient should be evaluated. If they are mild or nondistressing, no further interventions might be made. The documentation in the clinical record should reflect that a risk-benefit analysis favored continued maintenance of antipsychotic treatment despite mild tardive dyskinesia, to prevent the likelihood of relapse. However, if the symptoms are severe or distressing to the patient, treatment for the tardive dyskinesia should be considered. A large number of agents have been extensively studied for their therapeutic effects on tardive dyskinesia, and the results have been mixed (95). The general pattern in these studies has been for treatments to appear to be effective in open trials but to show no significantly greater efficacy than placebo in double-blind trials. Moreover, the amount of improvement in patients' symptoms has been neither substantial nor consistent. Several uncontrolled studies have evaluated clozapine as a treatment for tardive dyskinesia. Lieberman et al. (131) reviewed eight studies that monitored the outcome of tardive dyskinesia. Approximately 43% of the cases improved, suggesting that clozapine may be effective in reducing abnormal movements. Despite the fact that none of the trials was adequately controlled, conversion to clozapine is the preferred treatment option. It is not known whether risperidone may be similarly beneficial for patients with tardive dyskinesia. This seems less likely, as a case of tardive dyskinesia in a patient receiving risperidone has been reported (126). Among the more recent treatments that have been used and are currently being evaluated are vitamin E, amantadine, L-dopa, and selegiline, but these remain experimental (132–134). Largely on the basis of preclinical evidence, various agents have been suggested as having potentially preventive effects on development of tardive dyskinesia. These include lithium, vitamin E, L-dopa, amantadine, and selective MAO-B inhibitors, such as selegiline (132, 133, 135–137). Their preventive efficacy for tardive dyskinesia remains unproven.

(b) Other side effects

i) Seizures. Antipsychotic medications can lower the seizure threshold and result in the development of generalized grand mal seizures (138). The low-potency conventional antipsychotic medications and clozapine confer the greatest risk (see section III.C.1. b.2). The frequency of seizures is dose related, with higher doses associated with greater risk. The seizure rates are below 1% for all conventional antipsychotic medications at usual dose ranges (139). Patients with a history of an idiopathic or medication-induced seizure have a higher risk.

If a patient experiences a seizure, antipsychotic medication (with the exception of clozapine) should be withdrawn or the dose reduced by 50% until a neurologic evaluation is completed.

ii) Endocrine effects: galactorrhea and oligomenorrhea. All standard antipsychotic medications increase prolactin secretion by blocking the inhibitory actions of dopamine on lactotrophic cells in the pituitary. Risperidone can produce hyperprolactinemia comparable to that caused by typical compounds, whereas clozapine does not elevate prolactin beyond normal levels (140). The resultant hyperprolactinemia can lead to galactorrhea (secretion of liquid from the nipples) in 1% to 5% of patients and menstrual cycle changes (e.g., oligomenorrhea) in up to 20% of women. Reduction in medication dose may decrease the severity or alleviate these effects. When the antipsychotic dose must be maintained and galactorrhea is severe or for women with menstrual disturbances, low doses of bromocriptine (2–10 mg/day) or amantadine may be used (141).

iii) Weight gain. Weight gain occurs with most antipsychotic medications in up to 40% of treated patients (138). The most notable exception is molindone, which may not cause significant weight gain. The dose of antipsychotic medication may be reduced and efforts at dietary control initiated. There are few pharmacologic treatments with proven efficacy; one report suggests that amantadine may reverse antipsychotic-induced weight gain (141). An endocrine mechanism has not been established (138).

iv) Effects on sexual function.   Disturbances in sexual function can occur (142). For example, erectile dysfunction occurs in 23%–54% of men (114). Other effects can include ejaculatory disturbances in men and loss of libido or anorgasmia in women and men. In addition, with specific antipsychotic medications, including thioridazine and risperidone (103), retrograde ejaculation has been reported. These effects are mainly due to antiadrenergic and antiserotonergic effects. Dose reduction or discontinuation usually results in improvement or elimination of symptoms. Imipramine, 25–50 mg h.s., may be helpful for treating retrograde ejaculation induced by thioridazine (143). If dose reduction or a switch to an alternative medication is not feasible, yohimbine (an α_2 antagonist) or cyproheptadine (a 5-HT$_2$ antagonist) can be used (138).

v) Allergic and hepatic effects.   Cutaneous reactions occur infrequently with antipsychotic medications. Medication discontinuation or administration of an antihistamine is usually effective in reversing these symptoms. Photosensitivity also occurs infrequently and is most common with the low-potency phenothiazine medications; patients should be instructed to avoid excessive sunlight and/or use sunscreen (79). Also occurring with this class of medications are elevation of liver enzyme levels and cholestatic jaundice. Jaundice has been noted to occur in 0.1%–0.5% of patients taking chlorpromazine (79). This usually occurs within the first month after the initiation of treatment and generally requires discontinuation of treatment. Given the relative infrequency of antipsychotic-induced jaundice, other etiologies for jaundice should be evaluated before the cause is judged to be antipsychotic medication.

vi) Ophthalmologic effects.   Pigmentary retinopathies and corneal opacities can occur with chronic administration of the low-potency medications thioridazine and chlorpromazine, particularly at high doses (e.g., more than 800 mg/day of thioridazine). For this reason, patients maintained with these medications should have periodic ophthalmologic examinations (approximately every 2 years for patients with a cumulative treatment of more than 10 years). A maximum dose of 800 mg/day of thioridazine is recommended (138). With the increased use of high-potency medications in the past two decades, there has been virtually no reporting of this side effect (82).

vii) Hematologic effects.   Hematologic effects, including inhibition of leukopoiesis, can occur with use of antipsychotic medications. Such effects include a benign leukopenia and the more serious agranulocytosis. The best data exist for chlorpromazine, with which benign leukopenia occurs in up to 10% of patients and agranulocytosis occurs in 0.32% of patients (138).

(3) Implementation

Antipsychotic medications have a very high therapeutic index (86). Consequently, overdoses rarely are fatal unless they are complicated by preexisting medical problems or concurrent ingestion of alcohol or other medications. Symptoms of overdose are generally characterized by exaggerations of the adverse effects, with respiratory depression and hypotension presenting the greatest danger. Treatment is symptomatic and supportive and includes 1) inducing emesis and gastric lavage; 2) ensuring airway patency and maintenance of respiration; 3) maintaining blood pressure with intravenous fluids, plasma, concentrated albumin, and vasopressor agents; and 4) anticholinergic agents to counteract extrapyramidal signs (120).

"Sudden death"—described as "a natural death, occurring instantaneously, or within one hour of the onset of symptoms, in a patient who may or may not have known pre-existing disease but in whom the time and mode come unexpectedly"—has been reported to occur in patients receiving antipsychotic medications (144). However, the rate of sudden death has not been found to be higher in patients receiving psychotropic medication (including antipsychotic medications) than in the general U.S. population (144). Although psychotropic medication treatment could have a purely coincidental association with sudden death, as suggested by the lack of an abnormally high incidence, there are a number of possible causes of death for individuals who are receiving antipsychotic medications. These include heart arrhythmia caused by cardiac toxicity, hypotension, seizure, aspiration, asphyxiation, megacolon and paralytic ileus, heat stroke, malignant hyperthermia, neuroleptic malignant syndrome, and physical exhaustion. It has been suggested that the pharmacologic actions of psychotropic medications could interact with stress in psychotic and agitated patients to make them more vulnerable to cardiovascular and autonomic system complications (144). Consequently, efforts to reduce possible risk factors for such complications should be considered, particularly for agitated, physically debilitated, and elderly patients. These considerations include a) minimization of medication dose; b) judicious use of physical restraints; c) adequate hydration and attention to thermoregulation, particularly in hot weather; and d) attention to signs of emerging neuroleptic malignant syndrome (rigidity, hyperthermia, blood pressure variability). In light of these considerations, psychiatrists should use the minimum antipsychotic medication dose necessary, monitor patients' vital signs and neurologic status, and ensure adequate hydration and a well-ventilated, temperature-controlled treatment setting (144).

(a) Route of administration

Psychiatrists can administer antipsychotic medications in oral forms, as short-acting intramuscular preparations, or as long-acting depot preparations. Short-acting intramuscular medications reach a peak concentration 30–60 minutes after the medication is administered, whereas oral medications reach a peak in 2–3 hours (145). As a result, the calming effect of the antipsychotic may begin more quickly when the medication is administered parenterally. However, this calming effect on agitation is different from the true antipsychotic effect of these medications, which may require several days or weeks (84).

A single or twice-daily dose of an oral preparation will result in steady-state blood levels in 2–5 days (145). Long-acting depot antipsychotic medications (fluphenazine decanoate or enanthate and haloperidol decanoate in the United States) require at least 3 to 6 months to reach a steady state (146). As a result, they are seldom used during acute treatment, when the psychiatrist is adjusting the dose in accordance with therapeutic and side effects.

The advantage of depot medications has been best demonstrated in studies such as those conducted by Johnson (147) under conditions that resemble most closely those in community clinics. In these studies, patients with histories of poor compliance were included in the population and the amount of contact between patients and staff was limited. In the larger, more carefully controlled investigations (89, 148), patients with serious compliance problems—that is, the individuals most likely to benefit from treatment with depot medications—were commonly not included. The study by Hogarty et al. (148) also included a second year, during which patients receiving fluphenazine decanoate had a lower rate of relapse than those assigned to oral fluphenazine.

Depot medications are thought to be especially helpful in the maintenance phase. Janicak et al. (79) examined six studies that compared the risk of psychotic relapse in patients who were randomly assigned to receive either oral or depot medication. The longest of those studies (148) lasted 2 years and showed a relapse rate of 65% for patients taking oral medication and a rate of 40% for patients taking depot medication. Although the remaining five studies, all of which lasted 1 year or less, had inconsistent results, a meta-analysis of all six studies showed a significantly lower relapse rate in patients who received depot treatment (p<0.0002) (79).

(b) Dosage strategy

The effective dose of a conventional antipsychotic medication is closely related to its affinity for dopamine receptors (particularly D_2 receptors) and its tendency to cause extrapyramidal side effects (149, 150). Thus, high-potency medications have a greater affinity for dopamine receptors than do low-potency medications, and a much lower dose is required to treat psychosis. This can be expressed in terms of dose equivalence; e.g., 100 mg of chlorpromazine has an antipsychotic effect that is similar to that of 2 mg of haloperidol. The dose equivalencies of commonly prescribed medications are listed in table 1.

High-potency antipsychotic medications, such as haloperidol and fluphenazine, are more commonly prescribed than low-potency compounds (151). Although these medications have a greater tendency to cause extrapyramidal side effects than the low-potency medications, such as chlorpromazine and thioridazine, their side effects are easier to manage than the sedation and orthostatic hypotension associated with low-potency agents. High-potency medications can more safely be administered intramuscularly, since they seldom cause hypotension. In addition, because of sedation, orthostatic hypotension, and lethargy, the dose of a low-potency medication should be increased gradually, whereas an adequate dose of a high-potency medication can usually be achieved within a day or two. Finding the best dose of a conventional antipsychotic is complicated by a number of factors. Patients with schizophrenia demonstrate large differences in the dose of antipsychotic they can tolerate and the dose required for an antipsychotic effect. A patient's age may determine the appropriate dose; the elderly are frequently more sensitive to both the therapeutic and toxic effects of antipsychotics. In addition, it is difficult to determine dose by assessing antipsychotic effectiveness, since it may take many days at a therapeutic dose before there is an appreciable decrease in psychosis (83, 86).

A number of studies (reviewed in references 82 and 152) provide guidance about the usual doses required for acute treatment. Results of 19 controlled trials suggested that daily doses below 250 mg of chlorpromazine (or 5 mg of haloperidol or fluphenazine) are less adequate for many acutely psychotic patients than are moderate doses, between 300 and 600 mg. In the studies reviewed by Baldessarini et al. (152), response was typically measured by improvement in the score on the excitement, agitation, or psychosis subscale of the Brief Psychiatric Rating Scale (BPRS) (153), and the proportions of patients responding to low doses after 1 and 2–10 days were 38% and 50%, respectively; these rates compared unfavorably with the improvement rates of 61% and 56% among patients taking moderate doses for similar periods. Davis et al. (82) came to similar conclusions. They found that daily doses between 540 and 940 mg of chlorpromazine were optimal. The findings of clinical trials involve groups of patients; some individuals have optimal responses at doses above or below these optimal ranges. Many psychiatrists have treated acutely psychotic patients with high doses of high-potency antipsychotic medications during the first days of treatment. This treatment is based on the belief that higher doses result in a more rapid improvement than that resulting from moderate doses (154). However, Baldessarini et al. (152) found that high daily doses (more than 800 mg of chlorpromazine equivalents daily) were no more effective, or faster acting, on average than were moderate doses (500–700 mg/day). After 1 day, 50% of the patients treated with high doses responded, compared to 61% receiving moderate doses. After 2–10 days, high-dose treatment led to a slightly worse outcome: only 38% of those receiving high doses but 56% of those receiving moderate doses were improved. These studies indicate that higher doses are no more effective than normal doses, but they are associated with a greater incidence of side effects.

Controlled trials have provided similar information regarding the effect of medication dose on outcome during the maintenance phase. Baldessarini et al. (152) reviewed 33 randomized trials in which high doses (mean, 5200 mg/day of chlorpromazine equivalents) were compared to low doses (mean, 400 mg/day) during maintenance treatment. The lower doses were more effective in improving clinical state in over two-thirds of the trials. In addition, in 95% of the studies the higher doses resulted in greater neurologic side effects. Studies of doses less than 200 mg/day of chlorpromazine equivalents tended to show that such doses were less effective than higher doses.

An international consensus conference (155) made the reasonable recommendation of a reduction in antipsychotic dose of approximately 20% every 6 months until a minimal maintenance dose is reached. A minimal dose was considered to be as low as 2.5 mg of oral fluphenazine or haloperidol daily, 50 mg of haloperidol decanoate every 4 weeks, or 5 mg of fluphenazine decanoate every 2 weeks.

Concerns about the side effects of antipsychotic medications during maintenance and the risk of tardive dyskinesia led to several studies that focused on methods for treating patients with the lowest effective maintenance dose. A number of investigators (76, 156–158) have studied gradual reductions in the amounts of medication given to stabilized patients until the medications are completely discontinued. Each patient is then followed closely until there are signs of the beginning of a relapse. At that time, the patient's medication is reinstituted. To make this strategy work, patients and their families are trained to detect the early signs of impending psychotic breakdown.

Studies of the efficacy of the targeted medication approach have produced mixed results. Carpenter et al. (156) found that roughly one-half of the patients in each treatment group, both patients receiving targeted medication and those receiving continuous medication, were rehospitalized during a 2-year period. Herz et al. (76) found a nonsignificantly higher rate of reemergence of psychotic symptoms for intermittently treated patients (30%) than for patients maintained on medication regimens (16%) over 2 years. Jolley et al. (157) found a significant difference in the rates of psychotic symptom relapse between intermittent treatment (30%) and maintenance (7%); however, on the basis of their finding that over 70% of the relapses were preceded by prodromal dysphoric and neurotic symptoms, Jolley et al. suggested that targeted medication treatment may be appropriate for some patients, for example, those who relapse gradually and retain their insight and compliance during relapse.

A presumed advantage of targeted medication over continuous medication has been that it may cause less tardive dyskinesia and other side effects. However, the preceding described studies provide only mixed findings on whether this advantage exists or its magnitude. Jolley et al. (157) found significantly fewer extrapyramidal side effects and a trend toward less tardive dyskinesia after 1 year among patients treated intermittently. However, Herz et al. (76) found no differences in medication side effects between intermittent and maintenance groups after 2 years. Carpenter et al. (156) provided no data on side effects in their two treatment groups.

Another strategy involves using much lower doses of depot antipsychotic than are usually prescribed. Studies by three separate groups have compared low doses to high doses of fluphenazine decanoate. Initially, Kane et al. (159) found that patients receiving very low doses (mean, 2.5 mg every 2 weeks) were significantly more likely to relapse over the course of 1 year than were patients receiving standard doses (12.5–50.0 mg every 2 weeks) (56% versus 7%). In a subsequent report, Kane et al. (160) demonstrated that patients given a slightly higher dose (2.5–10.0 mg every 2 weeks) showed a nonsignificant difference in relapse after 1 year from patients given standard doses (24% versus 14%). Marder et al. (161) found no significant difference in relapse between low doses (mean, 5 mg every 2 weeks) and standard doses (25–50 mg every 2 weeks) after 1 year but did detect a significant difference in relapse between low doses and standard doses (70% versus 35%) after 2 years. Hogarty et al. (162) reported no difference in relapse rates between low doses (mean, 3.8 mg every 2 weeks) and standard doses (25 mg every 2 weeks) after 2 years. Collectively, these studies indicate that doses of fluphenazine decanoate in the range of 5–10 mg every 2 weeks may be as clinically effective as conventional doses of 25–50 mg every 2 weeks.

In consideration of a low-dose depot antipsychotic strategy, the beneficial side effect profile associated with the use of lower doses should also be considered. Kane et al. (159) found that low-dose users had fewer early signs of tardive dyskinesia after 1 year than did standard-dose users. In the Marder et al. study (161), lower doses were associated with significantly less discomfort (as measured with the SCL-90-R [163]), psychomotor retardation, and akathisia after 2 years. Hogarty et al. (162) reported that patients receiving minimal doses had less muscle rigidity, akathisia, and other side effects at 1 year and had greater improvements in instrumental and interpersonal role performances at 2 years.

(c) Medication interactions

A number of medication interactions can have clinically important effects for patients who are treated with antipsychotic medications (114). Certain heterocyclic antidepressants, most selective serotonin reuptake inhibitors (SSRIs), some β blockers, and cimetidine may increase plasma levels and increase side effects. On the other hand, barbiturates and carbamazepine decrease plasma levels.

b) Clozapine

(1) Goals and efficacy

Clozapine is an atypical antipsychotic medication that is distinguished from other antipsychotic medications by its lack of extrapyramidal side effects. However, it causes potentially fatal agranulocytosis in about 1% of patients.

One study by Shopsin et al. (164) compared clozapine to both chlorpromazine and a placebo in the treatment of chronically ill schizophrenic patients involuntarily hospitalized with acute symptom exacerbations. Although the placebo arm was discontinued because the patients were unable to remain in the 5-week study, the results indicated that clozapine was superior to chlorpromazine. The clozapine-treated patients, compared to the chlorpromazine-treated patients, had significantly greater reductions in psychotic symptoms (60% versus 25%), proportions with improved clinical ratings (90%–100% versus 75%), and proportions judged to be ready for discharge (70% versus 25%). Baldessarini and Frankenberg (101) reviewed 14 double-blind studies that compared clozapine with a conventional antipsychotic. They found that 9% more of the subjects taking clozapine had improved symptoms and that those patients' mean clinical ratings improved 13% more than did the ratings of the patients taking conventional antipsychotics, although neither difference was statistically significant. The researchers concluded that clozapine is at least as effective as conventional medications. Other reviewers (165–167) have noted that the advantages of clozapine are most apparent when the dose is over 300 mg/day.

Clinical trials with clozapine indicate that certain populations of patients with schizophrenia are likely to improve if their treatment is changed from a conventional antipsychotic to clozapine. The strongest evidence is for patients whose illness is refractory to conventional antipsychotic medications. A multicenter study by Kane et al. (168) defined treatment-resistant patients as those who had not responded to three different conventional antipsychotics before the study and then subsequently did not respond to a 6-week trial of haloperidol at the start of the study. Improvements in symptoms and global clinical ratings occurred in 30% of the patients treated with clozapine for 6 weeks, in contrast to only 4% of the patients treated with chlorpromazine.

Breier et al. (169) followed outpatients who had persistent positive or negative symptoms after treatment with conventional antipsychotics and who had residual symptoms after a 6-week trial of fluphenazine. The patients were treated for 1 year with clozapine, and outcome measures were compared with those in the year before clozapine treatment. After clozapine treatment, the patients had significantly fewer symptom relapses (20% versus 86%) and significantly fewer hospitalizations (8% versus 38%). In a crossover comparison of clozapine and fluphenazine, Pickar et al. (170) evaluated patients who had not responded to two different antipsychotics or had significant extrapyramidal side effects. The mean duration of moderate clozapine doses was 52 days, and the mean duration of optimal clozapine doses was 107 days; the mean duration of fluphenazine treatment was 46 days. Clozapine was more effective in reducing positive and negative symptoms for 38% of the patients; fluphenazine was more effective for only 5% of the patients.

Clozapine's effectiveness in a typical inpatient setting was evaluated in a randomized trial involving 202 patients with treatment-resistant schizophrenia (171). At the end of the 6-week clinical trial the proportion of patients who were judged to be improved was 30%. At the end of 12 weeks (29%) and at 1 year (33%) the proportions were similar. This descriptive epidemiologic study shows clinical practitioners the contrast between the greater external validity (generalizability) of the field trial and the greater internal validity of the short-term randomized clinical trial, although in this instance the data are quite consistent. Together the studies offer a spectrum of short- and long-term effectiveness of clozapine.

Clozapine has also been evaluated specifically in the treatment of patients who are unable to tolerate conventional antipsychotic medications because of side effects, particularly extrapyramidal symptoms and tardive dyskinesia. The only controlled trial involving this population was reported by Claghorn et al. (172), who studied patients with active psychotic symptoms and adverse neurologic reactions after treatment with at least two conventional antipsychotics. At the end of the 8-week randomized trial, the clozapine-treated patients had a 23% reduction in positive and negative symptoms, whereas the chlorpromazine-treated patients had a 15% reduction. Also, 58% of the chlorpromazine-treated patients but only 11% of the clozapine-treated patients had to drop out of the study because of extrapyramidal symptoms.

Support for clozapine's effectiveness in the stable or maintenance phase of treatment is based on a number of open-label studies. Meltzer et al. (167) studied patients who had previously not responded in at least three trials of different conventional antipsychotics. The rehospitalization rate after 1 year of treatment was 83% lower than that in the year before clozapine treatment. Miller et al. (173) found that the number and duration of hospitalizations among patients treated with clozapine for 2.5 years were significantly lower than those during an equal period before clozapine treatment. Breier et al. (169) also showed that, compared to the year preceding treatment, patients treated with clozapine had significantly fewer symptom relapses (mean, 0.3 versus 2.0) and hospitalizations (mean, 0.4 versus 1.3). All of these studies included patients who were treated with clozapine because they had not responded to previous treatments. Taken together, these studies provide some evidence that clozapine prevents relapse in stabilized patients. Moreover, each study found that a number of patients demonstrated improvements in social and occupational functioning. Although these studies are encouraging, they are limited since they included only clozapine responders who continued to take the medication and no other medication was compared to clozapine.

(2) Side effects

(a) Common, dose-related side effects

Clozapine is associated with sedation, weight gain, hypersalivation, tachycardia, orthostatic hypotension, and fever (166). The first three are extremely common, occurring in the majority of patients, particularly in the initial phase of treatment.

Clozapine is also associated with a dose-related risk of seizures. The overall seizure rate is 2.8%; with low-dose treatment (<300 mg/day) the risk is 1%, with medium doses (300–599 mg/day) the risk is 2.7%, and with high doses (>599 mg/day) the risk is 4.4%. The seizure risk for clozapine is also related to rapid increases in dose. Therefore, the rate of titration should not exceed the guidelines described in section III.C.1.b.3.

(b) Less common, idiosyncratic side effects

Clozapine causes agranulocytosis in approximately 1% of patients who receive it (174). Agranulocytosis is defined as a granulocyte count less than $500/mm^3$ (79). Although the danger of this life-threatening condition can be minimized by weekly blood monitoring, it remains higher than for any other antipsychotic medication. Agranulocytosis is usually reversible if treatment is discontinued immediately (175). Patients with agranulocytosis should not receive clozapine again. Through 1995, clozapine had been associated with 382 cases of agranulocytosis and 12 fatalities in the United States (in about 100,000 "starts" of clozapine treatment; Sandoz Pharmaceuticals Corp., personal communication).

When agranulocytosis develops, patients are given intensive treatment for the secondary complications, e.g., sepsis (176). Granulocyte colony stimulating factor has been used to accelerate granulopoietic function and shorten recovery time (176, 177).

There is also evidence that clozapine is less likely to cause tardive dyskinesia than other antipsychotic medications and may be an effective treatment for tardive dyskinesia and tardive dystonia (although clozapine is not a cure for tardive dyskinesia, it may allow time for recovery from tardive dyskinesia in some patients) (131, 178).

(3) Implementation

Clozapine treatment should not be initiated if the initial WBC count is less than $3500/mm^3$ or if the patient has a history of a myeloproliferative disorder or a history of clozapine-induced agranulocytosis or granulocytopenia.

It is recommended that treatment be initiated at a low dose (12.5 mg once or twice daily) and increased gradually (by no more than 25–50 mg/day) if tolerated, until a target dose is reached at the end of 2 weeks. Subsequent dose increases should be made in increments no greater than 100 mg and no more frequently than once or twice weekly (179).

Controlled trials provide only limited guidance regarding the optimal dose of clozapine for schizophrenia. Since there have been no trials in which patients were randomly assigned to different doses of clozapine, the only available data are based on studies in which psychiatrists used what they considered the most effective dose. Fleischhacker et al. (180) reviewed 16 controlled trials from Europe and the United States. The mean dose from the European trials was 283.7 mg/day, and the U.S. mean was 444 mg/day.

Some investigators have suggested measuring plasma levels of clozapine and achieving levels between 200 and 400 ng/ml (typically associated with a dose of 300–400 mg/day) (114). The clinical utility of plasma levels and the correlation of plasma levels with efficacy or side effects remain uncertain, however (181). Patients who are treated with clozapine should be started with an initial dose of 12.5–25.0 mg/day. At this dose they should be monitored for signs of orthostatic hypotension, tachycardia, sedation, and respiratory depression. The dose of clozapine should be gradually increased in 12.5–25.0-mg daily increments until a target dose is reached. Although most clozapine responders demonstrate clinical improvement during the first 6 weeks of treatment, others respond more slowly. Experts differ as to the appropriate length of a clozapine trial; some suggest trials of at least 6 months (165), and others suggest that trials should not exceed 2–4 months (182). Twelve-week empirical trials of clozapine appear to be adequate to determine whether a patient is likely to respond to this medication.

The elimination half-life of clozapine is approximately 12 hours, indicating that patients are likely to reach a steady-state plasma concentration after 1 week (183). SSRIs (e.g., fluoxetine, paroxetine), valproic acid, and nefazodone (184) may increase clozapine plasma levels. The concomitant use of medications such as carbamazepine can lower the WBC count and increase the potential danger of agranulocytosis; it should therefore be avoided. Some cases of respiratory or cardiac arrest have occurred among patients receiving benzodiazepines or other psychoactive medications concomitantly with clozapine. While no specific interaction between clozapine and benzodiazepines has been established, judicious use is advised when benzodiazepines or other psychotropic medications are administered with clozapine (179).

Since the side effects of clozapine in the initial and dose-adjustment phases may be severe in some patients, admission to the hospital may be justifiable for some patients (e.g., unstable patients who require rapid dose increases to a therapeutic level and have no social support system or patients prone to orthostatic hypotension or seizures).

Current guidelines (179) specify that the WBC count be checked before initiation of clozapine treatment, at least weekly for the duration of treatment, and weekly for 4 weeks after the termination of treatment. Patients are advised to report any sign of infection (e.g., sore throat, fever, weakness, or lethargy) immediately. The following are guidelines for action based on laboratory hematology results:

a. If the WBC count is <2000/mm^3 or the absolute neutrophil count (ANC) is <1000/mm^3,

- stop clozapine treatment immediately,
- check WBC and differential counts daily,
- consider bone marrow aspiration,
- consider protective isolation if granulopoiesis is deficient.

b. If the WBC count is 2000–3000/mm^3 or the ANC is 1000–1500/mm^3,

- stop clozapine treatment immediately,
- check the WBC and differential counts daily,

- monitor for signs of infection,
- clozapine may be resumed if no infection is present, the WBC count is >3000, and the ANC is >1500 (resume checking WBC count twice a week until it is >3500).

c. If the WBC count is 3000–3500/mm^3, if it falls by 3000/mm^3 over 1–3 weeks, or if immature forms are present, repeat the WBC count with a differential count. If the subsequent WBC count is 3000–3500 and the ANC is >1500/mm^3, repeat the WBC count with a differential count twice a week until the WBC count is >3500/mm^3. If a subsequent WBC count is <3000 or an ANC is <1500/mm^3, go to step a or b.

c) Risperidone

Risperidone is an antipsychotic medication from a chemical class that is different from that of either conventional antipsychotic medications or clozapine. Its distinct properties have been attributed to central antagonism of both serotonin and dopamine receptors.

(1) Goals and efficacy

Several studies provide evidence of risperidone's antipsychotic efficacy, and some suggest it may be more useful than conventional antipsychotic medications in treating negative symptoms. However, there are limitations in these data, including the fact that the largest trials compared multiple risperidone doses to a single dose of haloperidol (71, 103, 185, 186). Johnson and Johnson (187) have criticized the Risperidone Study Group trial (185), which did not control for prior medication history and had a relatively short washout period.

In double-blind studies comparing risperidone to standard antipsychotics or a placebo for the treatment of schizophrenia, Min et al. (188) compared risperidone doses of 5 and 10 mg/day to 5 and 10 mg/day of haloperidol, Ceskova and Svestka (189) compared 2–20 mg/day of risperidone to 2–20 mg/day of haloperidol, and Peuskens (185) compared 1–16 mg/day of risperidone to 10 mg/day of haloperidol. In all three medication trials, patients treated with risperidone for 8 weeks had reductions in positive and negative symptoms comparable to those for patients treated with haloperidol.

In a 6-week medication trial, Borison et al. (190) found symptom reductions in 60% of patients treated with risperidone (average dose, 9.7 mg/day) and only 25% of haloperidol-treated patients (average dose, 18 mg/day), although this difference was not statistically significant. In a 12-week trial comparing risperidone (mean dose, 12 mg/day) to haloperidol (mean dose, 10 mg/day), Claus et al. (102) found significantly greater improvement for the risperidone-treated patients on clinical ratings and on one symptom measure; 33% showed improvement in the total score on the Positive and Negative Syndrome Scale (PANSS) (191), compared to 24% of the patients taking haloperidol. Hoyberg et al. (192) compared risperidone (mean dose, 8.5 mg/day) to perphenazine (mean dose, 28 mg/day) in an 8-week trial. They also found significantly greater improvements in PANSS total score among risperidone-treated patients; symptom reductions were found in 78% of the patients taking risperidone but only 59% of the patients treated with perphenazine.

A large double-blind trial by Müller-Spahn et al. (186) was an 8-week international multisite study that compared 10 mg/day of haloperidol and 1, 4, 8, 12, or 16 mg/day of risperidone. Although 1 mg/day of risperidone was the least effective dose, 4, 8, and 12 mg/day of risperidone all proved to be more effective in reducing symptoms than 10 mg/day of haloperidol (which had efficacy comparable to that of 16 mg/day of risperidone).

Some evidence for the efficacy of risperidone at treating specifically positive or negative symptoms comes from a large double-blind study carried out in the United States (71) and Canada (103). In this 8-week trial, four doses of risperidone (2, 6, 10, and 16 mg/day) were compared to 20 mg/day of haloperidol or placebo. In the U.S. study, improvement in total PANSS score was seen among significantly greater proportions of patients treated with 6 and 16 mg/day of risperidone than among haloperidol-treated patients. PANSS scores for positive symptoms were significantly lower among patients treated with 6, 10, and 16 mg/day of risperidone or with haloperidol than among patients given placebo. PANSS scores for negative symptoms were significantly lower than for placebo-treated patients among the patients treated with 6 and 16 mg/day of risperidone but not for patients given other risperidone doses or haloperidol. The findings from the Canadian component of the trial were similar. On the total PANSS and the positive symptom subscale, all risperidone groups (except 2 mg/day), but not the haloperidol group, had significantly better scores than did the placebo group. On the PANSS negative symptom subscale, only 6 mg/day of risperidone was significantly superior to placebo. The authors of these studies concluded that there was strong evidence for the efficacy of risperidone in treating positive symptoms and a suggestion that risperidone may be more effective for negative symptoms than conventional antipsychotics.

Although the U.S.-Canadian trials showed that the most effective risperidone dose, 6 mg/day, was significantly more effective than the 20-mg/day dose of haloperidol, this trial may have given risperidone an unfair advantage since multiple risperidone doses were compared to only a single haloperidol dose. The findings from the U.S.-Canadian trials will need to be verified, particularly in studies that use haloperidol at other doses or use other antipsychotic medications.

Davis and Janicak (193) conducted a meta-analysis of five double-blind controlled trials. They found that risperidone given at daily doses of 6–12 mg was significantly more effective than typical doses of standard antipsychotics (e.g., haloperidol, 10–20 mg daily).

There have been no controlled trials providing information about the effectiveness of risperidone in preventing relapse during the stable phase of treatment. In an open clinical trial, Addington et al. (194) found that patients treated with risperidone for 1 year had a significant (20%) reduction in the number of days they were hospitalized, compared to the year before risperidone treatment.

(2) Side effects
Studies using multiple doses of risperidone (71, 103, 185) have shown that this medication causes a dose-related increase in extrapyramidal side effects. Several of these studies indicate that the severity of extrapyramidal side effects with risperidone is lower than with conventional antipsychotic medications. As mentioned previously, this evidence is limited by the fact that in the largest studies risperidone was compared to only a single dose of haloperidol: 10 mg/day in the study by Peuskens et al. (185) and 20 mg/day in the study by Chouinard et al. (103).

In the U.S.-Canadian study, patients who received 6 mg/day of risperidone—the most effective dose—required antiparkinsonian medications at about the same rate as patients who received placebo. In the Risperidone Study Group trial (185), the maximum increase in score on the Extrapyramidal Symptom Rating Scale (195), between baseline and treatment, was measured. The increases in scores were significantly greater in patients treated with 10 mg/day of haloperidol (mean increase, 5.1) than in patients treated with risperidone doses of 1, 4, 8, and 12 mg/day (mean increases of 1.1, 1.8, 2.7, and 3.2, respectively). Although 10 mg/day of haloperidol also caused more extrapyramidal side effects than did 16 mg/day of risperidone, the difference was not statistically significant.

Risperidone produces some drowsiness and orthostatic hypotension. The Risperidone Study Group (185) noted sedation in 33% of the patients treated with 8 mg/day of risperidone. By comparison, they observed sleepiness in 40% of the patients treated with 10 mg/day of haloperidol. Orthostatic dizziness was reported in 18% of the patients treated with risperidone and in 23% of those treated with haloperidol.

Other common side effects among patients treated with 8 mg/day of risperidone or 10 mg/day of haloperidol that were noted by the Risperidone Study Group included the following: weight gain in 34% and 25%, respectively; decreased sexual interest in 10% and 12%; and erectile dysfunction in 9% and 13%. Kopala and Honer (196) and Remington and Adams (197) each reported a case in which risperidone appeared to induce obsessive-compulsive symptoms.

Risperidone elevates prolactin levels, and as a result it may cause galactorrhea and menstrual disturbances. Several cases of neuroleptic malignant syndrome associated with risperidone have also been described and were reviewed by Marder (198). It is unknown whether risperidone is associated with the same risk of tardive dyskinesia as conventional antipsychotic medications.

(3) Implementation

The recommended procedures for starting risperidone treatment are the same as those for treating patients with conventional antipsychotics.

Studies comparing different doses of risperidone indicate that it is most effective at 4 to 6 mg daily (71, 103, 185). Higher doses may lead to extrapyramidal side effects without greater effectiveness.

Risperidone's effectiveness appears to be related to both the parent compound and a major metabolite, 9-hydroxyrisperidone (199). They have similar types of pharmacological activity and, therefore, probably produce similar therapeutic effects. Although risperidone itself has an elimination half-life of only 3 hours, its metabolite has an elimination half-life of about 24 hours. As a result, most patients can be managed with single daily doses of risperidone. However, since risperidone can cause orthostatic hypotension, twice-daily dosing may be useful during the titration phase and for patients who may be vulnerable to orthostatic changes, such as the elderly.

d) Newer antipsychotic medications

Olanzapine was approved by the U.S. Food and Drug Administration (FDA) in 1996, and sertindole and quetiapine are likely to be approved in 1997. The clinical data available on the safety and efficacy of these agents come from studies that were developed by the pharmaceutical companies in order to obtain FDA approval. Unfortunately, only a portion of these studies have been published to date and are available for review. The results that are available have been from comparisons of each new agent to placebo and, in some cases, to a conventional antipsychotic medication as well. These randomized controlled trials have demonstrated short-term efficacy of these three medications in the acute phase of schizophrenia. However, it remains unclear whether these medications have greater overall efficacy than traditional antipsychotic medications, greater efficacy in treating specifically negative or positive symptoms, or greater efficacy in treatment-resistant cases of schizophrenia. In addition, their long-term efficacy and safety are not yet clearly established. However, this relative lack of data must be viewed in the context of knowledge that 1) the FDA process involves extensive review of safety data—although neither the data nor the deliberations have been available for consideration—and 2) there is no reason to suspect that an antipsychotic medication with short-term efficacy would not also have long-term efficacy for patients with schizophrenia. All three newer antipsychotic medications appear to cause fewer extrapyramidal symptoms than conventional antipsychotic medications. Although these medications were developed with the goal of being atypical (clozapine-like) without causing agranulocytosis, they have not been studied sufficiently for researchers to determine the full extent of their clinical efficacy and safety. The possible advantages of these newer medications need to be balanced with their likely higher costs and their current availability only in short-acting oral form.

(1) Olanzapine

(a) Goals and efficacy

The efficacy of olanzapine was evaluated in a 6-week, double-blind comparison of three dose ranges of olanzapine—2.5–7.5 (low dose), 7.5–12.5 (medium dose), and 12.5–17.5 (high dose) mg/day—haloperidol (10–20 mg/day), and placebo involving 335 patients with acute episodes of schizophrenia (200). The middle and highest doses of olanzapine and haloperidol were significantly more effective than placebo, as measured by reduction in total BPRS score. Although the capacity of olanzapine to reduce negative symptoms was assessed, the results were inconclusive (the low and high doses, but not the middle dose, led to small decreases in symptoms).

The same authors (201) also reported results from a 6-week international, multi-center trial in which a single dose range of olanzapine (5–20 mg/day) was compared to a single dose range of haloperidol (5–20 mg/day) in 1,996 patients, most of whom had schizophrenia but some of whom had schizoaffective or schizophreniform disorder. Patients treated with olanzapine showed a significantly greater reduction in total BPRS symptoms (11% versus 8% reduction) and BPRS negative symptoms.

(b) Side effects

The most common side effects of olanzapine are sedation and a decrease in standing systolic blood pressure; olanzapine has also been associated with weight gain.

In the study reported by Beasley et al. (200), the low, medium, and high olanzapine doses were associated with decreases in parkinsonism and akathisia, whereas haloperidol was associated with increases when the patients were studied as a group. The high-dose olanzapine group was significantly more likely to receive antiparkinsonian medications on one or more occasions than the placebo patients (p<0.02) but were less likely to receive such medications than the haloperidol-treated patients (p<0.001). Data cited in the patient package insert for olanzapine indicate that on the basis of adverse events reports, patients taking medium- and high-dose olanzapine had statistically significantly more akathisia than patients taking placebo; the package insert also noted, however, that patients taking olanzapine (all doses) did not differ significantly from patients taking placebo in rates of akathisia and parkinsonism when these outcomes were determined by rating scales.

In addition, olanzapine has not been found to increase prolactin secretion levels above normal.

(c) Implementation

Olanzapine is an effective antipsychotic when administered in doses of 10–20 mg/day in the acute phase of schizophrenia. At this time there are no data on its use for treatment-resistant patients, for elderly patients, or in long-term treatment.

The manufacturer has recommended starting patients at 10 mg/day. Clinicians concerned about the potential for orthostatic hypotension, especially in the elderly, should start patients at 5 mg/day and gradually increase the dose by 5 mg/day until patients are receiving 10–20 mg/day. Since olanzapine is associated with weight gain, weight should be monitored and patients should be counseled about weight-control strategies.

(2) Sertindole

(a) Goals and efficacy

Sertindole has been evaluated in the acute phase of schizophrenia. In the first clinical study of efficacy, McEvoy et al. (202) compared sertindole to placebo in a 7-week randomized, double-blind trial involving 38 patients with schizophrenia or schizoaffective disorder. The doses were determined by the treating clinicians. The patients who received sertindole demonstrated significantly greater improvement in total BPRS and BPRS positive symptom scores than did the patients receiving placebo.

The efficacy of sertindole has also been evaluated in 205 patients with schizophrenia who received one of three doses of sertindole (8, 12, or 20 mg/day) or placebo (203). The patients who received 20 mg/day of sertindole, but not lower doses, had significantly more improvement than patients assigned to placebo.

Schulz et al. (204) reported the results of two large 8-week randomized, double-blind trials comparing three doses of sertindole (12, 20, and 24 mg/day) to three doses of haloperidol (4, 8, and 16 mg/day) and placebo in the treatment of patients with schizophrenia. Unfortunately, published information concerning the results of this trial is limited. However, it appears that both active medications were superior to placebo. Preliminary data suggest the possibility that sertindole has greater efficacy in treating negative symptoms than does placebo, although this needs to be further studied.

(b) Side effects

At the doses studied, sertindole appears to be relatively free of a tendency to produce extrapyramidal side effects. Moreover, sertindole caused only mild increases in prolactin levels; most treated patients had levels in the normal range. Sertindole also caused little or no sedation and anticholinergic side effects.

The most common side effects of sertindole were rhinitis and a decreased ejaculatory volume in men. In the study of van Kammen et al. (203), 17% of the men who received 20 mg of sertindole daily reported a decreased ejaculatory volume. This side effect is usually not associated with erectile disturbances, retrograde ejaculation, decreases in libido, or decreased fertility. Sertindole was also associated with orthostatic hypotension and tachycardia, particularly during the initial titration period.

Sertindole caused a dose-related lengthening in the QT interval (15–25 msec) on the ECG, which was not associated with clinically significant symptoms. Although these increases are relatively small and within the normal variation in QT interval that occurs daily, it raises a concern that patients receiving sertindole may be vulnerable to developing torsades des pointes, a potentially fatal ventricular arrhythmia. To date there are no documented cases of this arrhythmia among patients taking sertindole. Nevertheless, clinicians should be concerned when patients taking sertindole report episodes of dizziness or lightheadedness. (A newspaper report of a hearing of the FDA advisory committee cited several cases of sudden death that may have been associated with sertindole use. The significance of this report cannot be evaluated until data are available for review [205].)

(c) Implementation

Currently, sertindole has been studied only in patients with acute schizophrenia who can be considered treatment responsive. There are no controlled studies to indicate its effectiveness for patients whose disorders are refractory to conventional antipsychotics or in the long-term treatment of schizophrenia.

Because of its tendency to cause orthostatic hypotension, sertindole should be started at 4 mg/day and increased by 4 mg every 2 to 3 days. The effective dose for most patients is 12 to 24 mg daily (206). The utility of ECG monitoring for patients taking sertindole cannot be assessed on the basis of the available data.

Sertindole has a serum half-life of 1 to 4 days. This indicates that once-daily dosing will result in stable medication levels. This may also afford additional protection to patients who occasionally miss a dose.

(3) Quetiapine

(a) Goals and efficacy

The short-term efficacy of quetiapine for acute schizophrenia has been evaluated in two 6-week multicenter, randomized, double-blind placebo-controlled trials. An early study compared a low dose (up to 250 mg/day) and higher dose (up to 750 mg/day) of quetiapine to placebo in 109 patients with schizophrenia (207). Compared to placebo, any use of quetiapine was associated with a significantly greater reduction in total BPRS score, BPRS activation and thought disturbance subscale scores, and summary scores on the Scale for the Assessment of Negative Symptoms (SANS) (208). A second trial, comparing the same low and higher dose ranges of quetiapine to placebo in 190 patients with schizophrenia, had similar results (207). Use of any dose of quetiapine was again associated with significantly greater reductions in total BPRS score compared to placebo; the higher dose of quetiapine was significantly more effective than placebo in reducing scores on the BPRS subscales for thought disturbance, hostile/suspiciousness, activation, anxiety/depression, and anergia.

Quetiapine has also been investigated in two 6-week multicenter, randomized, double-blind trials in which patients treated with a conventional antipsychotic served as controls. Borison et al. (209) compared five fixed doses of quetiapine (75, 150, 300, 600, or 750 mg/day), haloperidol (12 mg/day), and placebo in 361 patients with schizophrenia. Quetiapine at all doses, as well as haloperidol, was more effective than placebo in reducing the total BPRS score and the score on the BPRS positive symptom cluster; the most effective dose of quetiapine was 300 mg/day. Quetiapine at 300 mg/day, but not haloperidol, was also significantly more effective than placebo in reducing the SANS summary score. In a trial comparing quetiapine (up to 750 mg/day) to chlorpromazine (up to 750 mg/day) in 201 subjects with schizophrenia, there were no significant differences between the two groups in reduction in total BPRS score, BPRS factor scores, or SANS summary score (207).

(b) Side effects

In all three placebo-controlled trials, quetiapine had no greater propensity to cause extrapyramidal side effects than did placebo. In the comparison of quetiapine and chlorpromazine, neither active medication was found to cause extrapyramidal side effects, making the results difficult to interpret (207).

The most common side effects of quetiapine are drowsiness, constipation, dry mouth, weight gain, and orthostatic hypotension. It does not elevate prolactin levels above the normal range.

(c) Implementation

Quetiapine has been used and found to be effective at doses between 150 and 800 mg/day. Since it has a half-life of 6.9 hours, it should be administered 2 to 3 times daily. Although the comparison of five fixed doses suggests that 300 mg/day may be the most effective dose (209), there is insufficient published information with which to make other prescribing recommendations.

2. Other medications

Various ancillary medications have been used to enhance the therapeutic efficacy of antipsychotic medications and to treat residual symptoms, including positive (210), negative (165, 211), and affective symptoms (212).

a) Lithium

(1) Goals and efficacy

Studies evaluating the antipsychotic properties of lithium alone indicate that it has limited effectiveness as monotherapy in schizophrenia and may be harmful for some patients. In a 3-week trial, Alexander et al. (213) reported modest improvements in psychotic symptoms in one-half of patients treated with lithium (mean blood level, 0.9 meq/liter). The majority of these improved patients relapsed within 2 weeks of lithium withdrawal. However, Shopsin et al. (214) found that patients with schizophrenia treated with 3 weeks of lithium therapy (mean blood level, 0.75 meq/liter) showed a significant (26%) worsening in BPRS score, compared with a significant (15%) improvement among chlorpromazine-treated patients.

When added to antipsychotic medications, lithium has been shown to augment the antipsychotic response, in general, as well as improve negative symptoms specifically. Growe et al. (215) compared the addition of lithium (serum levels maintained at 0.5–1.0 meq/liter) or placebo for 4 weeks to an antipsychotic regimen in a double-blind crossover trial. When treated with lithium, patients showed a significantly lower level of psychotic excitement than when treated with placebo. There were trends toward less seclusiveness and retardation as well. Small et al. (216) also studied the addition of lithium (levels maintained at 0.6–1.0 meq/liter) or placebo for 4 weeks to antipsychotics in a double-blind crossover trial. The addition of lithium was associated with significantly greater improvements, relative to placebo, in overt psychotic symptoms, excitement, mannerisms/posturing, irritability, cooperativeness, personal neatness, and social competence.

Lithium has also has been shown to have specific therapeutic benefits for schizophrenic patients with affective symptoms. Lerner et al. (217) investigated the addition of lithium (300 mg/day) or placebo for 6 weeks to a regimen of haloperidol for schizophrenic patients judged to have either elevated or nonelevated BPRS depression scores. Lithium produced significantly greater reductions in BPRS depression-anxiety scores in the depressed patients with schizophrenia than did placebo; the mean reduction for the lithium-treated patients was 26%. In the nondepressed patients with schizophrenia, there was no difference in impact on BPRS depression-anxiety ratings between the lithium and placebo conditions. Comparing the depressed patients with schizophrenia to the nondepressed patients with schizophrenia, lithium had a significantly greater ability to decrease thought disorder than did placebo. The requirement for haloperidol decreased the most among the lithium-treated depressed group (by a mean of 26.1 mg/day); no decrease in haloperidol requirement was noted among the placebo-treated depressed patients. Indirect evidence for the efficacy of lithium for schizophrenic patients with affective symptoms comes from several studies demonstrating that lithium plus antipsychotic medication is effective for patients with schizoaffective disorder (218–221).

(2) Side effects

The side effects of lithium include polyuria, polydipsia, weight gain, cognitive problems, tremor, sedation or lethargy, impaired coordination, gastrointestinal distress, hair loss, benign leukocytosis, acne, and edema. These have been reviewed in detail in the *Practice Guideline for the Treatment of Patients With Bipolar Disorder* (222; included in this volume). The combination of an antipsychotic medication and lithium may increase the possibility of the development of neuroleptic malignant syndrome. However, the evidence for this association comes mainly from some debated reports of cases or series of cases, rather than quantitative data. Most reported cases of neuroleptic malignant syndrome in patients treated with lithium plus antipsychotic medication have occurred in cases of high lithium levels associated with dehydration.

Estimates of the incidence of toxic reactions, in general, vary. Small et al. (216) found that 5% of patients developed a toxic reaction consisting of confusion and moderate memory loss while taking antipsychotic medication plus lithium (serum level, 0.6–1.0 meq/liter). However, in one study (214) the proportion of patients was considerably higher; over 50% of patients treated with lithium alone developed symptoms of a toxic-confusional state (mean level, 0.75 meq/liter; only one subject had a level above 1.0 meq/liter). No specific combination of medications is contraindicated, but psychiatrists should maintain an increased level of vigilance for signs of toxicity, particularly in the initial stage of treatment.

(3) Implementation

Generally, lithium is added to the antipsychotic medication that the patient is already receiving, after the patient has had an adequate trial of the antipsychotic medication but has reached a plateau in the level of response and residual symptoms persist. The dose of lithium is that required to obtain a blood level in the range of 0.8 to 1.2 meq/liter. Response to treatment usually appears promptly; a trial of 3 to 4 weeks is adequate for determining whether there is a therapeutic response, although some investigators have noted that improvements may emerge only after 12 weeks or more (223). Patients should be monitored for adverse effects that are commonly associated with lithium (e.g., polyuria, tremor) and with its interaction with an antipsychotic medication (e.g., extrapyramidal side effects, confusion, disorientation, other signs of neuroleptic malignant syndrome) (224), particularly during the initial period of combined treatment.

b) Benzodiazepines

(1) Goals and efficacy

Benzodiazepines have been evaluated as monotherapy for schizophrenia and as adjuncts to antipsychotic medications. Wolkowitz and Pickar (225) reviewed double-blind studies of benzodiazepines as monotherapy and found that positive effects (reductions in anxiety, agitation, global impairment, or psychotic symptoms) were reported in nine of 14 studies. Of studies examining specifically psychotic symptoms, six out of 10 showed greater efficacy for benzodiazepines than placebo. Few studies have compared benzodiazepines to antipsychotic medications; one that did (226) demonstrated that chlordiazepoxide is superior to placebo but inferior to chlorpromazine. The reviewers concluded that benzodiazepines by themselves may have mild antipsychotic efficacy in some patients.

Double-blind studies evaluating benzodiazepines as adjuncts to antipsychotic medications were also reviewed by Wolkowitz and Pickar (225). Seven of 16 studies showed some positive effect on anxiety, agitation, psychosis, or global impairment; five of 13 showed efficacy in treating psychotic symptoms specifically. The reviewers concluded that benzodiazepines may improve the response to antipsychotic medications.

Some studies indicate that the effectiveness of benzodiazepines as adjuncts to antipsychotic medications is limited to the acute phase and may not be sustained. Altamura et al. (227) found that clonazepam plus haloperidol, but not haloperidol alone or placebo, produced significant lowering of total BPRS scores after 1 week. This reduction, which was primarily due to decreases in anxiety and tension, disappeared by the end of the 4-week study. Csernansky et al. (228) also found that when alprazolam was added to antipsychotic medication there was a significant reduction in the BPRS withdrawal/retardation subfactor score after the first week, but this reduction disappeared by study end at week 5.

Wolkowitz and Pickar (225) suggested that benzodiazepines as adjuncts to antipsychotic medications may be most useful in the acute management of psychotic agitation. The efficacy for patients with prominent agitation was one of their most consistent findings, although none of the double-blind studies reviewed had evaluated this issue specifically. Some retrospective and open-label studies support the practice of adding a benzodiazepine to antipsychotic medication for this indication, and it has become a relatively common practice in many inpatient settings. Salzman et al. (229) reported that when lorazepam was added to antipsychotic medication for management of severe disruptive episodes, the mean dose and average number of doses of antipsychotic medication required were only half those needed when just antipsychotic medication was given.

(2) Side effects
Benzodiazepines have some limitations in schizophrenia. Their common side effects include sedation, ataxia, cognitive impairment, and a tendency to cause behavioral disinhibition in some patients. This last side effect can be a serious problem in patients who are being treated for agitation. Reactions to withdrawal from benzodiazepines can include psychosis and seizures. In addition, patients with schizophrenia are vulnerable to both abuse of and addiction to these agents.

(3) Implementation
A number of benzodiazepines have been evaluated, but few studies have compared the effectiveness of more than one. The studies reviewed by Wolkowitz and Pickar (225) provide little guidance regarding the selection of a specific medication. Although the studies of benzodiazepine monotherapy included more patients who improved with diazepam (67%) than with chlordiazepoxide (43%), this difference was not significant. In the absence of clear differences in the efficacy of different medications, other issues guide the choice of a benzodiazepine, including the available routes of administration, risk of respiratory arrest, and abuse potential. With these considerations in mind, many psychiatrists choose lorazepam, which can be administered intramuscularly, intravenously, or orally, has a limited propensity to cause respiratory arrest, and has less abuse potential than other shorter-acting medications.

The reviewed studies also provide little information regarding the most effective dose. The authors reported that studies with positive results used significantly higher doses of adjunctive benzodiazepines than studies with negative results (54.1 versus 22.0 mg/day of diazepam equivalents).

c) Anticonvulsants

(1) Goals and efficacy

There are no current indications for the use of the anticonvulsant medications carbamazepine and valproate in the treatment of schizophrenia alone. McElroy et al. (230) reviewed five available studies of valproate in schizophrenia and concluded that the evidence for efficacy is not compelling. One open trial of valproate as monotherapy showed reductions in psychotic symptoms in 70% of the patients. One open trial and one double-blind crossover study showed that the addition of valproate to antipsychotic medication significantly decreased psychotic and other psychiatric symptoms. However, none of these studies used operational criteria for the diagnosis of schizophrenia, and they may have included patients with affective or other neuropsychiatric conditions. In the two studies using operational criteria for the diagnosis of schizophrenia, valproate was either ineffective or deleterious.

Some studies have shown that the anticonvulsant medications may be useful adjuncts to antipsychotic medications for special patient populations, particularly those with EEG abnormalities suggestive of seizure activity and those with agitated/violent behavior. Neppe (231) conducted a double-blind crossover study of nonepileptic patients with temporal lobe EEG abnormalities who did not respond to antipsychotic medications alone; when carbamazepine was added to the antipsychotic medication, the level of aggression was only one-half of that when placebo was added.

In a retrospective study, Luchins (232) investigated adjunctive carbamazepine for violent patients with and without EEG abnormalities. In one part of the study, carbamazepine was added to the antipsychotic medication regimens of seven patients (six with schizophrenia and one with a mixed personality disorder) who had no EEG abnormalities. During carbamazepine treatment, there were 60% fewer aggressive episodes than in the period before or after the addition of carbamazepine. In the second part of this study, carbamazepine was added to the antipsychotic medication regimens of eight patients (six with schizophrenia, one with mild mental retardation, and one with an organic personality disorder) with EEG abnormalities. During the period of carbamazepine treatment, there were 37% fewer aggressive episodes than during the period before carbamazepine addition.

Okuma et al. (233) studied adjunctive carbamazepine use for schizophrenic patients with agitated/violent behavior who had responded poorly to antipsychotic medication alone. Adjunctive carbamazepine treatment produced moderate to marked improvement in more patients than did placebo (43% versus 28%), although this difference was not significant.

Anticonvulsants are effective in the treatment of patients with schizophrenia who have a concurrent seizure disorder (138). For these patients and for patients who have experienced a seizure while taking a medication that may have lowered the seizure threshold, e.g., clozapine, and who have a strong indication to continue, an anticonvulsant can be administered concurrently to prevent the recurrence of seizures.

(2) Side effects

There are generally no additional side effects from the combination of anticonvulsant and antipsychotic medications beyond those of the individual medications themselves. Carbamazepine is not recommended for use with clozapine, because of the potential of both medications to cause agranulocytosis.

(3) Implementation

These medications are generally used at the same therapeutic dose ranges and blood levels as for the treatment of seizure disorders. A complicating factor is the fact that both carbamazepine (234–236) and valproate (237) decrease the blood levels of antipsychotic medications by induction of hepatic enzymes.

d) Other medications

Reserpine, propranolol, clonidine, and calcium channel blockers have been added to existing antipsychotic medication regimens (238–240). Their potential utility is limited and requires further investigation. Given the availability of clozapine and risperidone and the potential use of lithium, benzodiazepines, and carbamazepine as adjunctive treatments, these should be preferentially used (165).

D. ELECTROCONVULSIVE THERAPY

1. Goals and efficacy

ECT has been studied in the acute phase of schizophrenia. In several studies of first-admission schizophrenic patients, ECT was found to be as effective as antipsychotic medications (241–244). One randomized study of first-admission patients conducted by May indicated that ECT was superior to either psychotherapy or milieu therapy alone, although it was not as effective as antipsychotic medication alone (245, pp. 235–236). On the other hand, virtually all studies of first-admission patients that compared the effects of ECT alone or antipsychotic medication alone with the combination of ECT and antipsychotic medication found that the combination was more effective than either treatment alone. In one study, ECT either with or without chlorpromazine was associated with more improvement than either fluphenazine alone (20 mg/day) or chlorpromazine alone (1 g/day) (242). Another study (246) showed greater short-term (1 to 3 weeks) improvement for patients treated with ECT plus chlorpromazine (400 mg/day) than for those given chlorpromazine alone; in later assessments (6 weeks, 6 months, 1 year) the therapies were equivalent. While ECT has been shown to produce fairly dramatic improvement in first-admission patients, it is not as effective for patients with chronic schizophrenia. Improvement in psychosis and return to the community is estimated at 50% to 70% for patients who have been ill for less than 1 year but is less than 20% for patients who have been continuously ill for more than 3 years (247–251).

Open clinical trials of schizophrenic patients, including those with "positive symptom psychosis" who did not respond to courses of antipsychotic medication alone, have yielded positive findings with ECT. The addition of ECT to continued treatment with antipsychotic medications, including thiothixene, fluphenazine, and molindone, enhanced treatment efficacy (252–254). The addition of ECT to clozapine for patients who did not respond to either traditional medication or a trial of clozapine alone has been reported to be safe and effective in a handful of cases (255).

The efficacy of maintenance ECT has not been studied adequately. However, it can be considered in the case of an ECT responder for whom pharmacologic prophylaxis alone has been ineffective or cannot be tolerated.

2. Side effects

The chief side effects of ECT are cognitive. Treatment is associated with a transient postictal confusional state and with a longer period of anterograde and retrograde memory interference. The memory impairment typically resolves in a few weeks after cessation of treatment, except for some recent autobiographical memories (at least with bilateral ECT) (256). Rarely, patients report more pervasive and persistent cognitive disruption, the basis of which is uncertain.

3. Implementation

The evaluation preceding ECT should consist of a psychiatric history and examination to verify the indication for this treatment, a general medical evaluation to identify risk factors (including history and physical examination, assessment of vital signs, hemogram, serum electrolyte measurements, and ECG), anesthesia evaluation addressing the nature and extent of anesthetic risk and the need for modification of medications or anesthetic technique, the obtaining of informed consent, and, finally, an evaluation that summarizes treatment indications and risks and suggests any indicated additional evaluative procedures, alterations in treatment, or modifications in ECT technique. Recent myocardial infarction, some cardiac arrhythmias, and some intracranial-space-occupying lesions are indications for caution and consultation, since ECT causes a transient rise in heart rate, cardiac workload, blood pressure, intracranial pressure, and blood-brain barrier permeability, which may not be tolerated by some patients with these conditions (257).

The available research studies have failed to show a difference in efficacy between unilateral nondominant-hemisphere ECT and bilateral ECT, although these studies are not definitive (258). In addition, there is significant disagreement among clinicians regarding the efficacy of these two types of ECT treatment. Unilateral ECT appears to cause less cognitive impairment than bilateral ECT. Factors that should influence the decision regarding the type of ECT include past response to ECT, urgency of the situation, and degree of cognitive impairment already present in the patient.

E. SPECIFIC PSYCHOSOCIAL INTERVENTIONS

As part of a comprehensive treatment approach, psychosocial interventions can improve the course of schizophrenia when integrated with psychopharmacologic treatments. These interventions can provide additional benefits for patients in such areas as relapse prevention, improved coping skills, better social and vocational functioning, and ability to function more independently. While pharmacotherapy deals with symptom suppression, psychosocial interventions may provide emotional support and address particular deficits associated with schizophrenia. Psychosocial treatments are interpersonal and call on various roles of the therapist: a manager to coordinate the services available within a treatment system, a teacher to provide education about the patient's disorder and how to cope with it, a friendly other to provide support and encouragement, a trained therapist to provide strategies for interpersonal enrichment, and a physician to provide biological treatments. These roles and therapeutic opportunities come in many forms and settings, e.g., individual, group, family. The choice of psychosocial approaches and particular interventions depends on the particular needs of a patient at various phases of the person's life and illness.

The goals and tasks of these treatments vary widely, depending on the individual patient, disorder, and life situation. The central components of psychosocial treatment are described under the earlier section on psychiatric management (section III.B). The overall goals are to minimize vulnerability and stress and to maximize adaptive capacities and functioning while enhancing social supports.

1. Individual therapy

Individual therapy has also frequently been referred to as "individual psychotherapy." It encompasses a range of interventions that may be useful in schizophrenia. The forms most commonly described are supportive and insight oriented. Although they are discussed in the literature as distinct entities, such categorizations are primarily useful for heuristic or research purposes. In practice, psychiatrists use a combination or synthesis of various approaches and strategies; these are determined by and individually tailored to each patient on the basis of that person's particular clinical condition, coping capacities, and preferences. The results of efficacy studies of psychotherapy are difficult to interpret. Earlier controlled outcome studies generally failed to demonstrate differential clinical/functional advantages of psychotherapy without medication over somatic therapies (245, 259, 260).

There is a body of literature examining the utility of including psychotherapy in a treatment regimen. For example, supportive, problem-solving techniques differentially reduced relapse and enhanced social and occupational functioning when added to medication for schizophrenia outpatients (77, 90, 261, 262). In the most definitive study to date, reality-oriented supportive strategies appeared to be as effective as, if not better than, insight-oriented treatment in terms of relapse and social/work adjustment (263, 264). Overall, the studies of the efficacy of psychotherapy are of variable quality, making generalizations hard to draw (265–268).

According to the clinical-descriptive literature, optimal individual therapy uses a variety of strategies (see section III.B) based on an empathetic, understanding, continuous interpersonal relationship. The goals and strategies of individual therapy are organized roughly by phase of illness. (See the sections on psychiatric management in each phase, sections IV.A.3 and IV.C.2.) Intensive exploratory techniques during the acute phase of psychosis can prolong disorganization or precipitate relapse (267, 269, 270). Exploratory therapy may be indicated for a small number of patients who have achieved a stable remission, demonstrated a solid therapeutic alliance, are compliant with maintenance medication, and have the capacity to tolerate and motivation to pursue insight-oriented work to control self-defeating behaviors, become more in touch with their feelings, and achieve emotional growth.

2. Family interventions

A guiding principle is that families should be involved and engaged in a collaborative treatment process to the greatest extent possible. Families are often the caretakers of patients and can benefit from education, guidance, and support, as well as training to help them manage in this role. Studies have shown that some family members, especially those who have little knowledge of the behavioral manifestations of schizophrenia, may be highly critical or overprotective of patients, and these behaviors may increase the likelihood of relapse (271–273). Often these behaviors stem from a lack of knowledge about the characteristics of the illness, such as deficit symptoms, which may be mistaken for laziness or willful withdrawal by the patient. The goals of family intervention include decreasing patient relapses, improving patient functioning, decreasing family burden, and improving family functioning. All approaches emphasize the value of family participation in treatment and stress the importance of working together in a collaborative endeavor. They have in common psychoeducation about the illness and its course, training in coping and problem-solving skills within the family, improved communication, and stress reduction. These interventions use practical educative and behavioral methods to elicit family participation and collaboration in treatment planning, goal setting, and service delivery. At times, the goal may be to help the situation by facilitating the patient's move toward independent living. It has not been demonstrated that any one of these approaches is superior to any of the others. The studies described all use somatic treatments in addition to the family interventions.

While the use of different variants of family management and the different types of control treatments makes it difficult to compare the results of the more than 10 controlled studies, relapse rates typically have been halved (274–286). The control treatments have included individual supportive therapy, intensive case management, and medication alone.

However, when a recently completed multisite study (Treatment Strategies for Schizophrenia, sponsored by the National Institute of Mental Health [NIMH]) used a less intensive, once-monthly variant of family management as a control condition for the more intensive family management approach, significant differences in relapse rates between the conditions were not found (287).

a) Adverse effects

An adverse effect of family management can be overstimulation of the patient from involvement in stressful family sessions while the patient is still in the acute phase, when florid symptoms are still intrusive and the ability to concentrate may be seriously compromised (288). The alliance with families can frequently be harmed when family interventions draw from the discredited theoretical approach that views family influences between childhood and the present as implicated in the *cause* of schizophrenia (289).

b) Implementation

The acute phase is the best time to engage the family in psychoeducational family meetings. When the patient is most ill, family members tend to be most motivated to reach out and make contact, ask questions, and seek information to reassure and guide them.

Families may be seen individually (275, 276) or in multiple-family groups (286, 290). It appears that the results with these two approaches are comparable, although McFarlane (290) found slightly better protection against relapse from the multiple-family groups in a controlled study. The practicing psychiatrist should remain flexible when considering the type of family intervention to offer, with patient and family preferences playing a large role.

3. Group therapy

The group therapies include a range of modalities, such as psychoeducation groups, group counseling, and group psychotherapy, with some groups providing a blend of these modalities. The goals of group therapy are enhancements of problem solving, goal planning, social interactions, and medication and side effect management (291). Kanas (292, 293) suggests that groups should focus on "here and now" issues and can be effective in increasing patients' coping skills, including the ability to cope with psychotic symptoms. In addition, group approaches may be particularly well suited for teaching individuals with schizophrenia interpersonal and coping skills and for providing a supportive social network for patients who tend to be socially isolated. Group therapy on a weekly basis is also a time-efficient way of monitoring patients for the onset of prodromal symptoms (76).

A number of publications have reviewed the evidence for the efficacy of group therapy in schizophrenia (265, 291, 294–300). As for individual therapy, the evidence for the efficacy of group therapy is not strong, possibly because of the serious methodological flaws in many of the studies. Most studies of outpatient and inpatient group therapy were conducted in the 1970s; there have been few recent studies. A number of well-controlled studies involving stable outpatients indicate that there is very modest evidence that group therapy can be effective in improving social adjustment (301–304). For hospitalized patients in the acute phase of illness, there is no evidence for the effectiveness of insight-oriented group psychotherapy and some evidence that it may be harmful (305). However, supportive groups may be useful in helping patients learn to cope with their symptoms, practice relating to others in a controlled environment, and develop a therapeutic alliance with the treatment team (293, 306, 307).

a) Adverse effects

There may be adverse effects if the group environment becomes overly stressful for patients and leads to a worsening of symptoms. Excessive affective expression, confrontation, and probing can all be overly stimulating, requiring that the therapist set limits and structure to avoid these situations. Patients who reject the idea of group therapy, even after adequate explanation of its potential benefits, should be provided with alternative treatment.

b) Implementation

The criteria for selection of patients for groups are derived from clinical experience; patients must have sufficient stability and enough reality testing that they can meaningfully participate (the exception may be persons who have previously been group members who may benefit from the support of the group while being stabilized after an acute episode). Exclusion criteria include constant preoccupation by hallucinations or delusions (especially paranoid), severe thought disorganization, and very poor impulse control. Higher-functioning outpatients may benefit from interaction-oriented group therapy, while poorly functioning patients who may be overstimulated may benefit more from group approaches that attempt to reprogram cognitive and behavioral deficits (308). There should be flexible use of adjunctive individual sessions, especially in times of crisis, for patients whose primary treatment mode is group therapy. It is generally recommended that a group should consist of six to eight patients (304). A larger number of patients can be assigned to a group if some members do not attend sessions regularly (309).

4. Specific programs for early intervention

Early intervention when prodromal symptoms appear can be effective in preventing relapse and rehospitalization, and it is part of psychiatric management.

Studies have shown that relapse is usually preceded by the appearance of prodromal symptoms, which may last a few days, several weeks, or more. The prodromal phase of relapse usually consists of moderate to severe dysphoric symptoms, such as tension and nervousness, eating less, difficulty concentrating and remembering, trouble sleeping, and depression, and it may also include mild psychotic symptoms and idiosyncratic behaviors (76, 157, 310–319). Such changes preceding relapse indicate either the emergence of new symptoms or increases in symptoms that were already present at baseline. In addition to symptoms, changes in observable behaviors are noted by some patients and families. Examples include social withdrawal, wearing makeup in excessive or bizarre ways, and loss of concern about one's appearance.

Four controlled studies have demonstrated that specific programs to educate patients and families about prodromal symptoms and early intervention when symptoms occur can be helpful in reducing relapse rates (69, 70, 76, 158, 320).

a) Adverse effects

Adverse effects of such treatment programs might result from too-frequent interventions prompted by the slightest increase of dysphoric symptoms in the patient. It is well known that many individuals with schizophrenia show some emotional lability, especially during times of stress, and may even develop mild transient psychotic symptoms. As Marder et al. (70) have pointed out, knowing the patient's symptomatic fluctuations over time helps the psychiatrist evaluate whether or not the appearance of dysphoric symptoms signals a prodromal episode and possible impending relapse. Increasing medication doses too frequently because of false positives may be harmful to patients since they may be overmedicated and experience adverse side effects. Also, psychiatrists, patients, and families should not unduly focus on watching for prodromal symptoms, since treatment should emphasize attention to improvement in symptoms and functioning and not solely on pathology.

b) Implementation

In order to implement a formal strategy for early intervention, patients and family members are educated about prodromal symptoms and behaviors, and regular monitoring should occur. Patients and families are able to call for assistance 24 hours a day, 7 days a week, and assertive outreach should be available for patients who do not have access to or will not cooperate with treatment. As stated in the section on group therapy (section III.E.3), group therapy can be a time-efficient modality by which to monitor patients weekly, and frequent monitoring may be important, since for some patients the prodromal phase may last only 1 week or less before full relapse.

F. OTHER SOCIAL AND COMMUNITY INTERVENTIONS

For most individuals the primary locus of ongoing treatment is the community, not the hospital. Many of these individuals have moderate to severe impairment in role functioning during the stable phase of the disorder and require integrated interventions while in the community.

1. Coordinating and supportive therapeutic community interventions

a) Case management

A common observation has been that patients often "fall through the cracks" between different community agencies or program elements and do not receive needed care. To remedy this situation, a case management function has been developed. Either several members of a team or one individual can be assigned to be the case manager, ensuring that patients receive coordinated, continuous, and comprehensive services. For example, the case manager may accompany a patient to a welfare agency, visit the home if a clinical appointment is missed, or convene a meeting of workers from different agencies serving the patient to formulate an overall treatment plan in conjunction with the psychiatrist.

Results of controlled studies of the effects of case management have yielded inconsistent findings, probably because of methodological problems in design, including 1) lack of specification of the case management intervention, 2) poor characterization of the patient population, 3) inadequacy of outcome measures, 4) inadequate length of the program, and 5) lack of specification of community context (321).

A major problem that has arisen in community mental health planning is that some public programs have developed case management services without having adequate treatment resources for optimal patient care.

Problems in implementation occur when case managers function independently and are not well integrated into the treatment team.

b) Program for Assertive Community Treatment (PACT)

The Program for Assertive Community Treatment (PACT) includes both case management and active treatment interventions by one team using a highly integrated approach. This program is designed specifically for the marginally adjusted and poorly functioning individual with schizophrenia to help prevent relapse and maximize social and vocational functioning. It uses an individually tailored treatment program in the community based on an assessment of each person's deficits in coping skills, assets, and requirements for community living (322, 323). Treatment takes place through teams working 24 hours a day, 7 days a week, and most treatment is delivered in patients' homes, neighborhoods, and places of work. Staff members assist patients in daily living tasks, such as clothes laundering, shopping, cooking, grooming, budgeting, and using transportation. In addition, patients are given sustained and intensive assistance in finding a job, schooling, or a sheltered workshop placement; staff maintain their contact with the patient after these placements to resolve crises and conflicts and to help prevent relapse. Staff also guide patients in constructive use of leisure time and in social skills.

The key elements in PACT are emphasizing the patients' strengths in adapting to community life (versus focusing on psychopathology); providing support and consultation to patients' natural support networks—families, employers, friends and peers, and community agencies; and assertive outreach to assure that patients remain in the treatment program. Medication compliance is emphasized, as well as ready access to a psychiatrist.

Controlled studies have shown the efficacy of PACT in reducing the length of hospitalizations and improving living conditions (278, 296, 323–326). There have been replications of these results in several U.S. locales and in other countries (327, 328).

Individuals with schizophrenia who are marginally functioning and/or poorly compliant with treatment may benefit from such a comprehensive approach. Others who are more able to function in the community and who are compliant with treatment do not need such extensive services. Furthermore, it is not clear which particular elements in the PACT program are most essential for positive outcomes.

Other public mental health systems have attempted to apply PACT principles, but unfortunately, many do not have adequate resources to carry out such a program. Creative reallocation of resources within a system can strengthen PACT programs (329, 330). Evidence is strongest for programs that closely follow the PACT model, including maintenance of a patient-staff ratio of approximately 10:1 (331).

c) Fairweather Lodge

This approach to community care was pioneered in the 1960s by George Fairweather (332) and his colleagues, who selected patients from inpatient units who appeared to be either compatible with or complementary to each other in symptoms and social functioning. A transitional model was used; patients initially received training in the hospital, they then moved to a supervised community residence, and finally they reached autonomy in a self-help community residence with only consultative assistance from the staff. In common with the other practical and structured methods of treatment and rehabilitation for schizophrenia, the lodge emphasized the patients' strengths and provided positive feedback for small improvements in clinical status and for cohesion and mutual support. After the lodge was shown to be efficacious in a major controlled study (333), dozens of replications were successfully implemented throughout the Western and Midwestern United States, usually in close liaison with state hospitals.

d) Psychosocial clubhouse

Founded by former mental patients who were lonely and without constructive activities after discharge from state hospitals in New York, the psychosocial clubhouse model was initiated at Fountain House in New York City after World War II. It quickly spread to other cities in the United States where the self-help and antistigma values were actively promoted. While professional staff maintained leadership in administrative and clinical decision making, their role was to encourage decision making and engagement in a therapeutic community by the "members" of the club. Activities of the club focus on recreational, vocational, and residential functions. The key to the clubhouse model is a transitional approach, whereby members gradually assume more and more responsibility and privileges in the areas of recreation, work, and residential supervision. The research data on the clubhouse model are weak but do suggest that it may lower rehospitalization rates and appears to succeed in helping members obtain, if not keep, jobs.

2. Rehabilitation

The growing recognition that a large proportion of persons with schizophrenia experience long-term disability, even when symptoms are adequately controlled by medication, has led to the development of the field of psychiatric rehabilitation, which aims to optimize the recovery of individuals with schizophrenia. This is accomplished through the use of the full array of biopsychosocial interventions, strengthening the supports and resources available in the community, a collaborative approach with patients and their natural caregivers, and an emphasis on function rather than symptoms. There is an attempt to improve and optimize performance in social, vocational, educational, and familial roles in order to achieve the highest quality of life and productivity attainable for individuals with schizophrenia.

a) Social skills training

Social skills training is defined by the use of behavioral techniques or learning activities that enable patients to acquire instrumental and affiliative skills in domains required to meet the interpersonal, self-care, and coping demands of community life (334). The goal of social skills training is to remedy specific deficits in patients' role functioning. Social skills training can be provided either individually or in groups. It is a highly structured approach that involves systematically teaching patients specific behaviors that are critical for success in social interactions. It can also include teaching patients how to manage antipsychotic medications, identify side effects, identify warning signs of relapse, negotiate medical and psychiatric care, express their needs to community agencies, and interview for a job. Skills are taught through a combination of the therapist's modeling (demonstration); patient role playing, usually to try out a particular skill in a simulated interaction; positive and corrective feedback to the patient; and homework assignments, by which the patient can practice a skill outside the training session.

The efficacy of social skills training for persons with schizophrenia is established (334–338). It is evident that individuals with schizophrenia can learn a wide variety of social and independent living skills. Follow-up evaluations of up to 1 year showed good retention of the skills that were taught earlier (335, 339–341).

The data supporting generalization of skills into the patients' natural environments are not strong. However, a few controlled studies have suggested modest improvement in social adjustment by schizophrenic individuals completing social skills training (342, 343). When patients attempted to document the use of skills learned in the clinic in their natural environments, the results suggested generalization, but much more research is needed (335).

There are several reports of controlled studies in which social skills training significantly reduced relapse rates and symptom levels (344, 345), but more research is needed to document the extent to which social skills training actually protects an individual from relapse. In fact, the Hogarty et al. study (275) showed a loss in prophylactic effect at 2-year follow-up.

Adverse reactions can occur when patients are asked to do homework assignments beyond their capacity and experience repeated failure. Patients with several cognitive disabilities may not be appropriate for social skills training and may experience failure in the training process itself. Repeated failure can be demoralizing and stressful for individuals, and therapists should set realistic goals and select patients who are appropriate for this rehabilitative approach.

Skills training can be implemented both in individual and in group settings with patients and/or their families. Patients selected for training should have moderate to severe deficits in social functioning; better-functioning patients require other approaches. Useful tools for teaching social skills are contained in teaching modules consisting of a trainer's manual, a participant's workbook, and demonstration videos (346).

b) Vocational rehabilitation

Most literature reviews in this area have concluded that there is no relationship between involvement in inpatient vocational programs and successful posthospitalization employment and that such programs may actually increase institutional dependency (347). Therefore, in general, vocational rehabilitation efforts should focus mainly on patients who are living in the community. The aim is to enable a patient to achieve the highest level of vocational functioning possible for that individual.

(1) Sheltered workshops
Sheltered workshops provide patients who are not ready for competitive employment with a shortened work day, decreased on-the-job pressure, simplified tasks, and a structured positive work environment, but they often do not help patients progress to competitive employment (348, 349). Sheltered workshops can be a viable long-term placement for some severely disabled individuals, but they should also be viewed as a beginning step in the rehabilitation process.

(2) Job support
Results of research studies suggest that ongoing job support is often necessary for long-term employment of patients with severe mental illness (350). Supported employment programs differ from transitional employment programs by providing vocational support on an ongoing basis. Such support may range from instruction about

personal hygiene and social skills to providing transportation and on-the-job support. Controlled studies have shown the efficacy of this method when the supported employment program is closely integrated with a comprehensive community support program or mental health center (351, 352). Some studies showed rates of over 50% for successful and enduring employment by persons with schizophrenia who were involved in supported employment while receiving psychiatric services from a continuing treatment team (353, 354).

(3) Job clubs

Job clubs have been used to help individuals with schizophrenia find a job. They provide training in filling out resumes, soliciting job leads, and going through job interviews; the methods used include skills training, role playing, and video feedback. Participants are helped in locating jobs, obtaining interviews, and following up after interviews. The goal is to find full- or part-time work consistent with the individual's interests, stamina, and previous work experience. Uncontrolled studies conducted in Department of Veterans Affairs (VA) facilities have shown that employment rates vary from 15% to 40% (355–357). The efficacy of job clubs has not been formally tested in settings outside the VA health care system.

(4) Boston University model

The Boston University model of psychiatric rehabilitation is a broad approach that addresses clients' needs in the areas of living, learning, and working. It involves extensive assessment of a client's ability to choose, get, and keep a job; development of a rehabilitation plan; and subsequent skills training (358). Recently this model has been widely disseminated, although it remains to be empirically validated (359). This program is probably not suitable for lower-functioning individuals with schizophrenia.

(5) Transitional employment

This modality was developed from the psychosocial clubhouse model of rehabilitation, which is based on the philosophy of self-help and empowerment. Members are asked to choose from among a variety of in-house jobs at the clubhouse—clerical, janitorial, kitchen, and tasks generated from contracts that the clubhouse has secured from private industry.

As the individual shows increasing amounts of stamina, self-confidence, work endurance, and productivity, opportunities are found in a variety of placements in community firms. Ideally, a graduate of transitional employment will ultimately enter full-time, competitive employment while continuing to use the supportive services available through dropping in at the clubhouse or attending self-help groups there. Research has indicated that transitional employment programs are effective in enabling individuals to secure employment (360), but they remain employed for only relatively short periods of time (361, 362). Negative effects can come from two sources in vocational rehabilitation: a) underexpectations and b) overexpectations. Adverse effects can be associated with sheltered or transitional employment that does not provide sufficient learning of the skills required for competitive employment in the community or that does not try to move individuals to higher levels of employment. This can lead to a form of "institutionalism" whereby patients remain "stuck," whether in a hospital, community sheltered workshop, or psychosocial clubhouse (353). Excessively high expectations may lead to placement in competitive employment of individuals who are too impaired symptomatically or cognitively or to insufficient ongoing support from a vocational expert and from the psychiatrist or psychiatric treatment team (223). When this occurs, the stressors from the workplace exceed the patient's vulnerability threshold, and relapse may occur. It is important to conduct a full psychiatric and vocational readiness evaluation, including discussion of options with patients, before implementing vocational rehabilitation.

c) Cognitive remediation and therapy

Two approaches to cognitive therapy have been used for patients with schizophrenia. One is remediation of the cognitive impairments evidenced by many individuals with schizophrenia, including distractibility, memory problems, lack of vigilance, attentional deficits, and limitations in planning and decision making. The belief behind such efforts is that remediating the underlying abnormal cognitive approaches will increase the ability of patients to profit from other therapeutic approaches and improve social and other aspects of functioning. The second approach to cognitive therapy used for patients with schizophrenia has been cognitive therapy interventions similar to those validated by Beck and his associates for depression (363–365).

The efficacy of remediation of neuropsychological deficits has been demonstrated in experimental trials (278, 366–368), but extended studies have not been carried out to correlate the improvement in information processing in laboratory tests with measures of psychopathology or social functioning. The durability of training effects has not been established (278). An exception has been the hierarchical program of cognitive behavior therapy for hospitalized patients with schizophrenia referred to as "integrated psychological therapy" (369), which links specific subprograms or curricula to corresponding cognitive and social deficits. Evaluations have shown that performance on various cognitive tests and on some global measures improves as a result of exposure to this treatment. However, these studies did not rigorously control for medication and other psychosocial influences on the subjects.

Several controlled and uncontrolled studies have extended Beck's cognitive therapy to schizophrenia, with encouraging clinical results, including reduction or removal of delusions and hallucinations (364, 370, 371). While cognitive therapy and remediation techniques appear promising, there have been no well-designed controlled studies demonstrating their efficacy. Furthermore, the techniques themselves are still undergoing modification. At this stage of development, they are not recommended for routine clinical use.

3. Self-help groups

Patients and their families are taking an increasingly active role in the treatment process. Their goals include increasing their influence on treatment planning and implementation, becoming less dependent on professionals, decreasing the stigma associated with mental illness, and working to achieve adequate support for treatment and research in mental illness. Consumer organizations fall into three major categories, each with its own membership, purpose, and philosophy (372). Patients and families should be informed about the existence of these organizations.

a) Patient organizations

The principal goal of these independent organizations, founded by patients themselves, is to advocate and work for the patient's right to exercise choice in the selection of treatment, including the possible choice of no treatment at all.

b) Self-help treatment organizations

These organizations are generally similar to the original prototype, Alcoholics Anonymous. The oldest and probably largest is Recovery Incorporated. Self-help methods are basically educational and cognitive. The efficacy of self-help groups has not been studied adequately.

c) Relative organizations

These groups are the largest of the three types and are made up mostly of parents of individuals with schizophrenia. They seek to improve services within organized psychiatry through education and advocacy. Specific groups are available for siblings and for families of children or adolescents with schizophrenia. Studies have suggested that helping families educate and empower themselves and helping them to become more involved in service delivery results in better outcomes for the mentally ill family members (373, 374).

d) Adverse effects

Adverse effects can result if individuals with schizophrenia deny themselves professional treatments that can be useful in preventing relapses and in maintaining and improving functioning. Such denial includes refusal to take medications or working to prevent the use of somatic treatments such as ECT, which in some situations may be the treatment of choice.

G. TREATMENT SETTINGS

Patients with schizophrenia may receive their care in a variety of settings. The choice of setting should be guided by the patient's clinical situation, patient and family preference, the requirements of the treatment plan, and the characteristics of available settings. Treatment settings vary with regard to the availability of different treatment capacities (e.g., general medical care, rehabilitative services); the degrees of support, structure, restrictiveness, and protection from harmful behaviors; the hours of operation; the capacity to care for severely agitated or psychotic patients; and overall milieu and treatment philosophy.

1. Commonly available treatment settings

a) Hospitals

Treatment in the hospital has the advantages of providing a safe, structured, and supervised environment and reducing stress on both patients and family members. It allows the psychiatrist to closely monitor the level of the patient's symptoms, the patient's level of functioning, reactions to treatment, and side effects of treatment.

Hospitalization is usually indicated for patients who are considered to pose a serious threat of harm to themselves or others or are so severely disorganized or under the influence of delusions or hallucinations that they are unable to care for themselves and need constant supervision. Efforts should be made to hospitalize such patients voluntarily. If patients refuse, they can be hospitalized involuntarily if their condition meets the criteria for involuntary admission of the local jurisdiction. Other indications for hospitalization include general medical or psychiatric problems that lead the psychiatrist to believe that outpatient treatment would be unsafe or ineffective (for example, if a patient's psychiatric status continues to deteriorate despite optimal care in the community). When it is uncertain whether the patient needs to be hospitalized, alternative treatment in the community, such as day hospitalization, home care, family crisis therapy, crisis residential care, or assertive community treatment (see section III.F.1.b), should be considered. Studies have shown that such alternatives to hospitalization for acutely ill patients can be at least as effective and sometimes more effective in terms of reducing symptoms, preserving role functioning, and reducing hospital readmission rates (323, 375–383).

Since a major aim of acute hospitalization is to facilitate rapid resolution of acute symptoms through the provision of a safe, nonstressful therapeutic environment, the hospital milieu should be organized to help achieve this goal. In consideration of the severe symptoms and cognitive impairment in acute schizophrenia, the hospital milieu should be highly structured; staff members should speak clearly and slowly; staff members should be clearly identifiable, wearing name tags with or without uniforms; calendars and clocks should be in evidence on the ward; and ward schedules should be posted in order to provide a clear-cut external structure for the patients, who often have disorganized and impaired reality testing (384).

For acutely ill patients whose psychotic symptoms respond rapidly to antipsychotic medication, a brief hospitalization followed by day hospitalization when indicated has been shown to be as effective as or more effective than longer-term hospitalization, with no increase in rehospitalization rate and better maintenance of role functioning and less family burden at 1- and 2-year follow-up (384, 385). There have been a number of randomized controlled studies comparing shorter and longer lengths of hospitalization. In the United States the duration of hospitalization in the study with the shortest hospital stay averaged 11 days, versus 60 days for the control group (385), while in England, Hirsch et al. (386) compared an average stay of 9 days with 14 days. Other studies had different lengths of shorter and longer hospitalizations, but the general conclusion from all of the studies was that longer hospitalization conferred no additional benefit over shorter hospitalization in such areas as symptoms, community adjustment, and readmission rate (387–396). Brief hospitalization is optimal only when there is a system of community care in place and patients are compliant with follow-up treatment. It allows for effective treatment in the least restrictive environment. Thus, when there is no longer a clear-cut need for the patient to remain in the hospital and community treatment is available and accessible, the psychiatrist should consider discharging the patient from the hospital. If adequate community treatment and support resources are not in place, patients should not be discharged until they have achieved sufficient remission to enable them to function in the community without such supports.

b) Long-term hospitalization

Before the introduction of clozapine, 10%–20% of individuals with schizophrenia remained severely psychotic and grossly impaired functionally despite optimal pharmacologic and conventional care (397). The degree to which this percentage has been decreased by the availability of clozapine and other agents is unclear, but there remains a group of patients who require long-term, supervised hospitalization for their safety and protection, as well as for the protection of the family and community (24, 25, 28).

The organization of the long-stay hospital ward, the training and use of its personnel, and the quality of care provided vary greatly and determine the therapeutic value of the hospital experience (398, 399). Studies have suggested that patients with treatment-resistant schizophrenia who require long-term hospitalization profit most from treatment programs that emphasize highly structured behavioral techniques, including a token economy, point systems, and skills training that can improve patients' functioning (400–404). Paradoxically, despite its demonstrated efficacy, the token economy is not often used in clinical settings (405, 406). Obstacles to its implementation include resistance by staff who hold tightly to traditional custodial methods, increased costs (for the reinforcers backing up the tokens), lack of support from administrators, and inadequate training of clinical staff.

c) Day hospitalization

Day hospitalization can be used as an immediate alternative to inpatient care for acutely psychotic patients or to continue stabilization after a brief hospital stay. As with all alternatives to inpatient care for acutely ill patients, the patient should not be considered at risk of harming self or others, should have the capacity to cooperate minimally in treatment, should have a significant other willing to provide care (a crisis residence can perform the same function), and should have access to appropriate community treatment resources. These alternatives, including day hospitalization, have the advantage of less disruption of the patient's life, treatment in a less restrictive environment, and avoidance of the stigma attached to psychiatric hospitalization.

Controlled studies have shown that day hospitalization is as least as effective as acute inpatient care, and in some studies more effective, in such areas as decreasing the rehospitalization rate and symptoms and better preserving role functioning (375, 376, 386, 407–415). While many of these studies included acutely ill patients with a variety of diagnoses, the majority of patients had a diagnosis of schizophrenia. It is likely, however, that some patients diagnosed with schizophrenia in those studies would not be so diagnosed according to the DSM-IV criteria.

The day hospital should be staffed in a manner similar to the staffing of the day shift on an acute inpatient service, with close coordination and involvement with family members and/or supervised residence staff. Brief overnight stays on inpatient units should be available when patients demonstrate severe exacerbation of symptoms.

d) Day treatment

Generally, day treatment programs are used to provide ongoing supportive care for marginally adjusted schizophrenic patients in the later part of the stabilization phase and the stable phase of illness, and they are usually not time limited. The goals are to provide structure, support, and treatment programs to help prevent relapse and to maintain and gradually improve social functioning. Many programs provide social skills and prevocational training. In contrast, day hospital programs are used in the acute and early stabilization phases and are time limited. While the staffing of day hospital programs is similar to that of inpatient hospital programs, day treatment programs generally have lower staff-to-patient ratios, fewer medical and nursing staff, and greater emphasis on recreational and prevocational activities.

Controlled studies comparing day treatment programs to outpatient treatment showed day treatment to have superior outcomes for chronic schizophrenic patients (416, 417). The better outcomes for day patients included a lower rehospitalization rate, greater symptom reduction, and greater improvement in social functioning. Linn et al. (418) conducted a prospective, randomized, controlled study comparing day treatment and outpatient medication management in 10 VA hospitals over a 2-year period. The study showed that day treatment patients had better social functioning and were less symptomatic than outpatients after 2 years. Six of the 10 day centers achieved significant reductions in both relapse rate and symptoms. The centers with successful outcomes had less use of individual and group therapy, less rapid patient turnover, more occupational therapy, and a more sustained, nonthreatening environment than was found in the poor-outcome centers. Linn et al. suggested that the programs with high turnovers and intensive psychotherapies may have had a higher relapse rate, but these two factors could not be sorted out in the analysis. The patients at greatest risk for relapse in these programs appeared to be those with motor retardation, emotional withdrawal, and anxiety.

e) Supportive housing

Supportive housing is a psychosocial support program widely used for patients who do not live with their families and would benefit from some supervision in their living arrangements. According to Budson (419), the most common types of residential facilities used currently are the following:

(1) Transitional halfway houses

A transitional halfway house is defined as a residential facility providing room and board and promoting socialization until suitable housing is available (420). It is used as a transitional facility between the hospital and the community for recovering patients.

(2) Long-term group residences

These facilities have on-site staff and are used for chronically functionally disabled individuals. The length of stay is indefinite, in contrast to the halfway house, where stays are usually 6 to 8 months.

(3) Cooperative apartments

No on-site staff are present in cooperative apartments, but there are regular visits by staff for oversight and guidance of residents.

(4) Intensive-care or crisis community residences

These facilities can be used to help prevent hospitalization or shorten the length of hospitalization. Usually there are on-site nursing personnel and counseling staff.

(5) Foster or family care

Some patients are placed in foster or family care in private homes. There is a concern that in some situations only a custodial function may be provided (421). Close supervision of foster families is necessary to assure that patients are in therapeutic environments.

(6) Board-and-care homes

These are generally proprietary rooming houses. As with family care, close monitoring and supervision is necessary since some of these facilities provide substandard environments for patients.

(7) Nursing homes

Nursing homes are suitable for some geriatric or medically disabled chronic patients but have been used inappropriately for other chronic patients to facilitate discharge, mainly from state hospitals. Various investigators have suggested that more developed activity programs and psychiatric supervision are needed to prevent declines in social functioning and self-care.

(8) Choice of residence

The transitional halfway house, the long-term group residence, the cooperative apartment, and intensive-care community residences are generally preferable for patients who need assistance in self-care and self-management, since they offer more professional supervision and care and are usually linked to psychiatric hospitals and/or community mental health programs (419). Studies have indicated that these programs can decrease rehospitalization and homelessness and increase social and vocational functioning and quality of life (422–424).

2. Factors affecting the choice of treatment setting

Patients should be treated in the least restrictive setting that is likely to prove safe and effective. Decisions regarding the site of care should be based on the following considerations:

a. Protection of the patient from harm to self or others.
b. The patient's need for external structure and support.
c. The patient's ability to cooperate with treatment.
d. The patient's need for a particular treatment or a particular intensity of treatment that may be available only in certain settings.
e. The patient's need for a specific treatment for a comorbid general medical or psychiatric condition.
f. The availability of psychosocial supports to facilitate the patient's receipt of treatment and to provide critical information to the psychiatrist about clinical status and response to treatments.
g. Patient and family preferences.

Patients should be moved from one level of care to another on the basis of these factors, with an ongoing assessment of their readiness and ability to benefit from a different level of care.

IV. FORMULATION AND IMPLEMENTATION OF A TREATMENT PLAN

Schizophrenia is a heterogeneous condition that has a varying course and outcome, is often chronic and disabling, has devastating effects on many aspects of the patient's life, and carries a high risk of suicide (approximately 10%) and other life-threatening conditions. The care of most patients with this disorder involves multiple efforts and a multidisciplinary team approach to reduce the frequency, duration, and severity of episodes, to reduce the overall morbidity and mortality of the disorder, and to improve psychosocial functioning, independence, and quality of life. Many patients require comprehensive and continuous care over the course of their lives with no limits as to duration of treatment (338, 425); however, early and high-quality biopsychosocial intervention can minimize morbidity and permit one-half or more of patients to function at more-normal levels in society with much less intensive treatment later in life (268, 426). Family members and other individuals who are actively involved in the patient's life should be engaged in a collaborative treatment effort.

The goals and strategies of treatment vary according to the phase and severity of illness. Therefore, the following sections are organized by phase of illness. Within each phase, guidelines for choosing among the various treatment options are presented.

Patients who are experiencing the first psychotic episode present special issues in terms of diagnostic evaluation and treatment decisions, which are further discussed in section V.A.1.

A. ACUTE PHASE

During the acute phase of psychotic exacerbation, the aim is to reduce acute symptoms and concomitantly improve role functioning. Engagement and collaboration with the patient, family members, and other natural caregivers should begin in this phase, when their motivation for participation in treatment is high, and continue throughout treatment. The main task for the clinician is to select and "titrate" the doses of both pharmacologic and psychosocial interventions in accordance with the symptoms and sociobehavioral functioning of the patient (427).

1. Assessment in the acute phase

Every patient should have a thorough initial workup, including complete psychiatric and general medical histories, where possible, and physical and mental status examinations. Interviews of family members or other individuals knowledgeable about the patient should be conducted routinely unless the patient objects, especially since many patients are unable to provide a reliable history at the first interview.

In order to exclude most general medical conditions that can contribute to psychotic symptoms, physical and mental status examinations, including a neurologic examination, are indicated. Ordinarily, a urine screen should be performed to assess recent use of alcohol or other substances, to alert the psychiatrist if the patient has been abusing drugs or alcohol (and indicate the presence of a substance-induced psychotic disorder), and to determine the need for detoxification. It may be useful to assess blood levels of antipsychotic medication to establish whether the patient had been taking his or her medication. Basic laboratory tests should be conducted and should include CBC, measurements of blood electrolytes and glucose, tests of liver, renal, and thyroid function, determination of HIV status, when indicated and permissible, and a syphilis test. Such tests have multiple purposes. In addition to establishing baselines for the administration of psychotropic medication, these tests examine the patient for illnesses that can mimic schizophrenia and illnesses that are often comorbid with schizophrenia and require modification of the treatment plan. Tests to assess other general medical needs of patients should be considered (laboratory studies, such as measurement of the human chorionic gonadotropin β subunit in women of childbearing age, Pap smear, mammogram, etc.) (428).

Patients with preexisting cardiac disease need to be carefully monitored for ECG abnormalities since antipsychotic medications, such as thioridazine and clozapine, can be cardiotoxic; such knowledge may also influence choice of medication for these patients (429). Other examinations may be necessary, depending on the particular medication that is to be used. If the results of the neurologic examination are normal and there is no indication of a neurologic disorder or history of severe head trauma, more-extensive diagnostic tests, such as EEG, computerized tomography (CT), or magnetic resonance imaging (MRI), are usually not indicated (430). Neuropsychological tests are generally not useful in making a diagnosis of schizophrenia during the acute phase.

Special attention should be paid to the presence of suicidal ideation, intent, or plan and the presence of command hallucinations, and precautions should be taken whenever there is any question about a patient's intent to commit suicide, since suicidal ideation is the best predictor of a subsequent suicide attempt in schizophrenia (431). Similar evaluations are necessary in considering the likelihood that the individual will harm someone else or engage in other forms of violence. The coexistence of substance abuse (432) significantly increases the risk of violent behavior. Because past behavior best predicts future behavior, families and friends are often helpful in determining the risk of a patient's harming self or others and in assessing the individual's ability to care for himself or herself.

A psychiatrist may see a patient who is in an acute psychotic state that renders the patient dangerous to self and others. Under these circumstances, it may be impossible to perform an adequate evaluation at the time of the initial evaluation. Given the relative safety of most antipsychotic medications, the psychiatrist may begin treatment with an appropriate medication, even in states where involuntary use of medication must be approved by a court, and perform the necessary evaluations as they become possible.

2. Choice of treatment setting in the acute phase

Patients should be cared for in the least restrictive setting that is likely to be safe and to allow for effective treatment. The psychiatrist should weigh the risks and the benefits of different settings on the basis of an evaluation of the condition of the patient, the need for particular treatments, family functioning, social supports, the preferences of the patient and family, and treatment resources that are available in the community.

Indications for hospitalization usually include the patient's being considered to pose a serious threat of harm to self or others or being unable to care for self and needing constant supervision. Other possible indications for hospitalization include general medical or psychiatric problems that make outpatient treatment unsafe or ineffective. Patients who cannot be adequately cared for in nonhospital settings should be hospitalized voluntarily if possible; however, involuntary hospitalizations are indicated if patients refuse and meet the requirements of the local jurisdiction. Alternative treatment settings, such as partial hospitalization, home care, family crisis therapy, crisis residential care, and assertive community treatment, should be considered for patients who do not need formal hospitalization for their acute episodes but require more-intensive services than can be expected in a typical outpatient setting (433).

3. Psychiatric management in the acute phase

In the acute phase, the specific treatment goals are to prevent harm, control disturbed behavior, suppress symptoms, effect a rapid return to the best level of functioning, develop an alliance with the patient and family, formulate short- and long-term treatment plans, and connect the patient with appropriate community care.

Psychosocial interventions in this phase aim at reducing overstimulating or stressful relationships, environments, or life events and at promoting relaxation or reduced arousal through simple, clear, coherent communications and expectations, a structured and predictable environment, low performance requirements, and tolerant, nondemanding, supportive relationships with the psychiatrist and other members of the treatment team.

The patient should be provided information on the nature and management of the illness that is appropriate to his or her ability to assimilate the information. The patient should also be encouraged to collaborate with the psychiatrist in adjusting the medication and other treatments provided. Ordinarily, a hospitalized patient should be provided with some information about the disorder and the medication(s) being used to treat it, including the benefits and side effects of the medication(s). The psychiatrist must realize that the degree of acceptance of medication and information about it varies according to the patient's cognitive capacity, the degree of the patient's denial of the illness, and efforts made by the psychiatrist to engage the patient and family in a collaborative treatment relationship (434).

The acute phase is also the best time for the psychiatrist to initiate a relationship with family members, who tend to be particularly concerned about the patient's disorder, disability, and prognosis during the acute phase and during hospitalization. Educational meetings, "survival workshops" that teach the family how to cope with schizophrenia, and referrals to local chapters of the Alliance for the Mentally Ill may be helpful. Manuals, workbooks, and videotapes are available to aid families in this process (273, 435–438). Active efforts to involve relatives in treatment planning and implementation are often a critical component of treatment.

4. Use of antipsychotic medications in the acute phase

The process for determining pharmacologic treatment in the acute phase is shown in figure 1. Antipsychotic medications are indicated for nearly all acute psychotic episodes in patients with schizophrenia. Treatment should start promptly because schizophrenia may be associated with a substantial risk of suicide and other dangerous behaviors. Although psychiatrists may find circumstances in which it is reasonable to delay treatment for several days—for example, to confirm the diagnosis or to determine whether the patient will have a rapid recovery when removed from environmental stressors—delaying treatment for longer periods may prolong the episode or truncate the patient's recovery. The evidence suggesting this comes from studies (reviewed by McGlashan and Johannessen [439]) associating longer durations of untreated psychosis in first-episode schizophrenia with poorer treatment response and long-term outcome.

Before treatment with antipsychotic medication is begun, the potential risks and benefits of the medication should, whenever possible, be discussed with the patient by the treating physician. The nature of this discussion will be affected by the patient's condition. However, even with thought-disordered and agitated patients, the provision of education regarding medications can have some degree of impact, especially if the clinician uses repetition, speaks slowly, uses audiovisual and pictorial aids, and engages other members of the treatment team to supply similar information. In some cases, it may be necessary to return to this topic many times in the course of a hospitalization as the patient's symptoms improve.

It is important for the psychiatrist to assess the ability of the patient to participate in the decision about medication treatment. For severely psychotic individuals, especially those who are grossly disorganized or have prominent suspiciousness, it may be difficult to have a meaningful exchange about medication treatment immediately. When an acutely psychotic patient refuses medication and is dangerous, the physician may consider administering it despite the patient's objection. In less emergent circumstances, the physician should assess the patient's competency to refuse medication. Depending on the local and state laws, the determination of competency may require a judicial hearing. When a patient refuses medication, it is often helpful to enlist family members as allies in helping the patient to accept medication. The use of involuntary treatment with medication may be an option, even in the absence of acute dangerousness, depending on the prevailing state laws (440).

Because of their efficacy and safety, the conventional antipsychotic medications and risperidone are reasonable first-line medications for patients in the acute phase

If a patient has a specific contraindication to any medication, remove that medication from the possibilities for that patient.

At each point in the algorithm, medications are chosen on the basis of
- Past response
- Side effects
- Patient preference
- Planned route of administration

GROUP 1: Conventional antipsychotic medications
GROUP 2: Risperidone
GROUP 3: Clozapine
GROUP 4: New antipsychotic medications—olanzapine, quetiapine

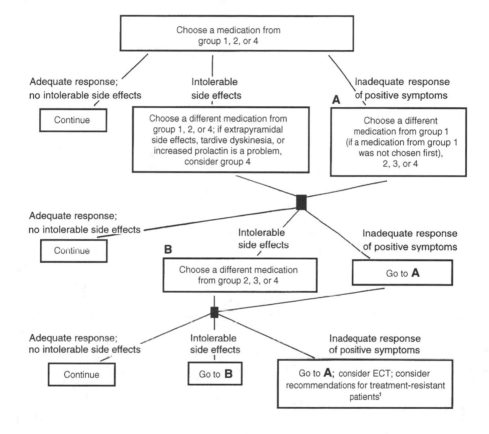

FIGURE 1. Pharmacologic Treatment of Schizophrenia in the Acute Phase.
[1]Given in section IV.D.

of schizophrenia. In choosing among these medications, the psychiatrist should consider the patient's past responses to treatment, the side effect profile (including subjective responses, such as a dysphoric response to a medication), patient preferences for a particular medication based on past experience, and intended route of administration.

Unfortunately, fewer data are available for the newer antipsychotic medications—olanzapine, sertindole, and quetiapine. All demonstrate efficacy in acute psychotic episodes and appear to cause fewer extrapyramidal symptoms than conventional antipsychotic agents at therapeutic doses. In addition, they do not appear to increase prolactin levels, making them potentially useful for women who develop irregular menses or galactorrhea while taking conventional antipsychotic medications. However, there is greater uncertainty regarding their safety and long-term efficacy and efficacy for special populations (such as treatment-resistant patients or those with predominantly negative symptoms). If results from additional controlled trials and the experience of clinicians continue to indicate advantages for the newer antipsychotic medications, then they may be appropriate first choices for acute patients. (Olanzapine has FDA approval. The recommendations for sertindole and quetiapine are pending FDA approval.) Acutely ill patients for whom these newer agents may be particularly useful as first-line treatments include those who are reluctant to take medication, sensitive to side effects, or experiencing a first episode (i.e., patients for whom there may be advantages to having a favorable initial experience with antipsychotic medication). The possible advantages of the newer antipsychotic medications need to be balanced with their likely higher costs, the lack of their availability in parenteral forms, and the more limited data currently available on their safety and efficacy. There are also currently few data on comparisons of the newer antipsychotic medications, making recommendations for choosing among them difficult.

The selection of an antipsychotic medication is frequently guided by the patient's tolerance of side effects. The management of potential side effects, including tardive dyskinesia, is discussed in detail in section III. Some patients find it difficult to tolerate the extrapyramidal side effects of high-potency antipsychotic medications. These individuals may experience discomforting side effects, particularly akathisia, at the doses that are necessary to treat their psychosis. Others may experience daytime drowsiness, dizziness, dry mouth, and constipation while taking low-potency medications and find that the side effects of high-potency medications are more easily treated. A mid-potency conventional medication, such as loxapine or molindone, may be preferable for a patient who finds both low- and high-potency medications difficult to tolerate. Newer antipsychotic medications, including risperidone (at 4–6 mg/day), olanzapine, sertindole, and quetiapine, appear to cause fewer extrapyramidal side effects at clinically effective doses. As a result, they may be useful for patients who experience these side effects while taking other medications; the apparent propensity of these agents to cause fewer extrapyramidal side effects should be balanced by their higher costs and as yet undetermined long-term therapeutic efficacy and safety (particularly for olanzapine, sertindole, and quetiapine). In addition, their lack of availability in parenteral form may limit their clinical utility, especially in the stable phase. Whether these newer antipsychotic medications have a lower propensity to cause tardive dyskinesia has not been adequately studied. The patient's vulnerability and attitudes regarding other potential side effects and their consequences also should be considered.

Before selecting an antipsychotic medication, the psychiatrist should also consider the preferred route of medication administration. If a patient is a candidate for a long-acting depot antipsychotic medication, the oral form of the depot medication (i.e., haloperidol or fluphenazine in the United States) is the logical choice. If the patient is agitated and the psychiatrist plans to use a short-acting intramuscular medication, a high-potency antipsychotic medication that is also available as an intramuscular medication will probably be preferred. As of late 1996, the newer antipsychotic medications (risperidone, olanzapine, sertindole, and quetiapine) were available only in short-acting, oral forms.

Long-acting depot medications are not usually prescribed for acute psychotic episodes because these medications take months to reach a stable steady state and are eliminated very slowly (146). As a result, the psychiatrist has relatively little control over the amount of medication the patient is receiving, and it is difficult to titrate the dose to control side effects and therapeutic effects. There may, however, be circumstances when it is useful to prescribe long-acting medications during acute treatment. For example, if a patient experiences an exacerbation of psychotic symptoms while receiving depot medications, it may be useful to continue the depot medication but supplement it with oral medication (146). Another indication may be involuntary administration of antipsychotic medication or sporadic compliance by the patient. Also, during the acute stage a psychiatrist may decide that the long-term plan for an individual will include depot medication. The transition from oral to depot medication can begin during the acute phase.

It is important to select a dose that is both effective and not likely to cause serious side effects (see section III.C.1). If a high-potency antipsychotic medication is selected, the effective daily dose is likely to be in the range of 5 to 20 mg of haloperidol or 300 to 1000 mg of chlorpromazine. For risperidone, the dose should be in the range of 4 to 6 mg; for olanzapine, 10 to 20 mg; for sertindole, 20 to 24 mg; the optimal dose range for quetiapine has yet to be established. Unless there is evidence that the patient is having uncomfortable side effects, the patient should be monitored at this range for at least 3 weeks. During this phase it may be important for psychiatrists to be patient and avoid the temptation to prematurely escalate the dose for patients who are responding slowly.

Titration of dose is an empirical process, and the psychiatrist should encourage input on the response of symptoms to each medication and dose from the patient, other members of the treatment team, and the family or other natural caregivers who are in a position to evaluate changes in the patient's clinical status from a longitudinal perspective. The psychiatrist can more sensitively titrate the dose by monitoring symptoms with convenient rating scales that quantify the severity of symptoms over time (441).

If the patient is not improving, it may be helpful to establish whether the lack of response can be explained by medication noncompliance, unusual medication metabolism, or poor absorption. If the patient has been treated with one of the medications for which there are adequate data (e.g., haloperidol), determination of the plasma concentration may be helpful. If noncompliance is a problem, discussion with the patient about the rationale for medication treatment can be helpful, as can administering the medication in liquid oral form or intramuscularly. Noncompliance is often associated with medication-induced side effects, particularly extrapyramidal side effects (74). If this is the case, treatment adherence may improve if the side effects are adequately managed.

If the patient is complying and has an adequate plasma concentration but is not responding, then alternative treatment methods should be considered. If the patient is able to tolerate a higher dose of antipsychotic medication without significant side effects, raising the dose for a finite period, such as 2 weeks, can be tried, although it is rarely beneficial. If this does not result in an adequate response, an antipsychotic medication from a different class should be considered. In most cases, patients who have a poor therapeutic response to one conventional antipsychotic medication also respond poorly to others (85). Nevertheless, it is the impression of many psychiatrists that some patients respond to another antipsychotic medication that is from a different class or has a different side effect profile. If the patient has not had a trial with a newer antipsychotic medication, such as risperidone, olanzapine, sertindole, or quetiapine, one of these may have advantages as the medication from a different class. Although there is no definitive evidence to date that the new antipsychotic medications are more effective than conventional antipsychotics in reducing positive and negative symptoms, they do appear to cause fewer extrapyramidal side effects at effective doses and, as a result, diminish secondary symptoms.

Monitoring the plasma levels of conventional antipsychotic medications may be helpful in the following circumstances: a) when a patient fails to respond to what is usually an adequate dose, b) when it is difficult for the psychiatrist to discriminate medication side effects (e.g., akathisia, akinesia) from symptoms of schizophrenia, c) when an antipsychotic medication is combined with another medication that may affect its pharmacodynamics, d) when the patient is very young or elderly or has a general medical condition that might alter the pharmacodynamics, and e) when noncompliance is suspected. Plasma levels are most useful for haloperidol.

A trial of clozapine should be considered for patients with schizophrenia who have positive symptoms or violent behavior that does not fully respond to an adequate trial of at least one other antipsychotic medication and for patients who experience intolerable side effects from at least two different antipsychotic medications from different classes. Clozapine should generally not be given to a patient who has a history of blood dyscrasia, has a cardiac arrhythmia, or is unable or unwilling to cooperate with the monitoring requirements.

5. Use of other medications in the acute phase

Other psychoactive medications are commonly added to antipsychotic medications when patients continue to demonstrate active psychotic symptoms despite adequate medication trials. However, the effectiveness of these adjuncts—lithium, carbamazepine, valproic acid, and benzodiazepines—for treatment-resistant patients has not been clearly demonstrated in controlled trials (reviewed in 442). Given the clear evidence supporting clozapine as an effective medication for this population (168), it is recommended that these adjunctive medications be reserved for treatment-resistant patients for whom clozapine is not appropriate (e.g., because of lack of efficacy, adverse effects, patient preference, or likely lack of compliance with the monitoring schedule). In addition, adjunctive medications are used to enhance response in patients who have inadequate responses (especially those with affective symptoms) and to reduce violent behavior.

Adjunctive medications are also commonly prescribed for comorbid conditions in schizophrenia. Antidepressants should be considered for patients with persistent depressive symptoms. Benzodiazepines may be helpful for managing both anxiety and agitation during the acute phase of treatment. The most agitated patients may benefit when an oral or a parenteral benzodiazepine is added to the antipsychotic medication. Lorazepam has the advantage of reliable absorption when it is administered either orally or parenterally (79). The combination of lorazepam and a high-potency antipsychotic medication has been found to be safer and more effective than large doses of antipsychotic medications in controlling excitement and motor agitation (443). Oral clonazepam has also been found to be helpful in similar circumstances (227).

Medications are used to treat extrapyramidal side effects (see table 2) and other side effects of antipsychotic medications (see section III). Decisions regarding the use of medications for side effects depend on the severity and degree of distress associated with the side effect and on consideration of other potential strategies, including lowering the dose of the antipsychotic medication or switching to a different antipsychotic medication. The following factors should be considered in decisions regarding the prophylactic use of antiparkinsonian medications: the propensity of the antipsychotic medication to cause extrapyramidal side effects, patient preferences, prior history of extrapyramidal side effects, other risk factors for extrapyramidal side effects (especially dystonia), and risk factors for and potential consequences of anticholinergic side effects.

6. Use of ECT in the acute phase

Catatonic and treatment-resistant schizophrenic patients may be candidates for ECT, as are patients with severe depression that cannot be managed with medication. While clozapine is the treatment of choice for patients who have not responded to conventional antipsychotics, those who are do not respond or are intolerant to clozapine may benefit from a trial of ECT (8 to 20 treatments), especially when affective symptoms are prominent (165). The available evidence suggests that antipsychotic medications should be continued during and after ECT when it is used in the treatment of schizophrenia (444). A trial of ECT may be useful for catatonic patients who do not respond to a trial of lorazepam, 1–2 mg i.v. or i.m. or 2–4 mg p.o., repeated as needed over 48–72 hours (445–448).

▶ B. STABILIZATION PHASE

During the stabilization phase, the aims of treatment are to minimize stress on the patient and provide support to minimize the likelihood of relapse, enhance the patient's adaptation to life in the community, and facilitate the continued reduction in symptoms and consolidation of remission.

Controlled trials provide relatively little guidance for medication treatment during this phase. If the patient has improved with a particular medication regimen, he or she should be monitored, whenever possible, while taking the same medication and dose for the next 6 months. Premature lowering of dose or discontinuation of medication during this phase may lead to a relatively rapid relapse.

Psychotherapeutic interventions remain supportive but may be less structured and directive than in the acute phase. Education about the course and outcome of the illness and about factors that influence the course and outcome, including treatment compliance, can begin in this phase for patients and continue for family members. Educational programs during this phase have been effective in teaching a wide range of schizophrenic patients medication self-management (e.g., benefits of maintenance antipsychotic medication, how to cope with side effects), symptom self-management (e.g., how to identify early warning signs of relapse, develop a relapse prevention plan, refuse illicit substances and alcohol), and basic conversation skills (339, 340, 449).

It is important that there be no gaps in service delivery, because patients are vulnerable to relapse and need support in adjusting to community life. Not uncommonly, problems in continuity of care arise when patients are discharged from hospitals to community care. It is desirable to arrange for linkage of services between hospital and community treatment before the patient is discharged from the hospital. Before discharge, a visit to a community residence and arrangement of an appointment with an outpatient psychiatrist are frequently beneficial. Patients should be helped to adjust to life in the community through realistic goal setting without undue pressure to perform at high levels vocationally and/or socially, since unduly ambitious expectations on the part of therapists (77), family members (272), or others, as well as an overly stimulating treatment environment (418), can be stressful to patients and can increase the risk of relapse. These principles also apply in the stable phase. Efforts should be made to actively involve family members in the treatment process. Other psychosocial treatments are discussed in section III.

▶ C. STABLE PHASE

Treatment during the stable phase is designed to optimize functioning and minimize the risk and consequences of relapse. Treatment may include psychosocial, pharmacologic, and other modalities reviewed in section III.

1. Assessment in the stable phase

Ongoing monitoring and assessment during the stable phase is necessary to determine whether the patient might benefit from alterations in his or her treatment program. This allows patients and those who interact with them to describe any changes in symptoms or functioning and raise questions about specific symptoms and side effects.

The goals of treatment during the stable phase are to ensure that the patient is maintaining or improving his or her level of functioning and quality of life, that increases in symptoms or relapses are effectively treated, and that monitoring for adverse treatment effects continues. Monitoring for adverse effects, including tardive dyskinesia, should be done at every opportunity, and results should be recorded at least every 6 months.

If the patient agrees, it may be helpful to maintain strong ties with individuals who interact with the patient frequently and would therefore be most likely to notice any resurgence of symptoms. However, the frequency of assessments by the psychiatrist or member of the team depends on the specific nature of the treatment and expected fluctuations of the illness. For example, patients given depot antipsychotic medications must be evaluated at least monthly, patients receiving clozapine must be evaluated weekly, and those who are going through potentially stressful changes in their lives should sometimes be assessed daily. Formal or standardized instruments that others can easily follow can be used for some assessments (450, 451), e.g., the Abnormal Involuntary Movement Scale (AIMS) (452) for monitoring tardive dyskinesia and the BPRS for monitoring psychopathology.

2. Psychiatric management and specific psychosocial treatments in the stable phase

Specific psychosocial treatment strategies (see section III.E) can be introduced as the patient's clinical status stabilizes. These strategies include reeducation in basic living skills, social skills training, cognitive rehabilitation, and beginning vocational rehabilitation. For patients with few or no positive and deficit symptoms, psychosocial interventions such as individual or group therapy may become more complex and ambitious, with higher expectations, especially if patients are compliant with treatment and have more than minimal stress tolerance. Patients with marked deficit states, however, require a continuation of more structured, supportive, and soothing strategies (36, 270, 449, 453–460). Involvement with family members should be ongoing (see section III.E.2).

Knowing a person's neuropsychological limitations and assets in the stable phase can be very helpful for treatment planning; for example, it has been documented that certain forms of memory and vigilance deficits may hinder patients' psychosocial adjustment (461, 462). Neurocognitive information is most helpful when it is collected during the stable phase of the illness. The treatment program should be organized to respond quickly when a patient, family member, or friend reports prodromal symptoms or exacerbations of schizophrenic symptoms in the patient. Early intervention using supportive therapeutic techniques and higher medication doses as indicated can be very helpful in reducing the likelihood of relapse and hospitalization. During prodromal episodes, patients and family members should be seen more frequently for treatment, monitoring, and support, and assertive outreach, including home visits, should be used when indicated (69, 76, 158). Specific training of patients and relatives in identifying and monitoring prodromal symptoms can be helpful in forestalling relapse (463). By the time the patient has fully relapsed and appears in an emergency room, it is usually too late to abort the psychotic episode and prevent hospitalization.

3. Use of antipsychotic medications in the stable phase

Once a patient reaches the stable phase, it is important for the psychiatrist to develop a long-term management plan that minimizes both side effects and the risk of relapse. For many patients, particularly those who have a history of poor adherence with treatment plans, long-acting depot medications may be preferable during this phase. Patients who receive depot antipsychotic medications tend to have a better long-term outcome than patients who receive oral medications. One disadvantage of using the newer antipsychotic medications (risperidone, olanzapine, sertindole, and quetiapine) in the stable phase is that they are not currently available in depot form.

Deciding on a dose of an antipsychotic medication during the stable phase is often difficult. For some stable patients, antipsychotic medications are actively suppressing psychotic symptoms. When medication treatment is discontinued or doses are significantly reduced, these individuals worsen almost immediately (76). For them, the maintenance dose can be titrated according to symptoms.

Other patients enter true remissions with minimal psychotic symptoms. Medications are prophylactic for these patients. If their medications are discontinued, these patients may do well for weeks or months before they relapse. For such a patient, decisions about the dose of maintenance antipsychotic medication can be difficult since it may be months before the psychiatrist will be able to evaluate the effect of a dose adjustment. Also, doses that are too high or too low may have serious effects on long-term community adjustment. Patients who are unstable because of medication doses that are too low will have difficulty sustaining gains that result from rehabilitation programs. Too high a dose can result in extrapyramidal side effects—particularly akinesia or akathisia—which can also impair community adjustment and reduce adherence. Akathisia can sometimes be tolerated for a period of time during the acute stage of treatment, but during the stable phase even subtle akathisia has the potential for impairing an individual's quality of life. During chronic treatment subtle akinesia can appear as decreased spontaneous movement, diminished conversation, apathy, and a disinclination to initiate any activity (111), making it particularly difficult to distinguish from the negative impairments of schizophrenia or the symptoms of depression.

The long-term efficacy of risperidone and the newer antipsychotic medications (olanzapine, sertindole, and quetiapine) has not been studied. However, on the basis of data and experience with other antipsychotic medications, it may be expected that agents that are effective in treating acute schizophrenia will also be effective in the stable phase. Use of risperidone or one of the newer antipsychotic medications may be useful for patients who experience extrapyramidal side effects while taking conventional antipsychotic medications and who are compliant with regimens of daily oral doses.

Lower doses of conventional antipsychotic medications may be associated with improved compliance, better subjective state, and perhaps better community adjustment. However, these advantages should be weighed against a somewhat greater risk of relapse and more frequent exacerbations of schizophrenic symptoms.

Dose reduction studies (reviewed by Schooler [464]) provide guidance for treating patients with the lowest effective dose of maintenance antipsychotic medication. Stable patients who do not have positive symptoms may be candidates for dose reductions. It is prudent to reduce the medication dose gradually as long as the patient remains stable, to a level of at least one-fifth the usual maintenance dose.

A patient who has had only one episode of positive symptoms and has had no symptoms during the following year of maintenance therapy may be considered for a trial period without medication. Medication discontinuation can also be considered for patients with multiple prior episodes who have remained stable for 5 years with no positive symptoms and who are compliant with treatment (155). Continuing antipsychotic medications indefinitely is recommended for patients with a history of serious suicide attempts or violent, aggressive behavior.

When a decision is made to discontinue antipsychotic medication, additional precautions should be taken to minimize the risk of a psychotic relapse. These precautions may include a gradual dose reduction over several months, more frequent visits, the use of early intervention strategies, or all of these safeguards. In this context, the psychiatrist should educate the patient and the family about early signs of relapse and collaborate to develop plans for action should these signs appear.

The treatment program should be organized to respond quickly when a patient, family member, or friend reports prodromal symptoms or behaviors or exacerbations of schizophrenic symptoms in the patient. Early intervention using supportive therapeutic techniques and increasing medication as indicated can be very helpful in reducing the likelihood of relapse and hospitalization. During prodromal episodes, patients and family members should be seen more frequently for treatment, monitoring, and support, and assertive outreach including home visits should be used when indicated.

4. ECT in the stable phase

Maintenance ECT should be considered for ECT responders for whom pharmacologic prophylaxis alone has been ineffective or cannot be tolerated.

D. SPECIAL ISSUES IN CARING FOR PATIENTS WITH TREATMENT-REFRACTORY ILLNESS

Treatment may be unsuccessful for a variety of reasons. Some patients may be unresponsive or only partially responsive to available treatments (i.e., treatment resistant); this is the case for 30% to 60% of schizophrenia patients (465). Up to 50% of patients experience serious side effects (138), and others are noncompliant with treatment. Refractoriness may be defined as persisting positive and negative psychotic symptoms with deficits in social functioning and bizarre behaviors that interfere with community adaptation (397).

Most patients who have not responded adequately to a trial of an antipsychotic medication should be given a trial of clozapine (168). Patients with severe extrapyramidal side effects or tardive dyskinesia despite a trial of one of the newer antipsychotic medications should also be considered for a trial of clozapine (98, 166).

For noncompliant patients, special efforts to enhance the therapeutic alliance should be made. It may be helpful to view patient noncompliance as a challenge to the patient-psychiatrist collaboration. Many schizophrenic patients and their families can be helped to enter into a therapeutic alliance and develop a partnership that enhances adherence to treatment and rehabilitation programs.

V. CLINICAL AND ENVIRONMENTAL FEATURES INFLUENCING TREATMENT

A. PSYCHIATRIC FEATURES

1. First episode

A patient with a first episode of symptoms characterizing schizophrenia may indeed be experiencing a schizophrenic episode or the onset of schizophreniform disorder, or he or she may be having an episode of another illness or disorder that can cause similar symptoms. The first step is to conduct the initial evaluation described in section IV.A.1. Observing a patient, even for a short while, often can provide clues to the nature of the diagnosis. It is important to establish not only whether the patient has had a previous psychiatric illness and subsequent response to treatment, but also whether he or she presents evidence of another general medical disorder (including substance-induced psychotic disorders, mood disorders, and psychotic disorders due to general medical conditions) that should be treated and that might be responsible for the psychotic symptoms.

Psychiatrists may experience pressure from patients and their families to discontinue antipsychotic medication after patients recover from a first episode of schizophrenia (466). Evidence (155) indicates that the rate of relapse after a first episode is relatively high and that continuation of medication can play an important role in relapse prevention. At least 1 year of maintenance treatment with antipsychotic medication is recommended for remitted patients after a first episode. Although this may be longer than current practice in many settings, this is recommended because the social deterioration and potential losses following a relapse may be severe. About 40% to 60% of untreated patients relapse within a year after recovery from the initial acute psychotic episode (91, 92).

Even when psychotic patients are not dangerous, the hospital is often the preferred setting for first-episode patients because they can be carefully observed for side effects of treatment with antipsychotic medications, including dystonia, akathisia, and neuroleptic malignant syndrome (224).

Unfortunately, the preceding recommendations can be followed only in an ideal situation. Often, with psychotic and possibly violent patients an adequate diagnostic interview or physical examination cannot be conducted. Nevertheless, no matter how agitated the patient, the admitting staff should do everything they can to make sure that the patient is not suffering from another disorder that requires emergency aid.

A single dose of an antipsychotic medication can produce frightening and at times dangerous side effects, so patients should be monitored closely. Neuroleptic malignant syndrome is a possible adverse reaction, as is acute dystonia, which can be both terrifying and painful. The phenothiazines can cause severe hypotension. In general, high-potency antipsychotic medications, such as haloperidol and fluphenazine, are more likely to cause dystonia. For young patients, in whom dystonia is more likely to occur, one might consider antiparkinsonian agents for prophylaxis.

2. Subtypes and deficit symptoms

The negative symptoms of the deficit state have been classified into primary and secondary categories (467). (The negative symptoms of schizophrenia are described in DSM-IV.) Primary symptoms are negative symptoms that are not due to concurrent positive psychotic symptoms, depressive symptoms, anxiety symptoms, or extrapyramidal side effects, specifically parkinsonism and akinesia.

Treatment of negative symptoms should begin with assessment of the patient for a variety of syndromes that can cause the appearance of negative symptoms (468). If a patient exhibits signs of extrapyramidal side effects, the dose of antipsychotic medication should be reduced to the minimally effective level. If signs of extrapyramidal side effects continue, a full trial of antiparkinsonian therapy should be administered to determine whether the negative symptoms improve. If symptoms of depression or anxiety are present, treatment of these symptoms with an antidepressant (see section V.A.4) or an anxiolytic should be considered. If the patient has persistent active psychotic symptoms that could cause negative symptom behaviors (e.g., paranoid delusions, auditory hallucinations), these should be the primary focus of treatment.

If negative symptoms persist in the absence or after adequate treatment of associated extrapyramidal side effects or depressive, anxiety, or positive symptoms, patients are presumed to have primary negative symptoms of the deficit state. There are no treatments with proven efficacy for primary negative symptoms. Clozapine and risperidone have been reported to be effective for negative symptoms (101, 103, 168, 198, 469). However, the evidence on which these claims are based is limited and leaves them open to question. Given the fact that clozapine and risperidone produce fewer extrapyramidal side effects and have potentially superior antipsychotic efficacy (this point has been proven with treatment-resistant patients given clozapine but has not yet been definitively demonstrated with risperidone), any improvement in negative symptoms that occurs with their use may be due to the reduction of secondary negative symptoms (470). Nevertheless, the fact that these medications do not appear to worsen primary negative symptoms by compounding them with secondary negative symptoms is a useful feature for patients who are sensitive to the extrapyramidal side effects and dysphoric effects of standard medications.

A variety of medications have been used for negative symptoms. The most extensively studied and promising agent appears to be L-dopa (132, 471–479). Most studies of dopamine agonists for treatment of negative symptoms have been relatively short term; the long-term effects are not known. One concern is that the therapeutic benefits may dissipate with sustained administration. Selegiline has been considered as a potential treatment for negative symptoms, for reasons along the same lines as those for more directly acting dopamine agonists, but there are no convincing data about efficacy.

3. Substance-related disorders

Substance-related disorders are an important factor in morbidity when they occur in conjunction with schizophrenia. Estimates of the incidence of concurrent substance abuse or dependency range as high as 40% of persons with schizophrenia, and the lifetime incidence is even higher: 60% in some studies (480). Substance-related disorders are associated with more frequent and longer periods of hospitalization and other negative outcomes, including homelessness, violence, incarceration, suicide, and HIV infection (17, 481, 482).

The goals of treatment for patients with such comorbidity are the same as those for treatment of schizophrenia without comorbidity but with the addition of the goals for substance abuse, e.g., harm reduction, abstinence, relapse prevention, and rehabilitation (483).

The presence of substance abuse or dependence is often overlooked or underestimated in individuals with schizophrenia, especially if such a patient is seen during an acute psychotic episode. Self-report is often unreliable, and so corroborating evidence from all sources should be sought; such sources include friends, family, community-based case managers, and treatment personnel (481, 484, 485). Laboratory tests, including liver function tests and urine and blood screens for abused substances, and screening instruments for substance use disorders, as described in the practice guideline on substance use disorders (483), can be helpful in detecting or suggesting substance or alcohol use (482, 485, 486). Many schizophrenic patients do not develop the full physiological dependence syndrome associated with alcohol or substance dependence (481). Because of this, psychiatrists are advised to be aware of other evidence of possible substance abuse in this population, such as homelessness, violence, medication noncompliance, frequent symptom exacerbations, financial problems, and family difficulties. The effects of abused substances on schizophrenic symptoms vary, making difficult the differentiation of substance-abuse-related symptoms from those related to functional psychosis or to both (18, 19, 487–492).

The key issue in providing treatment for this population is developing a dual disorder approach that integrates treatment of substance abuse and schizophrenia (493–495). Many programs are now providing this integration through interdisciplinary teams with expertise in the treatment of schizophrenia and substance abuse. Antipsychotic medications can be used in the usual doses, but patients should be informed that combining antipsychotic medication with alcohol or other substances may increase sedation and incoordination (496). In prescribing medications, the psychiatrist should take into account the potential for lowering of the seizure threshold by antipsychotic medications and for abuse of medications such as benzodiazepines and antiparkinsonian agents. Infrequently, antipsychotic medications can precipitate seizures during alcohol or benzodiazepine withdrawal (497). Disulfiram may pose some risk for schizophrenic patients who abuse alcohol since it can precipitate psychosis at high doses (498, 499). Since it has harmful physical effects when taken with alcohol, it should be used only for patients with reasonably good judgment, treatment compliance, and reality testing. Naltrexone, a promising medication that lowers the desire for alcohol and is used to treat opioid addiction, has not been studied definitively for patients with schizophrenia. Further study of the use of naltrexone with this population is needed.

Many dual diagnosis patients are noncompliant with any treatment, and therefore assertive outreach is especially important (17, 500).

Many psychiatrists use a group therapy approach, usually after patients have achieved stabilization of schizophrenic symptoms. However, the evidence for the efficacy of group therapy is inconclusive (501). The therapeutic approach should be an integrated one taking into account patients' cognitive deficits and limited tolerance for stress. Generally, groups should be supportive and educational in format (484, 502). The length and frequency of group sessions should be regulated according to the attention span and tolerance of the patients. Therapists should be active in keeping the group structured and focused and should limit the amount of stress by avoiding the direct confrontation of patients that is traditional in substance abuse programs. Patients should understand that they have two complex chronic disorders that together lead to a poorer prognosis than each would have separately. There is some evidence that supportive, accepting programs for these patients have better outcomes than confrontative ones. Patients who have not yet attained complete abstinence should be accepted into treatment, with abstinence as a treatment goal (484, 498, 502).

Most psychiatrists recognize the importance of motivational treatments for dually diagnosed persons. Such approaches reflect the belief that in order to harness clients' cooperation in the early stages of treatment, special efforts must be undertaken to engage them and help them see that their substance abuse is interfering with their ability to pursue personal goals (as opposed to psychiatrist-defined goals) (503). Several investigators have conceptualized motivational treatment as having stages (e.g., engagement, persuasion, active treatment, and relapse prevention), which differ in the clinical interventions that are appropriate (504, 505). Studies show that treatment programs with these characteristics can be effective in reducing substance abuse and in decreasing the frequency and severity of psychotic decompensations (482, 502, 506). Collaboration with family members is often helpful for both patients and family members (507–509).

Community-based self-help and support groups can be important in the recovery of individuals with substance use disorders. However, many individuals with schizophrenia are unable to make firm connections to groups such as Alcoholics Anonymous (AA) or Narcotics Anonymous (NA) because they lack social skills and have persistent positive and/or deficit symptoms of schizophrenia (498, 506). Furthermore, some of these programs are opposed to the use of any chemicals that alter brain function, whether they are alcohol or illicit drugs or prescribed medications, thus making it difficult for individuals with schizophrenia to participate. In some communities, self-help groups geared toward individuals with substance abuse disorders and schizophrenia (e.g., Double Recovery in the New York area) have been inaugurated.

4. Depressive symptoms

Depressive symptoms occur frequently as part of the psychopathology of schizophrenia (212, 510). When they are present at the syndromal level during the acute phase of the illness they may lead to a diagnosis of schizoaffective disorder; alternatively, they can occur after remission and be superimposed on the symptoms of residual schizophrenia (511). Generally, depressive symptoms that occur with acute psychotic symptoms are treated sequentially; that is, antipsychotic medications are used first to treat the acute psychosis. The addition of an antidepressant during the acute phase of the illness should be undertaken with caution as it can exacerbate psychotic symptoms (512, 513).

Depressive symptoms that persist beyond or develop after the remission of psychotic symptoms, termed "residual" or "secondary" (postpsychotic) depressive symptoms, have been shown to respond to antidepressant treatment (see review by Siris [212]). As with negative symptoms of the deficit state, secondary depression must be distinguished from other potentially causal conditions (e.g., general medical disorders, substance-induced conditions) (514, 515). The differential diagnosis includes concurrent substance abuse, extrapyramidal side effects (including akinesia and akathisia), demoralization, and situational reactions. Generally, treatment is indicated when the symptoms meet the syndromal criteria for major depressive disorder or are severe and causing significant distress or interfering with function (e.g., when accompanied by suicidal ideation) (516–519).

Tricyclic antidepressants have been the most extensively studied and are commonly used to treat residual and secondary depression in schizophrenia (see review by Siris [212]). They are used in the same doses that are used for major depressive disorder. Since blood levels of some antidepressants are elevated by the concomitant administration of antipsychotic medications, patients should be monitored closely for signs of toxicity, particularly during the dose-titration phase (520). Although the SSRIs may be used preferentially because of their better side effect profiles, there are few data on their use for treating depression in schizophrenia and potential interactions with antipsychotic medications.

Lithium has been used for the treatment of depressive symptoms in schizophrenia but has not been studied systematically (521).

5. Risk of suicide

Suicide is the leading cause of premature death among patients with schizophrenia (522). In their review of long-term follow-up studies, Caldwell and Gottesman (523) concluded that the lifetime incidence of completed suicide among patients with schizophrenia is 10% to 13%, and an estimated 18% to 55% of patients with schizophrenia make suicide attempts (518).

Studies of suicide in patients with schizophrenia have revealed a number of risk factors in common with those for the general population: being male, white, single, socially isolated, depressed or hopeless, unemployed, or chemically dependent and having a significant recent loss, personal history of suicide attempts, or family history of suicide. In addition, patients with schizophrenia may have specific risk factors, including being young, being within the first 6 years of the initial hospitalization, and having a high IQ, high aspirations, a high level of premorbid scholastic achievement, a chronic and deteriorating course with many exacerbations, or an awareness of loss of functional abilities (453, 523). Additional risk factors include the presence of suicidal ideas, command auditory hallucinations to kill oneself, and recent discharge from the hospital.

Many patients, of course, have one or more of these risk factors but do not complete or attempt suicide, while others may unexpectedly do so without prior evidence of significant risk. It is not possible to predict whether an individual patient will kill herself or himself. A significant proportion of suicides in schizophrenic patients occur during a period of remission after 5 to 10 years of illness (518), apparently reflecting a "hopeless awareness of their own pathology" (524) that may emerge without warning. Family members should be made aware of this possibility. Even with the best possible care, a small proportion of schizophrenic patients are likely to die by suicide. Nevertheless, it is essential that suicide risk be assessed initially and regularly as part of each patient's psychiatric evaluation. Suicidal ideas or threats should be judged in the context of a patient's history as provided by the patient and by relatives and the current therapist, if they are available (525). Patients considered at high risk for suicide should be hospitalized, and suicide precautions should be instituted. It is important to maximize the somatic treatment of psychosis and depression and address the patient's suicidality directly, with an empathic and supportive approach (526). There should be close monitoring of vulnerable patients during times of personal crisis, significant environmental changes (527), or heightened distress or depression during the course of illness (511). The frequency of outpatient visits may need to be increased during vulnerable periods, including recent discharge from the hospital (528–530).

6. Violent behavior

Violent behavior in schizophrenic patients is not infrequent; the rate may be under-reported and probably varies with the acuity and severity of psychosis (531–537). General risk factors for violence in schizophrenia include prior arrests; substance abuse; the presence of hallucinations, delusions, or bizarre behaviors (533); the presence of neurologic impairment (538); and being male, poor, unskilled, uneducated, or unmarried (539).

Identifying risk factors for violence and violent ideation is part of a standard psychiatric evaluation. In an evaluation with a potentially violent patient, the use of safety precautions (e.g., having additional staff) is essential (540). When a patient is found to pose a serious threat to other people, the psychiatrist must exercise his or her own best judgment, in accord with the legal requirements of the jurisdiction, to protect those people from foreseeable harm (541, 542). Patients found to be at imminent risk for violent behavior should be evaluated for hospitalization, and if indicated, precautions should be initiated on admission (543).

Effective management of aggression and assaultiveness in patients with schizophrenia can often be achieved through behavioral treatment and limit setting (540, 544). Antipsychotic medications are the mainstay of management; anticonvulsants, lithium, and high-dose propranolol have also been reported to have some utility (545). There have been anecdotal reports that clozapine can be beneficial.

Emergency management of violence in schizophrenia may include sedation, restraint, and seclusion. Sedation can be achieved with lorazepam, 1 or 2 mg i.m. repeated hourly as needed. Lorazepam, 1 or 2 mg i.m. or p.o., may also be combined with a 5-mg dose of haloperidol or other high-potency medication for sedation (229, 443). Rapid sedation may be achieved through administration of droperidol, 5–10 mg i.m. (525).

Initiation of seclusion or restraint is usually an emergency procedure and should be undertaken after less restrictive alternatives have failed or when they are considered to have a low probability of success. The physician should see a secluded or restrained patient as frequently as needed to monitor any changes in the patient's physical or mental status and to comply with local law. Release from seclusion or restraint can be graded, as risk of harm to self or others diminishes (540).

7. Psychosis-induced polydipsia

Compulsive water drinking (between 4 and 10 liters per day) associated with psychological disturbances and hyponatremia occurs in 6% to 20% of patients with chronic mental illnesses (546). The syndrome has been termed "psychosis-induced polydipsia" because it occurs most commonly in the most severely ill patients with schizophrenia.

The initial management of psychosis-induced polydipsia requires evaluation to rule out possible medical causes of polydipsia, e.g., diabetes mellitus, diabetes insipidus, chronic renal failure, hypocalcemia, and hypokalemia. Acute management involves water restriction and sodium replacement to prevent seizures and other consequences of severe hyponatremia (serum sodium <120 mmol/liter). For long-term management various medications, including lithium, phenytoin, and demeclocycline (600 to 1200 mg/day) have been used. There have been anecdotal reports that clozapine can be beneficial. Because the contribution of antipsychotic medications to the pathogenesis of psychosis-induced polydipsia is unknown, discontinuation of medication has also been used. The current recommended approach is to control psychosis and water intake. If the plasma sodium level is insufficient, replacement therapy and a loop diuretic should be considered.

B. DEMOGRAPHIC AND PSYCHOSOCIAL VARIABLES

1. Homelessness

Estimates of the prevalence of schizophrenia among the homeless have varied, ranging up to 12% (547). Goldfinger (547) concluded that there are at least 100,000 individuals who are homeless and suffering from schizophrenia in the United States. Factors that have been noted to contribute to the magnitude of homelessness among schizophrenic patients include deinstitutionalization (548), limitations of public funding, problems in service integration, and lack of low-cost housing (549). Substance and alcohol abuse contribute substantially to homelessness among schizophrenic patients. Many housing programs do not accept schizophrenic patients who abuse substances or alcohol, and substance abuse treatment is often lacking for these patients (549). In addition, the illness of schizophrenia may directly predispose individuals to housing difficulties through withdrawal, disorganization, and disruptive behaviors (547).

Homeless mentally ill persons are likely to have multiple impairments. Most lack basic health care, income, and any social support network. Services should include provision of appropriate housing, access to medical services, treatment of chemical dependency, income support and benefits, and rehabilitation and employment assistance (549). Services for this population should be comprehensive, continuous, accessible, and individualized (547).

Clinical care of homeless mentally ill patients involves four basic stages (550): a) introduction of services into the community, b) outreach, c) provision of treatment and other services during homelessness, and d) support in the transition to housing. In introducing services into the community, psychiatrists must be prepared to work with homeless patients in nonclinical environments, including streets, shelters, subways, bus terminals, and other public spaces. Active outreach is usually necessary in order to engage the homeless schizophrenic patient, and it is often performed by case managers. In discussing outreach to homeless schizophrenic patients, Goldfinger (547) stressed the importance of engagement. Homeless schizophrenic patients are often fearful and distrustful of the mental health system, and they can require a combination of patience, persistence, and understanding. Depending on the needs and wants of a particular patient, the provision of food, clothing, medical attention, or simply company can be indispensable in developing a therapeutic relationship. As noted by Goldfinger (547), such provisions document one's concern, demonstrate one's reliability, and acknowledge the importance of the homeless schizophrenic patient's needs.

Despite appropriate outreach efforts, some homeless mentally ill persons are so impaired that they remain unable to recognize their basic needs or avoid personal dangers. One program developed to address the treatment needs of this population was the Homeless Emergency Liaison Project (Project HELP), in which a mobile treatment team arranged for involuntary psychiatric emergency room evaluation of high-risk homeless patients (551). Involuntary hospitalization resulted from 93% of such evaluations, and 80% of all patients received the diagnosis of schizophrenia. At 2-year follow-up of 298 patients initially evaluated during the project, only 12% were found to be back living on the streets. Controlled studies are needed to further evaluate the efficacy of outreach, treatment, and support programs for homeless schizophrenic patients.

2. Cultural factors

Cultural factors are known to affect the course, diagnosis, and treatment of schizophrenia (552). Since studies have demonstrated that African Americans are more likely than other groups to be misdiagnosed as having schizophrenia when an affective disorder or organic brain syndrome is present (553, 554), particular care should be taken in diagnostic assessments of this group. Although inconclusive, some studies have suggested that Asian American patients may require lower doses of haloperidol and have higher serum levels of haloperidol after oral administration than do Caucasian patients (555). Psychiatrists should be aware of this possibility when administering antipsychotic medications to Asian Americans. Ethnic factors may confer a susceptibility to medication side effects in certain individuals. Schizophrenic patients of Jewish descent have been noted to be at greater risk for clozapine-induced agranulocytosis than other schizophrenic patients (556) and therefore may require close monitoring during clozapine treatment.

Cultural and ethnic factors may also confer susceptibility to illnesses that may coexist with schizophrenia. For example, high rates of alcoholism have been noted among some groups of American Indians (557). In addition, HIV infection is known to be particularly prevalent in some segments of the gay male population and among economically deprived African American and Hispanic populations who have a high incidence of substance abuse and dependence (558). Psychiatrists should be alert to such diagnostic possibilities when providing treatment for patients belonging to these groups.

3. Gender and pregnancy

There are numerous gender differences in the presentation and course of schizophrenia (37, 559). Men with schizophrenia have been noted to have a younger age at onset, a poorer premorbid history, more negative symptoms, a poorer response to neuroleptics, and a poorer overall course than women with schizophrenia (559). While such differences may be biologically mediated, psychosocial factors, including family and societal expectations, may also affect outcome. One study of inpatient family treatment showed that women with schizophrenia had lower pre- and postadmission levels of substance abuse and antisocial behavior, better responses to inpatient family intervention, and better occupational functioning at follow-up than did men (560). The authors of that study noted that social and occupational role demands may result in unrealistic family expectations of male schizophrenic patients, and this issue should be dealt with in treatment. In addition, they noted that traditional socialization practices may allow greater dependence on the family and greater acceptance of family treatment among female schizophrenic patients. Also, it has been observed that even after body weight is considered, women generally require lower doses of antipsychotic medication than men (561).

Studies of the use of psychotropic medications during pregnancy have focused on chlorpromazine and haloperidol. Use of those medications should be avoided unless the patient's psychosis places the mother and/or her fetus at significant risk, since antipsychotic medications cross the placenta. Even then, use of antipsychotic medication during the first trimester should be minimized or avoided if possible, especially between weeks 6 and 10. High-potency medications may be safer; the dose needs to be kept low, administration should be as brief as possible, and the medication should be terminated 5–10 days before anticipated delivery. Antiparkinsonian medication should also be avoided, especially for the first trimester (562–564).

4. Psychosocial stressors

A variety of stressors can precipitate the initial development or recurrence of symptoms in a vulnerable person (30, 34, 61, 62, 565). Stressors can be biological (e.g., physical illness, substance abuse) but more usually are psychosocial; such psychosocial stressors include stressful life events (e.g., interpersonal loss, leaving home, military service), sociocultural stress (e.g., poverty, homelessness, fragmented social network), or a distressing emotional climate (e.g., hostile and critical attitudes and overprotection by others in one's living situation) (36, 271, 273, 566–571). While schizophrenia can emerge or worsen in the absence of environmental influences, attention to stressors frequently helps to prevent relapse and/or maximize healthy functioning. Treatment strategies include preventing the development or accumulation of stressors and helping patients develop coping strategies that keep tension levels within manageable bounds.

5. Old age

With the overall increase in longevity, the number of older schizophrenic patients is expected to increase. The prevalence of schizophrenia in the elderly population is believed to be 1% (572). Ten percent of older schizophrenic patients have late-onset schizophrenia, i.e., onset of prodromal symptoms after age 45, while the other 90% had onset of symptoms during adolescence or early adulthood. Late-onset schizophrenia is more common in women than men, is typically of the paranoid type, and is characterized by better premorbid adjustment and a requirement for lower doses of antipsychotic medications than early-onset schizophrenia (573). As patients with early-onset schizophrenia reach middle and old age, their positive symptoms tend to become less severe and negative symptoms tend to increase (574).

Compared to younger patients, the geriatric patients show greater variability of response and greater sensitivity to medications (575). While an exaggerated response is more common in the elderly, some patients manifest diminished, idiosyncratic, and even paradoxical effects of medications. Older patients tend to have higher blood levels of antipsychotic medications than do younger subjects (576).

Elderly patients tend to be more sensitive to the therapeutic and toxic effects of antipsychotic medications, partly because of age-related decreases in dopamine and acetylcholine neurotransmission in the brain. This sensitivity is especially higher in older patients with structural brain abnormalities.

Side effects of antipsychotic medications that occur more frequently in older subjects include sedation, orthostatic hypotension, anticholinergic reactions, extrapyramidal symptoms (akathisia and parkinsonism but not acute dystonia), and tardive dyskinesia.

It is recommended that before an antipsychotic medication is prescribed for an elderly patient, a comprehensive medical, psychiatric, and psychosocial evaluation be performed. A baseline peripheral WBC count is useful for older patients being treated for the first time with antipsychotic medications, particularly phenothiazines, since they can lower the WBC count. If the pretreatment peripheral WBC count is low or if the patient is being treated with another medication that may also lower the count, the patient may be more safely treated with a nonphenothiazine antipsychotic medication.

All the commonly prescribed antipsychotic medications are equally efficacious for older patients with schizophrenia. Therefore, selection of an antipsychotic medication for use with the elderly should be based primarily on the following: a) the side effect profile of the particular medication, b) the potential adverse consequences of addition of a specific antipsychotic to a preexisting medication regimen or the effects on a concomitant physical illness, and c) the patient's previous therapeutic response to a specific antipsychotic medication (577).

The side effect profiles of individual antipsychotic medications differ considerably, and these differences may be important in prescribing a particular medication to a patient for whom the occurrence of a particular side effect might prove dangerous. Thus, for patients with preexisting parkinsonian symptoms, high-potency antipsychotic medications may worsen tremor and rigidity. On the other hand, high-potency antipsychotic medications (especially haloperidol), which have lower cardiovascular toxicity than low-potency antipsychotic medications, may be a better choice for patients with preexisting cardiovascular disorders. Low-potency antipsychotic medications (e.g., thioridazine) with marked anticholinergic activity should be avoided for patients with prostatic hypertrophy or glaucoma or those who are already taking other anticholinergics.

Only one medication should be started at a time, in order to minimize side effects and evaluate the effectiveness of a given medication. For the elderly patient with chronic schizophrenia whose compliance is unreliable, the long-acting depot form of fluphenazine or haloperidol can be administered intramuscularly every 2 to 4 weeks. Intramuscular injections for the thin, frail older patient with small muscle mass may, however, be painful, and absorption may be erratic and unpredictable. Intramuscular depot forms should therefore be avoided if possible, and liquid preparations should be used if pills or capsules cannot be swallowed. Subcutaneous decanoate injections may also be considered.

While there is wide variability in the doses required for the elderly, the starting doses of antipsychotic medications for older patients are often approximately one-quarter of those prescribed for younger adults. The dose should be increased gradually or decreased according to clinical response or development of side effects. Initially, antipsychotic medications may be given to elderly patients in divided doses (two or three times a day) because the patients may not be able to tolerate the side effects, such as a sudden decrease in blood pressure, that can result from one large daily dose.

For the geriatric patient with nighttime agitation, the daily dose should be given one or two hours before the disturbance usually occurs, to take advantage of the sedating effects of the medication.

The dose of antipsychotic medication for an older schizophrenic patient tends to correlate inversely with current age and with age at onset of illness. Thus, "old-old" patients and those with late-onset schizophrenia require lower doses than "young-old" patients and those with early-onset schizophrenia. Some older patients may need amounts comparable to those given to their younger counterparts. Intensely disturbed elderly patients may require higher doses than those given to less agitated older persons, and intramuscular injection may be necessary in emergency situations.

As chronically ill schizophrenic patients who have been taking antipsychotic medications for many years continue to age, their dose requirements often decrease. Doses must therefore be monitored and calibrated according to the clinical needs of the individual patient at different times.

Aging is associated with complete remission in social deficits in over one-quarter of schizophrenic patients, while another 40% show a marked improvement in symptoms, especially positive symptoms (28, 29, 578). This fact, coupled with the considerably greater risk of tardive dyskinesia in older patients, suggests that withdrawal of antipsychotic medication may deserve consideration for this patient population. On the other hand, discontinuation of antipsychotic medication is associated with a high incidence of psychotic relapse (577). In six double-blind controlled studies that included schizophrenic patients with a mean age greater than 45 years, the mean rate of relapse for the groups whose antipsychotic medication was withdrawn was 39.9% over an average 6-month follow-up period, while the relapse rate for the groups whose antipsychotic medication was maintained was 11.4% (577). In general, the rate of relapse is higher for abrupt antipsychotic medication discontinuation than for slow withdrawal. Tapering of antipsychotic medication may, therefore, be attempted very gradually, over weeks or even months, in order to avoid a full-blown relapse. The optimal goal for many patients is the use of the lowest effective dose of antipsychotic medication for maintenance.

Unfortunately, clozapine's potential for agranulocytosis, its potent anticholinergic effects, and its propensity to produce hypotension and sedation restrict its use with elderly patients. Low-dose clozapine may have a role in the treatment of selected elderly schizophrenic patients who are sensitive to the extrapyramidal symptoms induced by conventional antipsychotic medications. There is relative little experience with risperidone treatment for the elderly. The recommended starting dose of risperidone for this age group is 0.5 mg once or twice daily, to be increased (if necessary) very slowly to a maintenance dose that should not exceed 3 mg/day in most cases.

The treating psychiatrist should review the entire biopsychosocial situation to ensure that all general medical conditions are evaluated and treated appropriately, there is no unnecessary polypharmacy, and the patient has access to various available forms of social assistance.

6. Correctional settings

Individuals with schizophrenia should receive appropriate treatment that includes psychotropic medications and psychosocial and rehabilitation interventions. These modalities are often available in correctional units known as residential treatment units, intermediate-care units, and other similar settings. Persons with schizophrenia may become more symptomatic in a jail or prison because of a variety of factors, including the stress related to incarceration, removal from support systems, and inadequate mental health services within the correctional setting.

Such persons may manifest symptoms of withdrawal, disorganization, and/or disruptive behavior, which may result in a disciplinary infraction that leads to placement in a locked-down setting (generally 23 hours per day in a cell within units often called "administrative segregation" or "disciplinary segregation"). Persons with schizophrenia should generally not be placed in 23-hour/day lockdown for behaviors that directly result from the schizophrenia, because a) such an intervention is not likely to reduce the risk of the behaviors in question and b) such an intervention is likely to exacerbate the schizophrenic symptoms that are responsible for the behavior (579, 580).

C. CONCURRENT GENERAL MEDICAL CONDITIONS

As regards cardiovascular disorders, patients with symptomatic orthostatic hypotension should probably not be given low-potency antipsychotic medications. Patients with known cardiac disease, particularly a prolonged QT interval, should probably not be given phenothiazines, especially thioridazine. Patients with hepatic disease may have impaired metabolism of antipsychotic medications and are at risk for toxicity.

It is important to note that all antipsychotic medications lower the seizure threshold. Probably the one that lowers it the least is molindone (581). Patients with known seizure disorders should probably be treated with an anticonvulsant, such as valproate, while taking antipsychotic medications.

Patients with schizophrenia who also suffer from AIDS dementia appear to be more sensitive to the extrapyramidal side effects of antipsychotic medications than most other patients. For such patients, low-potency antipsychotic medications should be considered.

VI. RESEARCH DIRECTIONS

It is likely that schizophrenia is the final common pathway for a group of disorders with a variety of etiologies, courses, and outcomes. To provide more-precise diagnosis and prognosis and more-specific treatment approaches, it would be helpful if subgroups of patients with schizophrenia were identified.

With improved knowledge of the basic pathophysiology of the disorder it might be possible to develop biological tests for the presence of the disorder. At present, definitive diagnosis depends on descriptive behavioral and symptomatic information.

Genetic research could lead to the location of genes responsible for subtypes of the disorder, which would improve knowledge of the particular pathophysiology associated with a particular gene or combination of genes. Elucidating pathophysiology should enhance medication development. Furthermore, genetic research could be useful in providing better information regarding genetic counseling.

Improved knowledge of the functions of the many neurotransmitters in the brain would also enhance medication development.

The specific semi-independent symptom clusters described for schizophrenia include positive and negative symptoms, symptoms of thought disorganization, and cognitive deficits, such as deficits in attention, memory, and information processing. While these variables are not completely independent, it may be that the pathophysiologies underlying them are different. Understanding their specific pathophysiology could facilitate development of more-specific antipsychotic medications.

More-effective medications for positive, negative, and disorganized symptoms and cognitive deficits are needed, especially medications with fewer side effects. Currently, many patients respond only partially to treatment, and some have disorders that are refractory to treatment, even with the newer antipsychotic medications. Since they ensure compliance, development of depot medications would be useful for the newer antipsychotic medications.

There are few empirical data regarding the efficacy of individual and group treatments, and such studies should be undertaken with state-of-the-art research methods. Information about the timing and sequencing of particular psychosocial interventions is needed, as are development and improvement of treatments aimed at the specific deficits in schizophrenia, such as impairment in social skills and cognitive deficits. More precision is needed in specifying types of patients appropriate for specific treatment approaches at particular phases of the illness. Specific treatment approaches, such as social skills training and cognitive remediation, need to be improved to ensure that learning that takes place in the therapeutic environment can be applied in everyday situations. Regarding families, better methods are needed for assessing the needs of particular families and providing interventions appropriate to their needs.

The optimal dose ranges of antipsychotic medications for relapse prevention in the stable phase need better specification. Regarding medication discontinuation, there is no evidence-based data that offer guidance about when and for which types of patients maintenance medication can be withdrawn. Improved definition of prodromal symptoms and development of biological measures that may signal impending relapse would be useful in relapse prevention. Improved methods of teaching patients coping skills to deal with life stressors could make them less vulnerable to relapse.

Studies of interventions aimed at highly vulnerable individuals, such as those whose parents both have schizophrenia or those who have cognitive deficits, would be useful in determining whether the disorder can be prevented.

In the area of vocational rehabilitation, better assessment tools are needed to determine which individuals are suitable for which type of rehabilitative programs. Improved vocational rehabilitative strategies are needed, since the rates of success in vocational functioning for individuals with schizophrenia have not been high.

Improved methods of early detection and treatment of childhood schizophrenia are needed.

In the area of services research, better information is needed about the impacts of alternative approaches on the organization and financing of treatment for schizophrenia and about implementation of guidelines such as these.

VII. INDIVIDUALS AND ORGANIZATIONS THAT SUBMITTED COMMENTS

Christer Allgulander, M.D.
Ross J. Baldessarini, M.D.
Richard Balon, M.D.
Alan S. Bellack, Ph.D.
Cheston M. Berlin, Jr., M.D.
Charles H. Blackington, M.D., P.A.
Peter Buckley, M.D.
Daniel G. Carlson
Jerry Cott, Ph.D.
Francine Cournos, M.D.
Prakash Desai, M.D.
Leah Dickstein, M.D.
Wayne S. Fenton, M.D.
William A. Fisher, M.D.
Lois T. Flaherty, M.D.
Robert Freedman, M.D.
Marc Galanter, M.D.
Elizabeth Galton, M.D.
Rohan Ganguli, M.D.
Lorne K. Garrettson, M.D.
Steven Goldfinger, M.D.
Larry S. Goldman, M.D.
Marion Z. Goldstein, M.D.

Tracy R. Gordy, M.D.
Sheila Hafter Gray, M.D.
Maurice R. Green, M.D.
William M. Greenberg, M.D.
John G. Gunderson, M.D.
Laura Lee Hall, Ph.D.
Ellen Haller, M.D.
Edward Hanin, M.D.
Linda Hawkins, M.D.
Thomas W. Hester, M.D.
Thomas Horn, M.D.
John K. Hsiao, M.D.
Nalini V. Juthani, M.D.
John M. Kane, M.D.
Allen Kayser, M.D.
Howard D. Kibel, M.D.
R. A. Kimmich, M.D.
Ronald R. Koegler, M.D.
James Krajeski, M.D.
Timothy Kuehnel, Ph.D.
J. Steven Lamberti, M.D.
Anthony Lehman, M.D.
John Leunello, M.D.

Ronald L. Martin, M.D.
Robert McCarley, M.D.
Mark McGee, M.D.
Herbert Y. Meltzer, M.D.
Marsel Mesulam, M.D.
Jeffrey L. Metzner, M.D., P.C.
Loren R. Mosher, M.D.
Jerome A. Motto, M.D.
Kim T. Mueser, Ph.D.
Rodrigo A. Muñoz, M.D.
Henry A. Nasrallah, M.D.
John W. Newcomer, M.D.
Lewis A. Opler, M.D.
Glen N. Peterson, M.D.
Mark Rapaport, M.D.
Michelle Riba, M.D.
Vaughn I. Rickert, Psy.D.
Arthur Rifkin, M.D.
Judy S. Rivenbark, M.D.
Sadie Robertson
Pedro Ruiz, M.D.
W. G. Ryan, M.D.
M. Olwen Sanderson, M.D.

Randolph B. Schiffer, M.D.
Paul M. Schyve, M.D.
Robert H. Sebring, Ph.D.
Winston W. Shen, M.D.
David Shore, M.D.
George M. Simpson, M.D.
Hissam E. Soufi, M.D.
Leonard I. Stein, M.D.
Nada Stotland, M.D.
John Strauss, M.D.
Debbie Sundberg for the Texas
    Society of Psychiatric Physicians
Dale Svendsen, M.D.
Mauricio Tohen, M.D., Dr.P.H.
Ming Tsuang, M.D.
John G. Wagnitz, M.D., M.S.
Richard Weiner, M.D., Ph.D.
William D. Weitzel, M.D., P.S.C.
Linda J. Wilkerson
Dane Wingerson, M.D.
Carlos A. Zarate, Jr., M.D.
Julie Zito, Ph.D.
Howard V. Zonana, M.D.

American Academy of Clinical Psychiatrists
American Academy of Family Physicians
American Academy of Pediatrics
American Academy of Psychiatry and the Law
American Group Psychotherapy Association
American Medical Association
American Neurological Association
American Society for Adolescent Psychiatry
Department of Veterans Affairs
Joint Commission on Accreditation of Healthcare Organizations
National Alliance for the Mentally Ill
National Institute of Mental Health
Royal Australian and New Zealand College of Psychiatrists
Society of Adolescent Medicine
Washington State Psychiatric Association

VIII. REFERENCES

The following coding system is used to indicate the nature of the supporting evidence in the summary recommendations and references:

[A] *Randomized clinical trial.* A study of an intervention in which subjects are prospectively followed over time; there are treatment and control groups; subjects are randomly assigned to the two groups; both the subjects and the investigators are blind to the assignments.

[B] *Clinical trial.* A prospective study in which an intervention is made and the results of that intervention are tracked longitudinally; study does not meet standards for a randomized clinical trial.

[C] *Cohort or longitudinal study.* A study in which subjects are prospectively followed over time without any specific intervention.

[D] *Case-control study.* A study in which a group of patients is identified in the present and information about them is pursued retrospectively or backward in time.

[E] *Review with secondary data analysis.* A structured analytic review of existing data, e.g., a meta-analysis or a decision analysis.

[F] *Review.* A qualitative review and discussion of previously published literature without a quantitative synthesis of the data.

[G] *Other.* Textbooks, expert opinion, case reports, and other reports not included above.

1. American Psychiatric Association: Diagnostic and Statistical Manual of Mental Disorders, 4th ed (DSM-IV). Washington, DC, APA, 1994 [G]

2. McClellan J, Werry J: Practice parameters for the assessment and treatment of children and adolescents with schizophrenia. J Am Acad Child Adolesc Psychiatry 1994; 33:616–635 [G]

3. Karasu T, Waltzman S, Lindenmayer JP, Buckley P: The medical care of patients with psychiatric illness. Hosp Community Psychiatry 1980; 31:463–471 [G]

4. Bland RC, Parker JH, Orn H: Prognosis in schizophrenia: a ten-year follow-up of first admissions. Arch Gen Psychiatry 1976; 33:949–954 [C, E]

5. Tsuang MT, Woolson RF: Mortality in patients with schizophrenia, mania, depression and surgical conditions: a comparison with general population mortality. Br J Psychiatry 1977; 130:162–166 [C, D, E]

6. Tsuang MT, Woolson RF: Excess mortality in schizophrenia and affective disorders: do suicides and accidental death solely account for this excess? Arch Gen Psychiatry 1978; 35:1181–1185 [C, D, E]

7. Tsuang MT, Woolson RF, Fleming JA: Causes of death in schizophrenia and manic-depression. Br J Psychiatry 1980; 136:239–242 [E]

8. Tsuang MT, Woolson RF, Fleming JA: Premature deaths in schizophrenia and affective disorders: an analysis of survival curves and variables affecting the shortened survival. Arch Gen Psychiatry 1980; 37:979–983 [C, D, E]

9. Eaton WW, Day R, Kramer M: The use of epidemiology for risk factor research in schizophrenia: an overview and methodologic critique, in Handbook of Schizophrenia, vol 3: Nosology, Epidemiology and Genetics of Schizophrenia. Edited by Tsuang MT, Simpson JC. New York, Elsevier, 1988, pp 169–204 [E, G]

10. Dingman CW, McGlashan TH: Discriminating characteristics of suicides: Chestnut Lodge follow-up sample including patients with affective disorder, schizophrenia and schizoaffective disorder. Acta Psychiatr Scand 1986; 74:91–97 [C, D, E]

11. Tsuang MT: Suicide in schizophrenics, manics, depressives, and surgical controls: a comparison with general population suicide mortality. Arch Gen Psychiatry 1978; 35:153–155 [C, D, E]

12. McGlashan TH: A selective review of recent North American long-term followup studies of schizophrenia. Schizophr Bull 1988; 14:515–542 [F, G]

13. Docherty NM, DeRosa M, Andreasen NC: Communication disturbances in schizophrenia and mania. Arch Gen Psychiatry 1996; 53:358–364 [E]

14. McGlashan TH, Fenton WS: The positive/negative distinction in schizophrenia: review of natural history validators. Arch Gen Psychiatry 1992; 49:63–72 [F]

15. McGlashan TH, Fenton WS: Classical subtypes for schizophrenia: literature review for DSM-IV. Schizophr Bull 1991; 17:609–632 [F]

16. Fenton WS, McGlashan TH: Natural history of schizophrenia subtypes, I: longitudinal study of paranoid, hebephrenic, and undifferentiated schizophrenia. Arch Gen Psychiatry 1991; 48:969–977 [C, D]

17. Drake RE, Osher FC, Wallach MA: Alcohol use and abuse in schizophrenia: a prospective community study. J Nerv Ment Dis 1989; 177:408–414 [C, E]

18. Brady K, Anton R, Ballenger JC, Lydiard RB, Adinoff B, Selander J: Cocaine abuse among schizophrenic patients. Am J Psychiatry 1990; 147:1164–1167 [E, G]

19. Dixon L, Haas G, Weiden P, Sweeney J, Frances A: Acute effects of drug abuse in schizophrenic patients: clinical observations and patients' self-reports. Schizophr Bull 1990; 16:69–79 [G]

20. McGlashan TH, Krystal JH: Schizophrenia-related disorders and dual diagnosis, in Treatments of Psychiatric Disorders, 2nd ed, vol 1. Edited by Gabbard GO. Washington, DC, American Psychiatric Press, 1995, pp 1039–1074 [F, G]

21. Test MA, Wallisch LS, Allness DJ, Ripp K: Substance use in young adults with schizophrenic disorders. Schizophr Bull 1989; 15:465–476 [C, D, E]

22. Zisook S, Heaton R, Moranville J, Kuck J, Jernigan T, Braff D: Past substance abuse and clinical course of schizophrenia. Am J Psychiatry 1992; 149:552–553 [C, D, E]

23. Fenton WS, McGlashan TH: The prognostic significance of obsessive-compulsive symptoms in schizophrenia. Am J Psychiatry 1986; 143:437–441 [C, D]

24. Bleuler M: The Schizophrenic Disorders: Long-Term Patient and Family Studies. New Haven, Conn, Yale University Press, 1978 [E]

25. Huber G, Gross G, Schuttler R, Linz M: Longitudinal studies of schizophrenic patients. Schizophr Bull 1980; 6:592–605 [C, E]

26. Harding CM, Brooks GW, Ashikaga T, Strauss JS, Breier A: The Vermont longitudinal study of persons with severe mental illness, I: methodology, study sample, and overall status 32 years later. Am J Psychiatry 1987; 144:718–726 [C, D, E]

27. Tsuang MT, Woolson RF, Winokur G, Crowe RR: Stability of psychiatric diagnosis: schizophrenia and affective disorders followed up over a 30- to 40-year period. Arch Gen Psychiatry 1981; 38:535–539 [C, D, E]

28. Ciompi L: The natural history of schizophrenia in the long term. Br J Psychiatry 1980; 136:413–420 [E]

29. Ciompi L: Catamnestic long-term study on the course of life and aging of schizophrenics. Schizophr Bull 1980; 6:608–618 [D]

30. McGlashan TH, Fenton WS: Subtype progression and pathophysiologic deterioration in early schizophrenia. Schizophr Bull 1993; 19:71–84 [C, D]

31. Fenton WS, McGlashan TH: Prognostic scale for chronic schizophrenia. Schizophr Bull 1987; 13:277–286 [C, D, E]

32. Fenton WS, McGlashan TH: Sustained remission in drug-free schizophrenic patients. Am J Psychiatry 1987; 144:1306–1309 [C, D, E]

33. Fenton WS, McGlashan TH: Natural history of schizophrenia subtypes, II: positive and negative symptoms and long-term course. Arch Gen Psychiatry 1991; 48:978–986 [C, D]

34. McGlashan TH: Schizophrenia: psychosocial therapies and the role of psychosocial factors in its etiology and pathogenesis, in Psychiatry Update: The American Psychiatric Press Annual Review, vol 5. Edited by Frances AJ, Hales RE. Washington, DC, American Psychiatric Press, 1986, pp 96–111 [F, G]

35. McGlashan TH: Predictors of shorter-, medium-, and longer-term outcome in schizophrenia. Am J Psychiatry 1986; 143:50–55 [C, D, E]

36. McGlashan TH: The prediction of outcome in chronic schizophrenia, IV: the Chestnut Lodge follow-up study. Arch Gen Psychiatry 1986; 43:167–176 [C, D]

37. Bardenstein KK, McGlashan TH: Gender differences in affective, schizoaffective, and schizophrenic disorders: a review. Schizophr Res 1990; 3:159–172 [F]

38. McGlashan TH, Bardenstein KK: Gender differences in affective, schizoaffective, and schizophrenic disorders. Schizophr Bull 1990; 16:319–329 [C, D]

39. McGlashan TH, Williams PV: Predicting outcome in schizoaffective psychosis. J Nerv Ment Dis 1990; 178:518–520 [C, D]

40. Kendler KS, Gruenberg AM, Tsuang MT: Outcome of schizophrenic subtypes defined by four diagnostic systems. Arch Gen Psychiatry 1984; 41:149–154 [E]

41. Stephens JH, Astrup C, Mangrum JC: Prognostic factors in recovered and deteriorated schizophrenics. Am J Psychiatry 1966; 122:1116–1121 [C, D, E]

42. Stephens J: Long-term prognosis and follow-up in schizophrenia. Schizophr Bull 1978; 4:25–47 [C, D, E, F]

43. Vaillant GE: An historical review of the remitting schizophrenias. J Nerv Ment Dis 1964; 138:48–56 [C, D, E]

44. Vaillant GE: Prospective prediction of schizophrenic remission. Arch Gen Psychiatry 1964; 11:509–518 [C, D, E]

45. Stephens JH, Astrup C: Prognosis in "process" and "non-process" schizophrenia. Am J Psychiatry 1963; 119:945–952 [C, D, E]

46. Christensen JK: A 5-year follow-up study of male schizophrenics: evaluation of factors influencing success and failure in the community. Acta Psychiatr Scand 1974; 50:60–72 [C, E]

47. Faibish GM, Pokorny AD: Prediction of long-term outcome in schizophrenia. Dis Nerv Syst 1972; 33.304–309 [C, D, E]

48. Engelhardt DM, Rosen B, Feldman J, Engelhardt JA, Cohen P: A 15-year followup of 646 schizophrenic outpatients. Schizophr Bull 1982; 8:493–503 [C, D, E]

49. Strauss JS, Carpenter WT Jr: Prediction of outcome in schizophrenia, III: five-year outcome and its predictors. Arch Gen Psychiatry 1977; 34:159–163 [C, D, E]

50. World Health Organization: Schizophrenia: An International Follow-up Study. New York, John Wiley & Sons, 1979 [C, D, E]

51. Bromet E, Harrow M, Kasl S: Premorbid functioning and outcome in schizophrenics and nonschizophrenics. Arch Gen Psychiatry 1974; 30:203–207 [C, D, E]

52. Bromet E, Davis M, Schulz SC: Basic principles of epidemiologic research in schizophrenia, in Handbook of Schizophrenia, vol 3: Nosology, Epidemiology and Genetics of Schizophrenia. Edited by Tsuang MT, Simpson JC. New York, Elsevier, 1988 [D, E]

53. Levy L, Rowitz L: The Ecology of Mental Disorder. New York, Behavioral Publications, 1973 [G]

54. Fairs R, Dunham H: Mental Disorders in Urban Areas: An Ecological Study of Schizophrenia and Other Psychoses. New York, Hafner Press, 1960 [D, E]

55. Wyatt RJ, Alexander RC, Egan MF, Kirch DG: Schizophrenia: just the facts. Schizophr Res 1988; 1:3–18 [G]

56. Regier DA, Myers JK, Kramer M, Robins LN, Blazer DG, Hough RL, Eaton WW, Locke BZ: The NIMH Epidemiologic Catchment Area program: historical context, major objectives, and study population characteristics. Arch Gen Psychiatry 1984; 41:934–941 [D, E]

57. Robins LN, Helzer JE, Weissman MM, Orvaschel H, Gruenberg E, Burke JD Jr, Regier DA: Lifetime prevalence of specific psychiatric disorders in three sites. Arch Gen Psychiatry 1984; 41:949–958 [D, E]

58. McNeil TF: Obstetric factors and perinatal injuries, in Handbook of Schizophrenia, vol 3: Nosology, Epidemiology and Genetics of Schizophrenia. Edited by Tsuang MJ, Simpson JC. New York, Elsevier, 1988, pp 319–344 [G]

59. Pulver AE, Sawyer JW, Childs B: The association between season of birth and the risk for schizophrenia. Am J Epidemiol 1981; 114:735–749 [E, F]

60. Goldberg EM, Morrison SL: Schizophrenia and social class. Br J Psychiatry 1963; 109:785–802 [E, F]

61. Spring B: Stress and schizophrenia: some definitional issues. Schizophr Bull 1981; 7:24–33 [E, G]

62. Dohrenwend BP, Egri G: Recent stressful life events and episodes of schizophrenia. Schizophr Bull 1981; 7:12–23 [C, D, E]

63. Rupp A, Keith SJ: The costs of schizophrenia: assessing the burden. Psychiatr Clin North Am 1993; 16:413–423 [G]

64. Wyatt RJ, Henter I, Leary MC, Taylor E: An economic evaluation of schizophrenia—1991. Soc Psychiatry Psychiatr Epidemiol 1995; 30:196–205 [G]

65. Attkisson C, Cook J, Karno M, Lehman A, McGlashan TH, Meltzer HY, O'Connor M, Richardson D, Rosenblatt A, Wells K, Williams J, Hohmann AA: Clinical services research. Schizophr Bull 1992; 18:561–626 [F]

66. Outcasts on Main Street: Report of the Federal Task Force on Homelessness and Severe Mental Illness. Washington, DC, US Department of Health and Human Services, Interagency Council on the Homeless, 1992 [G]

67. Frank AF, Gunderson JG: The role of the therapeutic alliance in the treatment of schizophrenia: relationship to course and outcome. Arch Gen Psychiatry 1990; 47:228–236 [C]

68. Amador XF, Flaum M, Andreasen NC, Strauss DH, Yale SA, Clark SC, Gorman JM: Awareness of illness in schizophrenia and schizoaffective and mood disorders. Arch Gen Psychiatry 1994; 51:826–836 [D]

69. Herz MI, Lamberti JS, Scott R, O'Dell SP, Mustafa SI, McCartan L, Nix G: Early intervention strategy to prevent relapse in schizophrenia: a controlled study. Presented at the 149th Annual Meeting of the American Psychiatric Association, New York, May 4–9, 1996 [B]

70. Marder SR, Wirshing WC, Van Putten T, Mintz J, McKenzie J, Johnston-Cronk K, Lebell M, Liberman RP: Fluphenazine vs placebo supplementation for prodromal signs of relapse in schizophrenia. Arch Gen Psychiatry 1994; 51:280–287 [A]

71. Marder SR, Meibach RC: Risperidone in the treatment of schizophrenia. Am J Psychiatry 1994; 151:825–835 [A]

72. Herz MI: Prodromal symptoms and prevention of relapse in schizophrenia. J Clin Psychiatry 1985; 46:22–25 [F]

73. Weiden P, Rapkin B, Mott T, Zygmunt A, Goldman D, Horvitz-Lennon M, Frances A: Rating of Medication Influences (ROMI) scale in schizophrenia. Schizophr Bull 1994; 20:297–310 [G]

74. Van Putten T: Why do schizophrenic patients refuse to take their drugs? Arch Gen Psychiatry 1974; 31:67–72 [G]

75. Van Putten T, May PR: Subjective response as a predictor of outcome in pharmacotherapy: the consumer has a point. Arch Gen Psychiatry 1978; 35:477–480 [B]

76. Herz MI, Glazer WM, Mostert MA, Sheard MA, Szymanski HV, Hafez H, Mirza M, Vana J: Intermittent vs maintenance medication in schizophrenia: two-year results. Arch Gen Psychiatry 1991; 48:333–339 [A]

77. Hogarty GE, Goldberg SC: Drugs and sociotherapy in the aftercare of schizophrenic patients: one-year relapse rates. Arch Gen Psychiatry 1973; 28:54–64 [A]

78. Pardes H, Kaufmann CA, Pincus HA, West A: Genetics and psychiatry: past discoveries, current dilemmas, and future directions. Am J Psychiatry 1989; 146:435–443 [F]

79. Janicak PG, Davis JM, Preskorn SH, Ayd FJ Jr: Principles and Practice of Psychopharmacotherapy. Baltimore, Williams & Wilkins, 1993, pp 93–184 [G]

80. Laskey JJ, Klett CJ, Caffey EM Jr, Bennett JL, Rosenblum MP, Hollister LE: Drug treatment of schizophrenic patients: a comparative evaluation of chlorpromazine, chlorprothixene, fluphenazine, reserpine, thioridazine, and triflupromazine. Dis Nerv Syst 1962; 23:698–706 [A]

81. National Institute of Mental Health Psychopharmacology Service Center Collaborative Study Group: Phenothiazine treatment in acute schizophrenia. Arch Gen Psychiatry 1964; 10:246–261 [A]

82. Davis JM, Barter JT, Kane JM: Antipsychotic drugs, in Comprehensive Textbook of Psychiatry, 5th ed, vol 2. Edited by Kaplan HI, Sadock BJ. Baltimore, Williams & Wilkins, 1989, pp 1591–1626 [G]

83. Casey JF, Lasky JJ, Klett CJ, Hollister LE: Treatment of schizophrenic reactions with phenothiazine derivatives: a comparative study of chlorpromazine, triflupromazine, mepazine, prochlorperazine, perphenazine, and phenobarbital. Am J Psychiatry 1960; 117:97–105 [A]

84. Klein DF, Davis JM: Diagnosis and Drug Treatment of Psychiatric Disorders. Huntington, NY, Krieger, 1969 [G]

85. Kolakowska T, Williams AO, Ardern M, Reveley MA, Jambor K, Gelder MG, Mandelbrote BM: Schizophrenia with good and poor outcome, I: early clinical features, response to neuroleptics and signs of organic dysfunction. Br J Psychiatry 1985; 146:229–239 [D]

86. Baldessarini RJ: Drugs and the treatment of psychiatric disorders: psychosis and anxiety, in Goodman & Gilman's The Pharmacological Basis of Therapeutics, 9th ed. Edited by Hardman JG, Gilman AG, Limbird LE. New York, McGraw-Hill, 1996, pp 399–430 [G]

87. Davis JM: Overview: maintenance therapy in psychiatry, I: schizophrenia. Am J Psychiatry 1975; 132:1237–1245 [F]

88. Kane JM: Treatment programme and long-term outcome in chronic schizophrenia. Acta Psychiatr Scand (Suppl) 1990; 358:151–157 [F]

89. Schooler NR, Levine J, Severe JB, Brauzer B, DiMascio A, Klerman GL, Tuason VB: Prevention of relapse in schizophrenia: an evaluation of fluphenazine decanoate. Arch Gen Psychiatry 1980; 37:16–24 [A]

90. Hogarty GE, Ulrich RF, Mussare F, Aristigueta N: Drug discontinuation among long term, successfully maintained schizophrenic outpatients. Dis Nerv Syst 1976; 37:494–500 [C]

91. Kane JM, Rifkin A, Quitkin F, Nayak D, Ramos-Lorenzi J: Fluphenazine vs placebo in patients with remitted, acute first-episode schizophrenia. Arch Gen Psychiatry 1982; 39:70–73 [A]

92. Crow TJ, MacMillan JF, Johnson AL, Johnstone EC: The Northwick Park study of first episodes of schizophrenia, II: a randomised controlled trial of prophylactic neuroleptic treatment. Br J Psychiatry 1986; 148:120–127 [A]

93. Van Putten T, Marder SR: Behavioral toxicity of antipsychotic drugs. J Clin Psychiatry 1987; 48(Sept suppl):13–19 [F]

94. Cole JO, Davis JM: Antipsychotic drugs, in The Schizophrenic Syndrome. Edited by Bellak L, Loeb L. New York, Grune & Stratton, 1969, pp 478–568 [G]

95. American Psychiatric Association: Tardive Dyskinesia: A Task Force Report of the American Psychiatric Association. Washington, DC, APA, 1992 [F]

96. Arana GW, Santos AB: Anticholinergics and amantadine, in Comprehensive Textbook of Psychiatry, 6th ed, vol 2. Edited by Kaplan HI, Sadock BJ. Baltimore, Williams & Wilkins, 1995, pp 1919–1923 [G]

97. Gelenberg AJ: The catatonic syndrome. Lancet 1976; 1:1339–1341 [F]

98. Lieberman JA, Kane JM, Johns CA: Clozapine: guidelines for clinical management. J Clin Psychiatry 1989; 50:329–338 [F]

99. Ayd FJ Jr: A survey of drug-induced extrapyramidal reactions. JAMA 1961; 75:1054–1060 [D]

100. Casey DE: Neuroleptic drug-induced extrapyramidal syndromes and tardive dyskinesia. Schizophr Res 1991; 4:109–120 [G]

101. Baldessarini RJ, Frankenburg FR: Clozapine: a novel antipsychotic agent. N Engl J Med 1991; 324:746–754 [G]

102. Claus A, Bollen J, DeCuyper H, Eneman M, Malfroid M, Peuskens J, Heylen S: Risperidone versus haloperidol in the treatment of chronic schizophrenic inpatients: a multicentre double-blind comparative study. Acta Psychiatr Scand 1992; 85:295–305 [A]

103. Chouinard G, Jones B, Remington G, Bloom D, Addington D, MacEwan W, Labelle A, Beauclair L, Arnott W: A Canadian multicenter placebo-controlled study of fixed doses of risperidone and haloperidol in the treatment of chronic schizophrenic patients. J Clin Psychopharmacol 1993; 13:25–49 [A]

104. Goetz CG, Klawans HL: Drug-induced extrapyramidal disorders: a neuropsychiatric interface. J Clin Psychopharmacol 1981; 1:297–303 [G]

105. Braude WM, Barnes TRE, Gore SM: Clinical characteristics of akathisia: a systematic investigation of acute psychiatric inpatient admissions. Br J Psychiatry 1983; 143:139–150 [C]

106. Caroff S: The neuroleptic malignant syndrome. J Clin Psychiatry 1980; 41:79–83 [F]

107. Rupniak NM, Jenner P, Marsden CD: Acute dystonia induced by neuroleptic drugs. Psychopharmacology (Berl) 1986; 88:403–419 [F]

108. Chakos MH, Mayerhoff DI, Loebel AD, Alvir JM, Lieberman JA: Incidence and correlates of acute extrapyramidal symptoms in first episode of schizophrenia. Psychopharmacol Bull 1992; 28:81–86 [C]

109. Bollini P, Pampallona S, Orza MJ, Adams ME, Chalmers TC: Antipsychotic drugs: is more worse? a meta-analysis of the published randomized control trials. Psychol Med 1994; 24:307–316 [G]

110. Opler LA: Drug treatment of schizophrenia: old issues and new developments. Einstein Q J Biol Med 1991; 9:10–14 [F]

111. Rifkin A, Quitkin F, Klein DF: Akinesia: a poorly recognized drug-induced extrapyramidal behavioral disorder. Arch Gen Psychiatry 1975; 32:672–674 [F]

112. Van Putten T, May PRA: Akinetic depression in schizophrenia. Arch Gen Psychiatry 1978; 35:1101–1107 [E]

113. Gelenberg AJ: Treating extrapyramidal reactions: some current issues. J Clin Psychiatry 1987; 48(Sept suppl):24–27 [G]

114. van Kammen DP, Marder SR: Clozapine, in Comprehensive Textbook of Psychiatry, 6th ed, vol 2. Edited by Kaplan H, Sadock B. Baltimore, Williams & Wilkins, 1995, pp 1979–1987 [G]

115. Ayd FJ Jr: Early-onset neuroleptic-induced extrapyramidal reactions: a second survey, 1961–1981, in Neuroleptics: Neurochemical, Behavioral and Clinical Perspectives. Edited by Coyle JT, Enna SJ. New York, Raven Press, 1983, pp 75–92 [C]

116. Drake RE, Ehrlich J: Suicide attempts associated with akathisia. Am J Psychiatry 1985; 142:499–501 [G]

117. Fleischhacker WW, Roth SD, Kane JM: The pharmacologic treatment of neuroleptic-induced akathisia. J Clin Psychopharmacol 1990; 10:12–21 [F]

118. Rifkin A, Siris S: Drug treatment of acute schizophrenia, in Psychopharmacology: The Third Generation of Progress. Edited by Meltzer HY. New York, Raven Press, 1987, pp 1095–1101 [G]

119. Hanlon TE, Shoenrich C, Freinek W, Turek I, Kurland AA: Perphenazine benztropine mesylate treatment of newly admitted psychiatric patients. Psychopharmacologia 1966; 9:328–339 [A]

120. USP DI, 17th ed, vol 1: Drug Information for the Health Care Professional. Rockville, Md, United States Pharmacopeial Convention, 1997 [G]

121. Antipsychotic drugs, in Drug Evaluations Annual 1995. Chicago, American Medical Association, 1995, pp 261–287 [F]

122. Rosenberg MR, Green M: Neuroleptic malignant syndrome: a review of response to therapy. Arch Intern Med 1989; 149:1927–1931 [F]

123. Shader RI, Greenblatt DJ: A possible new approach to the treatment of neuroleptic malignant syndrome (editorial). J Clin Psychopharmacol 1992; 12:155 [G]

124. Rosebush PI, Stewart TD, Gelenberg AJ: Twenty neuroleptic rechallenges after neuroleptic malignant syndrome in 15 patients. J Clin Psychiatry 1989; 50:295–298; correction, 50:472 [B]

125. Tarsy D, Baldessarini RJ: Tardive dyskinesia. Am Rev Med 1984; 35:605–623 [F]

126. Woerner MG, Sheitman BB, Lieberman JA, Kane JM: Tardive dyskinesia induced by risperidone? (letter). Am J Psychiatry 1996; 153:843 [G]

127. Fenton WS, Wyatt RJ, McGlashan TH: Risk factors for spontaneous dyskinesia in schizophrenia. Arch Gen Psychiatry 1994; 51:643–650 [C]

128. Saltz BL, Woerner MG, Kane JM, Lieberman JA, Alvir JMJ, Bergmann KJ, Blank K, Koblenzer J, Kahaner K: Prospective study of tardive dyskinesia incidence in the elderly. JAMA 1991; 266:2402–2406 [C]

129. Ganzini L, Casey DE, Hoffman WF, Heintz RT: Tardive dyskinesia and diabetes mellitus. Psychopharmacol Bull 1992; 28:281–286 [A]

130. Woerner MG, Saltz BL, Kane JM, Lieberman JA, Alvir JM: Diabetes and development of tardive dyskinesia. Am J Psychiatry 1993; 150:966–968 [C]

131. Lieberman JA, Saltz BL, Johns CA, Pollack S, Borenstein M, Kane J: The effects of clozapine on tardive dyskinesia. Br J Psychiatry 1991; 158:503–510 [F]

132. Alpert M, Friedhoff AJ, Marcos LR, Diamond F: Paradoxical reaction to L-dopa in schizophrenic patients. Am J Psychiatry 1978; 135:1329–1332 [E]

133. Allen RM, Flemenbaum A: The effect of amantadine HCl on haloperidol-induced striatal dopamine neuron hypersensitivity. Biol Psychiatry 1979; 14:541–544 [A]

134. Szymanski S, Masiar S, Mayerhoff D, Loebel A, Geisler S, Pollack S, Kane J, Lieberman J: Clozapine response in treatment-refractory first-episode schizophrenia. Biol Psychiatry 1994; 35:278–280 [B]

135. Klawans HL, Weiner WJ, Nausieda PA: The effect of lithium on an animal model of tardive dyskinesia. Prog Neuropsychopharmacol 1977; 1:53–60 [G]

136. Lohr JB, Cadet JL, Lohr MA, Larson L, Wasli E, Wade L, Hylton R, Vidoni C, Jeste DV, Wyatt RJ: Vitamin E in the treatment of tardive dyskinesia: the possible involvement of free radical mechanisms. Schizophr Bull 1988; 14:291–296 [G]

137. Lohr JB, Cadet JL, Wyatt RJ, Freed WJ: Partial reversal of the iminodipropionitrile-induced hyperkinetic syndrome in rats by alpha-tocopherol (vitamin E). Neuropsychopharmacology 1988; 1:305–309 [G]

138. Kane JM, Lieberman JA (eds): Adverse Effects of Psychotropic Drugs. New York, Guilford Press, 1992 [G]

139. Devinsky O, Pacia SV: Seizures during clozapine therapy. J Clin Psychiatry 1994; 55(Sept suppl B):153–156 [C]

140. Lieberman JA: Understanding the mechanism of action of atypical antipsychotic drugs: a review of compounds in use and development. Br J Psychiatry 1993; 163(suppl 22):7–18; correction 1994; 164:709 [F]

141. Correa N, Opler LA, Kay SR, Birmaher B: Amantadine in the treatment of neuroendocrine side effects of neuroleptics. J Clin Psychopharmacol 1987; 7:91–95 [B]

142. Pollack MH, Reiter S, Hammerness P: Genitourinary and sexual adverse effects of psychotropic medication. Int J Psychiatry Med 1992; 22:305–327 [F]

143. Aizenberg D, Zemishlany Z, Dorfman-Etrog P, Weizman A: Sexual dysfunction in male schizophrenic patients. J Clin Psychiatry 1995; 56:137–141 [B, G]

144. American Psychiatric Association Task Force Report 27: Sudden Death in Psychiatric Patients: The Role of Neuroleptic Drugs. Washington, DC, APA, 1987 [F]

145. Dahl SG: Pharmacokinetics of antipsychotic drugs in man. Acta Psychiatr Scand (Suppl) 1990; 358:37–40 [G]

146. Marder SR, Hubbard JW, Van Putten T, Midha KK: The pharmacokinetics of long-acting injectable neuroleptic drugs: clinical implications. Psychopharmacology (Berl) 1989; 98:433–439 [E]

147. Johnson DAW: Observations on the use of long-acting depot neuroleptic injections in the maintenance therapy of schizophrenia. J Clin Psychiatry 1984; 5:13–21 [D]

148. Hogarty GE, Schooler NR, Ulrich R, Mussare F, Fero P, Herron E: Fluphenazine and social therapy in the aftercare of schizophrenic patients: relapse analyses of a two-year controlled study of fluphenazine decanoate and fluphenazine hydrochloride. Arch Gen Psychiatry 1979; 36:1283–1294 [A]

149. Seeman P, Lee T, Chau-Wong M, Wong K: Antipsychotic drug doses and neuroleptic/dopamine receptors. Nature 1976; 261:717–719 [G]

150. Creese I, Burt DR, Snyder SH: Dopamine receptor binding predicts clinical and pharmacologic potencies of antischizophrenic drugs. Science 1976; 192:481–483 [G]

151. Reardon GT, Rifkin A, Schwartz A, Myerson A, Siris SG: Changing pattern of neuroleptic dosage over a decade. Am J Psychiatry 1989; 146:726–729 [G]

152. Baldessarini RJ, Cohen BM, Teicher MH: Significance of neuroleptic dose and plasma level in the pharmacological treatment of psychoses. Arch Gen Psychiatry 1988; 45:79–90 [E]

153. Overall JE, Gorham DR: The Brief Psychiatric Rating Scale. Psychol Rep 1962; 10:799–812 [G]

154. Neborsky R, Janowsky D, Munson E, Depry D: Rapid treatment of acute psychotic symptoms with high- and low-dose haloperidol: behavioral considerations. Arch Gen Psychiatry 1981; 38:195–199 [E]

155. Kissling W (ed): Guidelines for Neuroleptic Relapse Prevention in Schizophrenia. Berlin, Springer-Verlag, 1991 [F, G]

156. Carpenter WT Jr, Heinrichs DW, Hanlon TE: A comparative trial of pharmacologic strategies in schizophrenia. Am J Psychiatry 1987; 144:1466–1470 [A]

157. Jolley AG, Hirsch SR, McRink A, Manchanda R: Trial of brief intermittent neuroleptic prophylaxis for selected schizophrenic outpatients: clinical outcome at one year. Br Med J 1989; 298:985–990 [A]

158. Pietzcker A, Gaebel W, Kopcke M, Linden M, Muller P, Muller-Spahn F, Schussler G, Tegeler J: A German multicentre study of the neuroleptic long term therapy of schizophrenic patients: preliminary report. Pharmacopsychiatry 1986; 19:161–166 [A, B]

159. Kane JM, Rifkin A, Woerner M, Reardon G, Sarantakos S, Schiebel D, Ramos-Lorenzi J: Low-dose neuroleptic treatment of outpatient schizophrenics. Arch Gen Psychiatry 1983; 40:893–896 [A]

160. Kane JM, Woerner M, Sarantakos S: Depot neuroleptics: a comparative review of standard, intermediate, and low-dose regimens. J Clin Psychiatry 1986; 47(May suppl):30–33 [F]

161. Marder SR, Van Putten T, Mintz J, Lebell M, McKenzie J, May PR: Low- and conventional-dose maintenance therapy with fluphenazine decanoate: two-year outcome. Arch Gen Psychiatry 1987; 44:518–521 [A]

162. Hogarty GE, McEvoy JP, Munetz M, DiBarry AL, Bartone P, Cather R, Cooley SJ, Ulrich RF, Carter M, Madonia MJ (Environmental/Personal Indicators in the Course of Schizophrenia Research Group): Dose of fluphenazine, familial expressed emotion, and outcome in

schizophrenia: results of a two-year controlled study. Arch Gen Psychiatry 1988; 45:797–805 [A]

163. Derogatis LR: SCL-90-R: Administration, Scoring, and Procedures Manual, II. Towson, Md, Clinical Psychometric Research, 1983 [G]

164. Shopsin B, Klein H, Aaronsom M, Collora M: Clozapine, chlorpromazine, and placebo in newly hospitalized, acutely schizophrenic patients: a controlled, double-blind comparison. Arch Gen Psychiatry 1979; 36:657–664 [A]

165. Meltzer HY: Treatment of the neuroleptic-nonresponsive schizophrenic patient. Schizophr Bull 1992; 18:515–542 [G]

166. Safferman A, Lieberman JA, Kane JM, Szymanski S, Kinon B: Update on the clinical efficacy and side effects of clozapine. Schizophr Bull 1991; 17:247–261 [E]

167. Meltzer HY, Burnett S, Bastani B, Ramirez LF: Effects of six months of clozapine treatment on the quality of life of chronic schizophrenic patients. Hosp Community Psychiatry 1990; 41:892–897 [B]

168. Kane J, Honigfeld G, Singer J, Meltzer H: Clozapine for the treatment-resistant schizophrenic: a double-blind comparison with chlorpromazine. Arch Gen Psychiatry 1988; 45:789–796 [A]

169. Breier A, Buchanan RW, Irish D, Carpenter WT Jr: Clozapine treatment of outpatients with schizophrenia: outcome and long-term response patterns. Hosp Community Psychiatry 1993; 44:1145–1149 [A, C]

170. Pickar D, Owen RR, Lutman RE, Konicki E, Gutierrez R, Rapaport MH: Clinical and biologic response to clozapine in patients with schizophrenia: crossover comparison with fluphenazine. Arch Gen Psychiatry 1992; 49:345–353 [A]

171. Zito JM, Volavka J, Craig TJ, Czobor P, Banks S, Vitrai J: Pharmacoepidemiology of clozapine in 202 inpatients with schizophrenia. Ann Pharmacother 1993; 27:1262–1269 [E]

172. Claghorn J, Honigfeld G, Abuzzahab FS, Wang R, Steinbook R, Tuason V, Klerman G: The risks and benefits of clozapine versus chlorpromazine. J Clin Psychopharmacol 1987; 7:377–384 [A]

173. Miller DD, Perry PJ, Cadoret R, Andreasen NC: A two and one-half year follow-up of treatment-refractory schizophrenics treated with clozapine (abstract). Biol Psychiatry 1992; 31 (March suppl):85A [E]

174. Alvir JM, Lieberman JA, Safferman AZ, Schwimmer JL, Schaaf JA: Clozapine-induced agranulocytosis: incidence and risk factors in the United States. N Engl J Med 1993; 329:162–167 [G]

175. Lieberman JA, Johns C, Kane JM, Rai K, Pisciotta AV, Saltz B, Howard A: Clozapine induced agranulocytosis: non-cross reactivity with other psychotropic drugs. J Clin Psychiatry 1988; 49:271–277 [F]

176. Mendelowitz D, Reynolds PJ, Andresen MC: Heterogeneous functional expression of calcium channels at sensory and synaptic regions in nodose neurons. J Neurophysiol 1995; 73:872–875 [A]

177. Lamberti JS, Bellnier TJ, Schwarzkopf SB, Schneider E: Filgrastim treatment of three patients with clozapine-induced agranulocytosis. J Clin Psychiatry 1995; 56:256–259 [B]

178. Lamberti JS, Bellnier T: Clozapine and tardive dystonia. J Nerv Ment Dis 1993; 181:137–138 [G]

179. Physicians' Desk Reference, 51st ed. Montvale, NJ, Medical Economics, 1997, pp 2377–2380 [G]

180. Fleischhacker WW, Hummer M, Kurz M, Kurzthaler I, Lieberman JA, Pollack S, Safferman AZ, Kane JM: Clozapine dose in the United States and Europe: implications for therapeutic and adverse effects. J Clin Psychiatry 1994; 55(Sept suppl B):78–81 [E]

181. Zarin DA, Pincus HA: Diagnostic tests with multiple possible thresholds: the case of plasma clozapine levels. J Practical Psychiatry Behav Health 1996; 2:183–185 [F]

182. Carpenter WT Jr, Conley RR, Buchanan RW, Breier A, Tamminga CA: Patient response and resource management: another view of clozapine treatment of schizophrenia. Am J Psychiatry 1995; 152:827–832 [F]

183. Ackenheil M: Clozapine—pharmacokinetic investigations and biochemical effects in man. Psychopharmacology (Berl) 1989; 99(suppl):S32–S37 [B]

184. Nemeroff CB, DeVane CL, Pollack BG: Newer antidepressants and the cytochrome P450 system. Am J Psychiatry 1996; 153:311–320 [F]

185. Peuskens J: Risperidone in the treatment of patients with chronic schizophrenia: a multinational, multi-centre, double-blind, parallel-group study versus haloperidol. Br J Psychiatry 1995; 166:712–726 [A]

186. Müller-Spahn F and the International Risperidone Research Group: Risperidone in the treatment of chronic schizophrenic patients: an international double-blind parallel-group study versus haloperidol. Clin Neuropharmacol 1992; 15(suppl 1):90A–91A [A]

187. Johnson AL, Johnson DAW: Peer review of "Risperidone in the treatment of patients with chronic schizophrenia: a multi-national, multi-centre, double-blind, parallel-group study versus haloperidol." Br J Psychiatry 1995; 166:727–733 [A]

188. Min SK, Rhee CS, Kim CE, Kang DY: Risperidone versus haloperidol in the treatment of chronic schizophrenic patients: a parallel group double-blind comparative trial. Yonsei Med J 1992; 34:179–190 [A]

189. Ceskova E, Svestka J: Double-blind comparison of risperidone and haloperidol in schizophrenic and schizoaffective psychoses. Pharmacopsychiatry 1993; 26:121–124 [A]

190. Borison RL, Pathiraja AP, Diamond BI, Meibach RC: Risperidone: clinical safety and efficacy in schizophrenia. Psychopharmacol Bull 1992; 28:213–218 [A]

191. Kay SR, Fiszbein A, Opler LA: The Positive and Negative Syndrome Scale (PANSS) for schizophrenia. Schizophr Bull 1987; 13:261–276 [G]

192. Hoyberg OJ, Fensbo C, Remvig J, Lingjaerde O, Sloth-Nielzsen M, Salvesen I: Risperidone versus perphenazine in the treatment of chronic schizophrenic patients with acute exacerbations. Acta Psychiatr Scand 1993; 88:395–402 [A]

193. Davis JM, Janicak PG: Efficacy and safety of the new antipsychotics. Lancet 1994; 343:476–477 [G]

194. Addington DE, Jones B, Bloom D, Chouinard G, Remington G, Albright P: Reduction of hospital days in chronic schizophrenic patients treated with risperidone: a retrospective study. Clin Ther 1993; 15:917–926 [D]

195. Chouinard G, Ross-Chouinard A, Annable L, Jones BD: Extrapyramidal Symptom Rating Scale. Can J Neurol Sci 1980; 7:233 [G]

196. Kopala L, Honer WG: Risperidone, serotonergic mechanisms, and obsessive-compulsive symptoms in schizophrenia (letter). Am J Psychiatry 1994; 151:1714–1715 [D]

197. Remington G, Adams M: Risperidone and obsessive-compulsive symptoms. J Clin Psychopharmacol 1994; 14:358–359 [D]

198. Marder SR: Clinical experience with risperidone. J Clin Psychiatry 1996; 57(Sept suppl):57–61 [F]

199. Borison RL, Diamond B, Pathiraja A, Meibach RC: Pharmacokinetics of risperidone in chronic schizophrenic patients. Psychopharmacol Bull 1994; 30:193–197 [D]

200. Beasley CM, Tollefson G, Tran P, Satterlee W, Sanger T, Hamilton S, Fabre L, Small J, Ereshefsky L, True J, Nemeroff C, Risch SC, Perry PJ, Potkin SG, Borison RL, James S, Meltzer HY, Iqbal N, Fann WE, Gewirtz GR, Landbloom R, Roy-Byrne PP, Tuason VB, Carman JS, Stokes PE, et al: Olanzapine versus placebo and haloperidol—acute phase results of the North American double-blind olanzapine trial. Neuropsychopharmacology 1996; 14:111–123 [A]

201. Tollefson GD, Beasley CM Jr, Tran PV, Street JS, Krueger JA, Tamura RN, Graffeo KA, Thieme ME: Olanzapine versus haloperidol in the treatment of schizophrenia and schizoaffective

and schizophreniform disorders: results of an international collaborative trial. Am J Psychiatry 1997; 154:457–465 [A]

202. McEvoy J, Borison R, Small J, van Kammen D, Meltzer H, Hamner M, Morris D, Shu V, Sebree T, Grebb J: The efficacy and tolerability of sertindole in schizophrenic patients: a pilot double-blind placebo controlled, dose ranging study. Schizophr Res 1993; 9:244 [A]

203. van Kammen DP, McEvoy JP, Targum SD, Kardatzke D, Sebree TB: A randomized controlled dose-ranging trial of sertindole in patients with schizophrenia. Psychopharmacology (Berl) 1996; 124:168–175 [A]

204. Schulz SZ, Zborowski J, Morris D, Sebree T, Wallin B: Efficacy, safety, and dose response of three doses of sertindole and three doses of haloperidol in schizophrenic patients. Schizophr Res 1996; 18:133 [A]

205. Burton TM: Risk vs benefit: FDA weighs antipsychotic. Wall Street Journal, Oct 14, 1996, pp B1, B4 [G]

206. Zimbroff DL, Kane JM, Tamminga CA, Daniel DG, Mack RJ, Morris DD, Sebree TB, Wallin BA, Kashkin KB, Sertindole Study Group: A controlled, dose-response study of sertindole and haloperidol in schizophrenia. Am J Psychiatry (in press) [B]

207. Hirsch SR, Link CG, Goldstein JM, Arvanitis LA: ICI 204,636: a new atypical antipsychotic drug. Br J Psychiatry 1996; 168 (suppl 29):45–56 [A]

208. Andreasen NC: Scale for the Assessment of Negative Symptoms (SANS). Iowa City, University of Iowa, 1983 [G]

209. Borison RL, Arvanitis LA, Miller BG: A comparison of five fixed doses of Seroquel (ICI-204,636) with haloperidol and placebo in patients with schizophrenia. Schizophr Res 1996; 18:132[A]

210. Christison GW, Kirch DG, Wyatt RJ: When symptoms persist: choosing among alternative somatic treatments for schizophrenia. Schizophr Bull 1991; 17:217–245 [E, F, G]

211. Carpenter WT Jr: The treatment of negative symptoms: pharmacological and methodological issues. Br J Psychiatry 1996; 168(suppl 29):17–22 [G]

212. Siris SG: Diagnosis of secondary depression in schizophrenia: implications for DSM-IV. Schizophr Bull 1991; 17:75–98 [F]

213. Alexander PE, van Kammen DP, Bunney WE Jr: Antipsychotic effects of lithium in schizophrenia. Am J Psychiatry 1979; 136:283–287 [B]

214. Shopsin B, Kim SS, Gershon S: A controlled study of lithium vs chlorpromazine in acute schizophrenics. Br J Psychiatry 1971; 119:435–440 [A]

215. Growe GA, Crayton JW, Klass DB, Evans H, Strizich M: Lithium in chronic schizophrenia. Am J Psychiatry 1979; 136:454–455 [A]

216. Small JG, Kellams JJ, Milstein V, Moore J: A placebo-controlled study of lithium combined with neuroleptics in chronic schizophrenic patients. Am J Psychiatry 1975; 132:1315–1317 [A]

217. Lerner Y, Mintzer Y, Schestatzky M: Lithium combined with haloperidol in schizophrenia patients. Br J Psychiatry 1988; 153:359–362 [A]

218. Biederman J, Lerner A, Belmaker RR: Combination of lithium carbonate and haloperidol in schizoaffective disorder. Arch Gen Psychiatry 1979; 36:327–333 [A]

219. Johnson G: Differential response to lithium carbonate in manic-depressive and schizoaffective disorders. Dis Nerv Syst 1970; 13:613–615 [A]

220. Prien RF, Cafe EM, Klett JC: A comparison of lithium carbonate and chlorpromazine in the treatment of excited schizo-affectives. Arch Gen Psychiatry 1972; 27:182–189 [A]

221. Carman JS, Bigelow LB, Wyatt RJ: Lithium combined with neuroleptics in chronic schizophrenic and schizoaffective patients. J Clin Psychiatry 1981; 42:124–128 [A]

222. American Psychiatric Association: Practice Guideline for the Treatment of Patients With Bipolar Disorder. Am J Psychiatry 1994; 151 (Dec suppl) [F]

223. Hogarty GE, McEvoy JP, Ulrich RF, DiBarry AL, Bartone P, Cooley S, Hammill K, Carter M, Munetz MR, Perel J: Pharmacotherapy of impaired affect in recovering schizophrenic patients. Arch Gen Psychiatry 1995; 52:29–41 [A]

224. Kaufmann C, Wyatt R: Neuroleptic malignant syndrome, in Psychopharmacology: The Third Generation of Progress. Edited by Meltzer HY. New York, Raven Press, 1987, pp 1421–1430 [G]

225. Wolkowitz OM, Pickar D: Benzodiazepines in the treatment of schizophrenia: a review and reappraisal. Am J Psychiatry 1991; 148:714–726 [B]

226. Hekimian LJ, Friedhoff AJ: A controlled study of placebo, chlordiazepoxide, and chlorpromazine with 30 male schizophrenic patients. Dis Nerv Syst 1967; 28:675–678 [A]

227. Altamura AC, Mauri MC, Mantero M, Brunetti M: Clonazepam/haloperidol combination therapy in schizophrenia: a double-blind study. Acta Psychiatr Scand 1987; 76:702–706 [A]

228. Csernansky JG, Riney SJ, Lombarozo L, Overall JE, Hollister LE: Double-blind comparison of alprazolam, diazepam and placebo for the treatment of negative schizophrenic symptoms. Arch Gen Psychiatry 1988; 45:655–659 [A]

229. Salzman C, Solomon D, Miyawaki E, Glassman R, Rood L, Flowers E, Thayer S: Parenteral lorazepam versus parenteral haloperidol for the control of psychotic disruptive behavior. J Clin Psychiatry 1991; 52:177–180 [A, B]

230. McElroy SL, Keck PE, Pope HG Jr: Sodium valproate: its use in primary psychiatric disorders. J Clin Psychopharmacol 1987; 7:16–24 [D]

231. Neppe VM: Carbamazepine as adjunctive treatment in nonepileptic chronic inpatients with EEG temporal lobe abnormalities. J Clin Psychiatry 1983; 44:326–331 [A]

232. Luchins D: Carbamazepine in violent non-epileptic schizophrenics. Psychopharmacol Bull 1987; 20:569–571 [B]

233. Okuma T, Yamashita I, Takahashi R, Itoh H, Otsuki S, Watanabe S, Sarai K, Hazama H, Inanaga K: A double-blind study of adjunctive carbamazepine versus placebo on excited states of schizophrenic and schizoaffective disorders. Acta Psychiatr Scand 1989; 80:250–259 [A]

234. Jann MW, Ereshefsky L, Saklad SR, Seidel DR, Davis CM, Burch NR, Bowden CL: Effect of carbamazepine on plasma haloperidol levels. J Clin Psychopharmacol 1985; 5:106–109 [B]

235. Fast DK, Jones BD, Kusalic M, Erickson M: Effect of carbamazepine on neuroleptic plasma levels and efficacy (letter). Am J Psychiatry 1986; 143:117–118 [B]

236. Raitasuo V, Lehtovaara R, Huttunen MO: Carbamazepine and plasma levels of clozapine (letter). Am J Psychiatry 1993; 150:169 [B]

237. Ishizaki T, Chiba K, Saito M, Kobayashi K, Iizuka R: The effects of neuroleptics (haloperidol and chlorpromazine) on the pharmacokinetics of valproic acid in schizophrenic patients. J Clin Psychopharmacol 1984; 4:254–261 [B]

238. Freedman R, Kirch D, Bell J, Adler LE, Pecevich M, Pachtman E, Denver P: Clonidine treatment of schizophrenia: double-blind comparison to placebo and neuroleptic drugs. Acta Psychiatr Scand 1982; 65:35–49 [A]

239. Pickar D, Wolkowitz OM, Doran AR, Labarca R, Roy A, Breier A, Narang PK: Clinical and biochemical effects of verapamil administration to schizophrenic patients. Arch Gen Psychiatry 1987; 44:113–118 [B]

240. van Kammen DP, Peters JL, van Kammen WB, Rosen J, Yao JK, McAdam D, Linnoila M: Clonidine treatment of schizophrenia: can we predict treatment response? Psychiatry Res 1989; 27:297–311 [C]

241. Baker AA, Bird G, Lavin NI, Thoripe JG: ECT in schizophrenia. J Ment Sci 1960; 106:1506–1511 [B]

242. Childers RT Jr: Comparison of four regimens in newly admitted female schizophrenics. Am J Psychiatry 1964; 120:1010–1011 [B]

243. King P: Chlorpromazine and electroconvulsive therapy in the treatment of newly hospitalized schizophrenics. J Clin Exp Psychopathol 1960; 21:101–105 [B]

244. Langsley DG, Enterline JD, Hickerson GX Jr: A comparison of chlorpromazine and EST in treatment of acute schizophrenic and manic reactions. Arch Neurol Psychiatry 1959; 81:384–391 [A]

245. May PRA: Treatment of Schizophrenia. New York, Science House, 1968 [A]

246. Smith K, Surphlis WRP, Gynther MD, Shimkunas A: ECT-chlorpromazine and chlorpromazine compared in the treatment of schizophrenia. J Nerv Ment Dis 1967; 144:284–290 [B]

247. Danziger L, Kendwall JA: Prediction of the immediate outcome of shock therapy in dementia praecox. Dis Nerv Syst 1946; 7:229–303 [G]

248. Kalinowsky LB: Electric convulsive therapy, with emphasis on importance of adequate treatment. Arch Neurol Psychiatry 1943; 50:652–660 [G]

249. Kalinowsky LB, Worthing HJ: Results with electroconvulsive therapy in 200 cases of schizophrenia. Psychiatr Q 1943; 17:144–153 [F]

250. Naidoo D: The effects of reserpine (Serpasil) on the chronic disturbed schizophrenic: a comparative study of rauwolfia alkaloids and electroconvulsive therapy. J Nerv Ment Dis 1956; 123:1–13 [A]

251. Ross JR, Malzberg B: A review of the results of the pharmacological shock therapy and the metrazol convulsive therapy in New York State. Am J Psychiatry 1939; 96:297–316 [G]

252. Friedel RO: The combined use of neuroleptics and ECT in drug resistant schizophrenic patients. Psychopharmacol Bull 1986; 22:928–930 [B]

253. Gujavarty K, Greenberg LB, Fink M: Electroconvulsive therapy and neuroleptic medication in therapy-resistant positive-symptom psychosis. Convulsive Therapy 1987; 3:185–195 [B]

254. Sajatovic M, Meltzer HY: The effect of short-term electroconvulsive treatment plus neuroleptics in treatment-resistant schizophrenia and schizoaffective disorder. Convulsive Therapy 1993; 9:167–176 [B]

255. Safferman AZ, Munne R: Combining clozapine with ECT. Convulsive Ther 1992; 8:141–143 [G]

256. Weiner RD, Rogers HJ, Davidson JR, Kahn EM: Effects of electroconvulsive therapy upon brain electrical activity. Ann NY Acad Sci 1986; 462:270–281 [A]

257. The Practice of Electroconvulsive Therapy: Recommendations for Treatment, Training, and Privileging: A Task Force Report of the American Psychiatric Association. Washington, DC, APA, 1990 [G]

258. Bagadia VN, Abhyankar RR, Doshi J, Pradhan PV, Shah LP: A double blind controlled study of ECT vs chlorpromazine in schizophrenia. J Assoc Physicians India 1983; 31:637–640 [A]

259. Grinspoon L, Ewalt JR, Shader RI: Schizophrenia. Pharmacotherapy and Psychotherapy. Baltimore, Williams & Wilkins, 1972 [B]

260. Karon BP, VandenBos GR: The consequences of psychotherapy for schizophrenic patients. Psychotherapy: Theory, Research, and Practice 1972; 9:111–119 [A]

261. Hogarty GE, Goldberg SC, Schooler NR, Ulrich RF: Drugs and sociotherapy in the aftercare of schizophrenic patients, II: two-year relapse rates. Arch Gen Psychiatry 1974; 31:603–608 [A]

262. Hogarty GE, Goldberg SC, Schooler NR: Drugs and sociotherapy in the aftercare of schizophrenic patients, III: adjustment of nonrelapsed patients. Arch Gen Psychiatry 1974; 31:609–618 [A]

263. Stanton AH, Gunderson JG, Knapp PH, Frank AF, Vannicelli ML, Schnitzer R, Rosenthal R: Effects of psychotherapy in schizophrenia, I: design and implementation of a controlled study. Schizophr Bull 1984; 10:520–563 [B]

264. Gunderson JG, Frank AF, Katz HM, Vannicelli ML, Frosch JP, Knapp PH: Effects of psychotherapy in schizophrenia, II: comparative outcome of two forms of treatment. Schizophr Bull 1984; 10:564–596 [B]

265. Mosher LR, Keith SJ: Psychosocial treatment: individual, group, family and community support approaches. Schizophr Bull 1980; 6:10–41 [F]

266. Gomes-Schwartz B: Individual psychotherapy of schizophrenia, in Schizophrenia: Treatment, Management and Rehabilitation. Edited by Bellack A. Orlando, Fla, Grune & Stratton, 1984, pp 307–335 [F]

267. Mueser KT, Berenbaum H: Psychodynamic treatment of schizophrenia: is there a future? Psychol Med 1990; 20:253–262 [G]

268. Lehman AF, Thompson JW, Dixon LB, Scott JE (eds): Schizophrenia: Treatment Outcomes Research. Schizophr Bull 1995; 21:561–675 [E, G]

269. Goldberg SC, Schooler NR, Hogarty GE, Roper M: Prediction of relapse in schizophrenic patients treated by drug and social therapy. Arch Gen Psychiatry 1977; 34:171–184 [A]

270. McGlashan TH, Nayfack B: Psychotherapeutic models and the treatment of schizophrenia: the records of three successive psychotherapists with one patient at Chestnut Lodge for eighteen years. Psychiatry 1988; 51:340–362 [G]

271. Kavanagh DJ: Recent developments in expressed emotion and schizophrenia. Br J Psychiatry 1992; 160:601–620 [F, G]

272. Vaughn CE, Leff JP: Patterns of emotional response in relatives of schizophrenic patients. Schizophr Bull 1981; 7:43–44 [G]

273. Mueser KT, Gingerich SL, Rosenthal CK: Familial factors in psychiatry. Current Opinion in Psychiatry 1993; 6:251–257 [G]

274. Hogarty GE, Anderson CM, Reiss DJ, Kornblith SJ, Greenwald DP, Javna CD, Madonia MJ: Family psychoeducation, social skills training, and maintenance chemotherapy in the aftercare treatment of schizophrenia, I: one-year effects of a controlled study on relapse and expressed emotion. Arch Gen Psychiatry 1986; 43:633–642 [A, B]

275. Hogarty GE, Anderson CM, Reiss DJ, Kornblith SJ, Greenwald DP, Ulrich RF, Carter M: Family psychoeducation, social skills training, and maintenance chemotherapy in the aftercare treatment of schizophrenia, II: two-year effects of a controlled study on relapse and adjustment. Arch Gen Psychiatry 1991; 48:340–347 [B]

276. Falloon IR, Boyd JL, McGill CW, Williamson M, Razani J, Moss HB, Gilderman AM, Simpson GM: Family management in the prevention of morbidity of schizophrenia: clinical outcome of a two-year longitudinal study. Arch Gen Psychiatry 1985; 42:887–896 [A, B]

277. Goldstein MJ, Rodnick EH, Evans JR, May PR, Steinberg MR: Drugs and family therapy in the aftercare of acute schizophrenics. Arch Gen Psychiatry 1978; 35:1169–1177 [A, B]

278. Penn DL, Mueser KT: Research update on the psychosocial treatment of schizophrenia. Am J Psychiatry 1996; 153:607–617 [F, G]

279. McFarlane WR, Stastny P, Deakins S: Family-aided assertive community treatment: a comprehensive rehabilitation and intensive case management approach for persons with schizophrenic disorders. New Dir Ment Health Serv 1992; 53 (spring):43–54 [F]

280. Tarrier N, Barrowclough C, Vaughn C, Bamrah JS, Porceddu K, Watts S, Freeman H: The community management of schizophrenia: a controlled trial of a behavioural intervention with families to reduce relapse. Br J Psychiatry 1988; 153:532–542 [A, B]

281. Tarrier N, Barrowclough C, Vaughn C, Bamrah JS, Porceddu K, Watts S, Freeman H: Community management of schizophrenia: a two-year follow-up of a behavioural intervention with families. Br J Psychiatry 1989; 154:625–628 [A, B]

282. Leff J, Kuipers L, Berkowitz R, Eberlein-Vries R, Sturgeon D: A controlled trial of social intervention in the families of schizophrenic patients. Br J Psychiatry 1982; 141:121–134 [B]

283. Leff J, Berkowitz R, Shavit N, Strachan A, Glass I, Vaughn C: A trial of family therapy v a relatives group for schizophrenia. Br J Psychiatry 1989; 154:58–66 [B]

284. Randolph ET, Eth S, Glynn SM, Paz GG, Leong GB, Shaner AL, Strachan A, Van Vort W, Escobar JI, Liberman RP: Behavioural family management in schizophrenia: outcome of a clinic-based intervention. Br J Psychiatry 1994; 164:501–506 [A]

285. Liberman RP, Lillie F, Falloon IR, Harpin RE, Hutchinson W, Stoute B: Social skills training with relapsing schizophrenics: an experimental analysis. Behav Modif 1984; 8:155–179 [A]

286. Vaughn CE, Snyder KS, Freeman W, Jones S, Falloon IR, Liberman RP: Family factors in schizophrenic relapse: a replication. Schizophr Bull 1982; 8:425–426 [B]

287. Schooler NR, Keith SJ, Severe JB, Matthews SM: Maintenance treatment of schizophrenia: a review of dose reduction and family treatment strategies. Psychiatr Q 1995; 66:279–292 [F]

288. Mueser KT, Glynn SM: Behavioral Family Therapy for Psychiatric Disorders. Needham Heights, Mass, Allyn & Bacon, 1995 [G]

289. Terkelsen KC: Schizophrenia and the family, II: adverse effects of family therapy. Fam Process 1983; 22:191–200 [E]

290. McFarlane WR: Multiple-family groups and psychoeducation in the treatment of schizophrenia. New Dir Ment Health Serv 1994; 62(summer):13–22 [F]

291. May PRA, Simpson GM: Schizophrenia: overview of treatment methods, in Comprehensive Textbook of Psychiatry, 3rd ed, vol 2. Edited by Kaplan HI, Freedman AM, Sadock BJ. Baltimore, Williams & Wilkins, 1980, pp 1192–1216 [F]

292. Kanas N: Group therapy with schizophrenic patients: a short-term, homogeneous approach. Int J Group Psychother 1991; 41:33–48 [G]

293. Kanas N: Group Therapy for Schizophrenic Patients. Washington, DC, American Psychiatric Press, 1996 [G]

294. Schooler NR, Keith SJ: The clinical research base for the treatment of schizophrenia. Psychopharmacol Bull 1993; 29:431–446 [F]

295. Kanas N: Group therapy with schizophrenics: a review of controlled studies. Int J Group Psychotherapy 1986; 36:339–351 [F]

296. Scott JE, Dixon LB: Psychological interventions for schizophrenia. Schizophr Bull 1995; 21:621–630 [G]

297. Keith SJ, Matthews SM: Group, family, and milieu therapies and psychosocial rehabilitation in the treatment of schizophrenic disorders, in Psychiatry 1982: The American Psychiatric Association Annual Review. Edited by Grinspoon L. Washington, DC, American Psychiatric Press, 1982, pp 166–177 [F]

298. Luborsky L, Singer B, Luborsky L: Comparative studies of psychotherapies: is it true that "Everybody has won and all must have prizes"?, in Evaluation of Psychological Therapies. Edited by Spitzer RL, Klein DF. Baltimore, Johns Hopkins University Press, 1976, pp 3–22 [F]

299. O'Brien CP: Group psychotherapy with schizophrenia and affective disorders, in Comprehensive Group Psychotherapy, 2nd ed. Edited by Kaplan HI, Sadock BJ. Baltimore, Williams & Wilkins, 1983, pp 242–249 [B]

300. Parloff MB, Dies RR: Group psychotherapy outcome research 1966–1975. Int J Group Psychother 1977; 27:281–319 [F]

301. Donlon PT, Rada RT, Knight SW: A therapeutic aftercare setting for "refractory" chronic schizophrenic patients. Am J Psychiatry 1973; 130:682–684 [B]

302. O'Brien CP, Hamm KB, Ray BA, Pierce JF, Luborsky L, Mintz J: Group vs individual psychotherapy with schizophrenics: a controlled outcome study. Arch Gen Psychiatry 1972; 27:474–478 [B]

303. Malm U: The Influence of Group Therapy on Schizophrenia. Acta Psychiatr Scand (Suppl) 1982; 297 [B]

304. Malm U: Group therapy, in Handbook of Schizophrenia, vol 4: Psychosocial Treatment of Schizophrenia. Edited by Herz MI, Keith SJ, Docherty JP. Amsterdam, Elsevier, 1990, pp 191–211 [F]

305. Kanas N, Rogers M, Kreth E, Patterson L, Campbell R: The effectiveness of group psychotherapy during the first three weeks of hospitalization: a controlled study. J Nerv Ment Dis 1980; 168:487–492 [B]

306. Kanas N: Group psychotherapy with schizophrenia, in Comprehensive Group Psychotherapy, 3rd ed. Edited by Kaplan HI, Sadock BJ. Baltimore, Williams & Wilkins, 1993, pp 407–418 [G]

307. Kibel HD: Group psychotherapy, in Less Time to Do More: Psychotherapy on the Short-Term Inpatient Unit. Edited by Leibenluft E, Tasman A, Green SA. Washington, DC, American Psychiatric Press, 1993, pp 89–109 [F]

308. Group therapy in schizophrenia, in Treatments of Psychiatric Disorders: A Task Force Report of the American Psychiatric Association, vol 2. Washington, DC, APA, 1989, pp 1529–1542 [F]

309. Stone WN: Group therapy for seriously mentally ill patients in a managed care system, in Effective Use of Group Therapy in Managed Care. Edited by MacKenzie KR. Washington, DC, American Psychiatric Press, 1995, pp 129–146 [G]

310. Herz MI, Melville C: Relapse in schizophrenia. Am J Psychiatry 1980; 137:801–805 [D]

311. Heinrichs DW, Carpenter WT Jr: Prospective study of prodromal symptoms in schizophrenic relapse. Am J Psychiatry 1985; 142:371–373 [D]

312. McCandless-Glimcher L, McKnight S, Hamera E, Smith BL, Peterson KA, Plumlee AA: Use of symptoms by schizophrenics to monitor and regulate their illness. Hosp Community Psychiatry 1986; 37:929–933 [C]

313. Subotnik KL, Nuechterlein KH: Prodromal signs and symptoms of schizophrenic relapse. J Abnorm Psychol 1988; 97:405–412 [D]

314. Jolley AG, Hirsch SR, Morrison E, McRink A, Wilson L: Trial of brief intermittent neuroleptic prophylaxis for selected schizophrenic outpatients: clinical and social outcome at two years. Br Med J 1990; 301:837–842 [A]

315. Kumar S, Thara R, Rajkumar S: Coping with symptoms of relapse in schizophrenia. Eur Arch Psychiatry Clin Neurosci 1989; 239:213–215 [D]

316. Tarrier N, Barrowclough C, Bamrah JS: Prodromal signs of relapse in schizophrenia. Soc Psychiatry Psychiatr Epidemiol 1991; 26:157–161 [C]

317. Marder SR, Mintz J, Van Putten T, Lebell M, Wirshing WC, Johnston-Cronk K: Early prediction of relapse in schizophrenia: an application of receiver operating characteristic (ROC) methods. Psychopharmacol Bull 1991; 27:79–82 [C]

318. Henmi Y: Prodromal symptoms of relapse in schizophrenic outpatients: retrospective and prospective study. Jpn J Psychiatry Neurol 1993; 47:753–775 [C, D]

319. Marder SR, Van Putten T, Mintz J, Lebell M, McKenzie J, Faltico G: Maintenance therapy in schizophrenia: new findings, in Drug Maintenance Strategies in Schizophrenia. Edited by Kane JM. Washington, DC, American Psychiatric Press, 1984, pp 31–49 [F]

320. Pietzcker A, Gaebel W, Kopcke W, Linden M, Muller P, Muller-Spahn F, Tegeler J: Intermittent versus maintenance neuroleptic long-term treatment in schizophrenia—2-year results of a German multicenter study. J Psychiatr Res 1993; 27:321–339 [A]

321. Baker F, Intagliata J: Case management, in Handbook of Psychiatric Rehabilitation. Edited by Liberman RP. Boston, Allyn & Bacon, 1992, pp 213–243 [G]

322. Stein LI, Diamond RJ, Factor RM: A system approach to the care of persons with schizophrenia, in Handbook of Schizophrenia, vol 4: Psychosocial Treatment of Schizophrenia. Edited by Herz MI, Keith SJ, Docherty JP. New York, Elsevier, 1990, pp 213–246 [G]

323. Stein LI, Test MA: Alternative to mental hospital treatment, I: conceptual model, treatment program, and clinical evaluation. Arch Gen Psychiatry 1980; 37:392–397 [B]

324. Group for the Advancement of Psychiatry: Implications for psychosocial interventions in patients with schizophrenia, in Beyond Symptom Suppression, Report 134. Washington, DC, American Psychiatric Press, 1992, pp 59–78 [F]

325. Burns BJ, Santos AB: Assertive community treatment: an update of randomized trials. Psychiatr Serv 1995; 46:669–675 [E]

326. Weisbrod BA, Test MA, Stein LI: Alternative to mental hospital treatment, II: economic benefit-cost analysis. Arch Gen Psychiatry 1980; 37:400–405 [G]

327. Hoult J: Community care of the acutely mentally ill. Br J Psychiatry 1986; 149:137–144 [F]

328. Test MA: Training in community living, in Handbook of Psychiatric Rehabilitation. Edited by Liberman RP. Needham Heights, Mass, Allyn & Bacon, 1992, pp 153–170 [F]

329. Stein LI: Wisconsin's system of mental health financing. New Dir Ment Health Serv 1989; 43:29–41 [G]

330. Stein LI: Innovating against the current. New Dir Ment Health Serv 1992; 56:5–22 [G]

331. Taube CA, Morlock L, Burns BJ, Santos AB: New directions in research on assertive community treatment. Hosp Community Psychiatry 1990; 41:642–646 [G]

332. Fairweather GW, Sanders DH, Maynard H, Cressler DL, Bleck DS: Community Life for the Mentally Ill. Chicago, Aldine, 1969 [A]

333. Fairweather GW, Sanders DH, Tornatzky LG: Creating Change in Mental Health Organizations. New York, Pergamon, 1974 [A]

334. Liberman RP, DeRisis WJ, Mueser KT: Social Skills Training for Psychiatric Patients. Needham Heights, Mass, Allyn & Bacon, 1989 [G]

335. Mueser KT, Wallace CJ, Liberman RP: New developments in social skills training. Behaviour Change 1995; 12:31–40 [G]

336. Benton MK, Schroeder HE: Social skills training with schizophrenics: a meta-analytic evaluation. J Consult Clin Psychol 1990; 58:741–747 [E]

337. Corrigan PW: Social skills training in adult psychiatric populations: a meta-analysis. J Behav Ther Exp Psychiatry 1991; 22:203–210 [E]

338. Liberman RP, Vaccaro JV, Corrigan PW: Psychiatric rehabilitation, in Comprehensive Textbook of Psychiatry, 6th ed. Edited by Kaplan HI, Sadock BJ. Baltimore, Williams & Wilkins, 1995, pp 2696–2717 [G]

339. Eckman TA, Wirshing WC, Marder SR, Liberman RP, Johnston-Cronk K, Zimmermann K, Mintz J: Technique for training schizophrenic patients in illness self-management: a controlled trial. Am J Psychiatry 1992; 149:1549–1555 [A]

340. Wallace CJ, Liberman RP, MacKain SJ, Blackwell G, Eckman TA: Effectiveness and replicability of modules for teaching social and instrumental skills to the severely mentally ill. Am J Psychiatry 1992; 149:654–658 [B]

341. Holmes MR, Hansen DJ, St Lawrence JS: Conversational skills training with aftercare patients in the community: social validation and generalization. Behav Ther 1984; 15:84–100 [B]

342. Wallace CJ, Liberman RP: Social skills training for schizophrenics: a controlled clinical trial. Psychiatry Res 1985; 15:239–247 [A]

343. Brown MA, Munford AM: Life skills training for chronic schizophrenics. J Nerv Ment Dis 1983; 17:1466–1476 [A]

344. Marder SR, Wirshing WC, Mintz J, McKenzie J, Johnston K, Eckman TA, Lebell M, Zimmerman K, Liberman RP: Two-year outcome of social skills training and group psychotherapy for outpatients with schizophrenia. Am J Psychiatry 1996; 153:1585–1592 [A]

345. Dobson DJ, McDougall G, Busheikin J, Aldous J: Effects of social skills training and social milieu treatment on symptoms of schizophrenia. Psychiatr Serv 1995; 46:376–380 [B]

346. Wallace CJ, Lieberman RP: Psychiatric rehabilitation, in Treatment of Psychiatric Disorders, 2nd ed. Edited by Gabbard GO. Washington, DC, American Psychiatric Press, 1995, pp 1019–1038 [G]

347. Bond GR, Boyer SL: Rehabilitation programs and outcomes, in Vocational Rehabilitation of Persons With Prolonged Psychiatric Disorders. Edited by Ciardiello JA, Bell MD. Baltimore, Johns Hopkins University Press, 1988, pp 231–263 [G]

348. Griffiths RD: Rehabilitation of chronic psychotic patients. Psychol Med 1974; 4:316–325 [B]

349. Weinberg JL, Lustig P: A workshop experience for post-hospitalization schizophrenics, in Rehabilitation Research. Edited by Wright GN, Trotter AB. Madison, University of Wisconsin, 1968, pp 72–78 [C]

350. Cook JA, Razzano L: Natural vocational supports for persons with severe mental illness: Thresholds Supported Competitive Employment Program. New Dir Ment Health Serv 1992; 56 (2):23–41 [G]

351. Drake RE, Becker DR, Biesanz JC, Torrey WC, McHugo GJ, Wyzik PF: Rehabilitative day treatment vs supported employment, I: vocational outcomes. Community Ment Health J 1994; 30:519–532 [A]

352. Drake RE, McHugo GJ, Becker DR, Anthony WA, Clark RE: The New Hampshire study of supported employment for people with severe mental illness. J Consult Clin Psychol 1996; 64:391–399 [A]

353. Bond GR: Vocational rehabilitation, in Handbook of Psychiatric Rehabilitation. Edited by Liberman RP. Needham Heights, Mass, Allyn & Bacon, 1992, pp 244–275 [G]

354. Danley KS, Sciarappa K, MacDonald-Wilson K: Choose-get-keep: a psychiatric rehabilitation approach to supported employment, in Effective Psychiatric Rehabilitation. Edited by Liberman RP. San Francisco, Jossey-Bass, 1992, pp 87–96 [G]

355. Jacobs HE, Kardashian S, Kreinbring RK, Ponder R, Simpson AS: A skills-oriented model for facilitating employment among psychiatrically disabled persons. Rehabilitation Counseling Bull 1984; 28:87–96 [B]

356. Mitchell J, Jacobs HE, Yen F: Costs and response rates in a community follow-up for a psychiatric vocational rehabilitation program. Rehabilitation Counseling Bull 1987; 31:273–277 [B]

357. Jacobs HE, Wissusik D, Collier R, Stackman D, Burkeman D: Correlations between psychiatric disabilities and vocational outcome. Hosp Community Psychiatry 1992; 43:365–369 [B]

358. Anthony WA, Howell J, Danley KS: Vocational rehabilitation of the psychiatrically disabled, in The Chronically Mentally Ill: Research and Services. Edited by Mirabi M. New York, Spectrum Publications, 1984, pp 215–237 [G]

359. Goering PN, Wasylenki DA, Farkas M, Lancee WJ, Ballantyne R: What difference does case management make? Hosp Community Psychiatry 1988; 39:272–276 [D]

360. Bond GR: Psychiatric vocational programs: a meta-analysis. Presented at the annual meeting of the International Association of Psychosocial Rehabilitation Services, Cleveland, 1986 [E]

361. Cook JA, Solomon M, Mock L: What happens after the first job placement? Programming for Adolescents With Behavioral Disorders 1989; 4:71–93 [uncoded]

362. Rutman I, Armstrong K: A comprehensive evaluation of transitional employment programs in the rehabilitation of chronically mentally disabled clients. Unpublished manuscript, 1985 [G]

363. Tarrier N, Harwood S, Yusopoff L, Beckett R, Baker A: Coping strategy enhancement (CSE): a method of treating residual schizophrenic symptoms. Behavioural Psychotherapy 1990; 18:283–293 [C]

364. Tarrier N, Beckett R, Harwood S, Baker A, Yusopoff L, Ugarteburu I: A trial of two cognitive-behavioral methods of treating drug-resistant residual psychotic symptoms in schizophrenic patients, I: outcome. Br J Psychiatry 1993; 162:524–532 [B]

365. Perris C: Cognitive Therapy of Schizophrenia. New York, Guilford Press, 1989 [B]

366. Green MF: Cognitive remediation in schizophrenia: is it time yet? Am J Psychiatry 1993; 150:178–187 [F]

367. Spaulding W, Sullivan M: From laboratory to clinic: psychological methods and principles in psychiatric rehabilitation, in Handbook of Psychiatric Rehabilitation. Edited by Liberman RP. Needham Heights, Mass, Allyn & Bacon, 1992, pp 30–55 [G]

368. Corrigan PW, Yudofsky SC (eds): Cognitive Remediation for Schizophrenia. Washington, DC, American Psychiatric Press, 1994 [B]

369. Brenner HD, Roder V, Hodel B, Kienzie N, Reed D, Liberman RP: Integrated Psychological Therapy for Schizophrenic Patients. Toronto, Hogrefe & Huber, 1994 [B]

370. Wykes T (ed): Psychological Treatments for Schizophrenia. Cambridge, England, Cambridge University Press (in press) [G]

371. Kingdon DG, Turkington D: Cognitive-Behavioral Therapy of Schizophrenia. New York, Guilford Press, 1994 [B]

372. Vine P, Beels CC: Support and advocacy groups for the mentally ill, in Handbook of Schizophrenia, vol 4: Psychosocial Treatment of Schizophrenia. Edited by Herz MI, Keith SJ, Docherty JP. New York, Elsevier, 1990, pp 387–405 [G]

373. Lam DH: Psychosocial family intervention in schizophrenia: a review of empirical studies. Psychol Med 1991; 21:423–441 [G]

374. Strachan A: Family intervention, in Handbook of Psychiatric Rehabilitation. Edited by Liberman RP. Needham Heights, Mass, Allyn & Bacon, 1992, pp 183–212 [G]

375. Wilder JF, Levin G, Zwerling I: A two-year follow-up evaluation of acute psychotic patients treated in a day hospital. Am J Psychiatry 1966; 122:1095–1101 [B]

376. Herz MI, Endicott J, Spitzer RL, Mesnikoff A: Day versus inpatient hospitalization: a controlled study. Am J Psychiatry 1971; 127:1371–1382 [B]

377. Langsley DG, Machotka P, Flomenhaft K: Avoiding mental hospital admission: a follow-up study. Am J Psychiatry 1971; 127:1391–1394 [B]

378. Pasamanick B, Scarpitti FR, Dinitz S: Schizophrenics in the Community. New York, Appleton-Century-Crofts, 1967 [B]

379. Fenton FR, Tessier L, Struening EL: A comparative trial of home and hospital psychiatric care: one-year follow-up. Arch Gen Psychiatry 1979; 36:1073–1079 [B]

380. Mosher LR, Menn A, Matthews SM: Soteria: evaluation of a home-based treatment for schizophrenia. Am J Orthopsychiatry 1975; 45:455–467 [B]

381. Ciompi L, Dauwalder HP, Maier C, Aebi E, Trutsch K, Kupper Z, Rutishauser C: The pilot project "Soteria Berne": clinical experiences and results. Br J Psychiatry 1992; 161(suppl 18):145–153 [B]

382. Sledge WH, Tebes J, Rakfeldt J: Acute respite care, in Emergency Mental Health Services in the Community. Edited by Phelan M, Strathdee G, Thornicroft G. Cambridge, England, Cambridge University Press, 1995, pp 233–258 [B]

383. Brook BD: Crisis hostel: an alternative to hospitalization for emergency patients. Hosp Community Psychiatry 1973; 24:621–624 [B]

384. Herz MI: Short-term hospitalization and the medical model. Hosp Community Psychiatry 1979; 30:117–121 [F]

385. Herz MI, Endicott J, Spitzer RL: Brief hospitalization: a two-year follow-up. Am J Psychiatry 1977; 134:502–507 [B]

386. Hirsch SR, Platt S, Knights A, Weyman A: Shortening hospital stay for psychiatric care: effect on patients and their families. Br Med J 1979; 1:442–446 [B]

387. Caffey EM, Jones RD, Diamond LS, Burton E, Bowen WT: Brief hospital treatment of schizophrenia: early results of a multiple-hospital study. Hosp Community Psychiatry 1968; 19:282–287 [B]

388. Caffey EM, Galbrecht CR, Klett CJ: Brief hospitalization and aftercare in the treatment of schizophrenia. Arch Gen Psychiatry 1971; 24:81–86 [B]

389. Glick ID, Hargreaves WA, Goldfield MD: Short vs long hospitalization: a prospective controlled study, I: the preliminary results of a one-year follow-up of schizophrenics. Arch Gen Psychiatry 1974; 30:363–369 [B]

390. Glick ID, Hargreaves WA, Raskin M, Kutner SJ: Short versus long hospitalization: a prospective controlled study, II: results for schizophrenic inpatients. Am J Psychiatry 1975; 132:385–390 [B]

391. Glick ID, Hargreaves WA, Drues J, Showstack JA: Short versus long hospitalization: a prospective controlled study, IV: one-year follow-up results for schizophrenic patients. Am J Psychiatry 1976; 133:509–514 [B]

392. Hargreaves WA, Glick ID, Drues J, Showstack JA, Feigenbaum E: Short vs long hospitalization: a prospective controlled study, VI: two-year follow-up results for schizophrenics. Arch Gen Psychiatry 1977; 34:305–311 [B]

393. Rosen B, Katzoff A, Carillo C, Klein DF: Clinical effectiveness of "short" vs "long" stay psychiatric hospitalization, I: inpatient results. Arch Gen Psychiatry 1976; 33:1316–1322 [B]

394. Mattes JA, Rosen B, Klein DF: Comparison of the clinical effectiveness of "short" versus "long" stay psychiatric hospitalization, II: results of a 3-year posthospital follow-up. J Nerv Ment Dis 1977; 165:387–394 [B]

395. Mattes JA, Rosen B, Klein DF, Millan D: Comparison of the clinical effectiveness of "short" versus "long" stay psychiatric hospitalization, III: further results of a 3-year post-hospital follow-up. J Nerv Ment Dis 1977; 165:395–402 [B]

396. Mattes JA, Klein DF, Millan D, Rosen B: Comparison of the clinical effectiveness of "short" versus "long" stay psychiatric hospitalization, IV: predictors of differential benefit. J Nerv Ment Dis 1979; 167:175–181 [B]

397. Brenner HD, Dencker SJ, Goldstein MJ, Hubbard JW, Keegan DL, Kruger G, Kulhanek F, Liberman RP, Malm U, Midha KK: Defining treatment refractoriness in schizophrenia. Schizophr Bull 1990; 16:551–561 [F]

398. Hall J, Baker R: Token economies and schizophrenia: a review, in Contemporary Issues in Schizophrenia. Edited by Kerr TA, Snaith RP. London, Gaskell, 1986, pp 410–419 [G]

399. Glynn SM, Mueser KT: Social learning programs, in Handbook of Psychiatric Rehabilitation. Edited by Liberman RP. Needham Heights, Mass, Allyn & Bacon, 1992 [G]

400. Paul GL, Lentz RJ: Psychological Treatment of Chronic Mental Patients: Milieu Versus Social-Learning Programs. Cambridge, Mass, Harvard University Press, 1977, p 214 [B]

401. Glynn SM: Token economy approaches for psychiatric patients: progress and pitfalls over 25 years. Behav Modif 1990; 14:383–407 [F]

402. Liberman RP: Behavior modification of schizophrenia: a review. Schizophr Bull 1972; 6:537–548 [G]

403. Mendotta A, Valdes LA, Beck NC: Implementing a comprehensive social learning program within a forensic psychiatric service of Fulton State Hospital, in Behavior Therapy in Psychiatric Hospitals. Edited by Corrigan PW, Liberman RP. New York, Springer, 1994, pp 61–78 [B]

404. Wong SE, Flanagan SG, Kuehnel TG, Liberman RP, Hunnicut R, Adams-Badgett J: Training chronic mental patients to independently practice personal grooming skills. Hosp Community Psychiatry 1988; 39:874–880 [B]

405. Boudewyns PA, Fry TJ, Nightingale T: Token economy programs in VA medical centers: where are they today? Behav Ther 1986; 9:126–127 [E]

406. Bellack AS, Mueser KT: A comprehensive treatment program for schizophrenia and chronic mental illness. Community Ment Health J 1986; 22:175–189 [B]

407. Herz MI, Endicott J, Gibbon M: Brief hospitalization: two year follow-up. Arch Gen Psychiatry 1979; 36:701–705 [B]

408. Washburn S, Vannicelli M, Longabaugh R, Scheff BJ: A controlled comparison of psychiatric day treatment and inpatient hospitalization. J Consult Clin Psychol 1976; 44:665–675 [B]

409. Creed F, Black D, Anthony P: Day hospital and community treatment for acute psychiatric illness: a critical appraisal. Br J Psychiatry 1989; 154:300–310 [F]

410. Creed F, Black D, Anthony P, Osborn M, Thomas P, Tomenson B: Randomised controlled trial of day patient versus inpatient psychiatric treatment. Br Med J 1990; 300:1033–1037 [B]

411. Creed F, Black D, Anthony P, Osborn M, Thomas P, Franks D, Polley R, Lancashire S, Saleem P, Tomenson B: Randomised controlled trial of day and in-patient psychiatric treatment, 2: comparison of two hospitals. Br J Psychiatry 1991; 158:183–189 [B]

412. Dick P, Cameron L, Cohen D, Barlow M, Ince A: Day and full time psychiatric treatment: a controlled comparison. Br J Psychiatry 1985; 147:246–249 [B]

413. Gudeman JE, Shore MF, Dickey B: Day hospitalization and an inn instead of inpatient care for psychiatric patients. N Engl J Med 1983; 308:749–753 [B]

414. Gudeman JE, Dickey B, Evans A, Shore MF: Four-year assessment of a day hospital-inn program as an alternative to inpatient hospitalization. Am J Psychiatry 1985; 142:1330–1333 [B]

415. Schene AH, van Wijngaarden B, Poelijoe NW, Gersons BP: The Utrecht comparative study on psychiatric day treatment and inpatient treatment. Acta Psychiatr Scand 1993; 87:427–436 [B]

416. Meltzhoff J, Blumenthal RL: The Day Treatment Center. Springfield, Ill, Charles C Thomas, 1966 [B]

417. Guy W, Gross M, Hogarty GE, Dennis H: A controlled evaluation of day hospital effectiveness. Arch Gen Psychiatry 1969; 20:329–338 [B]

418. Linn MW, Caffey EM Jr, Klett CJ, Hogarty GE, Lamb HR: Day treatment and psychotropic drugs in the aftercare of schizophrenic patients: a Veterans Administration cooperative study. Arch Gen Psychiatry 1979; 36:1055–1066 [B]

419. Budson RD: Models of supportive living: community residential care, in Handbook of Schizophrenia, vol 4: Psychosocial Treatment of Schizophrenia. Edited by Herz MI, Keith SJ, Docherty JP. New York, Elsevier, 1990, pp 317–338 [F]

420. Campbell RJ (ed): Psychiatric Dictionary, 7th ed. New York, Oxford University Press, 1996, pp 212, 311 [G]

421. Murphy HB, Engelsmann F, Tcheng-Laroche F: The influence of foster-home care on psychiatric patients. Arch Gen Psychiatry 1976; 33:179–183 [C]

422. Okin RL, Pearsall D: Patients' perceptions of their quality of life 11 years after discharge from a state hospital. Hosp Community Psychiatry 1993; 44:236–240 [C]

423. Okin RL, Borus JF, Baer L, Jones AL: Long-term outcome of state hospital patients discharged into structured community residential settings. Psychiatr Serv 1995; 46:73–78 [C]

424. Hawthorne WB, Fals-Stewart W, Lohr JB: A treatment outcome study of community-based residential care. Hosp Community Psychiatry 1994; 45:152–155 [C]

425. Bellack AS, Mueser KT: Psychosocial treatment for schizophrenia. Schizophr Bull 1993; 19:317–336 [F, G]

426. Harding C: Course types in schizophrenia: an analysis of European and American studies. Schizophr Bull 1988; 14:633–643 [E]

427. Kopelowicz A, Liberman RP: Biobehavioral treatment and rehabilitation of schizophrenia. Harvard Rev Psychiatry 1995; 3:55–64 [G]

428. American Psychiatric Association: Practice Guideline for Psychiatric Evaluation of Adults. Am J Psychiatry 1995; 152(Nov suppl):63–80 [F]

429. Gelenberg AJ, Bassuk EL, Schoonover SC (eds): The Practitioner's Guide to Psychoactive Drugs. New York, Plenum, 1990 [G]

430. McClellan RL, Eisenberg RL, Giyanani VL: Routine CT screening of psychiatric inpatients. Radiology 1988; 169:99–100 [D]

431. Young AS, Nuechterlein KH, Mintz J, Ventura J, Gitlin M, Liberman RP: Suicidal ideation and behavior in recent-onset schizophrenia. Unpublished manuscript, 1996 [C]

432. Taylor PJ, Monahan J: Dangerous patients or dangerous diseases? BMJ 1996; 312:967–969 [G]

433. Warner R, Wolleson C: Alternative acute treatment settings, in Practicing Psychiatry in the Community: A Manual. Edited by Vaccaro JV, Clark GH Jr. Washington, DC, American Psychiatric Press, 1996, pp 89–115 [G]

434. Schooler NR, Severe JB, Glick ID, Hargreaves WA, Keith SJ, Weiden P: Transition from acute to maintenance treatment: prediction of stabilization. Int Clin Psychopharmacol 1996; 11(suppl 2):85–91 [G]

435. Torrey WC: Psychiatric care of adults with developmental disabilities and mental illness in the community. Community Ment Health J 1993; 29:461–481 [G]

436. Hatfield AB: The National Alliance for the Mentally Ill: a decade later (editorial). Community Ment Health J 1991; 27:95–103 [G]

437. Falloon IR, Liberman RP: Interactions between drug and psychosocial therapy in schizophrenia. Schizophr Bull 1983; 9:543–544 [G]

438. Lefley HP, Johnson D (eds): Families as Allies in the Treatment of the Mentally Ill. Washington, DC, American Psychiatric Press, 1990 [G]

439. McGlashan TH, Johannessen JA: Early detection and intervention with schizophrenia: rationale. Schizophr Bull 1996; 22:201–222 [G]

440. Cournos F: Involuntary medication and the case of Joyce Brown. Hosp Community Psychiatry 1989; 40:736–740 [E]

441. Lukoff D, Liberman RP, Nuechterlein KH: Symptom monitoring in the rehabilitation of schizophrenic patients. Schizophr Bull 1986; 12:578–602 [F]

442. Wolkowitz OM: Rational polypharmacy in schizophrenia. Ann Clin Psychiatry 1993; 5:79–90 [F]

443. Salzman C, Green AI, Rodriguez-Villa F, Jaskiw GI: Benzodiazepines combined with neuroleptics for management of severe disruptive behavior. Psychosomatics 1986; 27(Jan suppl):17–22 [B]

444. Philbrick KL, Rummans TA: Malignant catatonia. J Neuropsychiatry Clin Neurosci 1994; 6:1–13 [C]

445. Fricchione G: Catatonia: a new indication for benzodiazepines? Biol Psychiatry 1989; 26:761–765 [G]

446. Rosebush PI, Hildebrand AM, Furlong BG, Mazurek MF: Catatonic syndrome in a general psychiatric inpatient population: frequency, clinical presentation, and response to lorazepam. J Clin Psychiatry 1990; 51:357–362 [B]

447. Fink M: Reply to Rosebush PI: The treatment of catatonia: benzodiazepines or ECT? (letter). Am J Psychiatry 1992; 149:1279–1280 [G]

448. Fink M, Sackeim HA: Convulsive therapy in schizophrenia? Schizophr Bull 1996; 22:27–39 [F, G]

449. Eckman TA, Liberman RP, Phipps CC, Blair KE: Teaching medication management skills to schizophrenic patients. J Clin Psychopharmacol 1990; 10:33–38 [G]

450. Wyatt RJ: Practical Psychiatric Practice: Forms and Protocols for Clinical Use. Washington, DC, American Psychiatric Press, 1993 [G]

451. Ventura J, Green MF, Shaner A, Liberman RP: Training and quality assurance in the use of the Brief Psychiatric Rating Scale: the "drift busters." Int J Methods Psychiatr Res 1993; 3:221–244 [B]

452. Guy W (ed): ECDEU Assessment Manual for Psychopharmacology: Publication ADM 76-338. Washington, DC, US Department of Health, Education, and Welfare, 1976, pp 534–537 [G]

453. Greenfeld D: The Psychotic Patient: Medication and Psychotherapy. New York, Free Press, 1985 [G]

454. Dingman CW, McGlashan TH: Psychotherapy, in A Clinical Guide for the Treatment of Schizophrenia. Edited by Bellack AS. New York, Plenum, 1989, pp 263–282 [F, G]

455. McGlashan TH, Keats CJ: Schizophrenia: Treatment, Process, and Outcome. Washington, DC, American Psychiatric Press, 1989 [G]

456. Coursey RD: Psychotherapy with persons suffering from schizophrenia: the need for a new agenda. Schizophr Bull 1989; 15:349–353 [G]

457. Fenton WS, McGlashan TH: Schizophrenia: individual psychotherapy, in Comprehensive Textbook of Psychiatry, 6th ed, vol 1. Edited by Kaplan HI, Sadock BJ. Baltimore, William & Wilkins, 1995, pp 1007–1018 [F, G]

458. Coursey RD, Keller AB, Farrell EW: Individual psychotherapy and persons with serious mental illness: the clients' perspective. Schizophr Bull 1995; 21:283–301 [F, G]

459. McGlashan TH: Intensive individual psychotherapy of schizophrenia. Arch Gen Psychiatry 1983; 40:909–920 [F]

460. McGlashan TH: Psychosocial treatments of schizophrenia: the potential of relationships, in Schizophrenia: From Mind to Molecule. Edited by Andreasen NC. Washington, DC, American Psychiatric Press, 1993, pp 189–215 [F, G]

461. Lewine RRJ: Psychological evaluation, in Schizophrenia: Treatment of Acute Psychotic Episodes. Edited by Levy ST, Ninan PT. Washington, DC, American Psychiatric Press, 1990, pp 45–60 [G]

462. Green MF: What are the functional consequences of neurocognitive deficits in schizophrenia? Am J Psychiatry 1996; 153:321–330 [F]

463. Liberman RP, Corrigan PW: Designing new psychosocial treatments for schizophrenia. Psychiatry 1993; 56:238–253 [G]

464. Schooler NR: Maintenance medication for schizophrenia: strategies for dose reduction. Schizophr Bull 1991; 17:311–324 [F, G]

465. Lieberman JA: Prediction of outcome in first-episode schizophrenia. J Clin Psychiatry 1993; 54(March suppl):13–17 [C]

466. Weber TT, McDaniel SH, Wynne LC: Helping more by helping less: family therapy and systems consultation. Psychotherapy 1987; 24(suppl 3):615–620 [F]

467. Carpenter WT Jr, Heinrichs DW, Wagman AMI: Deficit and nondeficit forms of schizophrenia: the concept. Am J Psychiatry 1988; 145:578–583 [E, G]

468. Carpenter WT, Heinrichs DW, Alphs LD: Treatment of negative symptoms. Schizophr Bull 1985; 11:440–452 [G]

469. Meltzer HY, Bastani B, Kwon KY, Ramirez LF, Burnett S, Sharpe J: A prospective study of clozapine in treatment-resistant schizophrenic patients, I: preliminary report. Psychopharmacology (Berl) 1989; 99(suppl):S68–S72 [B]

470. Lieberman JA, Safferman AZ, Pollack S, Szymanski S, Johns C, Howard A, Kronig M, Bookstein P, Kane JM: Clinical effects of clozapine in chronic schizophrenia: response to treatment and predictors of outcome. Am J Psychiatry 1994; 151:1744–1752 [F]

471. Buchanan FH, Parton RV, Warren JW: Double-blind trial of L-dopa in chronic schizophrenia. Aust NZ J Psychiatry 1975; 9:269–271 [A]

472. Gerlach J, Luhdorf K: The effect of L-dopa on young patients with simple schizophrenia, treated with neuroleptic drugs. Psychopharmacology (Berl) 1975; 44:105–110 [A]

473. Inanaga K, Nakazawa Y, Inoue K, Tachibana H, Oshima M, Kotorii T, Tanaka M, Ogawa N: Double-blind controlled study of L-dopa therapy in schizophrenia. Folia Psychiatr Neurol Jpn 1975; 29:123–142 [A]

474. Brambilla F, Scarone S, Ponzano M, Maffei C, Nobile P, Rovere C, Guastella A: Catecholaminergic drugs in chronic schizophrenia. Neuropsychobiology 1979; 5:185–200 [B]

475. Kay SR, Opler LA: L-Dopa in the treatment of negative schizophrenic symptoms: a single-subject experimental study. Int J Psychiatry Med 1985; 15:293–298 [B]

476. Angrist B, Santhanathan G, Gershon S: Behavioral effect of L-dopa in schizophrenic patients. Psychopharmacologia 1973; 31:1–12 [B]

477. Calil HM, Yesavage JA, Hollister LE: Low dose levodopa in schizophrenia. Communications in Psychopharmacology 1977; 1:593–596 [B]

478. Garfinkel PE, Stancer HC: L-Dopa and schizophrenia. Can J Psychiatry 1976; 21:27–29 [G]

479. Yaryura-Tobias JA, Diamond B, Merlis S: The action of L-dopa on schizophrenic patients (a preliminary report). Curr Ther Res 1970; 12:528–531 [B]

480. Mueser KT, Yarnold PR, Levinson DF, Singh H, Bellack AS, Kee K, Morrison RL, Yadalam KG: Prevalence of substance abuse in schizophrenia: demographic and clinical correlates. Schizophr Bull 1990; 16:31–56 [D, F]

481. Drake RE, Osher FC, Noordsy DL, Harlbut SC, Teague GB, Beaudett MS: Diagnosis of alcohol use disorders in schizophrenia. Schizophr Bull 1990; 16:57–67 [D]

482. Kivlahan DR, Heiman JR, Wright RC, Mundt JW, Shupe JA: Treatment cost and rehospitalization rate in schizophrenic outpatients with a history of substance abuse. Hosp Community Psychiatry 1990; 42:609–614 [C]

483. American Psychiatric Association: Practice Guideline for the Treatment of Patients With Substance Use Disorders: Alcohol, Cocaine, Opioids. Am J Psychiatry 1995; 152(Nov suppl):1–59 [F]

484. Salloum IM, Moss HB, Daley DC: Substance abuse and schizophrenia: impediments to optimal care. Am J Drug Alcohol Abuse 1991; 17:321–336 [F]

485. Searles J, Alterman A, Purtill JJ: The detection of alcoholism in hospitalized schizophrenics: a comparison of the MAST and the MAC. Alcohol Clin Exp Res 1990; 14:557–560 [D]

486. Brady K, Casto S, Lydiard RB, Malcom R, Arana G: Substance abuse in an inpatient psychiatric sample. Am J Drug Alcohol Abuse 1991; 17:389–397 [E]

487. Mitchell J, Vierkant AD: Delusions and hallucinations of cocaine abusers and paranoid schizophrenics: a comparative study. J Psychol 1991; 125:301–310 [D]

488. Castaneda R, Galanter M, Lifshutz H, Franko H: Effect of drugs of abuse on psychiatric symptoms among hospitalized schizophrenics. Am J Drug Alcohol Abuse 1991; 17:313–320 [D]

489. Turner W, Tsuang MT: Impact of substance abuse on the course and outcome of schizophrenia. Schizophr Bull 1990; 16:87–95 [G]

490. Sevy S, Kay SR, Opler LA, van Praag HM: Significance of cocaine history in schizophrenia. J Nerv Ment Dis 1990; 178:642–648 [E]

491. Fisch RZ: Trihexyphenidyl abuse: therapeutic implications for negative symptoms of schizophrenia? Acta Psychiatr Scand 1987; 75:91–94 [G]

492. Thornicroft G: Cannabis and psychosis: is there epidemiological evidence for an association? Br J Psychiatry 1990; 157:33–35 [F]

493. Drake RE, Noordsy DL, Ackerson T: Integrating mental health and substance abuse treatments for persons with chronic mental disorders: a model, in Double Jeopardy: Chronic Mental Illness and Substance Use Disorders. Edited by Lehman AF, Dixon LB. Chur, Switzerland, Harwood Academic, 1995, pp 251–264 [G]

494. Rosenthal RN, Hellerstein DJ, Miner CR: Integrated services for treatment of schizophrenic substance abusers: demographics, symptoms, and substance abuse patterns. Psychiatr Q 1992; 63:3–26 [F]

495. Weiss RD, Mirin SM, Frances RJ: Alcohol and drug abuse: the myth of the typical dual diagnosis patient. Hosp Community Psychiatry 1992; 43:107–108 [G]

496. Seppala T: Effect of chlorpromazine or sulpiride and alcohol on psychomotor skills related to driving. Arch Int Pharmacodyn Ther 1976; 223:311–323 [A]

497. Antipsychotic drugs, in Drug Evaluations Annual 1993. Chicago, American Medical Association, 1993, pp 251–277 [F]

498. Kofoed L, Kania J, Walsh T, Atkinson RM: Outpatient treatment of patients with substance abuse and coexisting psychiatric disorders. Am J Psychiatry 1986; 143:867–872 [B]

499. Kingsbury SJ, Salzman C: Disulfiram in the treatment of alcoholic patients with schizophrenia. Hosp Community Psychiatry 1990; 41:133–134 [G]

500. Smith CM, Pristach CA: Utility of the Self-Administered Alcoholism Screening Test (SAAST) in schizophrenic patients. Alcohol Clin Exp Res 1990; 14:690–694 [D]

501. Mueser KT, Noordsy DL: Group treatment for dually diagnosed clients: dual diagnosis of major mental illness and substance abuse disorder, II: recent research and clinical implications. New Dir Ment Health Serv 1996; 70:33–51 [F]

502. Hellerstein DJ, Meehan B: Outpatient group therapy for schizophrenic substance abusers. Am J Psychiatry 1987; 144:1337–1339 [B]

503. Drake RE, Mueser KT, Clark RE, Wallach MA: The course, treatment, and outcome of substance disorder in persons with severe mental illness. Am J Orthopsychiatry 1996; 66:42–51 [F]

504. Drake RE, Bartels SB, Teague GB, Noordsy DL, Clark RE: Treatment of substance abuse in severely mentally ill patients. J Nerv Ment Dis 1993; 181:606–611 [F]

505. Osher FC, Kofoed LL: Treatment of patients with psychiatric and psychoactive substance abuse disorders. Hosp Community Psychiatry 1989; 40:1025–1030 [G]

506. Drake RE, McHugo GJ, Noordsy DL: Treatment of alcoholism among schizophrenic outpatients: 4-year outcomes. Am J Psychiatry 1993; 150:328–329 [B]

507. Clark RE: Family support for people with dual disorders. New Dir Ment Health Serv 1996; 70:65–78 [F]

508. Dixon L, McNary S, Lehman A: Substance abuse and family relationships of persons with severe mental illness. Am J Psychiatry 1995; 152:456–458 [D]

509. Mueser KT, Gingerich SL: Coping With Schizophrenia: A Guide for Families. Oakland, Calif, New Harbinger Publications, 1994 [F]

510. Koreen AR, Siris SG, Chakos M, Alvir J, Mayerhoff D, Lieberman J: Depression in first-episode schizophrenia. Am J Psychiatry 1993; 150:1643–1648 [B]

511. McGlashan TH, Carpenter WT: Postpsychotic depression in schizophrenia. Arch Gen Psychiatry 1976; 33:231–239 [E]

512. Siris SG, van Kammen DP, Docherty JP: Use of antidepressant drugs in schizophrenia. Arch Gen Psychiatry 1978; 35:1368–1377 [F]

513. Kramer MS, Vogel WH, DiJohnson C, Dewey DA, Sheves P, Cavicchia S, Little P, Schmidt R, Kimes I: Antidepressants in "depressed" schizophrenic inpatients: a controlled trial. Arch Gen Psychiatry 1989; 46:922–928 [A]

514. Bartels SJ, Drake RE: Depressive symptoms in schizophrenia: comprehensive differential diagnosis. Compr Psychiatry 1988; 29:467–483 [G]

515. Siris SG: Akinesia and post-psychotic depression: a difficult differential diagnosis. J Clin Psychiatry 1987; 48:240–243 [G]

516. Drake RE, Cotton PG: Depression, hopelessness and suicide in chronic schizophrenia. Br J Psychiatry 1986; 148:554–559 [G]

517. Prasad AJ: Attempted suicide in hospitalized schizophrenics. Acta Psychiatr Scand 1986; 74:41–42 [B]

518. Roy A: Suicide in schizophrenia, in Suicide. Edited by Roy A. Baltimore, Williams & Wilkins, 1986, pp 97–112 [G]

519. Barnes TR, Curson DA, Liddle PF, Patel M: The nature and prevalence of depression in chronic schizophrenic in-patients. Br J Psychiatry 1989; 154:486–491 [B]

520. Siris SG, Rifkin AE, Reardon GT: Response of postpsychotic depression to adjunctive imipramine or amitriptyline. J Clin Psychiatry 1982; 43:485–486 [G]

521. van Kammen DP, Alexander PE, Bunney WE Jr: Lithium treatment in post-psychotic depression. Br J Psychiatry 1980; 136:479–485 [A]

522. Black DW, Fisher R: Mortality in DSM-III-R schizophrenia. Schizophr Res 1992; 7:109–116 [E]

523. Caldwell CB, Gottesman II: Schizophrenics kill themselves too: a review of risk factors for suicide. Schizophr Bull 1990; 16:571–589 [F]

524. Warnes H: Suicide in schizophrenia. Dis Nerv Syst 1968; 29 (May suppl):35–40 [F]

525. Slaby AE, Moreines R: Emergency room evaluation and management of schizophrenia, in Handbook of Schizophrenia, vol 4: Psychosocial Treatment of Schizophrenia. Edited by Herz MI, Keith SJ, Docherty JP. New York, Elsevier, 1990, pp 247–268 [G]

526. Drake RE, Bartels SJ, Torrey WC: Suicide in schizophrenia: clinical approaches, in Depression in Schizophrenics. Edited by Williams R, Dalby JT. New York, Plenum, 1989, pp 171–183 [G]

527. Nyman A, Jonsson H: Patterns of self-destructive behavior in schizophrenia. Acta Psychiatr Scand 1986; 73:252–262 [D]

528. Drake RE, Gates C, Whitaker A, Cotton PG: Suicide among schizophrenics: a review. Compr Psychiatry 1985; 26:90–100 [F]

529. Roy A: Depression, attempted suicide, and suicide in patients with chronic schizophrenia. Psychiatr Clin North Am 1986; 9:193–206 [F, G]

530. Roy A: Suicide in schizophrenia. Int Rev Psychiatry 1992; 4:205–209 [G]

531. Fottrell E: A study of violent behavior among patients in psychiatric hospitals. Br J Psychiatry 1980; 136:216–221 [D]

532. Shader RI, Jackson AH, Harmatz JS, Appelbaum PS: Patterns of violent behavior among schizophrenic inpatients. Dis Nerv Syst 1977; 38:13–16 [D]

533. Bartels SJ, Drake RE, Wallach MA, Freeman DH: Characteristic hostility in schizophrenic outpatients. Schizophr Bull 1991; 17:163–171 [G]

534. Zitrin A, Hardesty AS, Burdock EI, Drossman AK: Crime and violence among mental patients. Am J Psychiatry 1976; 133:142–149 [G]

535. Test MA, Knoedler WH, Allness DJ, Burke SS: Characteristics of young adults with schizophrenic disorders treated in the community. Hosp Community Psychiatry 1985; 36:853–858 [C]

536. Convit A, Isay D, Gadioma R, Volavka J: Underreporting of physical assaults in schizophrenic inpatients. J Nerv Ment Dis 1988; 176:507–509 [G]

537. Häfner H, Boker W: Crimes of Violence by Mentally Abnormal Offenders: A Psychiatric and Epidemiological Study in the Federal Republic of Germany. Cambridge, England, Cambridge University Press, 1982 [D]

538. Volavka J, Krakowski M: Schizophrenia and violence. Psychol Med 1989; 19:559–562 [F]

539. Glancy GD, Regehr C: The forensic psychiatric aspects of schizophrenia. Psychiatr Clin North Am 1992; 15:575–589 [G]

540. Tardiff K: Assessment and Management of Violent Patients, 2nd ed. Washington, DC, American Psychiatric Press, 1996 [G]

541. Simon RI: Clinical Psychiatry and the Law, 2nd ed. Washington, DC, American Psychiatric Press, 1992 [G]

542. American Psychiatric Association: Opinions of the Ethics Committee on the Principles of Medical Ethics, With Annotations Especially Applicable to Psychiatry. Washington, DC, APA, 1995 [G]

543. Appelbaum PS: The new preventive detention: psychiatry's problematic responsibility for the control of violence. Am J Psychiatry 1988; 145:779–785 [G]

544. Liberman RP, Blackwell G, Wallace CJ, Mintz J: Reducing relapse and rehospitalization in schizophrenic patients treated in a day hospital: a controlled study of skills training vs psychosocial occupational therapy. Presented at the 147th Annual Meeting of the American Psychiatric Association, Philadelphia, May 21–26, 1994 [B]

545. Silver JM, Yudofsky SC, Kogan M, Katz BL: Elevation of thioridazine plasma levels by propranolol. Am J Psychiatry 1986; 143:1290–1292 [B]

546. Riggs AT: A review of disorders of water homeostasis in psychiatric patients. Psychosomatics 1991; 32:133–148 [F]

547. Goldfinger SM: Homelessness and schizophrenia: a psychosocial approach, in Handbook of Schizophrenia, vol 4: Psychosocial Treatment of Schizophrenia. Edited by Herz MI, Keith SJ, Docherty JP. Amsterdam, Elsevier, 1990, pp 355–386 [G]

548. Bachrach LL: What we know about homelessness among mentally ill persons: an analytical review and commentary. Hosp Community Psychiatry 1992; 43:453–464 [G]

549. Schlenger WE, Kroutil LA, Roland EJ: Case management as a mechanism for linking drug abuse treatment and primary care: preliminary evidence from the ADAMHA/HRSA linkage demonstration. NIDA Res Monogr 1992; 127:316–330 [G]

550. Breakey WR, Susser E, Timms P: Services for the homeless mentally ill, in Measuring Mental Health Needs. Edited by Graham T, Brewin CR, Wing J. London, Gaskell/Royal College of Psychiatrists, 1992, pp 273–290 [F]

551. Cohen NL, Marcos LR: Outreach intervention models for the homeless mentally ill, in Treating the Homeless Mentally Ill: A Report of the Task Force on the Homeless Mentally Ill. Edited by Lamb RH, Bachrach LL, Kass FI. Washington, DC, American Psychiatric Association, 1992, pp 141–157 [G]

552. Karno M, Jenkins JH: Cross-cultural issues in the course and treatment of schizophrenia. Psychiatr Clin North Am 1993; 70:339–350 [G]

553. Cheetham RW, Griffiths JA: Errors in the diagnosis of schizophrenia in black and Indian patients. S Afr Med J 1981; 59 (3):71–75 [G]

554. Baker FM: A research agenda for the mental health concerns of African Americans. J Assoc Acad Minor Phys 1994; 5:74–76 [G]

555. Chang WH, Hwu HG, Chen TY, Lin SK, Lung FW, Chen H, Lin WL, Hu WH, Lin HN, Chien CP: Plasma homovanillic acid and treatment response in a large group of schizophrenic patients. Schizophr Res 1993; 10:259–265 [C]

556. Lieberman JA, Yunis J, Egea E, Canoso RT, Kane JM, Yunis EJ: HLA-B38, DR4, DQw3 and clozapine-induced agranulocytosis in Jewish patients with schizophrenia. Arch Gen Psychiatry 1990; 47:945–948 [B]

557. Thompson JW, Belcher JR, DeForge BR, Myers CP, Rosenstein MJ: Changing characteristics of schizophrenic patients admitted to state hospitals. Hosp Community Psychiatry 1993; 44:231–235 [D]

558. Cournos F, Guido JR, Coomaraswamy S, Meyer-Bahlburg H, Sugden R, Horwath E: Sexual activity and risk for HIV infection among patients with schizophrenia. Am J Psychiatry 1994; 151:228–232 [D]

559. Goldstein JM, Tsuang MT: Gender and schizophrenia: an introduction and synthesis of findings. Schizophr Bull 1990; 16:179–183 [F]

560. Haas GL, Glick ID, Clarkin JF, Spencer JH, Lewis AB: Gender and schizophrenia outcome: a clinical trial of an inpatient family intervention. Schizophr Bull 1990; 16:277–292 [B]

561. Szymanski S, Lieberman JA, Alvir JM, Mayerhoff D, Loebel A, Geisler S, Chakos M, Koreen A, Jody D, Kane J, Woerner M, Cooper T: Gender differences in onset of illness, treatment response, course, and biologic indexes in first-episode schizophrenic patients. Am J Psychiatry 1995; 152:698–703 [B]

562. Miller LJ: Clinical strategies for the use of psychotropic drugs during pregnancy. Psychiatry Med 1991; 9:275–298 [F]

563. Altshuler LL, Szuba MP: Course of psychiatric disorders in pregnancy. Neurol Clin 1994; 12:613–635 [F]

564. Goldberg HL, Nissim R: Psychotropic drugs in pregnancy and lactation. Int J Psychiatry Med 1994; 24:129–149 [F]

565. Zubin J, Spring B: Vulnerability—a new view of schizophrenia. J Abnorm Psychol 1977; 86:103–126 [G]

566. Beels CC, Gutwirth L, Berkeley J, Struening E: Measurements of social support in schizophrenia. Schizophr Bull 1984; 10:399–411 [G]

567. Doane JA, West KL, Goldstein MJ, Rodnick EH, Jones JE: Parental communication deviance and affective style: predictors of subsequent schizophrenia spectrum disorders in vulnerable adolescents. Arch Gen Psychiatry 1981; 38:679–685 [E, G]

568. Leff J, Vaughn C: The role of maintenance therapy and relatives' expressed emotion in relapse of schizophrenia: a two-year follow-up. Br J Psychiatry 1981; 139:102–104 [C, D, E]

569. Vaughn CE, Snyder KS, Jones S, Freeman WB, Falloon IR: Family factors in schizophrenic relapse: replication in California of British research on expressed emotion. Arch Gen Psychiatry 1984; 41:1169–1177 [C, D]

570. Hogarty GE: Depot neuroleptics: the relevance of psychosocial factors—a United States perspective. J Clin Psychiatry 1984; 45:36–42 [F]

571. Goldstein MJ. Family factors that antedate the onset of schizophrenia and related disorders: the results of a 15-year prospective longitudinal study. Presented at the Regional Symposium of the World Psychiatric Association, Helsinki, Finland, June 1984 [C, D, E]

572. Gurland BJ, Cross PS: Epidemiology of psychopathology in old age: some implications for clinical services. Psychiatr Clin North Am 1982; 5:11–26 [F]

573. Jeste DV, Harris MJ, Krull A, Kuck J, McAdams LA, Heaton R: Clinical and neuropsychological characteristics of patients with late-onset schizophrenia. Am J Psychiatry 1995; 152: 722–730 [F]

574. Belitsky R, McGlashan TH: The manifestations of schizophrenia in late life: a dearth of data. Schizophr Bull 1993; 19:683–685 [G]

575. Salzman C: Principles of psychopharmacology, in Verwoerdt's Clinical Geropsychiatry, 3rd ed. Edited by Bienenfeld D. Baltimore, Williams & Wilkins, 1990, pp 235–249 [G]

576. Marder SR, Davis JM, Janicak P: Clinical Use of Neuroleptic Plasma Levels. Washington, DC, American Psychiatric Press, 1993 [F]

577. Jeste DV, Lacro JP, Gilbert PL, Kline J, Kline N: Treatment of late-life schizophrenia with neuroleptics. Schizophr Bull 1993; 19:817–830 [F]

578. DeSisto MJ, Harding CM, McCormick RV, Ashikaga T, Brooks GW: The Maine and Vermont three-decade studies of serious mental illness, I: matched comparison of cross-sectional outcome. Br J Psychiatry 1995; 167:331–342 [A]

579. American Psychiatric Association Task Force Report 29: Psychiatric Services in Jails and Prisons: Report of the Task Force on Psychiatric Services in Jails and Prisons. Washington, DC, APA, 1989 [F]

580. Metzner JL: Guidelines for psychiatric services in prisons. Criminal Behav Ment Health 1993; 3:252–267 [G]

581. Oliver AP, Luchins DJ, Wyatt RJ: Neuroleptic-induced seizures: an in vitro technique for assessing relative risk. Arch Gen Psychiatry 1982; 39:206–209 [G]

PRACTICE GUIDELINE FOR THE
Treatment of Patients With Major Depressive Disorder
Second Edition

WORK GROUP ON MAJOR DEPRESSIVE DISORDER

T. Byram Karasu, M.D., Chair

Alan Gelenberg, M.D.
Arnold Merriam, M.D.
Philip Wang, M.D., Dr.P.H. (Consultant)

In this practice guideline, Part A includes treatment recommendations, and Part B includes data regarding the safety and efficacy of available treatments.

This practice guideline was first published in April 1993. This updated revision was approved in January 2000 and was published in *The American Journal of Psychiatry* in April 2000.

CONTENTS

GUIDE TO USING THIS PRACTICE GUIDELINE

This practice guideline uses available evidence to develop treatment recommendations for the care of adult patients with major depressive disorder. This guideline contains many sections, not all of which will be equally useful for all readers. The following guide is designed to help readers find the sections that will be most useful to them.

Part A contains the treatment recommendations for patients with major depressive disorder. Section I is the summary of treatment recommendations, which includes the main treatment recommendations, along with codes that indicate the degree of clinical confidence in each recommendation. Section II is a guide to the formulation and implementation of a treatment plan for the individual patient. This section includes all of the treatment recommendations. Section III, "Specific Clinical Features Influencing the Treatment Plan," discusses a range of clinical conditions that could alter the general recommendations discussed in Section II.

Part B, "Background Information and Review of Available Evidence," will be useful to understand, in detail, the evidence underlying the treatment recommendations of Part A. Section IV provides an overview of DSM-IV criteria, prevalence rates for major depressive disorder, and general information on its natural history and course. Section V is a structured review and synthesis of published literature regarding the available treatments for major depressive disorder.

Part C, "Future Research Needs," draws from the previous sections to summarize those areas in which better research data are needed to guide clinical decisions.

OVERVIEW OF GUIDELINE DEVELOPMENT PROCESS

This document is a practical guide to the management of major depressive disorder for adults over the age of 18 and represents a synthesis of current scientific knowledge and rational clinical practice. This guideline strives to be as free as possible of bias toward any theoretical posture, and it aims to represent a practical approach to treatment. Studies were identified through an extensive review of the literature by using MEDLARS for the period 1971–1999. The key words used were affective disorder, major depression, depressive disorder, seasonal affective disorder, melancholia, unipolar depression, endogenous depression, dysthymic disorder, dysthymia, postpartum depression, pseudodementia, antidepressant medications, tricyclic antidepressive agents, monoamine oxidase inhibitors, lithium, and electroconvulsive therapy and included the concepts of melancholia, neurotic depression, and major depression. In addition, the key words for the psychotherapy search were psychotherapy (not otherwise specified); behavior therapy, including aversive therapy, biofeedback (psychology), cognitive therapy, desensitization (psychologic), implosive therapy, and relaxation techniques (meditation); psychoanalytic therapy, including existentialism, free association, transactional analysis, psychotherapy (brief); and psychotherapy (group), including family therapy and marital therapy.

Major review articles and standard psychiatric texts were consulted. The Agency for Healthcare Policy Research Evidence Report on Treatment of Depression—Newer Pharmacotherapies (1) was reviewed in its entirety. Review articles and relevant clinical trials were reviewed in their entirety; other studies were selected for review on the basis of their relevance to the particular issues discussed in this guideline. Definitive standards are difficult to achieve, except in narrow circumstances in which multiple replicated studies and wide clinical opinion dictate certain forms of treatment. In other areas, the specific choice among two or more treatment options is left to the clinical judgment of the clinician.

The recommendations are based on the best available data and clinical consensus with regard to the particular clinical decision. The summary of treatment recommendations is keyed according to the level of confidence with which each recommendation is made. In addition, each reference is followed by a letter code in brackets that indicates the nature of the supporting evidence.

INTRODUCTION

This guideline seeks to summarize the specific forms of somatic, psychotherapeutic, psychosocial, and educational treatments that have been developed to deal with major depressive disorder. It begins at the point where the psychiatrist has diagnosed an adult patient as suffering from major depressive disorder, according to the criteria defined in DSM-IV, and has medically evaluated the patient to ascertain the presence of alcohol or substance use disorder or other somatic factors that may contribute to the disease process (e.g., hypothyroidism, pancreatic carcinoma) or complicate its treatment (e.g., cardiac disorders). The purpose of this guideline is to assist the physician faced with the task of implementing specific antidepressant treatment(s). It should be noted that many patients have coexisting conditions and their difficulties cannot be described with one DSM diagnostic category. The psychiatrist should consider, but not be limited to, the treatment guidelines for a single diagnosis. For patients found to have depressive symptoms within the context of bipolar disorder, the psychiatrist should refer to the *Practice Guideline for the Treatment of Patients With Bipolar Disorder* (2) (included in this volume).

This document concerns patients 18 years of age and older. Some comments regarding the treatment of major depressive disorders in children and adolescents can be found in section III.B.5., along with more definitive references.

PART A:
TREATMENT RECOMMENDATIONS FOR PATIENTS WITH MAJOR DEPRESSIVE DISORDER

I. SUMMARY OF TREATMENT RECOMMENDATIONS

Each recommendation is identified as falling into one of three categories of endorsement, indicated by a bracketed Roman numeral following the statement. The three categories represent varying levels of clinical confidence regarding the recommendation:

    [I] Recommended with substantial clinical confidence.
    [II] Recommended with moderate clinical confidence.
    [III] May be recommended on the basis of individual circumstances.

Successful treatment of patients with major depressive disorder is promoted by a thorough assessment of the patient [I]. Treatment consists of an acute phase, during which remission is induced; a continuation phase, during which remission is preserved; and a maintenance phase, during which the susceptible patient is protected against the recurrence of subsequent major depressive episodes. Psychiatrists initiating treatment for major depressive disorder have at their disposal a number of medications, a variety of psychotherapeutic approaches, electroconvulsive therapy (ECT), and other treatment modalities (e.g., light therapy) that may be used alone or in combination. The psychiatrist must determine the setting that will most likely ensure the patient's safety as well as promote improvement in the patient's condition [I].

A. PSYCHIATRIC MANAGEMENT
Psychiatric management consists of a broad array of interventions and activities that should be instituted by psychiatrists for all patients with major depressive disorder [I]. Regardless of the specific treatment modalities selected, it is important to continue providing psychiatric management through all phases of treatment. The specific components of psychiatric management that must be addressed for all patients include performing a diagnostic evaluation, evaluating safety of the patient and others, evaluating the level of functional impairments, determining a treatment setting, establishing and maintaining a therapeutic alliance, monitoring the patient's psychiatric status and safety, providing education to patients and families, enhancing treatment adherence, and working with patients to address early signs of relapse.

1. Choice of an initial treatment modality

In the acute phase, in addition to psychiatric management, the psychiatrist may choose between several initial treatment modalities, including pharmacotherapy, psychotherapy, the combination of medications plus psychotherapy, or ECT [I]. Selection of an initial treatment modality should be influenced by both clinical (e.g., severity of symptoms) and other factors (e.g., patient preference) (figure 1).

a. Antidepressant medication

If preferred by the patient, antidepressant medications may be provided as an initial primary treatment modality for mild major depressive disorder [I]. Antidepressant medications should be provided for moderate to severe major depressive disorder unless ECT is planned [I]. A combination of antipsychotic and antidepressant medications or ECT should be used for psychotic depression [I].

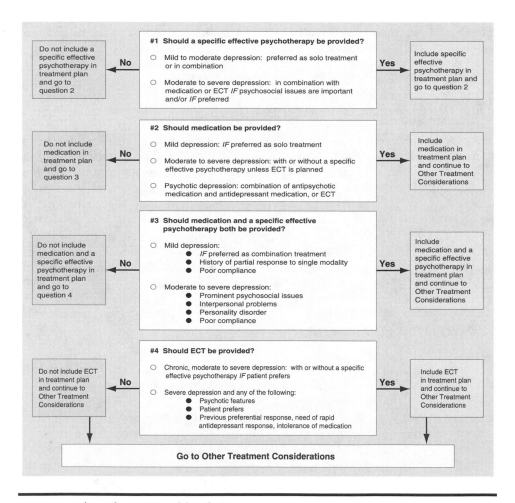

FIGURE 1. Choice of Treatment Modalities for Major Depressive Disorder.

b. Psychotherapy

A specific, effective psychotherapy alone as an initial treatment modality may be considered for patients with mild to moderate major depressive disorder [II]. Patient preference for psychotherapeutic approaches is an important factor that should be considered in the decision. Clinical features that may suggest the use of psychotherapeutic interventions include the presence of significant psychosocial stressors, intrapsychic conflict, interpersonal difficulties, or a comorbid axis II disorder [I].

c. Psychotherapy plus antidepressant medications

The combination of a specific effective psychotherapy and medication may be a useful initial treatment choice for patients with psychosocial issues, interpersonal problems, or a comorbid axis II disorder together with moderate to severe major depressive disorder [I]. In addition, patients who have had a history of only partial response to adequate trials of single treatment modalities may benefit from combined treatment. Poor adherence with treatments may also warrant combined treatment modalities.

d. Electroconvulsive therapy

ECT should be considered for patients with major depressive disorder with a high degree of symptom severity and functional impairment or for cases in which psychotic symptoms or catatonia are present [I]. ECT may also be the treatment modality of choice for patients in whom there is an urgent need for response, such as patients who are suicidal or refusing food and nutritionally compromised [II].

2. Choice of specific pharmacologic treatment

Antidepressant medications that have been shown to be effective are listed in table 1 [II]. The effectiveness of antidepressant medications is generally comparable between classes and within classes of medications. Therefore, the initial selection of an antidepressant medication will largely be based on the anticipated side effects, the safety or tolerability of these side effects for individual patients, patient preference, quantity and quality of clinical trial data regarding the medication, and its cost (see Section V.A.1.) [I]. On the basis of these considerations, the following medications are likely to be optimal for most patients: selective serotonin reuptake inhibitors (SSRIs), desipramine, nortriptyline, bupropion, and venlafaxine. In general, monoamine oxidase inhibitors (MAOIs) should be restricted to patients who do not respond to other treatments because of their potential for serious side effects and the necessity of dietary restrictions. Patients with major depressive disorder with atypical features are one group for whom several studies suggest MAOIs may be particularly effective; however, in clinical practice, many psychiatrists start with SSRIs in such patients because of the more favorable adverse effect profile.

a. Implementation

When pharmacotherapy is part of the treatment plan, it must be integrated with the psychiatric management and any other treatments that are being provided (e.g., psychotherapy) [I]. Once an antidepressant medication has been selected, it can be started at the dose levels suggested in table 1 [I]. Titration to full therapeutic doses generally can be accomplished over the initial week(s) of treatment but may vary depending on the development of side effects, the patient's age, and the presence of comorbid illnesses. Patients who have started taking an antidepressant medication should be carefully monitored to assess their response to pharmacotherapy as well as

TABLE 1. Commonly Used Antidepressant Medications (this list is representative, but not comprehensive)

Generic Name	Starting Dose (mg/day)[a]	Usual Dose (mg/day)
Tricyclics and tetracyclics		
Tertiary amine tricyclics		
Amitriptyline	25–50	100–300
Clomipramine	25	100–250
Doxepin	25–50	100–300
Imipramine	25–50	100–300
Trimipramine	25–50	100–300
Secondary amine tricyclics		
Desipramine[b]	25–50	100–300
Nortriptyline[b]	25	50–200
Protriptyline	10	15–60
Tetracyclics		
Amoxapine	50	100–400
Maprotiline	50	100–225
SSRIs[b]		
Citalopram	20	20–60[c]
Fluoxetine	20	20–60[c]
Fluvoxamine	50	50–300[c]
Paroxetine	20	20–60[c]
Sertraline	50	50–200[c]
Dopamine-norepinephrine reuptake inhibitors		
Bupropion[b]	150	300
Bupropion, sustained release[b]	150	300
Serotonin-norepinephrine reuptake inhibitors		
Venlafaxine[b]	37.5	75–225
Venlafaxine, extended release[b]	37.5	75–225
Serotonin modulators		
Nefazodone	50	150–300
Trazodone	50	75–300
Norepinephrine-serotonin modulator		
Mirtazapine	15	15–45
MAOIs		
Irreversible, nonselective		
Phenelzine	15	15–90
Tranylcypromine	10	30–60
Reversible MAOI-A		
Moclobemide	150	300–600
Selective noradrenaline reuptake inhibitor		
Reboxetine	—[d]	—[d]

[a]Lower starting doses are recommended for elderly patients and for patients with panic disorder, significant anxiety or hepatic disease, and general comorbidity.

[b]These medications are likely to be optimal medications in terms of the patient's acceptance of side effects, safety, and quantity and quality of clinical trial data.

[c]Dose varies with diagnosis; see text for specific guidelines.

[d]FDA approval is anticipated. When available, consult manufacturer's package insert or the Physician's Desk Reference for recommended starting and usual doses.

the emergence of side effects, clinical condition, and safety [I] (see figure 2). Factors to consider in determining the frequency of patient monitoring include the severity of illness, the patient's cooperation with treatment, the availability of social supports, and the presence of comorbid general medical problems. Visits should also be frequent enough to monitor and address suicidality and to promote treatment adherence. In practice, the frequency of monitoring during the acute phase of pharmacotherapy can vary from once a week in routine cases to multiple times per week in more complex cases.

b.   Failure to respond

If at least moderate improvement is not observed following 6–8 weeks of pharmacotherapy, a reappraisal of the treatment regimen should be conducted [I]. Section II.B.2.b. reviews options for adjusting the treatment regimen when necessary. Following any change in treatment, the patient should continue to be closely monitored. If there is not at least a moderate improvement in major depressive disorder symptoms after an additional 6–8 weeks of treatment, the psychiatrist should conduct another thorough review. An algorithm depicting the sequence of subsequent steps that can be taken for patients who fail to respond fully to treatment is provided in figure 3.

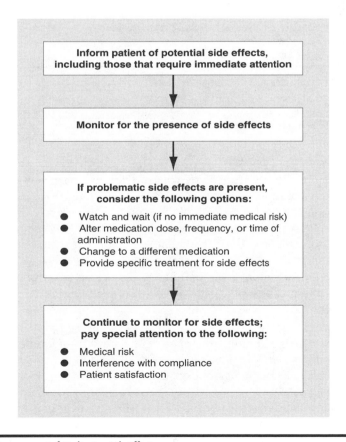

FIGURE 2. Management of Medication Side Effects.

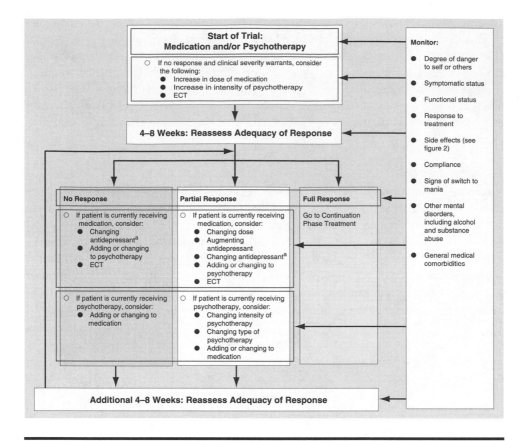

FIGURE 3. Acute Phase Treatment of Major Depressive Disorder.

[a]Choose either another antidepressant from the same class or, if two previous medication trials from the same class were ineffective, an antidepressant from a different class.

3. Choice of specific psychotherapy

Cognitive behavioral therapy and interpersonal therapy are the psychotherapeutic approaches that have the best documented efficacy in the literature for the specific treatment of major depressive disorder, although rigorous studies evaluating the efficacy of psychodynamic psychotherapy have not been published [II]. When psychodynamic psychotherapy is used as a specific treatment, in addition to symptom relief, it is frequently associated with broader long-term goals. Patient preference and the availability of clinicians with appropriate training and expertise in the specific approach are also factors in the choice of a particular form of psychotherapy.

a. Implementation

When psychotherapy is part of the treatment plan, it must be integrated with the psychiatric management and any other treatments that are being provided (e.g., medication treatment) [I]. The optimal frequency of psychotherapy has not been rigorously studied in controlled trials. The psychiatrist should take into account multiple factors when determining the frequency for individual patients, including the specific type and goals of psychotherapy, the frequency necessary to create and maintain a therapeutic relationship, the frequency of visits required to ensure treatment adherence, and the frequency necessary to monitor and address suicidality. The frequency of out-patient visits during the acute phase generally varies from once a week in routine cases to as often as several times a week.

Regardless of the type of psychotherapy selected, the patient's response to treatment should be carefully monitored [I].

If more than one clinician is involved in providing the care, it is essential that all treating clinicians have sufficient ongoing contact with the patient and with each other to ensure that relevant information is available to guide treatment decisions [I].

b. Failure to respond

If after 4–8 weeks of treatment at least a moderate improvement is not observed, then a thorough review and reappraisal of the diagnosis, complicating conditions and issues, and treatment plan should be conducted [I]. Figure 3 and section II.B.3.b. review the options to consider.

4. Choice of medications plus psychotherapy

In general, the same issues that influence the specific choice of medication or psychotherapy when used alone should be considered when choosing treatments for patients receiving combined modalities [I].

5. Assessing the adequacy of response

It is not uncommon for patients to have a substantial but incomplete response in terms of symptom reduction or improvement in functioning during acute phase treatments. It is important not to conclude the acute phase of treatment for such patients, as a partial response is often associated with poor functional outcomes. When patients are found to have not fully responded to an acute phase treatment, a change in treatment should be considered as outlined in figure 3 [II].

C. CONTINUATION PHASE

During the 16–20 weeks following remission, patients who have been treated with antidepressant medications in the acute phase should be maintained on these agents to prevent relapse [I]. In general, the dose used in the acute phase is also used in the continuation phase. Although there has been less study of the use of psychotherapy in the continuation phase to prevent relapse, there is growing evidence to support the use of a specific effective psychotherapy during the continuation phase [I]. Use of ECT in the continuation phase has received little formal study but may be useful in patients for whom medication or psychotherapy has not been effective in maintaining stability during the continuation phase [II]. The frequency of visits must be determined by the patient's clinical condition as well as the specific treatments being provided.

D. MAINTENANCE PHASE

Following the continuation phase, maintenance-phase treatment should be considered for patients to prevent recurrences of major depressive disorder [I]. Factors to consider are discussed in table 2 and in section II.D.

In general, the treatment that was effective in the acute and continuation phases should be used in the maintenance phase [II]. In general, the same full antidepressant medication doses are employed as were used in prior phases of treatment; use of low-

TABLE 2. Considerations in the Decision to Use Maintenance Treatment

Factor	Component
Risk of recurrence	Number of prior episodes; presence of comorbid conditions; residual symptoms between episodes
Severity of episodes	Suicidality; psychotic features; severe functional impairments
Side effects experienced with continuous treatment	
Patient preferences	

er doses of antidepressant medication in the maintenance phase has not been well studied. For cognitive behavioral therapy and interpersonal therapy, maintenance phase treatments usually involve a decreased frequency of visits (e.g., once a month).

The frequency of visits in the maintenance phase must be determined by the patient's clinical condition as well as the specific treatments being provided. The frequency required could range from as low as once every 2–3 months for stable patients who require only psychiatric management and medication monitoring to as high as multiple times a week for those in whom psychodynamic psychotherapy is being conducted.

E. DISCONTINUATION OF ACTIVE TREATMENT

The decision to discontinue active treatment should be based on the same factors considered in the decision to initiate maintenance treatment, including the probability of recurrence, the frequency and severity of past episodes, the persistence of dysthymic symptoms after recovery, the presence of comorbid disorders, and patient preferences [I]. In addition to the factors listed in table 2 and table 3, patients and their psychiatrists should consider the patient's response, in terms of both beneficial and adverse effects, to maintenance treatments.

Specific clinical features that will influence the general treatment are discussed in Section III.

TABLE 3. Risk Factors for Recurrence of Major Depressive Disorder

- Prior history of multiple episodes of major depressive disorder
- Persistence of dysthymic symptoms after recovery from an episode of major depressive disorder
- Presence of an additional, nonaffective psychiatric diagnosis
- Presence of a chronic general medical disorder

II. FORMULATION AND IMPLEMENTATION OF A TREATMENT PLAN

The following discussion regarding formulation and implementation of a treatment plan refers specifically to patients with major depressive disorder. For the treatment of patients found to have depressive symptoms within the context of bipolar disorder, readers should refer to the *Practice Guideline for the Treatment of Patients With Bipolar Disorder* (2) (included in this volume). The treatment recommendations that follow may have some relevance for patients who have depressive symptoms on the basis of other syndromes, such as dysthymia, although this cannot be fully established with the existing scientific literature.

The successful treatment of patients with major depressive disorders is promoted by an initial thorough assessment of the patient. Treatment then consists of an acute phase lasting a minimum of 6–8 weeks, during which remission is induced. Remission is defined as a return to the patient's baseline level of symptom severity and functioning and should not be confused with substantial but incomplete improvement. After achieving remission, the patient enters the continuation phase, which usually lasts 16–20 weeks, during which time the remission is preserved and relapse is prevented. Relapse is generally defined as the re-emergence of significant depressive symptoms or dysfunction following a remission. Patients who successfully complete the continuation phase without relapse then enter the maintenance phase of treatment. The goal during the maintenance phase is to protect susceptible patients against recurrence of subsequent major depressive episodes; the duration of the maintenance phase will vary depending on the frequency and severity of prior major depressive episodes.

Psychiatrists initiating treatment of an episode of major depressive disorder have at their disposal a number of medications, a variety of psychotherapeutic approaches, ECT, and other treatment modalities (e.g., light therapy). These various interventions may be used alone or in combination. The psychiatrist must determine the setting that will most likely ensure the patient's safety as well as promote improvement in the patient's condition.

A. PSYCHIATRIC MANAGEMENT

Psychiatric management consists of a broad array of interventions and activities that should be instituted by psychiatrists for all patients with major depressive disorder. The specific components of psychiatric management that must be addressed for all patients are described in more detail below.

1. Perform a diagnostic evaluation

Patients with major depressive disorder symptoms should receive a thorough diagnostic evaluation both to determine whether a diagnosis of depression is warranted and to reveal the presence of other psychiatric or general medical conditions. The general principles and components of a complete psychiatric evaluation have been outlined in the American Psychiatric Association's *Practice Guideline for Psychiatric Evaluation of Adults* (3) (included in this volume). These should include a history of the present illness and current symptoms; a psychiatric history, including symptoms of mania as well as a treatment history that particularly notes current treatments and responses to previous treatments; a general medical history and history of substance use disorders; a personal history (e.g., psychological development, response to life transitions, and major life events); a social, occupational, and family history; a review of the patient's medications; a review of systems; a mental status examination; a physical examination; and diagnostic tests as indicated.

2. Evaluate the safety of patient and others

A careful assessment of the patient's risk for suicide is crucial. Some components of an evaluation for suicidal risk are summarized in table 4. An assessment of the presence of suicidal ideation is essential, including the degree to which the patient intends to act on any suicidal ideation and the extent to which the patient has made plans for or begun to prepare for suicide. The availability of means for suicide should be inquired about and a judgment made concerning the lethality of those means. Clinical factors that may increase the likelihood of a patient acting on suicidal ideation should be assessed, including the presence of psychotic symptoms, severe anxiety, panic attacks, and alcohol or substance use. Whether a patient has a history of making previous suicide attempts and the nature of those attempts should be evaluated. Patients should also be asked about suicide in their family history and recent exposure to suicide or suicide attempts by others. A complete assessment of suicidal risk should be individualized to the particular circumstances of the patient and include an evaluation of the patient's strengths and motivation to seek help. Patients who are found to possess suicidal or homicidal ideation, intention, or plans require close monitoring. Measures such as hospitalization (involuntary when indicated) should be considered for those at significant risk. However, it should be kept in mind that the ability to predict suicide attempts and completed suicide is poor, with both many false positives (i.e., patients who appear more likely to make attempts or complete suicide but who do not) and false negatives (i.e., patients who appear less likely to make attempts or complete suicide but who do). For this reason, despite the best efforts of the psychiatrist, some patients may engage in self-harm or harm toward others.

3. Evaluate functional impairments

Major depressive disorder is frequently associated with functional impairments, and the presence, type(s), and severity of dysfunction should be evaluated. Impairments can include deficits in interpersonal relationships, work, living conditions, and other medical or health-related needs. Identified impairments in functioning should be addressed; for example, some patients may require assistance in scheduling absences from work or other responsibilities, whereas others may require encouragement to not make any major life changes while in a major depressive disorder state. Patients should also be encouraged to set realistic, attainable goals for themselves in terms of desirable levels of functioning.

TABLE 4. Components of an Evaluation for Suicidal Risk

- Presence of suicidal or homicidal ideation, intent, or plans
- Access to means for suicide and the lethality of those means
- Presence of psychotic symptoms, command hallucinations, or severe anxiety
- Presence of alcohol or substance use
- History and seriousness of previous attempts
- Family history of or recent exposure to suicide

4. Determine a treatment setting

Treatment settings for patients with major depressive disorder include a continuum of possible levels of care, from involuntary hospitalizations to day programs to ambulatory settings. In general, patients should be treated in the setting that is most likely to prove safe and effective. The psychiatrist should choose an appropriate site of treatment after evaluating the patient's clinical condition, including symptom severity, comorbidity, suicidality, homicidality, level of functioning, and available support system. The determination of a treatment setting should also include consideration of patients' ability to adequately care for themselves, provide reliable feedback to the psychiatrist, and cooperate with treatment of their major depressive disorder.

Patients who exhibit suicidal or homicidal ideation, intention, or a plan require close monitoring. Hospitalization is usually indicated for patients who are considered to pose a serious threat of harm to themselves or others. If patients refuse, they can be hospitalized involuntarily if their condition meets criteria for involuntary admission of the local jurisdiction. Severely ill patients who lack adequate social support outside of a hospital setting should be considered for admission to a hospital or intensive day program. Additionally, those patients who also have complicating psychiatric or general medical conditions or who have not responded adequately to outpatient treatment may need to be hospitalized.

The optimal treatment setting and the patient's ability to benefit from a different level of care should be reevaluated on an ongoing basis throughout the course of treatment.

5. Establish and maintain a therapeutic alliance

Regardless of the treatment modalities ultimately selected for patients, it is important for the psychiatrist to establish a therapeutic alliance with the patient. Major depressive disorder is often a chronic condition that requires patients to actively participate and adhere to treatment plans for long periods. Unfortunately, features of major depressive disorder may include poor motivation, pessimism over the effectiveness of treatments, decrements in cognition such as attention or memory, decreased self-care, and possibly intentional self-harm. In addition, successful treatment may require patients to tolerate side effects. For these reasons, a strong treatment alliance between patient and psychiatrist is crucial. To establish and maintain a therapeutic alliance with patients, it is important for psychiatrists to pay attention to the concerns of patients and their families as well as their wishes for treatment. Management of the therapeutic alliance should include awareness of transference and countertransference issues, even if these are not directly addressed in treatment.

6. Monitor the patient's psychiatric status and safety

As treatment progresses, different features and symptoms of the patient's illness may emerge or subside. Monitoring the patient's status for the emergence of changes in destructive impulses toward self or others is especially crucial; additional measures such as hospitalization or more intensive treatment should be considered for patients found to be at higher risk. The psychiatrist should be vigilant to changes in the patient's psychiatric status, including major depressive disorder symptoms as well as symptoms of other potential comorbid conditions. Significant changes in a patient's psychiatric status or the emergence of new symptoms may warrant a diagnostic reevaluation of the patient.

7. Provide education to the patient and, when appropriate, to the family

Education concerning major depressive disorder and its treatments should be provided to all patients. When appropriate, education should also be provided to involved family members. Specific educational elements may be especially helpful in some circumstances; for example, emphasizing that major depressive disorder is a real illness and that effective treatments are both necessary and available may be crucial for patients who attribute their illness to a moral defect or for family members who are convinced that there is nothing wrong with the patient. Education regarding available treatment options will help patients make informed decisions, anticipate side effects, and adhere to treatments.

8. Enhance treatment adherence

The successful treatment of major depressive disorder requires close adherence to treatment plans, in some cases for long or indefinite durations. Especially while symptomatic, patients with major depressive disorder may be poorly motivated, unduly pessimistic over their chances of recovery with treatment, suffering from deficits in memory, or taking less care of themselves. In addition, the side effects or requirements of treatments may lead to nonadherence. Particularly during the maintenance phase, euthymic patients may tend to undervalue the benefits of treatment and focus on the burdens of treatment. Psychiatrists should recognize these possibilities, encourage the patient to articulate any concerns regarding adherence, and emphasize the importance of adherence for successful treatment. Specific components of a message to patients that have been shown to improve adherence include emphasizing: 1) when and how often to take the medicine; 2) the need for at least 2–4 weeks before beneficial effects may be noticed; 3) the need to take medication even after feeling better; 4) the need to consult with the doctor before discontinuing medication; and 5) what to do if problems or questions arise (4). Some patients, particularly elderly patients, have been shown to have improved adherence when both the complexity of medication regimens and the costs of treatments are minimized. Severe or persistent problems of nonadherence may represent psychological conflicts or psychopathology for which psychotherapy should be considered. When family members are involved, they can also be encouraged to play a helpful role in improving adherence.

9. Work with the patient to address early signs of relapse

Given the chronic, episodic nature of major depressive disorder, exacerbations are common. Patients, as well as their families if appropriate, should be instructed about the significant risk of relapse. They should be educated to identify early signs and symptoms of new episodes. Patients should also be instructed to seek adequate treatment as early in the course of the new episode as possible to decrease the likelihood of a full-blown exacerbation or complications.

B. ACUTE PHASE

1. Choice of initial treatment modality

In the acute phase, in addition to psychiatric management, the psychiatrist may choose between several initial treatment modalities, including pharmacotherapy, psychotherapy, the combination of medications and psychotherapy, or ECT. A discussion of the potential role of other treatments (e.g., light therapy and St. John's wort) can be found in Section V. Selection of an initial treatment modality should be influenced by both clinical (e.g., severity of symptoms) and other factors (e.g., patient preference) (figure 1).

a. Antidepressant medications

When pharmacotherapy is part of the treatment plan, it must be integrated with the psychiatric management and any other treatments that are being provided (e.g., psychotherapy). Antidepressant medications can be used as an initial treatment modality by patients with mild, moderate, or severe major depressive disorder. Clinical features that may suggest that medications are the preferred treatment modality include history of prior positive response to antidepressant medications, severity of symptoms, significant sleep and appetite disturbances or agitation, or anticipation of the need for maintenance therapy. Other issues that may be important considerations in the decision to use antidepressant medication include patient preference or the lack of available adequate alternative treatment modalities. Patients with major depressive disorder with psychotic features require either the combined use of antidepressant and antipsychotic medications or ECT.

b. Psychotherapy

A specific, effective psychotherapy alone may be considered as an initial treatment modality for patients with mild to moderate major depressive disorder. Clinical features that may suggest the use of a specific psychotherapy include the presence of significant psychosocial stressors, intrapsychic conflict, interpersonal difficulties, or axis II comorbidity. Patient preference for psychotherapeutic approaches is an important factor that should be considered in the decision to use psychotherapy as the initial treatment modality. Pregnancy, lactation, or the wish to become pregnant may also be an indication for psychotherapy as an initial treatment.

c. Psychotherapy plus antidepressant medications

The combination of a specific effective psychotherapy and medication may be a useful initial treatment choice for patients with psychosocial issues, intrapsychic conflict, interpersonal problems, or a comorbid axis II disorder together with moderate to severe major depressive disorder. In addition, patients who have had a history of only partial response to adequate trials of single treatment modalities may benefit from combined treatment. Poor adherence with treatments may also warrant combined treatment with pharmacotherapy and psychotherapeutic approaches that focus on treatment adherence.

d. Electroconvulsive therapy

ECT should be considered for patients with major depressive disorder with a high degree of symptom severity and functional impairment as well as in cases in which psychotic symptoms or catatonia are present. ECT may also be the treatment modality of choice for patients in whom there is an urgent need for response, such as patients who are suicidal or who are refusing food and are nutritionally compromised. The presence of comorbid general medical conditions that preclude the use of antidepressant medications, a prior history of positive response to ECT, and patient preference are other important considerations that may influence the psychiatrist's decision to select ECT as a treatment modality.

TABLE 5. Factors to Consider in Choosing a First-Line Antidepressant Medication

- Anticipated side effects and their safety or tolerability
- History of prior response in patient or family member
- Patient preference
- Cost
- Quantity and quality of clinical trial data
- MAOIs: generally reserve for patients who do not respond to other treatments
- SSRIs or MAOIs: consider for patients with atypical symptoms

2. Choice of specific pharmacologic treatment

Antidepressant medications that have been shown to be effective are listed in table 1. The effectiveness of antidepressant medications is generally comparable between classes and within classes of medications. Therefore, the initial selection of an antidepressant medication will largely be based on the anticipated side effects, the safety or tolerability of these side effects for individual patients, patient preference, quantity and quality of clinical trial data regarding the medication, and its cost (table 5). On the basis of these considerations, the following medications are likely to be optimal agents for most patients: SSRIs, desipramine, nortriptyline, bupropion, and venlafaxine. Additional considerations that may influence the choice of antidepressant medication include a history of prior response to a medication and the presence of comorbid psychiatric or general medical conditions. For example, secondary amine tricyclic antidepressant medications may not be optimal in patients with cardiovascular conditions, cardiac conduction defects, closed angle glaucoma, urinary retention, or significant prostatic hypertrophy. SSRIs can carry a risk of sexual side effects and may be more expensive because of the lack of currently available generic preparations. Similarly, the specific side effect profiles and higher costs should be considerations in decisions regarding use of other newer antidepressant medications. In general, MAOIs should be restricted for patients who do not respond to other treatments because of their potential for serious side effects and the necessity of dietary restrictions. Patients with major depressive disorder with atypical features are one group for whom several studies suggest MAOIs may be particularly effective; however, in clinical practice, many psychiatrists start with SSRIs in such patients because of the more favorable adverse effect profile.

a. Implementation of pharmacotherapy

Once an antidepressant medication has been selected it can be started at doses suggested in table 1. Titration of the dose to full therapeutic doses generally can be accomplished over the initial week(s) of treatment but may vary depending on the development of side effects, the patient's age, and the presence of comorbid conditions. In elderly or medically frail patients, the starting and therapeutic doses should be reduced, generally to half of the usual adult doses.

Patients who have started taking an antidepressant medication should be carefully monitored to assess the response to pharmacotherapy as well as the emergence of side effects, clinical condition, and safety (see figure 2). There are limited clinical trial data to guide the decision regarding the frequency of monitoring patients during pharmacotherapy. Factors to consider when determining this frequency include the severity of illness, the patient's cooperation with treatment, the availability of social supports, and the presence of comorbid general medical problems. Visits should also be frequent enough to monitor and address suicidality and to promote treatment adherence. Experienced researchers have found that patients in clinical trials appear to benefit from monitoring once a week or more to enhance adherence rates and to avoid the demoralization that may occur before the onset of beneficial effects. In clinical practice, the frequency of monitoring during the acute phase of pharmacotherapy may vary from once a week in routine cases to multiple times per week in more complex cases. The method of monitoring may vary depending upon the clinical context (e.g., face-to-face visits, telephone contact, or contact with another clinician knowledgeable about the patient and the treatment modality).

Improvement with pharmacotherapy can be observed after 4–8 weeks of treatment. If at least a moderate improvement is not observed in this time period, reappraisal and adjustment of the pharmacotherapy should be considered.

b. Failure to respond

If at least moderate improvement is not observed following 4–8 weeks of pharmacotherapy, a reappraisal of the treatment regimen should be conducted. An algorithm depicting the sequence of subsequent steps that can be taken and possible outcomes for patients who do not respond fully to treatment is provided in figure 3. It is important to keep in mind when employing such algorithms that they are based largely on clinical experience and only limited clinical trial data.

First, patient adherence and pharmacokinetic/pharmacodynamic factors affecting treatment should be investigated, in some cases through determination of serum antidepressant medication levels. Following this review, the treatment plan can be revised by implementing one of several therapeutic options, including maximizing the initial medication treatment, switching to another non-MAOI antidepressant medication (table 1 and table 6), augmenting antidepressant medications with other agents or psychotherapy, by using an MAOI, or ECT (5).

Maximizing the initial treatment regimen is perhaps the most conservative strategy. For patients who have shown a partial response, particularly those with features of personality disorders, extending the antidepressant medication trial (e.g., by 2–4 weeks) may allow some patients to respond more fully (6). Use of higher antidepressant doses may be helpful for patients who have received only modest doses or for those who for pharmacodynamic reasons have low serum drug levels despite usual doses and adherence. Patients who have had their dose increased should be monitored for an increase in the severity of side effects.

Switching to a different non-MAOI antidepressant medication is a common strategy for treatment-refractory patients, especially those who have not shown at least partial response to the initial medication regimen. Patients can be switched to a non-MAOI antidepressant medication from the same pharmacologic class (e.g., from an SSRI to another SSRI) or to one from a different pharmacologic class (e.g., from an SSRI to a tricyclic antidepressant) (see table 1 and table 6) (5).

TABLE 6. Required Washout Times Between Antidepressant Trials

Antidepressant Change	Minimum Washout Period
To MAOI from drug with long-half-life metabolites (e.g., fluoxetine)	5 weeks
To MAOI from drug without long-half-life metabolites (e.g., tricyclic antidepressant, paroxetine, fluvoxamine, venlafaxine) or other MAOI	2 weeks
To non-MAOI antidepressant from MAOI	2 weeks

Augmentation of non-MAOI antidepressant medications may be helpful, particularly for patients who have had a partial response to antidepressant monotherapy. Options include adding a second non-MAOI antidepressant medication from a different pharmacologic class, taking care to avoid drug-drug interactions, or adding another adjunctive medication such as lithium, thyroid hormone, an anticonvulsant, or psychostimulants.

Adding, changing, or increasing the intensity of psychotherapy should be considered for patients with major depressive disorder who do not respond to medication treatment. Additional strategies for patients who do not respond adequately to treatment include switching to an MAOI after allowing sufficient time between medications to avoid hazardous interactions. ECT also remains perhaps the most effective therapy for treatment-resistant patients.

Following any change in treatment, the patient should continue to be closely monitored. If there is not at least a moderate improvement in major depressive disorder symptoms after an additional 4–8 weeks of treatment, the psychiatrist should conduct another thorough review. This reappraisal should include the following: verifying the patient's diagnosis and adherence; uncovering and addressing clinical factors that may be preventing improvement, such as the presence of comorbid general medical conditions or psychiatric conditions (e.g., alcohol or substance abuse); and uncovering and addressing psychosocial issues that may be impeding recovery. If no new information is uncovered to explain the patient's lack of adequate response, other treatment options should be considered, including obtaining a consultation and possibly ECT.

3. Choice of a specific psychotherapy

Cognitive behavioral therapy and interpersonal therapy have the best-documented effectiveness in the literature for the specific treatment of major depressive disorder. When psychodynamic psychotherapy is used as a specific treatment, in addition to symptom relief, it is frequently associated with broader long-term goals. Patient preference and the availability of clinicians with appropriate training and expertise in specific psychotherapeutic approaches are also factors in the choice of a particular form of psychotherapy. Other clinical factors influencing the type of psychotherapy employed are the stage and severity of the major depressive disorder episode. For example, although some data suggest that cognitive behavioral therapy alone may be effective for patients with moderate to severe major depressive disorder, most such patients will require medication. In general, the choice among psychotherapeutic approaches is dependent on patient preference, with particular regard to whether the goals are mainly symptomatic improvement versus broader psychosocial goals.

During the initial phases of treatment for patients with moderate to severe major depressive disorder, psychiatric management will have to include support and psychoeducation for the patient and the family, permission for the patient to excuse himself or herself from duties impossible to perform, and assistance regarding the making or postponing of major personal and business decisions. Some patients at this stage may not have the emotional energy or cognitive ability required for insight-oriented psychotherapy. If indicated, this may be initiated later in the course of recovery.

a. Implementation

When psychotherapy is part of the treatment plan, it must be integrated with the psychiatric management and any other treatments that are being provided (e.g., medication treatment). The optimal frequency of psychotherapy has not been rigorously studied in controlled trials. The psychiatrist should take into account multiple factors when determining the frequency for individual patients, including the specific type and goals of the psychotherapy, the frequency necessary to create and maintain a therapeutic relationship, the frequency of visits required to ensure treatment adherence, and the frequency necessary to monitor and address suicidality. Also affecting the frequency of psychotherapy visits are the severity of illness, the patient's cooperation with treatment, the availability of social supports, cost, geographic accessibility, and presence of comorbid general medical problems. The frequency of outpatient visits during the acute phase generally varies from once a week in routine cases to as often as several times a week. Transference-focused treatments tend to require more frequent and regular visits.

Regardless of the type of psychotherapy selected, the patient's response to treatment should be carefully monitored. If after 4–8 weeks of treatment at least a moderate improvement is not observed, then a thorough review and reappraisal of the treatment plan should be conducted.

There are no definitive studies to determine when it is preferable to have the psychiatrist provide all treatments (sometimes referred to as the "integrated" model) versus when it might be preferable to have a different clinician provide the psychotherapy, with the psychiatrist providing the psychiatric management and the medication (sometimes referred to as "split" treatment). The expertise of the psychiatrist in providing the desired type of psychotherapy and the preferences of the patient are frequently factors in the decision. The integrated treatment model provides for better coordination of care. Lower costs have been used as a rationale in support of the split-treatment model. However, it is not clear that the costs of that model are actually lower than for the integrated model (7).

If the split model is used, it is essential that the psychiatrist who is providing the psychiatric management and the medication treatment meets with the patient frequently enough to monitor his or her care. It is also essential that the two (or more) treating clinicians have sufficient ongoing contact to ensure that relevant information is available to guide treatment decisions.

b. Failure to respond

The patient's condition and response to therapeutic interventions should be carefully monitored from the outset of psychotherapy. If the patient's condition fails to stabilize or is deteriorating, reassessment is indicated (8). If after 4–8 weeks of treatment at least a moderate improvement is not observed, then a thorough review and reappraisal of the diagnosis, complicating conditions and issues, and treatment plan should be conducted. In many cases, the treatment plan can be revised by the addition or substitution of pharmacotherapy (see figure 3). Following any revision or refinement of treatment, the patient should continue to be closely monitored. If there continues to not be at least a moderate improvement in major depressive disorder symptoms after an additional 4–8 weeks of treatment, another thorough review, reappraisal, and revision of the treatment plan should be conducted.

4. Choice of medications plus psychotherapy

There are relatively few empirical data from clinical trials to help guide the selection of particular antidepressant medications and psychotherapeutic approaches for individuals who will receive the combination of both modalities. In general, the same issues that influence these decisions when choosing a monotherapy will apply, and the same doses of antidepressant medication and the same frequency and course of psychotherapy should be used for patients receiving combination modality treatments as those employed for patients receiving them as a monotherapy.

Patients receiving combined antidepressant medication and psychotherapy should also be monitored closely for treatment effect, side effects, clinical condition, and safety. If after 4–8 weeks there is not at least a moderate improvement, a thorough review should be conducted, including of the patient's adherence and pharmacokinetic/pharmacodynamic factors affecting treatment. The treatment plan can be revised by using many of the same therapeutic options described for patients who have not responded to treatment with either modality alone. Following any change in treatment, the patient should continue to be monitored, and if there is not at least a moderate improvement in major depressive disorder symptoms after an additional 4–8 weeks of treatment, another thorough review should be conducted. Other treatment options should be considered, including clinical consultation or possibly ECT.

5. Assessing the adequacy of treatment response

The goal of acute phase treatment for major depressive disorder is to return patients to their baseline levels of symptomatic and functional status. However, it is not uncommon for patients to have a substantial but incomplete response in terms of symptom reduction or improvement in functioning during acute phase treatment. It is important not to conclude the acute phase of treatment for such patients, as a partial response is often associated with poor functional outcomes.

Identifying patients who have not had a complete response to treatment and formally assessing the extent to which patients have returned to their baseline may be aided by the use of structured measures of depression symptom severity and functional status. When patients are found to have not fully responded to an acute phase treatment, a change in treatment should be considered, as outlined in figure 3.

▶ C. CONTINUATION PHASE

During the 16–20 weeks following remission, patients who have been treated with antidepressant medications in the acute phase should be maintained with these agents to prevent relapse. In general, the dose used in the acute phase is also used in the continuation phase. Some psychiatrists combine a decrease in the dose with careful monitoring in the continuation phase; however, there are no data to support the effectiveness of this approach. Although there has been less study of the use of psychotherapy in the continuation phase to prevent relapse, there is growing evidence to support the use of a specific effective psychotherapy during the continuation phase. Use of ECT in the continuation phase has received little formal study. The frequency of visits must be determined by the patient's clinical condition as well as the specific treatments being provided.

During the continuation phase, the frequency of visits may vary. For stable patients in whom the visits are for the purpose of providing psychiatric management, the frequency could be once every 2–3 months. For other patients, such as those in whom active psychotherapy is being conducted, the frequency required may be as high as multiple times a week. If maintenance-phase treatment is not indicated for patients who remain stable following the continuation phase, patients may be considered for discontinuation of treatment. If treatment is discontinued, patients should be carefully monitored for relapse, and treatment should be promptly reinstituted if relapse occurs.

▶ D. MAINTENANCE PHASE

On average, 50%–85% of patients with a single episode of major depressive disorder will have at least one more episode. Therefore, following the continuation phase, maintenance phase treatment should be considered for patients to prevent recurrences of major depressive episodes. Factors that should be considered when deciding whether to use maintenance treatment are summarized in table 2.

In general, the treatment that was effective in the acute and continuation phases should be used in the maintenance phase. In general, the same full antidepressant medication doses are employed as were used in prior phases of treatment; use of lower doses of antidepressant medication in the maintenance phase has not been well studied. For cognitive behavioral therapy and interpersonal therapy, maintenance-phase treatments usually involve a decrease in frequency of visits (e.g., once a month). Psychodynamic psychotherapy usually continues at the same frequency in the effort to explore the role of axis II disorders or other psychological factors in predisposing to depressive episodes.

Although the effectiveness of combinations of antidepressant medication and psychotherapy in the maintenance phase has not been well studied, such combinations may be an option for some patients. Patients who exhibit repeated episodes of moderate or severe major depressive disorder despite optimal pharmacologic treatment or patients who are medically ineligible for such treatment may be maintained with periodic ECT. There has been little formal study of other treatment modalities in the maintenance phase.

Similar to the continuation phase, the frequency of visits may vary in the maintenance phase. The frequency required could range from as low as once every several months for stable patients who require only psychiatric management and medication monitoring to as high as once or twice per week for those in whom psychodynamic psychotherapy is being conducted. Maintenance ECT is usually administered monthly; individuals for whom this is insufficient may find treatment at more frequent intervals to be beneficial. The optimal length of maintenance treatment is not known and may also vary depending on the frequency and severity of recurrences, tolerability of treatments, and patient preferences. For some patients, maintenance treatment may be required indefinitely.

E. DISCONTINUATION OF ACTIVE TREATMENT

The precise timing and method of discontinuing psychotherapy and pharmacotherapy for depression have not been systematically studied. The decision to discontinue maintenance treatment should be based on the same factors considered in the decision to initiate maintenance treatment, including the probability of recurrence, the frequency and severity of past episodes, the persistence of depressive symptoms after recovery, the presence of comorbid disorders, and patient preferences. In addition to the factors listed in table 2 and table 3, patients and their psychiatrists should consider the patient's response, both in terms of beneficial and adverse effects, to maintenance treatments.

When the decision is made to discontinue or terminate psychotherapy in the maintenance phase, the manner in which this is done should be individualized to the patient's needs and will depend on the type of psychotherapy, duration, and intensity of treatment. For example, maintenance treatment with cognitive behavioral therapy may have been of a preplanned length and not require extensive time for termination; on the other hand, a long-term psychodynamic psychotherapy may require greater time and attention to the termination process.

When the decision is made to discontinue maintenance pharmacotherapy, it is best to taper the medication over the course of at least several weeks. Such tapering may allow for the detection of emerging symptoms or recurrences when patients are still partially treated and therefore more easily returned to full therapeutic intensity. In addition, such tapering can help minimize the risks of antidepressant medication discontinuation syndromes (9). Discontinuation syndromes are problematic because their symptoms include disturbances of mood, energy, sleep, and appetite and can be mistaken for or mask signs of relapse (10). Discontinuation syndromes have been found to be more frequent after discontinuation of medications with shorter half-lives, and patients maintained on short-acting agents should be given even longer, more gradual tapering (11).

After the discontinuation of active treatment, patients should be reminded of the potential for a depressive relapse. Early signs of major depressive disorder should be reviewed, and a plan for seeking treatment in the event of recurrence of symptoms should be established. Patients should continue to be monitored over the next several months to identify those in whom a relapse has occurred. If a patient suffers a relapse upon discontinuation of medication, treatment should be promptly reinitiated. In general, the previous treatment regimen to which the patient responded in the acute and continuation phase should be considered. Patients who relapse following discontinuation of antidepressant medication therapy should be considered to have suffered from another major depressive disorder episode and should receive another round of adequate acute phase treatment followed by continuation phase treatment and possibly maintenance phase treatment.

III. SPECIFIC CLINICAL FEATURES INFLUENCING THE TREATMENT PLAN

▶ A. PSYCHIATRIC FEATURES

1. Suicide risk

Patients with major depressive disorder are at greater risk for suicide. Suicide risk should be assessed initially and over the course of treatment. If the patient has suicidal ideation, intention, or a plan, close surveillance is necessary. Factors to be considered in determining the nature and intensity of treatment include (but are not limited to) the nature of the doctor-patient alliance, the availability and adequacy of social supports, access to and lethality of suicide means, and past history of suicidal behavior. The risk of suicide in some patients recovering from major depressive disorder increases transiently as they develop the energy and capacity to act on self-destructive plans made earlier in the course of their illness. Clinicians must be aware of the risk of suicide throughout the course of treatment. However, the prediction of suicide attempts or suicide completion for any given patient is extremely difficult, with both many false positives (patients who appear to be at greater risk of making attempts or completing suicide but who do not) and false negatives (patients who appear to be at decreased risk but who ultimately do make attempts or complete suicide). Therefore, even with the best possible care, a small proportion of patients with major depressive disorder are likely to die by suicide.

2. Psychotic features

Major depressive disorder with psychotic features carries a higher risk of suicide than does major depressive disorder uncomplicated by psychosis (12), and it constitutes a risk factor for recurrent major depressive disorder. Major depressive disorder with psychotic features responds better to treatment with a combination of an antipsychotic medication and an antidepressant medication than to treatment with either component alone (13). Lithium augmentation is helpful in some patients who have not responded to combined antidepressant-antipsychotic medication treatment (14). ECT is highly effective in major depressive disorder with psychotic features and may be considered a first-line treatment for this disorder (15).

3. Catatonic features

Catatonic features may occur in the context of mood disorders and are characterized by at least two of the following manifestations: motoric immobility, as evidenced by catalepsy or stupor; extreme agitation; extreme negativism; peculiarities of voluntary movement, as evidenced by posturing, stereotyped movements, mannerisms, or grimacing; and echolalia or echopraxia (16). Catatonia often dominates the presentation and may be so severe as to be life-threatening, compelling the consideration of urgent biological treatment. Immediate relief may often be obtained by the intravenous administration of benzodiazepines such as lorazepam or amobarbital. For patients who show some relief, continued oral administration of lorazepam, diazepam, or amobarbital may be helpful. Concurrent antidepressant medication treatments should be considered. When relief is not immediately obtained by administering barbiturates or benzodiazepines, the urgent provision of ECT should be considered. The efficacy of ECT, usually apparent after a few treatments, is well documented; ECT may initially be administered daily. After the catatonic manifestations are relieved, treatment may be continued with antidepressant medications, lithium, antipsychotics, or a combination of these compounds, as determined by the patient's condition.

4. Atypical features

Atypical major depressive disorder features include vegetative symptoms of reversed polarity (i.e., increased rather than decreased sleep, appetite, and weight), marked mood reactivity, sensitivity to emotional rejection, phobic symptoms, and a sense of severe fatigue that creates a sensation of leaden paralysis or extreme heaviness of the arms or legs (17). Patients need not have all of these features to be diagnosed as having atypical major depressive disorder (18). There is some overlap between patients with atypical major depressive disorder and patients with anergic bipolar major depressive disorder. Although tricyclic antidepressant medications yield response rates of only 35%–50% in patients with atypical major depressive disorder, several other antidepressant classes have been found to be more effective, yielding response rates of 55%–75% (comparable to the response rate of typical forms of major depressive disorder to tricyclic therapy) (19, 20). Results of several studies suggest that SSRIs, MAOIs, and possibly bupropion may be more effective treatments for atypical major depressive disorder (21–23). The presence and severity of specific symptoms as well as safety considerations should help guide the choice of treatment for atypical major depressive disorder. For example, if a patient does not wish to, cannot, or is unlikely to adhere to the dietary and medication precautions associated with MAOI treatment, the use of an alternative antidepressant medication is indicated; on the other hand, bupropion may be anxiogenic and not preferred in cases where anxiety predominates.

5. Alcohol or substance abuse or dependence

Because of the frequent comorbidity of major depressive disorder and alcohol or other substance abuse, the psychiatrist should make every effort to obtain a detailed history of the patient's substance use. If there is suspicion that there is a problem in this area, the clinician should consider questioning a collateral for confirmation. If the patient is found to have a substance use disorder, a program to secure abstinence should be regarded as a principal priority in the treatment. A patient suffering from major depressive disorder with comorbid addiction is more likely to require hospitalization, more likely to attempt suicide, and less likely to comply with treatment than is a patient with major depressive disorder of similar severity not complicated by this factor. Some alcohol- and chemical-abusing patients reduce their consumption of these substances upon remediation of an underlying major depressive disorder, making the recognition and treatment of major depressive disorder doubly important for such individuals.

It is advisable, if other factors permit, to detoxify patients before initiating antidepressant medication therapy. Identifying the patients that should be started on a regimen of antidepressant medication therapy earlier, after initiation of abstinence, is difficult. A positive family history of major depressive disorder, a history of major depressive disorder preceding alcohol or other substance abuse, or a history of major depressive disorder during periods of sobriety raises the likelihood that the patient would benefit from antidepressant medication treatment, which may then be started earlier in treatment.

Concurrent drug abuse, especially with stimulant drugs, predisposes the patient to toxic interactions with MAOIs, although there have been few reports of such events (24). Benzodiazepines and other sedative hypnotics carry the potential for abuse or dependence and should be used cautiously except as part of a detoxification regimen. Benzodiazepines have also been reported to contribute to major depressive disorder symptoms. Hepatic dysfunction and hepatic enzyme induction frequently complicate pharmacotherapy of patients with alcoholism and other substance abuse; these conditions may require careful monitoring of blood levels (if available), therapeutic effects, and side effects to avoid either psychotropic medication intoxication or inadequate treatment.

6. Comorbid panic or other anxiety disorder

Panic disorder complicates major depressive disorder in 15%–30% of the cases (25). Individuals with symptoms of both disorders manifest greater degrees of impairment than do patients with major depressive disorder only. In major depressive disorder with comorbid anxiety or panic disorder, both the major depressive disorder symptoms and anxiety symptoms have been shown to respond to antidepressant medication treatment (26). Although there is some evidence that MAOIs may be more effective than other classes for patients with major depressive disorder and anxiety symptoms (25), therapy should first be initiated with a non-MAOI agent because of the somewhat greater complications associated with MAOIs. Tricyclic antidepressant medications and SSRIs may initially worsen rather than alleviate anxiety and panic symptoms; these medications should therefore be introduced at a low dose and slowly increased when used to treat such patients. Bupropion has been reported as ineffective in the treatment of panic disorder (27). Alprazolam may sometimes be used with benefit in conjunction with antidepressant medications; in general, benzodiazepines should not be used as the primary pharmacologic agent for patients with major depressive disorder and anxiety symptoms, especially patients with more severe forms of major depressive disorder.

Obsessive-compulsive symptoms are also more common in patients with major depressive disorder episodes. Clomipramine and the SSRIs have demonstrated efficacy in the management of obsessive-compulsive symptoms in addition to also being effective antidepressant medications (28, 29). Such agents may be used to good effect when obsessive symptoms accompany an episode of major depressive disorder.

7. Major depressive disorder–related cognitive dysfunction (pseudodementia)

Major depressive disorder is routinely accompanied by signs and symptoms of cognitive inefficiency. Some patients have both major depressive disorder and dementia, while others have major depressive disorder that causes cognitive impairment (i.e., pseudodementia). In the latter case, the treatment of the major depressive disorder should reverse the signs and symptoms of cognitive dysfunction. Many patients complain that their thoughts are slowed and their capacity to process information is reduced; they also display diminished attention to their self-care and to their environment. Transient cognitive impairments, especially involving attention, concentration, and memory storage and retrieval, are demonstrable through neuropsychological testing (30). In extreme examples, especially in the elderly, these complaints and deficits are so prominent that patients may appear demented. Major depressive disorder–related cognitive dysfunction is a reversible condition that resolves with treatment of the underlying major depressive disorder. Several clinical features help differentiate major depressive disorder pseudodementia from true dementia. When performing cognitive tasks, pseudodemented patients generally exert relatively less effort but report more incapacity than do demented patients. The latter group, especially in more advanced stages, typically neither recognize nor complain of their cognitive failures, since insight is impaired; in comparison, pseudodemented patients characteristically complain bitterly that they cannot think or cannot remember. Major depressive disorder pseudodementia lacks the signs of cortical dysfunction (i.e., aphasia, apraxia, agnosia) encountered in degenerative dementia, such as Alzheimer's disease (31). It is vital that individuals with major depressive disorder–related cognitive disturbance not be misdiagnosed and thereby denied vigorous antidepressant medication treatment or ECT.

8. Dysthymia

Antidepressant medications have been found to be effective in the treatment of dysthymia and chronic major depressive disorder, including tricyclic antidepressants, SSRIs, other newer agents, and MAOIs; unfortunately, there is little evidence from clinical trials regarding the relative efficacies of particular agents (1, 32, 33). In general, the manner in which antidepressive agents are implemented for dysthymia is similar to that for episodes of major depressive disorder; responses to antidepressant medications by patients with dysthymia and chronic major depressive disorder have been shown to be comparable to the responses by patients with major depressive disorder episodes (34).

Psychotherapy, including interpersonal therapy, cognitive behavioral therapy, cognitive therapy, and behavior therapy, has also been shown to be effective in treating patients with dysthymia and chronic major depressive disorder, although responses have been somewhat smaller than when these modalities are used to treat patients with major depressive disorder (34, 35). Individuals with chronic major depressive disorder may also be considered for psychodynamic psychotherapy in order to examine psychological factors that may maintain the depressed disposition. The combination of psychotherapy and medication has been shown to be more effective than medication alone in patients with dysthymia (36–38).

Double depression is the term used to describe the common condition of a patient with chronic dysthymia who suffers the additional burden of a more severe and pervasive episode of major depressive disorder. Antidepressant medication treatment has been shown to reverse not only the acute major depressive disorder episode but also the underlying chronic dysthymia (39).

9. Comorbid personality disorders

People with any of a variety of personality disorders, including obsessive-compulsive, avoidant, dependent, and borderline disorders, are prone to episodes of major depressive disorder (40). Clinical experience indicates that patients with narcissistic personality disorder are also particularly vulnerable to episodes of major depressive disorder. Patients with major depressive disorder who meet criteria for borderline personality disorder frequently exhibit atypical features, including mood reactivity, and may be more likely to respond to MAOIs and SSRIs than to tricyclic antidepressants (41). Patients with virtually any form of personality disorder exhibit less satisfactory antidepressant medication treatment response, in terms of both social functioning and residual major depressive disorder symptoms, than do individuals without personality disorders (42). Psychodynamic psychotherapy, including psychoanalysis, may be beneficial in modifying the personality disorder in selected patients. Antisocial personality traits tend to interfere with treatment adherence and development of a psychotherapeutic relationship.

10. Seasonal major depressive disorder

Some individuals suffer annual episodes of major depressive disorder with onset in the fall or early winter, usually at the same time each year. Some of these patients suffer manic or hypomanic episodes as well. The major depressive disorder episodes frequently have atypical features such as hypersomnia and overeating. The entire range of treatments for major depressive disorder may also be used to treat seasonal affective disorder, either in combination with or as an alternative to light therapy. As a primary form of treatment, light therapy may be recommended as a time-limited trial (43), primarily in outpatients with clear seasonal patterns. In patients with more severe forms of seasonal major depressive disorder, its use is considered adjunctive to psychopharmacologic intervention.

B. DEMOGRAPHIC AND PSYCHOSOCIAL VARIABLES

1. Major psychosocial stressors

Major depressive disorder may follow a substantial adverse life event, especially one that involves the loss of an important human relationship or life role. Major depressive disorder episodes following life stresses are no less likely than other depressive episodes to either require or benefit from antidepressant medication treatment. Nonetheless, attention to the relationship of both prior and concurrent life events to the onset, exacerbation, or maintenance of major depressive disorder symptoms is an important aspect of the overall treatment approach. A close relationship between a life stressor and major depressive disorder suggests the potential utility of a psychotherapeutic intervention coupled, as indicated, with somatic treatment.

2. Bereavement

Bereavement is a particularly severe stressor and is commonly accompanied by the signs and symptoms of major depressive disorder. Historically, such depressive manifestations have been regarded as normative, and presentations otherwise diagnosable as major depressive disorder are therefore diagnosed in DSM-IV as uncomplicated bereavement when they begin within the first 3 months of the loss (44). Data indicate that almost one-quarter of bereaved individuals meet the criteria for major depressive disorder at 2 months and again at 7 months and that many of these people continue to do so at 13 months (45). Individuals with more prolonged major depressive disorder manifestations tend to be younger and to have a history of prior episodes of major depressive disorder. Antidepressant medications or psychotherapy should be used when the reaction to a loss is particularly prolonged and psychopathology and functional impairment persist.

3. Family distress

The recognition of a problem in the family setting is important in that such a situation constitutes an ongoing stressor that may hamper the patient's response to treatment. Ambivalent, abusive, rejecting, or highly dependent family relationships may particularly predispose an individual to major depressive disorder. Such families should be evaluated for family therapy, which may be used in conjunction with individual and pharmacologic therapies. Even for instances in which there is no apparent family dysfunction, it is important to provide the family with education about the nature of the illness and to enlist the family's support and cooperation.

4. Cultural factors

Specific cultural variables may hamper the accurate assessment of major depressive disorder symptoms. An appreciation by the therapist of cultural variables is critical in the accurate diagnosis of major depressive disorder and in the selection and conduct of psychotherapy and pharmacotherapy. There is evidence that the expression of major depressive disorder symptoms may vary among cultures, especially the tendency to manifest somatic and psychomotor symptoms (46). Ethnic groups may also differ in their pharmacotherapeutic responses to antidepressant medications (47, 48). The language barrier has also been shown to severely impede accurate psychiatric diagnosis and effective treatment (49, 50).

5. Children and adolescents

The clinical presentation of depression in children and adolescents can differ significantly from that of adults and will vary with the child's age. Younger children may exhibit behavioral problems such as social withdrawal, aggressive behavior, apathy, sleep disruption, and weight loss. Adolescents may present with somatic complaints, self-esteem problems, rebelliousness, poor performance in school, or a pattern of engaging in risky or aggressive behavior. A careful assessment of the risk of suicide is necessary and should include an evaluation of risk factors such as recent loss or termination of a relationship, especially by suicide, disciplinary action, or alcohol or other substance abuse. A variety of informants should be used in the evaluation, including parents and teachers.

While a review of medication treatment studies (1) and a number of treatment recommendations (51) for children and adolescents are available, the evidence base for guiding treatment decisions for youth with major depressive disorder is quite limited. As a result, treatment decisions are frequently based on clinical consensus and the extrapolation of data from adults. It is important to be aware, however, that the extrapolation of adult data to children and adolescents is fraught with problems. For example, medications shown to be effective in adults have not always been found to be effective in children, and medications shown to be safe in adults have raised some serious safety concerns in children.

6. Older age

Considerations that go into choosing among psychotherapy, pharmacotherapy, and ECT for the elderly are essentially the same as for younger patients (52). The elderly typically display more vegetative signs and cognitive disturbance and complain less of subjective dysphoria than do their younger counterparts; major depressive disorder may consequently be misattributed to physical illness, dementia, or the aging process itself. It is recognized, however, that major depressive disorder and general medical illness frequently coexist in this age group, and those undergoing their first major depressive disorder episode in old age should be regarded as possibly harboring an as yet undiagnosed neurological or other general medical disorder that is responsible for the major depressive disorder condition. Some medications commonly prescribed for the elderly (e.g., β blockers) are thought to be risk factors for the development of major depressive disorder. The clinician should carefully assess whether a given agent contributed to the major depressive disorder before prematurely altering what may be a valuable medication regimen. Major depressive disorder is a common complication of cerebral infarction, especially in the anterior left hemisphere (53).

Although elderly patients typically require a lower oral dose than younger patients to yield a particular blood level and tolerate a given blood level less well, the blood levels at which antidepressant medications are maximally effective appear to be the same as for younger patients (54). Elderly patients are particularly prone to orthostatic hypotension and cholinergic blockade; for this reason, fluoxetine, sertraline, bupropion, desipramine, and nortriptyline are frequently chosen rather than amitriptyline, imipramine, and doxepin. Weight loss may be especially problematic in the elderly. When this is the case, it might be beneficial to use an antidepressant that causes weight gain (see table 7). Although the role of stimulants for antidepressant monotherapy is very limited, these compounds have some role in apathetic major depressive disorder in elderly patients with complicating general medical conditions. ECT should be considered for many of these patients. A recent study has shown that antidepressant medication (nortriptyline) or interpersonal therapy are effective maintenance therapies for elderly patients with recurrent major depressive disorder; a trend toward superior response was observed for combined pharmacotherapy and psychotherapy compared to pharmacotherapy alone (52).

7. Gender and pregnancy

The risks of certain adverse effects from treatments may also differ by gender. Caution is advised in the prescription of trazodone to men because of the risk of priapism. Older men are at risk for prostatic hypertrophy, making them particularly sensitive to medication effects on the bladder outlet. While both men and women may experience decreased libido or anorgasmia while taking SSRIs, men may also experience ejaculatory dysfunction. Some women who are taking birth control pills require higher

TABLE 7. Potential Treatments for Side Effects of Antidepressant Medications

Side Effect	Antidepressant(s) Associated With Effect	Treatment
Cardiovascular		
Orthostatic hypotension	Tricyclic antidepressants; trazodone; nefazodone; MAOIs	Lower dose; discontinue medication; fludrocortisone; add salt to diet
Reduced cardiac output	Tricyclic antidepressants	Discontinue medication
Arrhythmias	Tricyclic antidepressants	Discontinue medication
Hypertension	Venlafaxine	Lower dose; discontinue medication
Hypertensive crisis	MAOIs	Discontinue medication; intravenous phentolamine
Increase in cholesterol	Mirtazapine	Lower dose; discontinue medication
Anticholinergic		
Dry mouth	Tricyclic antidepressants; reboxetine	Pilocarpine oral rinse; gum; candy
Constipation	Tricyclic antidepressants; reboxetine	Hydration; bulk laxatives
Urinary hesitancy	Tricyclic antidepressants; reboxetine	Bethanechol
Visual changes	Tricyclic antidepressants; reboxetine	Pilocarpine eye drops
Delirium	Tricyclic antidepressants	Discontinue medication; antipsychotic medication
Sedation	Tricyclic antidepressants; trazodone; nefazodone; mirtazapine	Bedtime dosing
Weight gain	Tricyclic antidepressants; mirtazapine; MAOIs	Lower dose; change to secondary amine (if tricyclic antidepressant required); discontinue medication
Nausea, vomiting	SSRIs; bupropion, sustained release; venlafaxine, extended release	Lower dose; discontinue medication
Insomnia	SSRIs; bupropion; reboxetine	Lower dose; discontinue medication; morning dosing; trazodone at bedtime
Activation	SSRIs; venlafaxine	Lower dose; discontinue medication
Neurologic		
Myoclonus	Tricyclic antidepressants; MAOIs	Lower dose; discontinue medication; clonazepam
Extrapyramidal symptoms; tardive dyskinesia	Amoxapine; SSRIs	Lower dose; discontinue medication
Seizures	Bupropion; amoxapine	Lower dose; discontinue medication; antiepileptic medication
Headaches	SSRIs; bupropion	Lower dose; discontinue medication
Sexual side effects		
Arousal, erectile dysfunction	Paroxetine; venlafaxine	Lower dose; discontinue medication; sildenafil; yohimbine; ginkgo; methylphenidate; dextroamphetamine; pemoline
	Tricyclic antidepressants; SSRIs	Lower dose; discontinue medication; sildenafil; yohimbine; ginkgo; bethanechol; neostigmine
Orgasm dysfunction	SSRIs; venlafaxine	Lower dose; discontinue medication; granisetron; amantadine; cyproheptadine; sildenafil
	MAOIs; tricyclic antidepressants	Lower dose; discontinue medication; cyproheptadine; amantadine
Priapism	Trazodone	Discontinue medication; surgical correction
Serotonin syndrome	SSRIs; MAOIs; venlafaxine	Discontinue medication
Agranulocytosis	Mirtazapine	Discontinue medication; monitor white blood cell count, granulocyte colony-stimulating factor

doses of tricyclic antidepressant medications because of the induction of the hepatic enzymes responsible for medication metabolism.

The diagnostic assessment for women, in particular, should include a detailed inquiry regarding reproductive life history, including menstruation, menopause, birth control, and abortions. History of experiences of sexual and physical abuse, post-traumatic stress disorder, and treatment, if any, should be obtained.

Major depressive disorder occurring during pregnancy is a difficult therapeutic problem. Women of childbearing potential in psychiatric treatment should be carefully counseled as to the risks of becoming pregnant while taking psychotropic medications. Whenever possible, a pregnancy should be planned in consultation with the psychiatrist so that medication may be discontinued before conception if feasible. Antidepressant medication treatment should be considered for pregnant women who have major depressive disorder, as well as for those women who are in remission from major depressive disorder, receiving maintenance medication, and deemed to be at high risk for a recurrence if the medication is discontinued. The risks of treatment with medications must be weighed against the risks of alternative treatments, as well as the risks to the woman if the major depressive disorder is not effectively treated. These risks have recently been reviewed (55).

Specific concerns about the risks of untreated major depressive disorder in pregnancy include the possibility of low birth weight secondary to poor maternal weight gain (or frank weight loss). Suicidality, as well as the potential for long-term hospitalization, marital discord, the inability to engage in appropriate obstetrical care, and difficulty caring for other children must also be considered.

The considerations for the use of psychotherapy during pregnancy are identical to those relevant to nonpregnant patients, with the caveat that the risks of a delay in effectiveness may need to be considered in the context of the mother's safety as well as the safety of her fetus.

Wisner et al. reviewed the risks associated with the use of antidepressant medications during pregnancy (55). Potential risks that should be considered include intrauterine death, morphologic teratogenicity, growth impairment, behavioral teratogenicity, and neonatal toxicity. Wisner et al. also reviewed the limitations of the available database and the basic principles to be used in treating pregnant women with antidepressants. In particular, dose requirements change during pregnancy because of changes in volume of distribution, hepatic metabolism, protein binding, and gastrointestinal absorption. Although clinicians need to keep abreast of new data as they become available, at this time there is no evidence that tricyclic antidepressants, fluoxetine, or newer SSRIs cause either intrauterine death or major birth defects. However, in one large study (56), three or more minor physical anomalies occurred more commonly in infants exposed to fluoxetine than in a comparison group. This study also demonstrated that fetuses exposed to fluoxetine after 25 weeks' gestation had lower birth weights, which were associated with lower maternal weight gain.

The area of behavioral teratogenicity remains the major area of concern when prescribing psychoactive medications to pregnant women. Both tricyclic antidepressants and fluoxetine have been studied, and the results provide no evidence for effects on cognitive function, temperament, or general behavior. However, replication studies, as well as data regarding other newer antidepressants, are needed.

Neonatal withdrawal syndromes have been reported in babies exposed, in utero, to tricyclic antidepressants, fluoxetine, and sertraline. Given these data, it is recommended that consideration be given to using either a tricyclic antidepressant or an SSRI that has been studied in pregnant women. If a tricyclic antidepressant is to be used, nortriptyline should be particularly considered because of its relatively low anticholinergic effects, long history of use, and well-studied relationship between plasma concentration and therapeutic effect (55). When antidepressants are used, maternal weight gain should be carefully monitored, and consideration should be given to gradually tapering the medication 10–14 days before the expected date of delivery. If this is done, and the woman is considered to be at risk from her major depressive disorder, the medication can be restarted following delivery, although the dose should be readjusted to that required before pregnancy. In selected cases not responding to or unsuitable for medication, for patients with major depressive disorder with psychotic features, or for individuals electing to use this modality as a matter of preference after having weighed the relative risks and benefits, ECT may be used as an alternative treatment; the current literature supports the safety for mother and fetus, as well as the efficacy of ECT during pregnancy (57).

Several major depressive disorder conditions may follow childbirth (58). The transient 7–10-day depressive condition referred to as postpartum blues typically is too mild to meet the criteria for major depressive disorder and does not require medication. It is optimally treated by reassuring the patient of its brief nature and favorable outcome. Puerperal psychosis is a more severe disorder complicating 1–2 per 1,000 births; more than one-half of the episodes of this type meet the criteria for major depressive disorder (59), and many patients who have had episodes of this type ultimately prove to have bipolar disorder. Major depressive disorder, and especially major depressive disorder with psychotic features, can seriously interfere with the new mother's ability to provide physically and emotionally appropriate care for her baby. The woman's parenting skills for both the newborn baby and any other children in her care must be carefully assessed. Women with postpartum psychotic major depressive disorder may have homicidal impulses toward the newborn; for this reason, careful assessment of homicidal as well as suicidal ideation, intention, or plans is important. Women whose maintenance antidepressant medication treatment was discontinued during pregnancy appear to be particularly at risk for recurrence of major depressive disorder; such individuals should have their medications restored after delivery, in the absence of a contraindication.

Major depressive disorder in the postpartum period should be treated according to the same principles delineated for other types of major depressive disorder. However, when a woman decides to nurse, the potential benefits to the mother of using antidepressant medications should be balanced against the potential risks to the newborn inherent in the possibility of receiving some antidepressant in the breast milk; mothers should be counseled regarding the relative risks and benefits when making treatment decisions (60, 61).

8. Family history

The presence of a positive family history of recurrent major depressive disorder increases the chances that the patient's own illness will be recurrent and that the patient will not fully recover between episodes.

The presence in a depressed patient of a positive family history of bipolar disorder or acute psychosis probably increases the chances that the patient's own major depressive disorder is a manifestation of bipolar rather than unipolar disorder and that antidepressant medication therapy may incite a switch to mania (62). Patients with such a family history should be particularly closely questioned regarding a prior history of mania or hypomania, since lithium used alone or in conjunction with another antidepressant medication is particularly likely to exert a beneficial effect in patients with bipolar disorder who have a major depressive episode. Patients with major depressive disorder with a family history of bipolar disorder should be carefully observed for signs of a switch to mania during antidepressant medication treatment.

C. TREATMENT IMPLICATIONS OF CONCURRENT GENERAL MEDICAL DISORDERS

1. Asthma

Individuals with asthma who receive MAOIs should be cautioned regarding interactions with sympathomimetic bronchodilators, although other antiasthma agents appear to be safe. Other antidepressant medications may be used for patients with asthma without fear of interaction.

2. Cardiac disease

The presence of specific cardiac conditions complicates or contraindicates certain forms of antidepressant medication therapy, notably use of tricyclic agents; the cardiac history should therefore be carefully explored before the initiation of medication treatment. Although tricyclic antidepressants have been used effectively to treat major depressive disorder in patients with some forms of ischemic heart disease (63), psychiatrists should take particular care in using tricyclics for patients with a history of ventricular arrhythmia, subclinical sinus node dysfunction, conduction defects (including asymptomatic conduction defects), prolonged QT intervals, or a recent history of myocardial infarction (64–70). SSRIs, bupropion, and ECT appear to be safer for patients with preexisting cardiac disease, although the latter may require consultation with a specialist and treatment modification before use (63, 71–77). MAOIs do not adversely affect cardiac conduction, rhythm, or contraction but may induce orthostatic hypotension and also run the risk of interacting adversely with other medications that may be taken by such patients. There is anecdotal evidence that trazodone may induce ventricular arrhythmias, but the agent appears to be safe for the overwhelming majority of patients.

A depressed patient with a history of any cardiac problem should be monitored for the emergence of cardiac symptoms, ECG changes, or orthostatic blood pressure decrements. Consultation with the patient's cardiologist before and during antidepressant medication treatment may be advisable and is especially advisable during any treatment for a patient who has recently had a myocardial infarction.

3. Dementia

Treatment of major depressive disorder in the cognitively impaired patient requires the involvement of clinicians in the patient's pharmacotherapy, supervision, and monitoring; this involvement may entail education of home health aides, nursing home providers, and others. Individuals with dementia are particularly susceptible to the toxic effects of muscarinic blockade on memory and attention. Therefore, individuals suffering from dementia generally do best when given antidepressant medications with the lowest possible degree of anticholinergic effect, e.g., bupropion, fluoxetine, sertraline, trazodone, and, of the tricyclic agents, desipramine or nortriptyline. Alternatively, some patients do well given stimulants in small doses. ECT is also effective in major depressive disorder superimposed on dementia, and it should be used if medications are contraindicated, not tolerated, or if immediate resolution of the major depressive disorder episode is medically indicated (such as when it interferes with the patient's acceptance of food). Practitioners should be aware that a transient worsening of the patient's cognitive status may occur in such cases (72, 75, 78).

4. Epilepsy

Although many antidepressant medications lower the seizure threshold and theoretically exert a dose-dependent adverse effect on seizure control in patients with major depressive disorder with epilepsy, major depressive disorder in patients with seizure disorders can usually be safely and effectively managed according to the same principles outlined for patients without seizures. Consideration should be given to concomitant prescription of an antiepileptic (or elevating the dose of an existing antiepileptic).

5. Glaucoma

Medications with anticholinergic potency may precipitate acute narrow-angle glaucoma in susceptible individuals (i.e., those with shallow anterior chambers) (79). Patients with glaucoma receiving local miotic therapy may be treated with antidepressant medications, including those possessing anticholinergic properties, provided that their intraocular pressure is monitored during antidepressant medication treatment. Agents lacking anticholinergic activity (bupropion, sertraline, fluoxetine, and trazodone) avoid this liability.

6. Hypertension

Antihypertensive agents and tricyclic antidepressant medications may interact to either intensify or counteract the effect of the antihypertensive therapy. The action of antihypertensive agents that block alpha receptors (e.g., prazosin) may be intensified by antidepressant medications that block these same receptors, notably the tricyclic antidepressants and trazodone. Tricyclic antidepressants may antagonize the therapeutic actions of guanethidine, clonidine, or α-methyldopa. Concurrent antihypertensive treatment, especially with diuretics, increases the likelihood that tricyclic antidepressants, trazodone, or MAOIs will induce symptomatic orthostatic hypotension. β Blockers, especially propranolol, may be a cause of major depressive disorder in some patients; individuals who have become depressed after initiation of treatment with one of these medications should be changed to another antihypertensive regimen. Dose-dependent elevations in blood pressure with venlafaxine are usually mild, although more severe elevations have been observed (80), making this agent less preferable in patients with hypertension.

7. Obstructive uropathy

Prostatism and other forms of bladder outlet obstruction are relative contraindications to the use of antidepressant medication compounds with antimuscarinic effects. Benzodiazepines, trazodone, and MAOIs may also retard bladder emptying. The antidepressant medications with the least propensity to do this are SSRIs, bupropion, and desipramine.

8. Parkinson's disease

Amoxapine, an antidepressant medication with dopamine-receptor blocking properties, should be avoided for patients who have Parkinson's disease. Lithium may in some instances induce or exacerbate parkinsonian symptoms. Bupropion, in contrast, exerts a beneficial effect on the symptoms of Parkinson's disease in some patients but may also induce psychotic symptoms, perhaps because of its agonistic action in the dopaminergic system (81). MAOIs (other than selegiline, also known as L-deprenyl, a selective type B MAOI recommended in the treatment of Parkinson's disease) may adversely interact with L-dopa products (82). Selegiline loses its specificity for MAO-B in doses greater than 10 mg/day and may induce serotonin syndrome when given in higher doses in conjunction with serotonin-enhancing antidepressant medications. Major depressive disorder, which occurs to some degree in 40%–50% of patients with Parkinson's disease, may be related to the alterations of serotonergic and noradrenergic systems that occur in this disorder. There is no evidence favoring any particular antidepressant medication from the standpoint of therapeutic efficacy in patients with Parkinson's disease complicated by major depressive disorder. The theoretical benefits of the antimuscarinic effects of some of the tricyclic agents in the treatment of patients with major depressive disorder with Parkinson's disease are offset by the memory impairment that may result. ECT exerts a transient beneficial effect on the symptoms of idiopathic Parkinson's disease in many patients (83).

PART B:
BACKGROUND INFORMATION AND REVIEW OF AVAILABLE EVIDENCE

IV. DISEASE DEFINITION, EPIDEMIOLOGY, NATURAL HISTORY, AND COURSE

DSM-IV criteria for major depressive episode and major depressive disorder are listed in table 8.

▶ A. SPECIFIC FEATURES OF DIAGNOSIS

1. Severity
An episode of major depressive disorder may be classified as mild, moderate, or severe. Mild episodes are characterized by little in the way of symptoms beyond the minimum required to make the diagnosis and by minor functional impairment. Moderate episodes are characterized by the presence of symptoms in excess of the bare diagnostic requirements and by greater degrees of functional impairment. Severe episodes are characterized by the presence of several symptoms in excess of the minimum requirements and by the symptoms' marked interference with social and/or occupational functioning. In the extreme, afflicted individuals may be totally unable to function socially or occupationally or even to feed or clothe themselves or to maintain minimal personal hygiene. The nature of the symptoms, such as suicidal ideation and behavior, should also be considered in assessing severity.

TABLE 8. DSM-IV Criteria for Major Depressive Episode and Major Depressive Disorder

Diagnosis	Criterion/Symptom Description
Major depressive episode	A. At least five of the following symptoms have been present during the same 2-week period and represent a change from previous functioning; at least one of the symptoms is either 1) depressed mood or 2) loss of interest or pleasure (do not include symptoms that are clearly due to general medical condition or mood-incongruent delusions or hallucinations)
	1. Depressed mood most of the day, nearly every day, as indicated either by subjective report (e.g., feels sad or empty) or observation made by others (e.g., appears tearful)
	2. Markedly diminished interest or pleasure in all, or almost all, activities most of the day, nearly every day (as indicated either by subjective account or observation made by others)
	3. Significant weight loss when not dieting or weight gain (e.g., a change of more than 5% of body weight in a month), or decrease or increase in appetite nearly every day
	4. Insomnia or hypersomnia nearly every day
	5. Psychomotor agitation or retardation nearly every day (observable by others, not merely subjective feelings of restlessness or being slowed down)
	6. Fatigue or loss of energy nearly every day
	7. Feelings of worthlessness or excessive or inappropriate guilt (which may be delusional) nearly every day (not merely self-reproach or guilt about being sick)
	8. Diminished ability to think or concentrate, or indecisiveness, nearly every day (either by subjective account or as observed by others)
	9. Recurrent thoughts of death (not just fear of dying), recurrent suicidal ideation without a specific plan, or a suicide attempt or specific plan for committing suicide
	B. The symptoms do not meet criteria for a mixed episode
	C. The symptoms cause clinically significant distress or impairment in social, occupational, or other important areas of functioning
	D. The symptoms are not due to the direct physiological effects of a substance (e.g., a drug of abuse, a medication) or a general medical condition (e.g., hypothyroidism)
	E. The symptoms are not better accounted for by bereavement, i.e., after the loss of a loved one, the symptoms persist for longer than 2 months or are characterized by marked functional impairment, morbid preoccupation with worthlessness, suicidal ideation, psychotic symptoms, or psychomotor retardation
Major depressive disorder, single episode	A. Presence of a single major depressive episode
	B. The major depressive episode is not better accounted for by schizoaffective disorder and is not superimposed on schizophrenia, schizophreniform disorder, delusional disorder, or psychotic disorder not otherwise specified
	C. There has never been a manic episode, a mixed episode, or a hypomanic episode
Major depressive disorder, recurrent	A. Presence of two or more major depressive episodes (each separated by at least 2 months in which criteria are not met for a major depressive episode)
	B. The major depressive episodes are not better accounted for by schizoaffective disorder and are not superimposed on schizophrenia, schizophreniform disorder, delusional disorder, or psychotic disorder not otherwise specified
	C. There has never been a manic episode, a mixed episode, or a hypomanic episode

2. Melancholia

The melancholic subtype is a severe form of major depressive disorder with characteristic somatic symptoms, and it is believed to be particularly responsive to pharmacotherapy and ECT.

3. Psychotic features

Major depressive disorder may be accompanied by hallucinations or delusions; these may be congruent or noncongruent with the depressive mood.

4. Dysthymia

The differential diagnosis of dysthymia and major depressive disorder is particularly difficult, since the two disorders share similar symptoms and differ primarily in duration and severity. Usually major depressive disorder consists of one or more discrete major depressive episodes that can be distinguished from the person's usual functioning, whereas dysthymia is characterized by a chronic mild depressive syndrome that has been present for at least 2 years. If the initial onset of what appears to be dysthymia directly follows a major depressive episode, the appropriate diagnosis is major depressive disorder in partial remission. The diagnosis of dysthymia can be made following major depressive disorder only if there has been a full remission of the major depressive episode that has lasted at least 6 months before the development of dysthymia.

People with dysthymia frequently have a superimposed major depressive disorder, and this condition is often referred to as double major depressive disorder. Patients with double major depressive disorder are less likely to have a complete recovery than are patients with major depressive disorder without dysthymia.

B. EPIDEMIOLOGY

The Epidemiologic Catchment Area study indicates that major depressive disorder has a 1-month prevalence of 2.2% and a lifetime prevalence of 5.8% in Americans 18 years and older (84). Other studies estimate the lifetime prevalence to be as high as 26% for women and 12% for men. The illness is 1.5 to 3 times as common among those with a first-degree biological relative affected with the disorder as among the general population. Major depressive disorder is frequently accompanied by comorbid conditions. For example, in one study of patients with major depressive disorder under the care of psychiatrists in the U.S., 84% had at least one comorbid condition: 61% had a co-occurring axis I condition, 30% a comorbid axis II condition, and 58% a comorbid axis III condition (85). Frequently a major depressive episode follows a psychosocial stressor, particularly death of a loved one, marital separation, or the ending of an important relationship. Childbirth sometimes precipitates a major depressive episode. Patients with major depressive disorder identified in psychiatric settings tend to have episodes of greater severity and to have recurrent forms of major depressive disorder and also are more likely to have other mental disorders than are subjects from the community and primary care settings.

C. NATURAL HISTORY AND COURSE

The average age at onset is the late 20s, but the disorder may begin at any age. The symptoms of major depressive disorder typically develop over days to weeks. Prodromal symptoms, including generalized anxiety, panic attacks, phobias, or depressive symptoms that do not meet the diagnostic threshold, may occur over the preceding several months. In some cases, however, a major depressive disorder may develop suddenly (e.g., when associated with severe psychosocial stress). The duration of a major depressive episode is also variable. Untreated, the episode typically lasts 6 months or longer. Some patients with major depressive disorder will eventually have a manic or hypomanic episode and will then be diagnosed as having bipolar disorder.

1. Recurrence

Although some people have only a single episode of major depressive disorder, with full return to premorbid functioning, it is estimated that from 50% to 85% of the people who have such an episode will eventually have another episode, at which time the illness will meet the criteria for recurrent major depressive disorder (86). People with major depressive disorder superimposed on dysthymia are at greater risk for having recurrent episodes of major depressive disorder than those without dysthymia.

The course of recurrent major depressive disorder is variable. Some people have episodes separated by many years of normal functioning, others have clusters of episodes, and still others have increasingly frequent episodes as they grow older.

2. Interepisode status

Functioning usually returns to the premorbid level between episodes. In 20%–35% of the cases, however, there are persistent residual symptoms and social or occupational impairment. Patients who continue to meet the criteria for a major depressive episode throughout the course of the disturbance are considered to have the chronic type, whereas those who remain symptomatic are considered to be in partial remission.

3. Seasonal pattern

A seasonal pattern of major depressive disorder is characterized by a regular temporal relationship between the onset and remission of symptoms and particular periods of the year (e.g., in the northern hemisphere, regular appearance of symptoms between the beginning of October and the end of November and regular remission from mid-February to mid-April). Patients should not receive this diagnosis if there is an obvious effect of seasonally related psychosocial stressors, e.g., seasonal unemployment.

4. Complications

The most serious complications of a major depressive episode are suicide and other violent acts. Other complications include marital, parental, social, and vocational difficulties (87). The illness, especially in its recurrent and chronic forms, may cause distress for other individuals in the patient's social network, e.g., children, spouse, and significant others. If the patient is a parent, the disorder may affect his or her ability to fulfill parental role expectations (88). Major depressive disorder episodes are associated with occupational dysfunction, including unemployment, absenteeism, and decreased work productivity (89). Major depressive disorder may also complicate recovery from other medical illnesses. Major depressive disorder has been demonstrated to be a major risk factor in the post-myocardial-infarction period.

V. REVIEW AND SYNTHESIS OF AVAILABLE EVIDENCE

Successful treatment of patients with major depressive disorder is promoted by a thorough assessment of the patient's symptoms; past general medical and psychiatric history; psychological makeup and conflicts; life stressors; family, psychosocial, and cultural environment; and preference for specific treatments or approaches.

The psychiatrist's task is both to effect and to maintain improvement. Treatment consists of an acute phase, during which remission is induced; a continuation phase, during which remission is preserved; and a maintenance phase, during which the susceptible patient is protected against the recurrence of subsequent major depressive disorder episodes. Psychiatrists initiating treatment of a major depressive disorder episode have at their disposal a number of medications, a variety of psychosocial approaches, ECT, and light therapy. These various interventions may be used alone or in combination. Furthermore, the psychiatrist must decide whether to conduct treatment on an outpatient, partial hospitalization, or inpatient basis.

▶ A. ACUTE PHASE SOMATIC TREATMENTS

1. Antidepressant medications

a. Goals

The goal of treatment with antidepressant medications in the acute phase is the remission of major depressive disorder symptoms. For cases of first-episode major depressive disorder uncomplicated by comorbid general medical illness or by special features such as atypical, psychotic, or bipolar symptoms, many antidepressant medications are available. Systematic data from clinical trials regarding the relative efficacy of different antidepressant medications are lacking. For most patients, antidepressant medications approved by the Food and Drug Administration (FDA) are generally considered equally effective, with response rates in clinical trials ranging from 50% to 75% of patients. However, among some subgroups of patients with major depressive disorder, efficacy may differ. Antidepressant medications also differ in their potential to cause particular side effects. Antidepressant medications have been grouped as follows: 1) tricyclic antidepressant medications, which for the purposes of this review also include the tetracyclic antidepressant medication maprotiline; 2) SSRIs, which include fluoxetine, sertraline, paroxetine, fluvoxamine, and citalopram; 3) other antidepressant medications, including bupropion, nefazodone, trazodone, venlafaxine, mirtazapine, and reboxetine (for which FDA approval is anticipated); and 4) MAOIs, which include phenelzine, tranylcypromine, and isocarboxazid.

b. Efficacy

Quantitative reviews of the efficacy of antidepressant medications for major depressive disorder have been performed, including the recent *Evidence Report on Treatment of Depression—Newer Pharmacotherapies* (1). This study examined 315 trials, lasting 6 weeks or longer, of newer pharmacotherapies for patients with depressive disorders. Additional details concerning the evidence of antidepressant medication efficacy that may be beyond the scope of this guideline can be obtained from such reviews.

Interpreting data from clinical trials on the efficacy of pharmacotherapy for major depressive disorder can be complicated by several issues. First, it is important to consider whether and what type of comparison group was used (e.g., placebo or active agent). In trials of antidepressant medication treatments, high placebo response rates could explain observed treatment effects in poorly controlled trials as well as make detection of true treatment effects difficult in well-controlled trials. It is also important to consider both whether trials were blinded and whether in "blinded" trials, medication side effects could reveal the identity of active agents. Issues related to the outcomes measured in trials are important as well. A variety of different outcome measures are employed, and a report of "efficacy" could refer to symptom reduction (e.g., reduction in the frequency or severity of major depressive disorder symptoms), response (e.g., reduction in major depressive disorder symptoms below a threshold), or prevention of relapse. Data often come from short-term (6- to 12-week) efficacy trials that may not reveal whether treatments are effective over the medium- and long-term. Lastly, it is important to consider whether publication bias against reporting of negative studies could affect the perception of overall treatment effectiveness.

1) Tricyclic antidepressants

Since the first trial in which a tricyclic compound (imipramine) was shown to improve major depressive disorder symptoms (90), hundreds of subsequent randomized controlled trials have demonstrated the efficacy of this class as a treatment for major depressive disorder (1). Heterocyclic antidepressant medications, including tricyclics and tetracyclics, have been found to be statistically significantly superior to placebo in approximately 75% of studies (91); several reviews suggest that approximately 50%–75% of patients with major depressive disorder treated with heterocyclic antidepressant medications respond compared to 25%–33% treated with placebo (92–95). The efficacy of individual agents and subclasses of tricyclics (e.g., secondary amines or tertiary amines) appears to be comparable.

Results of some investigations have suggested that tricyclic antidepressants may possess superior efficacy among subgroups of patients with severe major depressive disorder symptoms (91, 96–99). Some studies have also suggested that in major depressive disorder marked by melancholic features, tricyclic antidepressants may be additionally effective (100, 101) as well as superior to SSRIs (102, 103); however, not all research supports these findings (104).

2) Selective serotonin reuptake inhibitors

SSRIs currently available include fluoxetine, sertraline, paroxetine, fluvoxamine, and citalopram. A large body of literature containing approximately 50 randomized, placebo-controlled trials supports the premise that SSRIs are superior to placebo in the treatment of major depressive disorder. In over 50 investigations the effectiveness of SSRIs has been compared to that of other antidepressant medications, mainly tricyclic antidepressants; in these trials, SSRIs have generally had comparable efficacy to antidepressant medications from other classes (1, 105, 106). In general, significant differences in efficacy between individual SSRIs have not been observed.

There is some evidence that SSRIs may be more effective than tricyclic antidepressants for subgroups of patients with atypical symptoms of major depressive disorder (e.g., mood reactivity, hypersomnia, hyperphagia, and hypersensitivity to rejections) (23). SSRIs have also been shown to be helpful for some patients who have not responded to tricyclic antidepressants (107).

3) Other antidepressant medications

Several other antidepressant medications are available that differ structurally or in their pharmacologic action from medications in the categories just described. Trazodone is the medication from this group for which the most data on efficacy exists. In most trials, trazodone has had superior efficacy relative to placebo; however, its efficacy relative to other antidepressant medications remains controversial. Although data from some controlled trials suggest comparable efficacy to tricyclic antidepressants (108, 109), other investigations suggest trazodone may possess inferior efficacy relative to other antidepressant medications (1, 110, 111), particularly in subgroups with severe major depressive disorder symptoms or prominent psychomotor retardation (112, 113).

Nefazodone has an analogous structure to trazodone but somewhat different pharmacologic properties. In controlled trials, nefazodone has had superior efficacy to placebo; in five trials, nefazodone has been found to have comparable efficacy to tricyclic antidepressants (1, 114, 115). Some studies suggest that nefazodone may have an optimal therapeutic dose range corresponding to approximately 300–600 mg/day (115, 116).

Bupropion appears to inhibit the reuptake of both norepinephrine and dopamine, although its mechanism of action remains unclear. Trial data have shown that bupropion is superior to placebo (117) and generally comparable in efficacy to both tricyclic antidepressants (1, 118–121) and SSRIs (122).

Venlafaxine and mirtazapine appear to act through inhibition of reuptake of both norepinephrine and serotonin. Both have been demonstrated to be superior to placebo; venlafaxine and mirtazapine have each been shown in four trials to possess generally comparable efficacy to tricyclic antidepressants (1, 110, 123–128). Results from one trial suggest a positive relationship between the effective dose of venlafaxine and the severity of major depressive disorder—favorable responses were achieved with lower doses in milder major depressive disorders, whereas higher doses were more efficacious in severe major depressive disorder (129).

Reboxetine is a new selective noradrenaline reuptake inhibitor for which approval from the FDA is expected. In four trials, reboxetine has been shown to be more effective than placebo; in 6 trials against active treatment, reboxetine has been found to possess at least comparable effectiveness as tricyclic antidepressants and SSRIs (1, 130).

4) Monoamine oxidase inhibitors

MAOIs that have been used as antidepressant medications include phenelzine, tranylcypromine, and isocarboxazid. MAOIs have also been shown in multiple trials to be effective treatments for major depressive disorder. Although some earlier comparisons employing lower doses of MAOIs found tricyclic antidepressants to be superior, MAOIs are now considered to have comparable efficacy to tricyclic antidepressants for typical cases of major depressive disorder (131–136). There are no significant differences in efficacy among the MAOIs.

Results of several investigations suggest that MAOIs may be particularly effective in treating subgroups of patients with major depressive disorder with atypical features such as reactive moods, reversed neurovegetative symptoms, and sensitivity to rejection (19, 137, 138). MAOIs have also been shown to be effective treatments for some patients who have failed other antidepressant medication trials (132, 136, 139, 140).

c. Side effects

The severity of side effects from antidepressant medications in clinical trials has been assessed both through the frequency of reported side effects and through the frequency of treatment dropout. The likelihood of different side effects varies between classes of antidepressant medications, between subclasses, and between individual agents. Prominent and clinically relevant side effects associated with particular classes, subclasses, and individual medications are reviewed in table 7.

1) Tricyclic antidepressants

i. Cardiovascular effects

Tricyclic antidepressants can cause a number of cardiovascular side effects through α-adrenergic blockade, including tachycardia or orthostatic hypotension. Side effects such as orthostatic hypotension may in turn lead to events such as dizziness, falls, or fractures. Secondary amines such as nortriptyline or desipramine cause less α-adrenergic blockade and may offer advantages over tertiary amines (69). Salt depletion, whether voluntary or a result of diuretic treatment, may contribute to orthostatic hypotension. If there is no medical contraindication, patients with symptomatic orthostatic hypotension should be cautioned against extreme dietary salt restriction.

Tricyclic antidepressant medications act similarly to class I antiarrhythmic agents such as quinidine, disopyramide, and procainamide by prolonging cardiac repolarization and depressing fast sodium ion channels (141). Both secondary and tertiary amines have been documented to suppress ventricular premature depolarizations (64, 67). Combinations of tricyclic antidepressants with other class I antiarrhythmic agents can exert additive toxic effects on cardiac conduction; patients with ventricular arrhythmias taking another class I antiarrhythmic agent who require tricyclic medication therapy should be under careful medical supervision. Tricyclic antidepressants may also provoke arrhythmias in patients with subclinical sinus node dysfunction; for example, in patients with tachyarrhythmias, treatment with tricyclic antidepressants may on occasion provoke bradyarrhythmias (65). Among patients with preexisting but asymptomatic conduction defects, such as interventricular conduction delay and bundle-branch block, tricyclic antidepressants may induce symptomatic conduction defects and symptomatic orthostatic hypotension (69). Individuals with prolonged QT intervals, whether preexistent or medication-induced, are predisposed to the development of ventricular tachycardia (70). It has also been reported that patients with normal pretreatment ECG results may develop atriventricular block that reverts to normal after discontinuation of antidepressant medication treatment (69).

For most patients, tricyclic antidepressants exert no appreciable effect on ventricular ejection fraction (142); rarely (and usually in patients with marked baseline disturbances of myocardial function), tricyclic antidepressants may exert a deleterious effect on ejection fraction (66, 68).

ii. Anticholinergic side effects

All tricyclic antidepressant medications have some degree of antimuscarinic action; tertiary amine tricyclic antidepressants produce the most anticholinergic side effects, whereas the newer secondary amines, desipramine and nortriptyline, have less antimuscarinic activity. The most common undesirable consequences of muscarinic blockade are dry mouth, impaired ability to focus at close range, constipation, urinary hesitation, tachycardia, and sexual dysfunction. Although patients can develop some degree of tolerance to anticholinergic side effects, these symptoms may require treatment if they cause substantial dysfunction or interfere with adherence. Impaired visual accommodation may be counteracted through the use of pilocarpine eye drops. Urinary hesitation may be treated by prescribing bethanechol, 200 mg/day (in divided doses to avoid symptoms of cholinergic excess, principally abdominal cramps, nausea, and diarrhea). Dry mouth may be counteracted by advising the patient to use sugarless gum or candy or by prescribing an oral rinse of 1% pilocarpine used three or four times daily; oral bethanecol may also be effective. Constipation is best dealt with through adequate hydration and the use of bulk laxatives. Antidepressant medications with anticholinergic side effects should be avoided in patients with cognitive impairment, narrow-angle glaucoma, or prostatic hypertrophy. Tricyclic antidepressants may also precipitate anticholinergic delirium, particularly in patients who are elderly or medically compromised.

iii. Sedation

Tricyclic antidepressants also have affinity for histaminergic receptors and produce varying degrees of sedation. In general, tertiary amines cause greater sedation, whereas secondary amines cause less. Sedation often attenuates in the first weeks of treatment, and patients experiencing only minor difficulty from this side effect should be encouraged to allow some time to pass before changing antidepressant medications. Patients with major depressive disorder with insomnia may benefit from sedation when their medication is given as a single dose before bedtime.

iv. Weight gain

Tricyclic antidepressants have the capacity to induce weight gain possibly through their histaminergic properties. The degree of weight gain appears to vary by agent (e.g., greater weight gain with amitriptyline and less with desipramine), be dose dependent, and be reversible with cessation of tricyclic antidepressant therapy.

v. Neurological effects

Tricyclic antidepressants can induce mild myoclonus (143). Since this may be a sign of toxicity, the clinician may wish to check the blood level (if available) to ensure that it is not excessive. If the level is nontoxic and the myoclonus is not symptomatic, the agent may be continued without a change in dose. If the myoclonus is symptomatic and the blood level is within the recommended range, the patient may be treated with clonazepam at a dose of 0.25 mg t.i.d. Alternatively, the antidepressant medication may be changed. A toxic confusional state has been identified in some patients with high blood levels of tricyclic antidepressant medications, and it responds to simply lowering the dose (144). Amoxapine, a tricyclic antidepressant with antipsychotic properties, can also cause extrapyramidal side effects and tardive dyskinesia. In overdoses, tricyclic antidepressants can precipitate seizures.

vi. Medication interactions

Medications that induce hepatic microsomal enzymes, such as carbamazepine or barbiturates, will cause a decrease in serum tricyclic antidepressant level. On the other hand, drugs such as antipsychotic medications or SSRIs can reduce the metabolism and clearance of tricyclic antidepressants and raise tricyclic antidepressant levels. Tricyclic antidepressants can also alter the pharmacokinetics or pharmacodynamics of other medications; for example, tricyclic antidepressants can cause a lowering of valproate levels and reduce the activity of clonidine. Therefore adjustments in medication doses may be necessary when tricyclic antidepressants are administered concomitantly with other drugs for which there is an interaction. Potentially dangerous interactions, including hypertensive crises, can develop when tricyclic antidepressants are administered with MAOIs, norepinephrine, or epinephrine.

2) Selective serotonin reuptake inhibitors

i.   Gastrointestinal

SSRIs cause nausea, vomiting, and diarrhea to a greater extent than tricyclic antidepressant medications (145). These adverse events are generally dose dependent and tend to dissipate over the first few weeks of treatment.

ii.   Activation/insomnia

In some patients, SSRIs may precipitate or exacerbate restlessness, agitation, and sleep disturbances. These side effects often attenuate with time. Anxiety may be minimized by introducing the agent at a low dose; insomnia may be effectively treated by the addition of trazodone, up to 100 mg at bedtime.

iii. Sexual side effects

Although loss of erectile or ejaculatory function in men and loss of libido and anorgasmia in both sexes may be complications of virtually any antidepressant medication, these side effects appear to be more common with SSRIs. The psychiatrist should ascertain whether the sexual dysfunction is a result of the antidepressant medication or the underlying major depressive disorder. If sexual dysfunction is determined to be a side effect of the antidepressant medication, a variety of strategies are available, including continuing treatment to assess whether the dysfunction will disappear with time, lowering the dose, discontinuing the antidepressant, or substituting another antidepressant such as bupropion (table 7) (146). Specific pharmacologic treatments that can be added for arousal or erectile dysfunction include sildenafil, yohimbine, or neostigmine; specific medications that can be added for orgasm dysfunction include sildenafil, cyproheptadine, or amantadine (147).

iv. Neurological effects

SSRIs can initially exacerbate both migraine headaches and tension headaches. These effects tend to be transient and improve within the first few weeks of treatment. There is some suggestion that with continued treatment, SSRIs may then actually help prevent and treat migraine headaches (148, 149). SSRIs have also been associated with extrapyramidal reactions, including akathisia, dystonia, parkinsonism, and tardive dyskinesia (150, 151). The occurrence of such extrapyramidal symptoms is generally very low but may be higher in older patients, especially those with Parkinson's disease.

v.   Effects on weight

Fluoxetine has been shown to cause an initial reduction in weight but this tends be gained back subsequently (152). The literature differs as to whether patients taking SSRIs beyond the acute phase do (153) or do not (154) experience weight gain as a medication side effect.

vi. Serotonin syndrome

SSRI use has been associated with the rare development of a syndrome due to an excess of serotonergic activity. Features of serotonin syndrome include abdominal pain, diarrhea, flushing, sweating, hyperthermia, lethargy, mental status changes, tremor and myoclonus, rhabdomyolysis, renal failure, cardiovascular shock, and possibly death (155, 156). Although serotonin syndrome can occur with the use of SSRIs alone, it is usually associated with the simultaneous use of multiple serotonergic agents such as SSRIs together with MAOIs, fenfluramine, or dexfenfluramine.

vii. Drug interactions

As previously described, there can be a potentially lethal interaction between SSRIs and MAOIs: serotonin syndrome. It has been suggested that at least five half-lives elapse between the time an SSRI is stopped and an MAOI is started; for fluoxetine discontinuation, this corresponds to waiting approximately 5 weeks before starting an MAOI, whereas for discontinuation of other SSRIs it corresponds to waiting approximately 1 week before starting an MAOI (157). A 2-week waiting period has been suggested after discontinuing an MAOI before starting an SSRI.

SSRIs can also have variable effects on hepatic microsomal enzymes and therefore cause both increases and decreases in the blood levels of other medications.

3) Other antidepressant medications

i. Trazodone

The most common side effect with trazodone is sedation; this side effect may allow trazodone to be used to advantage in patients with initial insomnia. Trazodone can also cause cardiovascular side effects including orthostasis. Although trazodone does not prolong cardiac conduction, there have been case reports of cardiac arrhythmias developing during trazodone treatment (158, 159). Trazodone can cause sexual side effects, including erectile dysfunction in men; in rare instances, this may lead to irreversible priapism requiring surgical correction (160).

ii. Nefazodone

Side effects observed with nefazodone treatment include dry mouth, nausea, and constipation. Although nefazodone lacks anticholinergic properties, blurred vision has been noted. Nefazodone may also cause sedation and orthostasis but not as severe as that observed with trazodone. Nefazodone is known to inhibit hepatic microsomal enzymes and can raise levels of concurrently administered medications such as certain antihistamines, benzodiazepines, and digoxin.

iii. Bupropion

Neurologic side effects have been observed with bupropion treatment including headaches, tremors, and seizures. Risks of seizures can be reduced by avoiding high doses (e.g., using less than 450 mg/day), using divided dosing schedules (e.g., three times a day), and avoiding bupropion use in patients with risk factors for seizures. Bupropion also possesses dopaminergic activity and has been associated with the development of psychotic symptoms, including delusions and hallucinations. For these reasons, bupropion should be used cautiously in patients with psychotic disorders. Other side effects observed with bupropion treatment include insomnia and gastrointestinal upset.

iv. Venlafaxine

The side effects of venlafaxine have been likened to those seen with SSRIs, including nausea and vomiting, sexual dysfunction, and activation; like the side effects seen with SSRIs, those with venlafaxine can attenuate with continued use. Venlafaxine can also cause an increase in blood pressure. Because this increase is dose related, venlafaxine-induced hypertension may respond to dose reduction.

v. Mirtazapine

The most common side effects from mirtazapine include sedation, dry mouth, and weight gain. These tend to occur early and may attenuate with continued treatment. Mirtazapine has also been shown to increase serum cholesterol levels in some patients

(161). Although agranulocytosis has been observed to occur in patients taking mirtazapine, its occurrence has been very rare. Routine monitoring of a patient's WBC count is not needed, although checking may be advisable in patients with signs or symptoms of infection.

vi. Reboxetine

The most frequently reported side effects in trials of reboxetine have been dry mouth, constipation, increased sweating, insomnia, urinary hesitancy/retention, impotence, tachycardia, and vertigo (162). In clinical trials done to date, few serious adverse events have been reported among patients treated with reboxetine.

4) Monoamine oxidase inhibitors

i. Hypertensive crises

A hypertensive crisis can occur when a patient taking an MAOI ingests large amounts of tyramine or other pressor amines in foods or medications. This reaction is characterized by the acute onset of severe headache, nausea, neck stiffness, palpitations, profuse perspiration, and confusion, possibly leading to stroke and death (163). Dietary restrictions include avoiding such foods as aged cheeses or meats, fermented products, yeast extracts, fava or broad beans, and overripe or spoiled foods. The list of medications that must be avoided includes all sympathomimetic and stimulant drugs as well as over-the-counter decongestants and cold remedies.

Some clinicians have recommended that patients carry nifedipine and, at the outset of a possible hypertensive crisis, take an oral dose of 10 mg before proceeding to the hospital (164); this practice has not been approved by the FDA, and further study of the safety and efficacy of this strategy is needed (165). Definitive treatment of hypertensive crises usually involves intravenous administration of phentolamine in an emergency room setting.

ii. Serotonin syndrome

This syndrome most commonly occurs when MAOIs are taken in close proximity to other serotonergic agents (166). When patients are being switched from an SSRI with a short half-life to an MAOI, a waiting period of at least 2 weeks is needed between the discontinuation of one medication and the initiation of the other. When switching from fluoxetine to an MAOI, a waiting period of at least 5 weeks is needed before the MAOI is started. The serotonin syndrome may also occur when venlafaxine is administered soon after an MAOI (167).

iii. Cardiovascular effects

Orthostatic hypotension is commonly seen during MAOI treatment. Possible treatments for this side effect include the addition of salt to increase intravascular volume or use of the steroid fludrocortisone. MAOI use can also be associated with the development of peripheral edema, which may be helped by the use of support stockings.

iv. Weight gain

Weight gain is also commonly seen in patients treated with MAOIs. The likelihood of this side effect appears to vary with the agent used, with most weight gain seen with tranylcypromine and the least with phenelzine.

v. Sexual side effects

Sexual side effects seen with MAOI therapy include anorgasmia, decreased libido, and erectile or ejaculatory dysfunction. Sexual side effects may diminish over time or with reductions in MAOI doses.

vi. Neurological effects

MAOI treatment can also be accompanied by headaches and insomnia; these side effects may diminish over time with continued use. Other neurological effects seen with MAOI use include sedation, myoclonic jerks, paresthesias, and, rarely, peripheral neuropathy.

d. Implementation

Typical starting doses and typical effective adult dose ranges that have been used in short-term efficacy trials of antidepressant medications appear in table 1. Initial doses should be incrementally raised as tolerated until a presumably therapeutic dose is reached. For some antidepressant medications, the exact relationships between doses and major depressive disorder symptom response have not been rigorously investigated with fixed-dose studies, and minimum effective doses have not been clearly established; for other antidepressant medications, studies have failed to show dose-response relationships (168–170). Therefore, the initial doses and usual adult doses in table 1 are intended to serve as general guidelines, and actual doses may vary from individual to individual. In general, older, medically frail, or patients with decreased ability to metabolize and clear antidepressant medications will require lower doses; in such patients, reduction of initial and therapeutic doses to 50% of usual adult doses is often recommended. Doses will also be affected by the side effect profile of medications and the patient's ability to tolerate these.

In short-term efficacy trials, all antidepressant medications appear to require 4–6 weeks to achieve their maximum therapeutic effects (171, 172) (although some patients may show partial improvement by as soon as the end of the first week [173]). Therefore, adequacy of response cannot be judged until after this period of time. Patients should be alerted to this and instructed to continue taking their antidepressant medications throughout this initial period.

For some medications, particularly the tricyclic antidepressants nortriptyline, desipramine, and imipramine, blood drug levels have been shown to correlate with both efficacy and side effects. Although in most cases, monitoring of serum antidepressant medication levels is not necessary, in some circumstances this can be very useful. These circumstances can include when patients have not responded to adequate doses of an antidepressant medication given for adequate durations; when patients are particularly vulnerable to the toxic effects of a medication and require the lowest possible effective dose; when there are concerns about patient adherence; and when there is concern that drug-drug interactions are adversely affecting antidepressant medication levels.

Some antidepressant medications, especially tricyclics, can be associated with significant morbidity and potentially mortality in overdose. Ingestion of a 10-day supply of a tricyclic agent administered at a dose of 200 mg/day is often lethal. Early on in treatment, it is prudent to dispense only small quantities of such antidepressant medications and keep in mind the possibility that patients can hoard medications over time. Alternatively, in patients who are suicidal it may be preferable to employ agents that are safer in overdose such as the SSRIs, trazodone, nefazodone, bupropion, venlafaxine, or mirtazapine.

2. Failure to respond to pharmacotherapy in the acute phase

Adequate treatment with an antidepressant medication for at least 4–8 weeks is necessary before concluding that a patient is not responsive or only partially responsive to a particular medication (172). Initial treatment with antidepressant medication fails to achieve a satisfactory response in approximately 20%–30% of patients with major depressive disorder; poor treatment response has been found to be not just the result of inadequate treatment but also a consequence of inappropriate diagnoses, failure to appreciate and remedy coexisting general medical conditions, psychiatric disorders, or complicating psychosocial factors, and nonadherence (174). For these reasons a first step in the care of a patient who has not responded to medication should be a review and reappraisal of the diagnosis, adherence, and neglected contributing factors, including general medical problems, alcohol or substance abuse or dependence, other psychiatric disorders, and general psychosocial issues impeding recovery. In cases where nonadherence or complicating psychosocial stressors are prominent, the addition of psychotherapy may be effective in enhancing response (152).

For patients whose treatment failure is not readily attributable to inappropriate diagnoses, poor adherence, or complicating conditions, a variety of therapeutic options are available, including maximizing the initial treatment, switching to another non-MAOI agent, augmenting antidepressant medications with other medications or psychotherapy, using an MAOI, and ECT (5). Empirical data concerning the relative efficacies of these strategies are limited.

a. Maximizing initial treatments

There is little evidence to support extending antidepressant medication trials beyond 6 weeks in patients who have shown no response. However, for patients who have shown a partial response, particularly those with features of personality disorders and prominent psychosocial stressors, extending the antidepressant medication trial (e.g., by 2–4 weeks) may allow up to one-third of patients to respond more fully (6).

Use of higher antidepressant medication doses is another strategy to maximize an initial treatment regimen, especially for patients who have received only modest doses or those who for pharmacodynamic reasons have low serum drug levels despite adequate doses and adherence. Unfortunately, with the exception of nortriptyline, therapeutic windows for serum drug levels of most antidepressant medications are unknown. In addition, the strategy of increasing doses is often limited by the occurrence of more frequent and severe side effects.

b. Switching to a different non-MAOI agent

With the introduction of many newer antidepressant medications, switching to a different non-MAOI antidepressant medication has been a common strategy for patients who have failed a trial of pharmacotherapy. A few trials have been conducted in which patients who failed an initial antidepressant medication were switched to a non-MAOI antidepressant medication from the same pharmacologic class (e.g., from one tricyclic antidepressant to another) or to one from a different pharmacologic class (e.g., from a tricyclic antidepressant to an SSRI). Although results from these trials have been variable, up to 50% of patients have been found to respond to a second non-MAOI antidepressant medication trial (5). Data regarding the types of treatment-refractory patients who are most likely to benefit from particular switching strategies are limited. Although their use in this context has not been extensively evaluated, mood stabilizers such as carbamazepine and valproic acid have demonstrated some benefit in the treatment of medication-resistant major depressive disorder (175, 176).

c. Augmenting antidepressant medications with other treatments

Antidepressant medication augmentation strategies often consist of the use of multiple non-MAOI antidepressant medications. An SSRI in combination with a tricyclic agent, such as desipramine, has been reported to induce a rapid antidepressant medication response (50). However, SSRIs added to a tricyclic antidepressant medication may cause an increased blood level and delayed elimination of the tricyclic medication, predisposing the patient to tricyclic medication toxicity unless the dose of the tricyclic is reduced (177).

Lithium is another medication commonly used as an adjunct; other agents in use are thyroid hormone and stimulants. Lithium is felt by many experienced clinicians to be the most effective adjunct; it is reported to be useful in up to 50% of antidepressant medication nonresponders and is usually well tolerated (178). The interval before full response to adjunctive lithium is said to be in the range of several days to 3 weeks. The blood level required in this context has not yet been determined. If effective and well tolerated, lithium should be continued for the duration of treatment of the acute episode. Lithium may also increase the antidepressant medication effectiveness of carbamazepine (179). Thyroid hormone supplementation, even in euthyroid patients, may increase the effectiveness of antidepressant medication treatment (180). The dose proposed for this purpose is 25 µg/day of triiodothyronine, increased to 50 µg/day in a week or so in the event of continued nonresponse. The duration of treatment required has not been well studied. Case reports suggest that stimulant medications may be effective adjuncts to antidepressant medication therapy (181, 182). There are no clear guidelines regarding the length of time stimulants should be coadministered.

A rarely used strategy is the combined use of a tricyclic antidepressant medication and an MAOI. This combination has been shown to be effective in alleviating some severe medication-resistant major depressive disorders; however, the risk of toxic interactions necessitates careful monitoring (183, 184). The combined use of MAOIs and other antidepressant medications has in some circumstances led to serious untoward reactions characterized by delirium, hyperthermia, hyperreflexia, myoclonus, and death; the reaction is sometimes referred to as the serotonin syndrome and is thought to be the result of overly enhanced serotonergic transmission. Use of an MAOI in combination with a tricyclic antidepressant should probably not be considered until all other strategies for treatment-refractory patients have been exhausted; psychiatrists and patients choosing to use an MAOI and tricyclic antidepressant should be well acquainted with the potential hazards and carefully weigh the relative risks and benefits of such a strategy.

Data indicating the relative efficacies of the various adjunctive treatments are generally lacking.

d. Using a monoamine oxidase inhibitor

The role of MAOIs in major depressive disorder has largely become that of a treatment for patients who have failed other pharmacotherapies. Studies have demonstrated the effectiveness of MAOIs in patients who have failed to respond to other antidepressant medications, particularly tricyclic antidepressants (185). However, the effectiveness of MAOIs relative to other strategies for treatment-resistant patients remains unclear. Great care must be taken when switching patients from another antidepressant medication to an MAOI and from an MAOI to other antidepressant medications because of the persistence of the effects of discontinued medications and their metabolites and the potential for toxic interactions. For example, if the clinician chooses to discontinue a monoamine uptake blocking antidepressant medication and substitute an MAOI, toxic interactions can best be avoided by allowing a 1–2-week washout period between medication trials. The long half-life of the SSRI fluoxetine and its metabolites necessitates a 5-week washout period before the use of an MAOI.

e. Using ECT

ECT has the highest rate of response of any form of antidepressant treatment and should be considered in virtually all cases of moderate or severe major depressive disorder not responsive to pharmacologic intervention. Even medication-resistant patients may show at least a 50% likelihood of a satisfactory response to ECT (186). ECT may also be the strategy of choice for patients with major depressive disorder with psychotic symptoms who have not responded to an antidepressant medication plus antipsychotic medication. ECT is generally considered to be safer than many forms of combination antidepressant medication treatment, although data to support this are lacking. There is growing use of ECT combined with antidepressant medication to potentiate response, although only a small amount of data supporting this practice presently exists (72, 187–191). The safety of combining lithium and ECT has been questioned, although there are conflicting data (72, 192–195).

3. Electroconvulsive therapy

a. Efficacy

ECT has been shown in controlled clinical trials to have efficacy that is superior to placebo, simulated ECT, and antidepressant medication therapy (196). The proportion of patients with major depressive disorder who respond to ECT is high, with 80%–90% of those treated showing improvement (197). Results of several studies indicate that ECT can be effective in over half of patients with major depressive disorder who have failed antidepressant medication therapy (198–200).

The report of the APA Task Force on Electroconvulsive Therapy identified patient populations for whom ECT may be particularly beneficial and indicated (72, 201). ECT should be considered as the treatment choice for severe major depressive disorder when it is coupled with psychotic features, catatonic stupor, severe suicidality, or food refusal leading to nutritional compromise, as well as in other situations (such as pregnancy or when a particularly rapid antidepressant response is required). ECT is also indicated as a first-line treatment for patients who have previously shown a positive response to this treatment modality or who prefer it. It should be considered for all patients with functional impairment whose illness has not responded to medication or who have a medical condition that precludes the use of an antidepressant medication.

b. Side effects

ECT is generally a very safe treatment. However, although risks of morbidity and mortality in general do not exceed those associated with anesthesia alone, some types of serious medical conditions may have an increased risk with ECT as well as with other treatment modalities (72, 202–204). The chief side effects of ECT are cognitive. Treatment is associated with a transient postictal confusional state and with a longer period of anterograde and retrograde memory interference. The anterograde memory impairment, which has been difficult to disentangle from the memory deficits accompanying major depressive disorder itself, typically resolves in a few weeks after cessation of treatment (205). Some degree of retrograde amnesia, particularly for recent memories, may continue, at least for patients receiving bilateral ECT (72, 206–209). Rarely, patients report more pervasive and persistent cognitive disruption, the basis of which is uncertain (210).

ECT may have cardiovascular side effects, mediated by changes on the autonomic nervous system. ECT can cause a transient rise in heart rate, cardiac workload, and blood pressure, which may have deleterious effects on patients with cardiovascular disease, including recent myocardial infarction, congestive heart failure, and cardiac arrhythmias (211). The presence of significant cardiovascular disease in candidates for ECT is an indication for caution and general medical or cardiology consultation.

ECT has also been associated with a transient rise in intracranial pressure and blood-brain barrier permeability (212). For these reasons, patients with evidence of increased intracranial pressure or cerebrovascular fragility are at substantially greater risk and should only receive ECT after careful general medical, neurological, or neurosurgical evaluation (72, 78).

c. Implementation

The evaluation preceding ECT should consist of a psychiatric history and examination to verify the indication for this treatment, a general medical evaluation to define risk factors (including medical history and physical examination with cognitive assessment, vital signs, and any specifically indicated laboratory tests), anesthesia evaluation addressing the nature and extent of anesthetic risk and the need for modification of medications or anesthetic technique, the obtaining of informed consent, and, finally, an evaluation that summarizes treatment indications and risks and suggests any indicated additional evaluative procedures, alterations in treatment, or modifications in ECT technique (72). In assessing cases with indications for caution (e.g., recent myocardial infarction, cardiac arrhythmias, and intracranial-space-occupying lesions) the relative risks and benefits should be carefully weighed in collaboration with an anesthesiologist and a general medical physician, cardiologist, or neurologist, as the case requires.

ECT may be administered either bilaterally or unilaterally. Compared to bilateral treatment, unilateral placement induces less cognitive interference in most patients, but in some cases it is also less effective (213). When unilateral treatment is used, stimuli that are only marginally above seizure threshold exhibit a less satisfactory antidepressant medication effect than those of higher intensity, although this effect must be balanced against the cognitive interference evoked by grossly suprathreshold stimulation. In the event that unilateral treatment is initiated and the patient does not respond satisfactorily to the initial six treatments, bilateral treatment should be considered. Stimulus parameters vary from patient to patient but should be titrated to induce an adequate generalized seizure, which is typically at least 15–25 seconds in duration (72, 214, 215).

The total course of treatment should be such that maximal remission of symptoms is achieved, i.e., the patient fully recovers or reaches a plateau; typically this involves six to 12 treatments and generally does not exceed 20 treatments (72, 216). ECT is typically administered every other day; less frequent administration has been associated with less cognitive impairment but also a prolonged period until onset of action (217).

Patients should be maintained on antidepressant medication therapy or lithium following acute response to ECT (218). Patients who do not respond to such maintenance medication therapies may require maintenance ECT treatment (219).

4. Light therapy

Although several trials conducted during the 1980s demonstrated that bright light therapy was more effective than a dim-light control condition, some questions have been raised concerning the adequacy of the study designs (220). However, recent trials with more adequate control conditions have also demonstrated the effectiveness of bright light therapy over nonlight control conditions (221–223). On the basis of limited trial data, bright light therapy has been suggested as a first-line treatment in subsyndromal winter "blues" and as an adjunct in chronic major depressive disorder or dysthymia with seasonal exacerbations. Patients with history of reactivity to ambient light, hypersomnia, atypical negative symptoms, and overeating of sweet food in the afternoon have also been considered candidates for favorable response to light treatment. On the other hand, studies of the role of light therapy in premenstrual dysphoria or in older patients with nonseasonal major depressive disorder with advanced sleep phase disorder yielded equivocal results.

Side effects of light therapy include headache, eye strain, irritability, insomnia, and occasionally hypomania, which declines by decrease of exposure time and/or distance to light. Although patients with retinal diseases or ordinary photosensitivity, systemic lupus erythematosus, and history of skin cancer are vulnerable, none of these conditions is an absolute contraindication for light therapy. Each condition would require the attention and consultative supervision of the appropriate specialist if the light therapy is to be conducted.

A 10,000-lux intensity light box slanted toward the patient's face for 30 minutes/day either once or in two divided times is the preferred short-term treatment procedure. Timing may be designed to secure adherence. The late-night application is discouraged as it may cause insomnia. Duration of treatment is titrated according to the patient's reaction. Patients usually show improvement within 1 week, but at times the full response manifests over several weeks.

Patients who are responsive may be given light therapy at each episode of recurrence, presumably without any diminished efficacy. Prophylactic use of light therapy administered in the late fall and early winter is being explored. Combining light therapy with an antidepressant medication may potentiate the effectiveness of each agent. Such an approach may be useful if either or both therapies cannot be used in full therapeutic doses. The potential photosensitizing effect of antidepressant medications should be considered, and patients receiving both treatments should be advised to take appropriate precautions.

5. St. John's wort

St. John's wort is a whole plant product with antidepressant medication properties. Since it is not regulated as a drug by the FDA, preparations lack standardization regarding their contained ingredients and composition as well as potency.

A recent review of 14 short-term, double-blind (although the distinctive taste of St. John's wort extract may have caused some unblinding) trials conducted in outpatients with mild to moderate major depressive disorder symptoms demonstrated that St. John's wort had efficacy superior to placebo and generally comparable to low-dose tricyclic treatment (e.g., amitriptyline, 30–150 mg/day) (1). The proportion experiencing any side effect was lower among those taking St. John's wort than tricyclics (25% versus 40%) (1).

Although the doses of St. John's wort used in trials ranged between 300 and 1800 mg/day, differences in extract preparations make dose comparisons and the identification of optimal doses difficult. The combined use of St. John's wort with MAOIs is contraindicated. The safety and efficacy of the combined use of St. John's wort with other antidepressant medications is not known.

B. ACUTE PHASE PSYCHOSOCIAL INTERVENTIONS

1. Goals

There are a range of psychosocial interventions that may be useful in the acute treatment of major depressive disorder. Although various therapeutic approaches are discussed here and in the literature as distinct entities, such separate categorizations are primarily useful for heuristic or research purposes. In practice, psychiatrists use a combination or synthesis of various approaches and strategies; these in turn are determined by and individually tailored to each patient on the basis of that person's particular conditions and coping capacities. In actual application the techniques and the therapist-patient relationship are powerfully intertwined.

2. Efficacy

Evaluating the efficacy of psychotherapeutic approaches for major depressive disorder can be complicated by several problems. For some types of psychotherapeutic interventions, few or no clinical trials have been conducted. Those that have been conducted have compared psychotherapy to a variety of control conditions such as waiting lists, other forms of psychotherapy, medications, placebos, or no control group, making comparisons of the observed treatment effect sizes between trials difficult. Some trials have not examined the effects of psychotherapy exclusively among patients with major depressive disorder and may not have examined or adequately assessed, specifically, improvement in major depressive disorder as an outcome. In other trials, the nature of the psychotherapeutic intervention has involved a poor protocol or has been poorly described, thereby making generalization of the study results to psychotherapeutic approaches used in practice difficult.

a. Cognitive behavioral therapy

Cognitive behavioral therapy (also considered to include cognitive psychotherapy) maintains that irrational beliefs and distorted attitudes toward the self, the environment, and the future perpetuate depressive affects. The goal of cognitive behavioral therapy is to reduce depressive symptoms by challenging and reversing these beliefs and attitudes (224).

In the two decades since it was first evaluated as a treatment for major depressive disorder, cognitive behavioral therapy has been extensively studied in over 80 controlled trials. Based on different subsets of these trials, several meta-analytic studies have quantified the efficacy of cognitive behavioral therapy. Effect sizes for cognitive behavioral therapy compared to no treatment or minimal treatment have been fairly robust (generally near or above 1 standard deviation in the outcome measure) (53, 225–228). However, estimates from meta-analyses of the effectiveness of cognitive behavioral therapy relative to other treatments have been more inconsistent, probably because of differences in the criteria that were used to include or exclude trials (e.g., characteristics of study populations, interventions or control conditions, or outcome measures used). For example, some meta-analyses have concluded that effect sizes for cognitive behavioral therapy are larger than for pharmacotherapy (225–231), whereas others suggest they are equally effective (232). Effect sizes for cognitive behavioral therapy have generally been at least as large as, and in some cases larger than, for other forms of psychotherapy such as behavior therapy, interpersonal therapy, or brief dynamic psychotherapy (231).

There have been suggestions on the basis of individual clinical trials that the efficacy of cognitive behavioral therapy may differ on the basis of the severity of major depressive disorder. In subanalyses of the National Institute of Mental Health (NIMH) Treatment of Depression Collaborative Research Program study, cognitive behavioral therapy was observed to be less effective than imipramine plus clinical management among individuals with severe depression (defined as scores ≥20 on the Hamilton Rating Scale for Depression or ≤50 on the Global Assessment of Functioning); there was also a trend for cognitive behavioral therapy to be less effective than interpersonal therapy (233). No differences were observed between cognitive behavioral therapy, interpersonal therapy, imipramine plus clinical management, or placebo plus clinical management among less severely depressed subjects. Other trials have failed to show a differential responses to treatments on the basis of initial symptom severity possibly because of lack of statistical power (230, 234).

Several studies have used clinical trial data to identify other characteristics of patients that may be associated with differential response to cognitive behavioral therapy. Factors suggested as being associated with poor response to cognitive behavioral therapy include unemployment, male gender, comorbidity, dysfunctional attitudes, and several laboratory test values (e.g., abnormal sleep EEG results, increased hypothalamic-pituitary-adrenocortical activity, and increased T_4 (235–238). On the other hand, results from several analyses have suggested that cognitive behavioral therapy may be more effective than other treatments for depressed individuals with personality disorders (42, 239).

b. Behavior therapy

Behavior therapy of major depressive disorder is based on theoretical models drawn from behavior theory (240) and social learning theory (241). Specific behavior therapy techniques include activity scheduling (155, 242), self-control therapy (243), social skills training (244), and problem solving (245).

Although the efficacy of behavior therapy has been examined in a substantial number of trials, relatively few have employed random assignments and adequate control arms. Two meta-analyses that covered 10 of these trials have concluded that behavior therapy is superior to wait listing (observed in seven of eight trials) (92, 231). Results of individual clinical trials have suggested that behavior therapy may be superior in efficacy to brief dynamic psychotherapy (246, 247) and generally comparable in efficacy to cognitive therapy (248–251) or pharmacotherapy (252).

One post hoc examination of clinical trial data found that response to behavior therapy may be more likely in patients with less initial severity of major depressive disorder symptoms (253), whereas other studies have not (254–256). Among depressed adolescents, parental involvement has been found to predict response to behavior therapy (257).

c. Interpersonal therapy

Interpersonal therapy focuses on losses, role disputes and transitions, social isolation, deficits in social skills, and other interpersonal factors that may impact on the development of depression (258). Interpersonal therapy attempts to intervene by facilitating mourning and promoting recognition of related affects, resolving role disputes and transitions, and overcoming deficits in social skills to permit the acquisition of social supports.

In one trial conducted among depressed psychiatric patients, interpersonal therapy was found to be superior to nonscheduled controls and comparable to other active treatments, including cognitive therapy or antidepressant medication (231). In the NIMH Treatment of Depression Collaborative Research Program study, interpersonal therapy was also reported to be more effective than placebo plus clinical management and comparable to cognitive behavioral therapy or imipramine plus clinical management (42). However, in subanalyses, interpersonal therapy, cognitive behavioral therapy, and imipramine plus clinical management were no different from placebo plus clinical management among those with mild depression severity (defined as scores of

<20 on the Hamilton depression rating scale or >50 on the Global Assessment of Functioning); among those with more severe major depressive disorder, both interpersonal therapy and imipramine plus clinical management were more effective than either cognitive behavioral therapy or placebo plus clinical management (233, 259). A controlled trial of interpersonal therapy has also been conducted demonstrating the effectiveness of interpersonal therapy among depressed primary care patients (260). After 8 months, the proportions of patients treated with interpersonal therapy, nortriptyline, or usual care that achieved remission were 46%, 48%, and 18%, respectively.

Some recent studies have also suggested possible subgroups in whom interpersonal therapy may show differential efficacy. In one trial conducted among HIV-positive patients with major depressive disorder, significantly greater improvement was observed following interpersonal therapy than supportive therapy (261). In a subsequent study among depressed HIV-positive patients, greater improvements were observed after interpersonal therapy or interpersonal therapy plus imipramine than supportive psychotherapy or cognitive behavioral therapy (262). On the other hand, post hoc analyses of clinical trial data suggest that there may be an interaction between type of psychotherapy and dimensions of personality. Two such analyses have found that patients with major depressive disorder with personality disorders, particularly avoidant personality pathology, may be less responsive to interpersonal therapy than cognitive therapy (42, 263). Conversely, interpersonal therapy has been proposed to be more effective than cognitive therapy for patients with major depressive disorder with obsessive personality traits and for patients who are single and noncohabitating (264).

d. Psychodynamic psychotherapy

The term "psychodynamic psychotherapy" encompasses a number of psychotherapeutic interventions that may be brief or long-term in duration (265–267). These interventions share a basis in psychodynamic theories regarding the etiologic nature of psychological vulnerability, personality development, and symptom formation as shaped by developmental deficit and conflict occurring during the life cycle from earliest childhood forward (268–272). Some of these theories focus predominantly on conflicts related to guilt, shame, interpersonal relationships, the management of anxiety, and repressed or unacceptable impulses. Others are more focused on developmental psychological deficits produced by inadequacies or problems in the relationship between the child and emotional caretakers, resulting in problems of self-esteem, a sense of psychological cohesiveness, and emotional self-regulation (271, 273–277).

Psychodynamic psychotherapy is most often of longer-term duration than other psychotherapies and is usually associated with goals beyond that of immediate symptom relief. These goals are usually associated with an attempt to modify the underlying psychological conflicts and deficits that increase the patient's vulnerability to major depressive affect and the development of major depressive disorder. Psychodynamic psychotherapy is therefore much broader than most other psychotherapies, encompassing both current and past problems in interpersonal relationships, self-esteem, and developmental conflicts associated with anxiety, guilt, or shame. Time-limited, structured psychodynamic psychotherapy may focus more on understanding the psychological basis of the presenting symptoms or on a selected underlying conflict. It is often combined with psychopharmacologic intervention to reduce the major depressive disorder episode, which is consistent with the common belief that major depressive disorder is a biopsychosocial phenomenon. Sometimes a goal of psychodynamic psychotherapy, brief or extended, may be to help the patient accept or adhere to necessary pharmacotherapy (8).

Determining the efficacy of psychodynamic psychotherapy as a single modality in the treatment of major depressive disorder is complicated by two problems. First, many trials of psychodynamic psychotherapy for depression have included patients with conditions that would not meet DSM-IV criteria for major depressive disorder. Second, variations of psychodynamic psychotherapy have served in many studies as a nonspecific comparison treatment to other psychotherapeutic interventions; as a result, details of the psychodynamic psychotherapy employed have been poorly defined. Results of two meta-analyses suggest that brief psychodynamic psychotherapy for the treatment of major depressive disorder is more effective than a waiting list control condition but probably less effective than other forms of psychotherapy (92, 231). In one of these meta-analyses involving six trials (92), the proportions of patients considered to be responders to brief psychodynamic psychotherapy, cognitive therapy, interpersonal therapy, and behavioral therapy were 35%, 47%, 52%, and 55%, respectively. Research on the efficacy of combined pharmacotherapy and brief psychodynamic psychotherapy (278, 279) is also limited and inconclusive.

Although psychodynamic psychotherapy appears to be used widely in clinical practice, the efficacy of long-term psychodynamic psychotherapy in the acute phase of major depressive disorder has not been adequately studied in controlled trials.

e. Marital therapy and family therapy

Marital and family problems are common in the course of mood disorders, and comprehensive treatment often demands that these problems be assessed and addressed. Marital and family problems may be a consequence of major depressive disorder but may also increase vulnerability to major depressive disorder and in some instances retard recovery (280, 281). Techniques for using marital/family approaches for the treatment of major depressive disorder have been developed, including behavioral approaches (280), a psychoeducational approach, and a strategic marital therapy approach (9). Family therapy has also been used in the inpatient treatment of patients with major depressive disorder (282).

Studies of the efficacy of marital or family therapy, either as a primary or adjunctive treatment, have been conducted among patients with depressive symptoms and not among patients with, specifically, major depressive disorder. Based on data from 17 clinical trials of marital therapy, two reviews have concluded that it is an effective means for reducing major depressive disorder symptoms and risk of relapse (283, 284). Results from individual studies suggest that the efficacy of marital therapy and its effectiveness relative to other psychotherapies may depend on whether marital distress is present. In one study, a greater proportion of depressed subjects with marital distress responded to marital therapy than cognitive therapy (88% versus 71%); on the other hand, among depressed subjects without marital distress, a greater proportion responded to cognitive therapy than marital therapy (85% versus 55%) (285). In another study conducted among depressed subjects with marital discord, marital therapy and cognitive behavioral therapy were both equally effective and more effective than a wait list condition (286).

f. Group therapy

Specific types of psychotherapy for which there are some data to support that they may be effective in the treatment of depression when administered in a group format include cognitive behavioral therapy (287–289) and interpersonal therapy (290–291).

Although there have been meta-analyses of the relative effectiveness of psychotherapeutic approaches conducted in a group format versus an individual format, these have not specifically involved studies of patients with rigorously defined major depressive disorder (292–295).

On the basis of very limited controlled study, supportive group therapy has also been suggested to be useful in the treatment of major depressive disorder. For example, one recent study conducted among depressed outpatients found that a mutual support group and cognitive behavioral therapy in a group format were equally effective in reducing depressive symptoms among depressed outpatients (287). In another study of patients with mild to moderate major depressive disorder who were also HIV positive, treatment with structured supportive group therapy plus placebo yielded similar decreases in depressive symptoms as structured group therapy plus fluoxetine (296). Individuals experiencing bereavement or such common stressors as chronic illness may particularly benefit from the example of others who have successfully dealt with the same or similar challenges. Survivors are offered the opportunity to gain enhanced self-esteem by making themselves models for others, and they offer newer patients successful role models.

Medication maintenance support groups may also offer benefits, although data from controlled trials among patients with major depressive disorder are lacking. Such groups provide information to the patient and to family members regarding prognosis and medication issues, thereby providing a psychoeducational forum that makes a chronic mental illness understandable in the context of a medical model.

The efficacy of self-help groups led by lay members (297) in the treatment of major depressive disorder has not been well studied. However, one recent investigation of group therapies found that a higher proportion of depressed outpatients had remitted following treatment in groups led by professionals than in groups led by nonprofessionals (287). The possibility that self-help support groups comprising individuals with major depressive disorder may serve a useful role by enhancing the support network and self-esteem of participating patients and their families requires future study.

3. Side effects

In general, psychotherapeutic treatments are relatively safe and well tolerated interventions. Psychotherapeutic approaches that may employ exposure to unpleasant situations (e.g., behavior therapy, cognitive behavioral therapy) may initially increase distress in patients. Psychotherapy that requires considerable time or patience to practice frequent exercises may be poorly tolerated.

One imperfect measure of the relative side effects and tolerability of psychotherapy can be obtained from the dropout rates in clinical trials; however, many other factors can also affect these rates (e.g., other burdens of the research trial, specific features of the clinical management provided). In the NIMH Treatment of Depression Collaborative Research Program, dropout rates during 16 weeks of treatment with interpersonal therapy, cognitive behavioral therapy, imipramine plus clinical management, or placebo plus clinical management were 23%, 32%, 33%, and 40%, respectively (259).

4. Implementation

There can be a variety of methods for conducting psychotherapeutic interventions, both between and within specific types of psychotherapy.

Clinical considerations and other patient factors should be considered in determinations of the nature and intensity of psychosocial interventions. Generally, dynamic psychotherapy is conducted in a less directive manner than behavioral psychotherapy; transference considerations and the patient's freedom to associate into unexpected material are taken into account. More behaviorally oriented psychotherapy on the other hand may be conducted in a more structured manner and require patients to be instructed in practice exercises and monitoring techniques.

There are little data available on optimal length of psychosocial interventions. In many trials, cognitive behavioral therapy has been delivered in approximately 12 weekly sessions and interpersonal therapy has been delivered in 16–20 weekly sessions. In a subanalysis of one clinical trial, cognitive behavioral therapy delivered in 16 weeks was more effective than cognitive behavioral therapy delivered in 8 weeks among those with severe major depressive disorder (298).

▶ C. PSYCHOTHERAPY COMBINED WITH PHARMACOTHERAPY

Several reviews of trials of the combination of psychotherapy and pharmacotherapy for patients with mild to moderate major depressive disorder have failed to find the combination to be superior to either treatment modality alone (92, 299). On the other hand, among patients with severe or recurrent major depressive disorder, the combination of psychotherapy (including interpersonal therapy, cognitive behavioral therapy, behavior therapy, or brief dynamic therapy) and pharmacotherapy has been found to be superior to treatment with a single modality in individual studies (38, 300–304) and a meta-analysis (305).

Results from a series of recent studies provide indirect evidence that for patients who have had only a partial response to pharmacotherapy, adding a course of cognitive behavioral therapy may be an effective strategy for preventing relapse (306–309).

▶ D. CONTINUATION TREATMENT

The continuation phase of treatment is generally considered to be the 16–20 weeks after achieving full remission. The goal of continuation treatment is to prevent relapse in the vulnerable period immediately following symptomatic recovery. Several studies have shown that if antidepressant medications are discontinued following recovery, approximately 25% of patients will relapse within 2 months (92, 310, 311). There is evidence that patients who do not completely recover during acute treatment have a significantly higher risk of relapse than those who have no residual symptoms and are especially in need of treatment in later phases (312).

Although randomized controlled trials of antidepressant medications in the continuation phase are limited, the available data indicate that patients treated for a first episode of uncomplicated major depressive disorder who exhibit a satisfactory response to an antidepressant medication should continue to receive a full therapeutic dose of that agent for at least 16–20 weeks after achieving and maintaining full remission (1, 313, 314).

There is some evidence that patients who are given cognitive behavioral therapy in the acute phase have a lower rate of relapse than those who receive then discontinue antidepressant medications in the acute phase and an equivalent relapse rate to those who take antidepressant medication in the continuation phase (234). There have also been a few recent studies of treatment with psychotherapeutic interventions administered in the continuation phase. One study found that among patients who responded to acute treatment with cognitive therapy, those who continued this treatment over 2 years had lower relapse rates than those who did not have continuation treatment (315). Results from a series of studies (307, 309, 316) suggest that cognitive behavioral therapy may be an effective continuation treatment following antidepressant medication therapy for preventing relapse (306).

When treatments are ultimately tapered and discontinued after the continuation phase, patients should be carefully monitored during and immediately after discontinuation to ensure that remission is stable. Patients who have had multiple prior episodes of major depressive disorder should be considered for maintenance medication treatment.

E. MAINTENANCE TREATMENT

Major depressive disorder is, for many, a recurrent disorder. Among those suffering from an episode of major depressive disorder, between 50% and 85% will go on to have at least one lifetime recurrence, usually within 2 or 3 years (310). Factors that have been found to be associated with a higher risk of recurrence appear in table 2. Factors that have been found to be associated with increased severity of subsequent episodes include a history of a prior episode complicated by serious suicide attempts, psychotic features, or severe functional impairment.

Among the therapeutic options available for maintenance treatment, antidepressant medications have received the most study. There have been over 20 trials of pharmacotherapy in the maintenance phase and results from these have generally demonstrated the effectiveness of antidepressant medication for relapse prevention (317); these trials have mainly been of tricyclic antidepressant medications (318, 319), although six trials involved newer antidepressant medications (1). Information to assist in the full range of clinical decisions regarding medication use in the maintenance phase is more limited. Results from one study suggest that full doses are superior to lower doses in the maintenance phase, despite the fact that lower doses are less likely to produce side effects (320).

There have been fewer investigations of the effectiveness of psychotherapy in the maintenance phase. In one study, maintenance cognitive therapy delivered over 2 years was as effective as maintenance medication for recurrent major depressive disorder (228). Another report suggests the interpersonal psychotherapy during the maintenance phase may be effective in lengthening the interepisode interval in some less severely ill patients not receiving medication (318).

The combined use of psychotherapy, such as cognitive behavioral therapy, cognitive therapy, or interpersonal therapy, and pharmacotherapy in the maintenance phase has also been considered by investigators, and some results suggest that the combination of antidepressant medications plus psychotherapy may be additionally effective in preventing relapse over treatment with single modalities (307, 318, 319, 321, 322).

ECT has also been used in the maintenance phase, although evidence for its benefits comes largely from case reports (197, 219, 323, 324). The optimal frequency and duration of maintenance phase ECT treatments has not been well studied.

The timing and method of discontinuing maintenance treatment has not been systematically studied. However, the risk of cholinergic rebound observed with abrupt discontinuation of some antidepressant medications together with concerns about major depressive disorder recurrences after the discontinuation of any antidepressant medication argue in favor of gradual tapering (325).

PART C:
FUTURE RESEARCH NEEDS

Notable progress has been made in our understanding of major depressive disorder and its treatment, including the introduction of a variety of therapeutic agents and treatment modalities. However, many issues remain regarding how to optimally use these treatments to achieve the best health outcomes for patients with major depressive disorder. The following are a few of the types of research questions that require future study.

VI. ANTIDEPRESSANT MEDICATIONS

In terms of the use of antidepressant medications during the acute, continuation, and maintenance phases of treatment, many important questions remain.

1. What are the specific clinical indications for the use of particular antidepressant medications?
2. What are the relative efficacies of different antidepressant medications?
3. What are the relationships between antidepressant blood levels and response?
4. What are the relative risks of toxicities (e.g., cardiotoxicity) and adverse effects for different antidepressant medications?
5. What should the duration of treatment be before a patient is considered medication-resistant, and does this duration vary among agents?
6. Does the combination of antidepressants from different pharmacologic classes (e.g., SSRIs and tricyclic antidepressants) offer greater efficacy than administration of single agents?
7. What are the comparative efficacies of different antidepressant medications in the continuation and maintenance phases?
8. What are the long-term side effects of chronic use of specific antidepressant medications?
9. What is the required duration of maintenance treatment with antidepressants?
10. What are indications for a trial of discontinuation of maintenance treatment?

VII. PSYCHOTHERAPY

Many issues concerning the use of psychotherapy in the treatment of major depressive disorder during the acute, continuation, and maintenance phases also require clarification. The disparity between the widespread use of psychodynamic psychotherapy in practice, and the complete lack of rigorous studies of its efficacy, must be addressed. In particular, there is a critical need to design and implement rigorous, controlled studies to evaluate the efficacy and effectiveness of psychodynamic psychotherapy for the treatment of patients with major depressive disorder.

In addition, the following are critical issues:

1. What are the relative efficacies of different psychotherapeutic approaches in the acute phase of treatment?
2. What components or aspects of specific psychotherapeutic approaches are responsible for efficacy? What common elements of all effective psychotherapeutic approaches are responsible for efficacy?
3. What are the indications (e.g., subtypes of depressive disorders) for use of various forms of psychotherapy?
4. What are the efficacies of particular psychotherapeutic approaches in the continuation and maintenance phases of treatment?
5. Is the use of multiple forms of psychotherapy, either concurrently or sequentially, effective?
6. What are the optimal frequencies of psychotherapeutic contact for the various forms of psychotherapy in the acute, continuation, and maintenance phases?

VIII. ECT

Regarding ECT, additional research is needed to clarify several important issues.

1. What are indications for initial treatment with bilateral electrode placement?
2. After how many unilateral treatments without satisfactory response should a switch from unilateral to bilateral electrode placement be made?
3. Can the efficacy or tolerability of ECT be increased with adjunctive antidepressant and antipsychotic agents?
4. What are the indications and best methods for providing maintenance ECT?

IX. OTHER TREATMENT MODALITIES

In addition to research on the treatments covered above, additional rigorous investigation is needed to answer questions concerning other therapeutic modalities.

1. What are the indications, relative efficacies, and safety of specific treatments such as lithium or thyroid hormone as adjuncts to antidepressant medications for nonresponders?
2. Is light therapy effective as an adjunct in nonseasonal major depressive disorder or as a primary treatment for seasonal major depressive disorder in the maintenance phase?

X. INDIVIDUALS AND ORGANIZATIONS THAT SUBMITTED COMMENTS

David A. Adler, M.D.
Carl Bell, M.D.
Dan G. Blazer II, M.D., Ph.D.
Philip Boyce, M.D.
David S. Brody, M.D.
Robert M. Chaflin, M.D.
Margaret J. Dorfman, M.D.
Peter Ellis, Ph.D.
Aaron H. Fink, M.D.
Michael Gales, M.D.
Linda Gochfeld, M.D.
David A. Gorelick, M.D., Ph.D.
James A. Greene, M.D.
Diane Keddy, M.S., R.D.
Sidney H. Kennedy, M.D.
Donald F. Klein, M.D.

James H. Kocsis, M.D.
K. Roy Mackenzie, M.D.
John C. Markowitz, M.D.
David A. Moltz, M.D.
Vaughn I. Rickert, Psy.D.
Peter Ross
Teresa A. Rummans, M.D.
Henry L. Shapiro, M.D.
Don Smith
   Michael Thase, M.D.
Richard Weiner, M.D., Ph.D.
Josef H. Weissberg, M.D.
Myrna M. Weissman, Ph.D.
Rhonda Whitson, R.R.A.
William M. Zurhellen, M.D.

American Academy of Psychoanalysis
American Association of Community Psychiatrists
American College of Emergency Physicians
American Dietetic Association
American Society of Clinical Psychopharmacology, Inc.
Black Psychiatrists of America
Royal Australian & New Zealand College of Psychiatrics
Society for Adolescent Medicine

XI. REFERENCES

The following coding system is used to indicate the nature of the supporting evidence in the references:

[A]   *Randomized clinical trial.* A study of an intervention in which subjects are prospectively followed over time; there are treatment and control groups; subjects are randomly assigned to the two groups; both the subjects and the investigators are blind to the assignments.

[B]   *Clinical trial.* A prospective study in which an intervention is made and the results of that intervention are tracked longitudinally; study does not meet standards for a randomized clinical trial.

[C]   *Cohort or longitudinal study.* A study in which subjects are prospectively followed over time without any specific intervention.

[D] *Case-control study.* A study in which a group of patients and a group of control subjects are identified in the present and information about them is pursued retrospectively or backward in time.

[E] *Review with secondary analysis.* A structured analytic review of existing data, e.g., a meta-analysis or a decision analysis.

[F] *Review.* A qualitative review and discussion of previously published literature without a quantitative synthesis of the data.

[G] *Other.* Textbooks, expert opinion, case reports, and other reports not included above.

1. Agency for Healthcare Policy Research: Evidence Report on Treatment of Depression—Newer Pharmacotherapies. San Antonio Evidence-Based Practice Center. Washington, DC, AHCPR, Evidence-Based Practice Centers, 1999 [F]

2. American Psychiatric Association: Practice Guideline for the Treatment of Patients With Bipolar Disorder. Am J Psychiatry 1994; 151(Dec suppl) [G]

3. American Psychiatric Association: Practice Guideline for Psychiatric Evaluation of Adults. Am J Psychiatry 1995; 152(Nov suppl):63–80 [G]

4. Lin EHB, von Korff M, Katon W, Bush T, Simon GE, Walker E, Robinson P: The role of the primary care physician in patients' adherence to antidepressant therapy. Med Care 1995; 33:67–74 [B]

5. Thase ME, Rush AJ: Treatment-resistant depression, in Psychopharmacology: The Fourth Generation of Progress. Edited by Bloom F, Kupfer DJ. New York, Raven Press, 1995, pp 1081–1097 [F]

6. Frank E, Kupfer DJ: Axis II personality disorders and personality features in treatment-resistant and refractory depression, in Treatment Strategies for Refractory Depression. Edited by Roose SP, Glassman AH. Washington, DC, American Psychiatric Press, 1990, pp 207–221 [F]

7. Goldman W, McCulloch J, Cuffel B, Zarin DA, Suarez A, Burns BJ: Outpatient utilization patterns of integrated and split psychotherapy and pharmacotherapy for depression. Psychiatr Serv 1998; 49:477–482 [G]

8. Gray SH: Developing practice guidelines for psychoanalysis. J Psychother Pract Res 1996; 5:213–227 [F]

9. Coyne JC: Strategic therapy, in Affective Disorders and the Family: Assessment and Treatment. Edited by Clarkin JF, Haas GL, Glick JD. New York, Guilford, 1988, pp 89–113 [F]

10. Lejoyeux M, Ades J: Antidepressant discontinuation: a review of the literature. J Clin Psychiatry 1997; 58(suppl 7):11–16 [F]

11. Coupland NJ, Bell CJ, Potokar JP: Serotonin reuptake inhibitor withdrawal. J Clin Psychopharmacol 1996; 16:356–362 [D]

12. Glassman AH, Roose SP: Delusional depression. Arch Gen Psychiatry 1981; 38:424–427 [E]

13. Spiker DG, Weiss JC, Dealy RS, Griffin SJ, Hanin I, Neil JF, Perel JM, Rossi AJ, Soloff PH: The pharmacological treatment of delusional depression. Am J Psychiatry 1985; 142:430–436 [A]

14. Price LH, Conwell Y, Nelson JC: Lithium augmentation of combined neuroleptic-tricyclic treatment in delusional depression. Am J Psychiatry 1983; 140:318–322 [E]

15. Kantor SJ, Glassman AH: Delusional depression: natural history and response to treatment. Br J Psychiatry 1977; 131:351–360 [E]

16. Fink M, Taylor MA: Catatonia: a separate category for DSM-IV? Integrative Psychiatry 1991; 7:2–10 [G]

17. Liebowitz MR, Quitkin FM, Stewart JW, McGrath PJ, Harrison WM, Markowitz JS, Rabkin JG, Tricamo E, Goetz DM, Klein DF: Antidepressant specificity in atypical depression. Arch Gen Psychiatry 1988; 45:129–137 [A]

18. Davidson JR, Miller R, Turnbull CD, Sullivan JL: Atypical depression. Arch Gen Psychiatry 1982; 39:527–534 [G]

19. Quitkin FM, Harrison W, Stewart JW, McGrath PJ, Tricamo E, Ocepek-Welikson K, Rabkin JG, Wager SG, Nunes E, Klein DF: Response to phenelzine and imipramine in placebo non-responders with atypical depression: a new application of the crossover design. Arch Gen Psychiatry 1991; 48:319–323 [A]

20. Quitkin FM, Stewart JW, McGrath PJ, Liebowitz MR, Harrison WM, Tricamo E, Klein DF, Rabkin JG, Markowitz JS, Wager SG: Phenelzine versus imipramine in the treatment of probable atypical depression: defining syndrome boundaries of selective MAOI responders. Am J Psychiatry 1988; 145:306–311 [A]

21. Goodnick PJ: Acute and long-term bupropion therapy: response and side effects. Ann Clin Psychiatry 1991; 3:311–313 [C]

22. Goodnick PJ, Extein I: Bupropion and fluoxetine in depressive subtypes. Ann Clin Psychiatry 1989; 1:119–122 [C]

23. Pande AC, Birkett M, Fechner-Bates S, Haskett RF, Greden JF: Fluoxetine versus phenelzine in atypical depression. Biol Psychiatry 1996; 40:1017–1020 [A]

24. Sands BF, Ciraulo DA: Cocaine drug-drug interactions. J Clin Psychopharmacol 1992; 12:49–55 [G]

25. Grunhaus L: Clinical and psychobiological characteristics of simultaneous panic disorder and major depression. Am J Psychiatry 1988; 145:1214–1221 [G]

26. Schatzberg AF, Ballenger JC: Decisions for the clinician in the treatment of panic disorder: when to treat, which treatment to use, and how long to treat. J Clin Psychiatry 1991; 52:26–31 [G]

27. Sheehan DV, Davidson JR, Manschreck T, Van Wyck Fleet J: Lack of efficacy of a new antidepressant (bupropion) in the treatment of panic disorder with phobias. J Clin Psychopharmacol 1983; 3:28–31 [C]

28. Clomipramine Collaborative Study Group: Clomipramine in the treatment of patients with obsessive-compulsive disorder. Arch Gen Psychiatry 1991; 48:730–738 [A]

29. Jenike MA, Buttolph L, Baer L, Ricciardi J, Holland A: Open trial of fluoxetine in obsessive-compulsive disorder. Am J Psychiatry 1989; 146:909–911 [A]

30. Stoudemire A, Hill C, Gulley LR, Morris R: Neuropsychological and biomedical assessment of depression-dementia syndromes. J Neuropsychiatry Clin Neurosci 1989; 1:347–361 [C]

31. Caine ED: Pseudodementia: current concepts and future directions. Arch Gen Psychiatry 1981; 38:1359–1364 [G]

32. Akiskal HS, Rosenthal TL, Haykal RF, Lemmi H, Rosenthal RH: Characterological depressions: clinical and sleep EEG findings separating subaffective dysthymias from character spectrum disorders. Arch Gen Psychiatry 1980; 37:777–783 [B]

33. Howland RH: Pharmacotherapy of dysthymia: a review. J Clin Psychopharmacol 1991; 11:83–92 [G]

34. Keller MD, Hanks DL, Klein DN: Summary of the DSM-IV mood disorders field trial and issue overview. Psychiatr Clin North Am 1996; 19:1–28 [F]

35. Thase ME, Reynolds CF, Frank E, Simons AD: Response to cognitive-behavioral therapy in chronic depression. J Psychotherapy Practice and Research 1994; 3:204–214 [B]

36. Conte HR, Karasu TB: A review of treatment studies of minor depression 1980–1981. Am J Psychother 1992; 46:58–74 [F]

37. Frances AJ: An introduction to dysthymia. Psychiatr Annals 1993; 23:607–608 [F]

38. Keller MD, McCullough JP, Rush AJ, Klein DF, Schatzberg AF, Gelenberg J, Thase ME: Nefazodone HCl, cognitive behavioral analysis system of psychotherapy and combination therapy for the acute treatment of chronic depression, in 1999 Annual Meeting New Research Program and Abstracts. Washington, DC, American Psychiatric Association, 1999, p 178 [A]

39. Kocsis JH, Frances AJ, Voss CB, Mann JJ, Mason BJ, Sweeney J: Imipramine treatment for chronic depression. Arch Gen Psychiatry 1988; 45:253–257 [A]

40. Shea MT, Glass DR, Pilkonis PA, Watkins J, Docherty JP: Frequency and implications of personality disorders in a sample of depressed outpatients. J Personal Disord 1987; 1:27–42 [C]

41. Parsons B, Quitkin FM, McGrath PJ, Stewart JW, Tricamo E, Ocepek-Welikson K, Harrison W, Rabkin JG, Wager SG, Nunes E: Phenelzine, imipramine, and placebo in borderline patients meeting criteria for atypical depression. Psychopharmacol Bull 1989; 25:524–534 [A]

42. Shea MT, Pilkonis PA, Beckham E, Collins JF, Elkin I, Sotsky SM, Docherty JP: Personality disorders and treatment outcome in the NIMH Treatment of Depression Collaborative Research Program. Am J Psychiatry 1990; 147:711–718 [A]

43. Rosenthal NE, Sack DA, Carpenter CJ, Parry BL, Mendelson WB, Wehr TA: Antidepressant effects of light in seasonal affective disorder. Am J Psychiatry 1985; 142:163–170 [C]

44. American Psychiatric Association: Diagnostic and Statistical Manual of Mental Disorders, 4th ed. Washington, DC, APA, 1994 [G]

45. Zisook S, Shuchter SR: Depression through the first year after the death of a spouse. Am J Psychiatry 1991; 148:1346–1352 [C]

46. Escobar JI, Gomez J, Tuason VB: Depressive phenomenology in North and South American patients. Am J Psychiatry 1983; 140:47–51 [C]

47. Escobar JI, Tuason VB: Antidepressant agents: a cross-cultural study. Psychopharmacol Bull 1980; 16:49–52 [C]

48. Marcos LR, Cancro R: Psychopharmacotherapy of Hispanic depressed patients: clinical observations. Am J Psychother 1982; 36:505–512 [F]

49. Marcos LR, Uruyo L, Kesselman M, Alpert M: The language barrier in evaluating Spanish-American patients. Arch Gen Psychiatry 1973; 29:655–659 [C]

50. Nelson JC, Mazure CM, Bowers MBJ, Jatlow PI: A preliminary, open study of the combination of fluoxetine and desipramine for rapid treatment of major depression. Arch Gen Psychiatry 1991; 48:303–307 [C]

51. American Academy of Child and Adolescent Psychiatry: Practice Parameters for the Assessment and Treatment of Children and Adolescents With Depressive Disorders. Washington, DC, AACAP, 1998 [G]

52. Reynolds CF, Frank E, Perel JM, Imber SD, Cornes C, Miller MD, Mazumdar S, Houck PR, Dew MA, Stack JA, Pollock BG, Kupfer DJ: Nortriptyline and interpersonal psychotherapy as maintenance therapies for recurrent major depression: a randomized controlled trial in patients older than 59 years. JAMA 1999; 281:39–45 [A]

53. Robinson RG, Starkstein SE: Current research in affective disorders following stroke. J Neuropsychiatry Clin Neurosci 1990; 2:1–14 [F]

54. Nelson JC, Jatlow PI, Mazure CM: Rapid desipramine dose adjustment using 24-hour levels. J Clin Psychopharmacol 1987; 7:72–77 [C]

55. Wisner KL, Gelenberg AJ, Leonard H, Zarin D, Frank E: Pharmacologic treatment of depression during pregnancy. JAMA 1999; 282:1264–1269 [F]

56. Chambers CD, Johnson KA, Dick LM, Felix RJ, Jones KL: Birth outcomes in pregnant women taking fluoxetine. N Engl J Med 1996; 335:1010–1015 [B]

57. Nurnberg HG: An overview of somatic treatment of psychosis during pregnancy and postpartum. Gen Hosp Psychiatry 1989; 11:328–338 [G]

58. Gitlin MJ, Pasnau RO: Psychiatric syndromes linked to reproductive function in women: a review of current knowledge. Am J Psychiatry 1989; 146:1413–1422 [G]

59. Brockington IF, Cernik KF, Schofield EM, Downing AR, Francis AF, Keelan C: Puerperal psychosis: phenomena and diagnosis. Arch Gen Psychiatry 1981; 38:829–833 [C]

60. Ananth J: Side effects in the neonate from psychotropic agents excreted through breast feeding. Am J Psychiatry 1978; 135:801–805 [E]

61. Altshuler LL, Cohen L, Szuba MP, Burt VK, Gitlin M, Mintz J: Pharmacologic management of psychiatric illness during pregnancy: dilemmas and guidelines. Am J Psychiatry 1996; 153: 592–606 [E]

62. Akiskal HS, Walker P, Puzantian VR, King D, Rosenthal TL, Dranon M: Bipolar outcome in the course of depressive illness: phenomenologic, familial, and pharmacologic predictors. J Affect Disord 1983; 5:115–128 [A]

63. Nelson JC, Kennedy JS, Pollock BG, Laghrissi-Thode F, Narayan M, Nobler MS, Robin DW, Gergel I, McCafferty J, Roose S: Treatment of major depression with nortriptyline and paroxetine in patients with ischemic heart disease. Am J Psychiatry 1999; 156:1024–1028 [A]

64. Bigger JT, Giardina EG, Perel JM, Kantor SJ, Glassman AH: Cardiac antiarrhythmic effect of imipramine hydrochloride. N Engl J Med 1977; 296:206–208 [E]

65. Connolly SJ, Mitchell LB, Swerdlow CD, Mason JW, Winkle RA: Clinical efficacy and electrophysiology of imipramine for ventricular tachycardia. Am J Cardiol 1984; 53:516–521 [E]

66. Dalack GW, Roose SP, Glassman AH: Tricyclics and heart failure (letter). Am J Psychiatry 1991; 148:1601 [E]

67. Giardina EG, Barnard T, Johnson L, Saroff AL, Bigger JT, Louie M: The antiarrhythmic effect of nortriptyline in cardiac patients with ventricular premature depolarizations. J Am Coll Cardiol 1986; 7:1363–1369 [E]

68. Glassman AH, Johnson LL, Giardina EG, Walsh BT, Roose SP, Cooper TB, Bigger JT: The use of imipramine in depressed patients with congestive heart failure. JAMA 1983; 250:1997–2001 [C]

69. Roose SP, Glassman AH, Giardina EG, Walsh BT, Woodring S, Bigger JT: Tricyclic antidepressants in depressed patients with cardiac conduction disease. Arch Gen Psychiatry 1987; 44:273–275 [A]

70. Schwartz P, Wolf S: QT interval prolongation as predictor of sudden death in patients with myocardial infarction. Circulation 1978; 57:1074–1077 [E]

71. Applegate RJ: Diagnosis and management of ischemic heart disease in the patient scheduled to undergo electroconvulsive therapy. Convuls Ther 1997; 13:128–144 [F]

72. The Practice of Electroconvulsive Therapy: Recommendations for Treatment, Training, and Privileging: A Task Force Report of the American Psychiatric Association. Washington, DC, APA, 1990 [E]

73. Dolinski SY, Zvara DA: Anesthetic considerations of cardiovascular risk during electroconvulsive therapy. Convuls Ther 1997; 13:157–164 [E]

74. Rayburn BK: Electroconvulsive therapy in patients with heart failure or valvular heart disease. Convuls Ther 1997; 13:145–156 [F]

75. Weiner RD, Coffey CE, Krystal AD: Electroconvulsive therapy in the medical and neurologic patient, in Psychiatric Care of the Medical Patient, 2nd ed. Edited by Stoudemire A, Fogel B. Greenberg D. New York, Oxford University Press, 1999 [F]

76. Roose SP, Dalack GW, Glassman AH, Woodring S, Walsh BT, Giardina EGV: Cardiovascular effects of bupropion in depressed patients with heart disease. Am J Psychiatry 1991; 148:512–516 [C]

77. Roose SP, Glassman AH, Giardina EG, Johnson L, Walsh BT, Bigger JT: Cardiovascular effects of imipramine and bupropion in depressed patients with congestive heart failure. J Clin Psychopharmacol 1987; 7:247–251 [A]

78. Krystal AD, Coffey CE: Neuropsychiatric considerations in the use of electroconvulsive therapy. J Neuropsychiatry Clin Neurosci 1997; 9:283–292 [F]

79. Lieberman E, Stoudemire A: Use of tricyclic antidepressants in patients with glaucoma. Psychosomatics 1987; 28:145–148 [G]

80. Thase ME: Effects of venlafaxine on blood pressure: a meta-analysis of original data on 3744 depressed patients. J Clin Psychiatry 1998; 59:502–508 [E]

81. Goetz CG, Tanner CM, Klawans HL: Bupropion in Parkinson's disease. Neurology 1984; 34:1092–1094 [C]

82. Monoamine oxidase inhibitors for depression. Med Lett Drugs Ther 1980; 22:58–60 [G]

83. Andersen K, Balldin J, Gottfries CG, Granerus AK, Modigh K, Svennerholm L, Wallin A: A double-blind evaluation of electroconvulsive therapy in Parkinson's disease with on-off phenomena. Acta Neurol Scand 1987; 76:191–199 [A]

84. Regier DA, Boyd JH, Burke JD Jr, Rae DS, Myers JK, Kramer M, Robins LN, George LK, Karno M, Locke BZ: One-month prevalence of mental disorders in the United States: based on five Epidemiologic Catchment Area sites. Arch Gen Psychiatry 1988; 45:977–986 [A]

85. Pincus HA, Zarin DZ, Tanielian TL, Johnson JL, West JC, Petit AR, Marcus SC, Kessler RC, McIntyre JS: Psychiatric patients and treatments in 1997: findings from the American Psychiatric Practice Research Network. Arch Gen Psychiatry 1999; 56:442–449 [C]

86. Mueller TI, Leon AC, Keller MB, Solomon DA, Endicott J, Coryell W, Warshaw M, Maser JD: Recurrence after recovery from major depressive disorder during 15 years of observational follow-up. Am J Psychiatry 1999; 156:1000–1006 [B]

87. Klerman GL, Weissman MM: The course, morbidity and costs of depression. Arch Gen Psychiatry 1992; 49:831–834 [G]

88. Keller MD, Beardslee WR, Dorer DJ, Lavori PW, Samuelson H, Klerman GL: Impact of severity and chronicity of parental affective illness on adaptive functioning and psychopathology in children. Arch Gen Psychiatry 1986; 43:930–937 [B]

89. Mintz J, Mintz LI, Arruda MJ, Hwang SS: Treatments of depression and the functional capacity to work. Arch Gen Psychiatry 1992; 49:761–768 [G]

90. Kuhn R: The treatment of depressive states with G22355 (imipramine hydrochloride). Am J Psychiatry 1958; 115:459–464 [B]

91. Brotman AW, Falk WE, Gelenberg AJ: Pharmacologic treatment of acute depressive subtypes, in Psychopharmacology: The Third Generation of Progress. Edited by Meltzer HY. New York, Raven Press, 1987, pp 1031–1040 [F]

92. Depression Guideline Panel: Clinical Practice Guideline Number 5: Depression in Primary Care, Treatment of Major Depression: HHS Publication 93-0551. Rockville, Md, Agency for Health Care Policy and Research, 1993 [E]

93. Klein DF, Gittelman R, Quitkin FM, Rifkin A: Diagnosis and Drug Treatment of Psychiatric Disorders: Adults and Children, 2nd ed. Baltimore, Md, Williams & Wilkins, 1980 [G]

94. Klerman GL, Cole JO: Clinical pharmacology of imipramine and related antidepressant compounds. Int J Psychiatry 1967; 3:267–304 [F]

95. Potter WZ, Manji HK, Rudorfer MV: Tricyclics and tetracyclics, in American Psychiatric Press Textbook of Psychopharmacology, 2nd ed. Edited by Schatzberg AF, Nemeroff CB. Washington, DC, American Psychiatric Press, 1998, pp 199–218 [F]

96. Coryell W, Turner R: Outcome and desipramine therapy in subtypes of non-psychotic major depression. J Affect Disord 1985; 9:149–154 [B]

97. Fairchild CJ, Rush AJ, Vasavada N, Giles DE, Khatami M: Which depressions respond to placebo? Psychiatry Res 1986; 18:217–226 [B]

98. Joyce PR, Paykel ES: Predictors of drug response in depression. Arch Gen Psychiatry 1989; 46:89–99 [F]

99. Stewart JW, Quitkin FM, Liebowitz MR, McGrath PJ, Harrison WM, Klein DF: Efficacy of desipramine in depressed outpatients: response according to Research Diagnostic Criteria diagnoses and severity of illness. Arch Gen Psychiatry 1989; 40:220–227 [A]

100. Paykel ES: Depressive typologies and response to amitriptyline. Br J Psychiatry 1972; 120:147–156 [B]

101. Raskin A, Crook TA: The endogenous-neurotic distinction as a predictor of response to antidepressant drugs. Psychol Med 1976; 6:59–70 [G]

102. Danish University Antidepressant Group: Paroxetine: a selective serotonin reuptake inhibitor showing better tolerance but weaker antidepressant effect than clomipramine in a controlled multicenter study. J Affect Disord 1990; 18:289–299 [A]

103. Perry PJ: Pharmacotherapy for major depression with melancholic features: relative efficacy of tricyclic versus selective serotonin reuptake inhibitor antidepressants. J Affect Disord 1996; 39:1–6 [F]

104. Paykel ES: Treatment of depression: the relevance of research for clinical practice. Br J Psychiatry 1989; 155:754–763 [F]

105. Anderson IM, Tomenson BM: Treatment discontinuation with selective serotonin reuptake inhibitors compared with tricyclic antidepressants: a meta-analysis. Br Med J 1995; 310:1433–1438 [E]

106. Rickels K, Schweizer E: Clinical overview of serotonin reuptake inhibitors. J Clin Psychiatry 1990; 51:9–12 [F]

107. Delgado PL, Price LH, Charney DS, Heninger GR: Efficacy of fluvoxamine in treatment-refractory depression. J Affect Disord 1988; 15:55–60 [B]

108. Golden RN, Brown TM, Miller H, Evans DL: The new antidepressants. NC Med J 1988; 49:549–554 [F]

109. Schatzberg AF: Trazodone: a 5-year review of antidepressant efficacy. Psychopathology 1987; 20(suppl 1):48–56 [F]

110. Cunningham LA, Borison RL, Carman JS, Chouinard G, Crowder JE, Diamond BI, Fischer DE, Hearst E: A comparison of venlafaxine, trazodone, and placebo in major depression. J Clin Psychopharmacol 1994; 14:99–106 [A]

111. Weisler RH, Johnston JA, Lineberry CG, Samara B, Branconnier RJ, Billow AA: Comparison of bupropion and trazodone for the treatment of major depression. J Clin Psychopharmacol 1994; 14:170–179 [A]

112. Klein HE, Muller N: Trazodone in endogenous depressed patients: a negative report and a critical evaluation of the pertaining literature. Prog Neuropsychopharmacol Biol Psychiatry 1985; 9:173–186 [B]

113. Shopsin B, Cassano GB, Conti L: An overview of new second generation antidepressant compounds: research and treatment implications, in Antidepressants: Neurochemical, Behavioral and Clinical Perspectives. Edited by Enna SJ, Malick J, Richelson E. New York, Raven Press, 1981, pp 219–251 [F]

114. Feighner JP, Pambakian R, Fowler RC, Boyer WF, D'Amico MF: A comparison of nefazodone, imipramine, and placebo in patients with moderate to severe depression. Psychopharmacol Bull 1989; 25:219–221 [A]

115. Fontaine R, Ontiveros A, Elie R, Kensler TT, Roberts DL, Kaplita S, Ecker JA, Faludi G: A double-blind comparison of nefazodone, imipramine, and placebo in major depression. J Clin Psychiatry 1994; 55:234–241 [A]

116. Mendels J, Reimherr F, Marcus RN, Roberts DL, Francis RJ, Anton SF: A double-blind, placebo-controlled trial of two dose ranges of nefazodone in the treatment of depressed outpatients. J Clin Psychiatry 1995; 56(suppl 6):30–36 [A]

117. Pitts WM, Fann WE, Halaris AE, Dressler DM, Sajadi C, Snyder S, Ilaria RL: Bupropion in depression: a tri-center placebo-controlled study. J Clin Psychiatry 1983; 44(5, part 2):95–100 [A]

118. Chouinard G: Bupropion and amitriptyline in the treatment of depressed patients. J Clin Psychiatry 1983; 44:121–129 [A]

119. Davidson J, Miller R, Van Wyck Fleet J, Strickland R, Manberg P, Allen S, Parrott R: A double-blind comparison of bupropion and amitriptyline in depressed patients. J Clin Psychiatry 1983; 44:115–117 [B]

120. Feighner J, Hendrickson G, Miller L, Stern W: Double-blind comparison of doxepin versus bupropion in outpatients with a major depressive disorder. J Clin Psychopharmacol 1986; 6:27–32 [A]

121. Mendels J, Amin MM, Chouinard G, Cooper AJ, Miles JE, Remick RA, Saxena B, Secunda SK, Singh AN: A comparative study of bupropion and amitriptyline in depressed outpatients. J Clin Psychiatry 1983; 44:118–120 [A]

122. Feighner JP, Gardner EA, Johnston JA, Batey SR, Khayrallah MA, Ascher JA, Lineberry CG: Double-blind comparison of bupropion and fluoxetine in depressed outpatients. J Clin Psychiatry 1991; 52:329–335 [A]

123. Claghorn JL, Lesem MD: A double-blind placebo-controlled study of Org 3770 in depressed outpatients. J Affect Disord 1995; 34:165–171 [A]

124. Guelfi JD, White C, Hackett D, Guichoux JY, Magni G: Effectiveness of venlafaxine in patients hospitalized with major depression and melancholia. J Clin Psychiatry 1995; 56:450–458 [A]

125. Holm KJ, Markham A: Mirtazapine: a review of its use in major depression. CNS Drugs 1999; 57:607–631 [F]

126. Kasper S: Clinical efficacy of mirtazapine: a review of meta-analyses of pooled data. Int Clin Psychopharmacol 1995; 10(suppl 4):25–35; correction, 1996; 11:153 [F]

127. Schweizer E, Feighner J, Mandos LA, Rickels K: Comparison of venlafaxine and imipramine in the acute treatment of major depression in outpatients. J Clin Psychiatry 1994; 55:104–108 [A]

128. Zivkov M, DeJongh G: Org 3770 versus amitriptyline: a 6-week randomized, double-blind multicentre trial in hospitalized depressed patients. Human Psychopharmacology 1995; 10:173–180 [B]

129. Kelsey JE: Dose-response relationship with venlafaxine. J Clin Psychopharmacol 1996; 16(suppl 2):21S–28S [A]

130. Montgomery SA: Reboxetine: additional benefits to depressed patients. J Psychopharmacol 1997; 11(4 suppl):S9–S15 [F]

131. Davidson J, Raft D, Pelton S: An outpatient evaluation of phenelzine and imipramine. J Clin Psychiatry 1987; 48:143–146 [B]

132. Himmelhoch JM, Thase ME, Mallinger AG, Houck P: Tranylcypromine versus imipramine in anergic bipolar depression. Am J Psychiatry 1991; 148:910–916 [A]

133. McGrath PJ, Stewart JW, Harrison W, Wager S, Quitkin FM: Phenelzine treatment of melancholia. J Clin Psychiatry 1986; 47:420–422 [B]

134. Quitkin FM, Rifkin A, Klein DF: Monoamine oxidase inhibitors: a review of antidepressant effectiveness. Arch Gen Psychiatry 1979; 36:749–760 [F]

135. Thase ME, Trivedi MH, Rush AJ: MAOIs in the contemporary treatment of depression. Neuropsychopharmacology 1995; 12:185–219 [E]

136. White K, Razani J, Cadow B, Gelfand R, Palmer R, Simpson G, Sloane RB: Tranylcypromine vs nortriptyline vs placebo in depressed outpatients: a controlled trial. Psychopharmacology (Berl) 1984; 82:259–262 [B]

137. Quitkin FM, McGrath PJ, Stewart JW, Harrison W, Tricamo E, Wager SG, Ocepek-Welikson K, Nunes E, Rabkin JG, Klein DF: Atypical depression, panic attacks, and response to imipramine and phenelzine: a replication. Arch Gen Psychiatry 1990; 47:935–941 [A]

138. Zisook S, Braff DL, Click MA: Monoamine oxidase inhibitors in the treatment of atypical depression. J Clin Psychopharmacol 1985; 5:131–137 [A]

139. Himmelhoch JM, Fuchs CZ, Symons BJ: A double-blind study of tranylcypromine treatment of major anergic depression. J Nerv Ment Dis 1982; 170:628–634 [A]

140. Thase ME, Mallinger AG, McKnight D, Himmelhoch JM: Treatment of imipramine-resistant recurrent depression, IV: a double-blind crossover study of tranylcypromine for anergic bipolar depression. Am J Psychiatry 1992; 149:195–198 [A]

141. Stoudemire A, Atkinson P: Use of cyclic antidepressants in patients with cardiac conduction disturbance. Gen Hosp Psychiatry 1988; 10:389–397 [G]

142. Veith RC, Raskind MA, Caldwell JH, Barnes RF, Gumbrecht G, Ritchie JL: Cardiovascular effects of tricyclic antidepressants in depressed patients with chronic heart disease. N Engl J Med 1982; 306:954–959 [A]

143. Garvey MJ, Tollefson GD: Occurrence of myoclonus in patients treated with cyclic antidepressants. Arch Gen Psychiatry 1987; 44:269–272 [E]

144. Preskorn SH, Jerkovich GS: Central nervous system toxicity of tricyclic antidepressants: phenomenology, course, risk factors, and role of therapeutic drug monitoring. J Clin Psychopharmacol 1990; 10:88–95 [E]

145. Frazer A: Antidepressants. J Clin Psychiatry 1997; 58:9–25 [F]

146. Walker PW, Cole JO, Gardner EA, Hughes AR, Johnston JA, Batey SR, Lineberry CG: Improvement in fluoxetine-associated sexual dysfunction in patients switched to bupropion. J Clin Psychiatry 1993; 54:459–465 [B]

147. Pollack MH, Rosenbaum JF: Management of antidepressant-induced side effects: a practical guide for the clinician. J Clin Psychiatry 1987; 48:3–8 [G]

148. Doughty MJ, Lyle WM: Medications used to prevent migraine headaches and their potential ocular adverse effects. Optom Vis Sci 1995; 72:879–891 [F]

149. Hamilton JA, Halbreich U: Special aspects of neuropsychiatric illness in women: with a focus on depression. Annu Rev Med 1993; 44:355–364 [F]

150. Gerber PE, Lynd LD: Selective serotonin-reuptake inhibitor-induced movement disorders. Ann Pharmacother 1998; 32:692–698 [E]

151. Leo RJ: Movement disorders associated with the serotonin selective reuptake inhibitors. J Clin Psychiatry 1996; 57:449–454 [E]

152. Marcus ER, Bradley SS: Combination of psychotherapy and psychopharmacotherapy with treatment-resistant inpatients with dual diagnoses. Psychiatr Clin North Am 1990; 13:209–214 [E]

153. Bouwer CD, Harvey BH: Phasic craving for carbohydrate observed with citalopram. Int Clin Psychopharmacol 1996; 11:273–278 [B]

154. Michelson D, Amsterdam JD, Quitkin FM, Reimherr F, Rosenbaum JF, Zajecka J, Sundell KL, Kim Y, Beasley CM Jr: Changes in weight during a 1-year trial of fluoxetine. Am J Psychiatry 1999; 156:1170–1176 [A]

155. Lewinsohn PM, Antonuccio DA, Steinmetz-Breckinridge J, Teri L: The Coping With Depression Course: A Psychoeducational Intervention for Unipolar Depression. Eugene, Ore, Castalia Publishing, 1984 [F]

156. Metz A, Shader RI: Adverse interactions encountered when using trazodone to treat insomnia associated with fluoxetine. Int Clin Psychopharmacol 1990; 5:191–194 [G]

157. Beasley CM Jr, Masica DN, Heiligenstein JH, Wheadon DE, Zerbe RL: Possible monoamine oxidase inhibitor-serotonin uptake inhibitor interaction: fluoxetine clinical data and preclinical findings. J Clin Psychopharmacol 1993; 13:312–320 [F]

158. Vitullo RN, Wharton JM, Allen NB, Pritchett EL: Trazodone-related exercise-induced nonsustained ventricular tachycardia. Chest 1990; 98:247–248 [G]

159. Aronson MD, Hafez H: A case of trazodone-induced ventricular tachycardia. J Clin Psychiatry 1986; 47:388–389 [G]

160. Thompson JW Jr, Ware MR, Blashfield RK: Psychotropic medication and priapism: a comprehensive review. J Clin Psychiatry 1990; 51:430–433 [F]

161. Davis R, Wilde MI: Mirtazapine: a review of its pharmacology and therapeutic potential in the management of major depression. CNS Drugs 1996; 5:389–402 [F]

162. Mucci M: Reboxetine: a review of antidepressant tolerability. J Psychopharmacol 1997; 11(4 suppl):S33–S37 [F]

163. Gardner DM, Shulman KI, Walker SE, Tailor SAN: The making of a user friendly MAOI diet. J Clin Psychiatry 1996; 57:99–104 [F]

164. Schenk CH, Remick RA: Sublingual nifedipine in the treatment of hypertensive crisis associated with monoamine oxidase inhibitors (letter). Ann Emerg Med 1989; 18:114–115 [B]

165. Grossman E, Messerli FH, Grodzicki T, Kowey P: Should a moratorium be placed on sublingual nifedipine capsules given for hypertensive emergencies and pseudoemergencies? JAMA 1996; 276:1328–1331 [F]

166. Sternbach H: The serotonin syndrome. Am J Psychiatry 1991; 148:705–713 [F]

167. Gelenberg AJ: Serotonin syndrome update. Biological Therapies in Psychiatry Newsletter 1997; 20:33–34 [F]

168. Beasley CM Jr, Sayler ME, Cunningham GE, Weiss AM, Masica DN: Fluoxetine in tricyclic refractory major depressive disorder. J Affect Disord 1990; 20:193–200 [B]

169. Jenner PN: Paroxetine: an overview of dosage, tolerability, and safety. Int Clin Psychopharmacol 1992; 6(suppl 4):69–80 [F]

170. Montgomery SA, Pedersen V, Tanghoj P, Rasmussen C, Rioux P: The optimal dosing regimen for citalopram—a meta-analysis of nine placebo-controlled studies. Int Clin Psychopharmacol 1994; 9(suppl 1):35–40 [E]

171. Quitkin FM, Rabkin JG, Markowitz JM, Stewart JW, McGrath PJ, Harrison W: Use of pattern analysis to identify true drug response. Arch Gen Psychiatry 1987; 44:259–264 [A]

172. Quitkin FM, Rabkin JG, Ross D, McGrath PJ: Duration of antidepressant drug treatment: what is an adequate trial? Arch Gen Psychiatry 1984; 41:238–245 [G]

173. Katz MM, Koslow SH, Maas JW, Frazer A, Bowden CL, Casper R, Croughan J, Kocsis J, Redmond E Jr: The timing, specificity and clinical prediction of tricyclic drug effects in depression. Psychol Med 1987; 17:297–309 [C]

174. Guscott R, Grof P: The clinical meaning of refractory depression: a review for the clinician. Am J Psychiatry 1991; 148:695–704 [G]

175. Cullen M, Mitchell P, Brodaty H, Boyce P, Parker G, Hickie I, Wilhem K: Carbamazepine for treatment-resistant melancholia. J Clin Psychiatry 1991; 52:472–476 [C]

176. Hayes SG: Long-term use of valproate in primary psychiatric disorders. J Clin Psychiatry 1989; 50:35–39 [E]

177. Rosenstein DL, Takeshita J, Nelson JC: Fluoxetine-induced elevation and prolongation of tricyclic levels in overdose (letter). Am J Psychiatry 1991; 148:807 [E]

178. Price LH, Charney DS, Heninger GR: Variability of response to lithium augmentation in refractory depression. Am J Psychiatry 1986; 143:1387–1392 [C]

179. Kramlinger KG, Post RM: The addition of lithium to carbamazepine: antidepressant efficacy in treatment-resistant depression. Arch Gen Psychiatry 1989; 46:794–800 [C]

180. Prange AJ, Loosen PT, Wilson IC, Lipton MA: The therapeutic use of hormones of the thyroid axis in depression, in The Neurobiology of Mood Disorders. Edited by Post R, Ballenger J. Baltimore, Williams & Wilkins, 1984, pp 311–322 [E]

181. Feighner JP, Herbstein J, Damlouji N: Combined MAOI, TCA, and direct stimulant therapy of treatment-resistant depression. J Clin Psychiatry 1985; 46:206–209 [G]

182. Wharton RN, Perel JM, Dayton PG, Malitz S: A potential clinical use for methylphenidate (Ritalin) with tricyclic antidepressants. Am J Psychiatry 1971; 127:1619–1625 [E]

183. Razani J, White KL, White J, Simpson G, Sloane RB, Rebal R, Palmer R: The safety and efficacy of combined amitriptyline and tranylcypromine antidepressant treatment: a controlled trial. Arch Gen Psychiatry 1983; 40:657–661 [A]

184. Young JPR, Lader MH, Hughes WC: Controlled trial of trimipramine, monoamine oxidase inhibitors, and combined treatment in depressed outpatients. Br Med J 1979; 2:1315–1317 [A]

185. Devlin MJ, Walsh BT: Use of monoamine oxidase inhibitors in refractory depression, in American Psychiatric Press Review of Psychiatry, vol 9. Edited by Tasman A, Goldfinger SM, Kaufmann CA. Washington, DC, American Psychiatric Press, 1990, pp 74–90 [F]

186. Prudic J, Sackeim HA: Refractory depression and electroconvulsive therapy, in Treatment Strategies for Refractory Depression. Edited by Roose SP, Glassman AH. Washington, DC, American Psychiatric Press, 1990, pp 111–128 [G]

187. El-Ganzouri A, Ivankovich AD, Braverman B, McCarthy R: Monoamine oxidase inhibitors: should they be discontinued preoperatively? Anesth Analg 1985; 64:592–596 [B]

188. Klapheke MM: Combining ECT and antipsychotic agents: benefits and risks. Convuls Ther 1993; 9:241–255 [F]

189. Klapheke MM: Electroconvulsive therapy consultation: an update. Convuls Ther 1997; 13:227–241 [F]

190. Lauritzen L, Odgaard K, Clemmesen L, Lunde M, Ohrstrom J, Black C, Bech P: Relapse prevention by means of paroxetine in ECT-treated patients with major depression: a comparison with imipramine and placebo in medium-term continuation therapy. Acta Psychiatr Scand 1996; 94:241–251 [A]

191. Nelson JP, Benjamin L: Efficacy and safety of combined ECT and tricyclic antidepressant therapy in the treatment of depressed geriatric patients. Convuls Ther 1989; 5:321–329 [E]

192. Penney JF: Concurrent and close temporal administration of lithium and ECT. Convuls Ther 1990; 6:139–145 [D]

193. Hill GE, Wong KC, Hodges MR: Potentiation of succinylcholine neuromuscular blockade by lithium carbonate. Anesthesiology 1976; 44:439–442 [E]

194. Jha AK, Stein GS, Fenwick P: Negative interaction between lithium and electroconvulsive therapy—a case control study. Br J Psychiatry 1996; 168:241–243 [D]

195. Lippman SB, Tao CA: Electroconvulsive therapy and lithium: safe and effective treatment. Convuls Ther 1993; 9:54–57 [G]

196. Janicak PG, Davis JM, Gibbons RD, Ericksen S, Chang S, Gallagher P: Efficacy of ECT: a meta-analysis. Am J Psychiatry 1985; 142:297–302 [E]

197. Weiner RD: Electroconvulsive therapy, in Treatments of Psychiatric Disorders. Edited by Gabbard GO. Washington, DC, American Psychiatric Press, 1995, pp 1237–1262 [F]

198. Devanand DP, Sackeim HA, Prudic J: Electroconvulsive therapy in the treatment resistant patient. Psychiatr Clin North Am 1991; 14:905–923 [F]

199. Avery D, Winokur G: The efficacy of electroconvulsive therapy and antidepressants in depression. Biol Psychiatry 1977; 12:507–523 [F]

200. Paul SM, Extein I, Calil HM, Potter WZ, Chodoff P, Goodwin FK: Use of ECT with treatment-resistant depressed patients at the National Institute of Mental Health. Am J Psychiatry 1981; 138:486–489 [B]

201. The Practice of Electroconvulsive Therapy: Recommendations for Treatment, Training, and Privileging: A Task Force Report of the American Psychiatric Association. Washington, DC, APA, 1990 [F]

202. Abrams R: The mortality rate with ECT. Convuls Ther 1997; 13:125–127 [G]

203. Fink M: Efficacy and safety of induced seizures (ECT) in man. Compr Psychiatry 1978; 19:1–18 [F]

204. Gomez J: Subjective side-effects of ECT. Br J Psychiatry 1975; 127:609–611 [B]

205. Stoudemire A, Hill CD, Morris R, Dalton ST: Improvement in depression-related cognitive dysfunction following ECT. J Neuropsychiatry Clin Neurosci 1995; 7:31–34 [B]

206. McElhiney MC, Moody BJ, Steif BL, Prudic J, Devanand DP, Nobler MS, Sackeim HA: Autobiographical memory and mood: effects of electroconvulsive therapy. Neuropsychology 1995; 9:501–517 [A]

207. Sobin C, Sackeim HA, Prudic J, Devanand DP, Moody BJ, McElhiney MC: Predictors of retrograde amnesia following ECT. Am J Psychiatry 1995; 152:995–1001 [A]

208. Squire LR, Slater PC, Miller PL: Retrograde amnesia and bilateral electroconvulsive therapy: long-term follow-up. Arch Gen Psychiatry 1981; 38:89–95 [C]

209. Weiner RD, Rogers HJ, Davidson JR, Squire LR: Effects of stimulus parameters on cognitive side effects. Ann NY Acad Sci 1986; 462:315–325 [B]

210. Squire LR, Slater PC: Electroconvulsive therapy and complaints of memory dysfunction: a prospective three-year follow-up study. Br J Psychiatry 1983; 142:1–8 [B]

211. Dec GW Jr, Stern TA, Welch C: The efforts of electroconvulsive therapy on serial electrocardiograms and serum cardiac enzyme values: a prospective study of depressed hospitalized inpatients. JAMA 1985; 253:2525–2529 [B]

212. Abrams R: Electroconvulsive Therapy, 3rd ed. New York, Oxford University Press, 1997 [G]

213. Sackeim HA, Prudic J, Devanand DP, Kiersky JE, Fitzsimons L, Moody BJ, McElhiney MC, Coleman EA, Settembrino JM: Effects of stimulus intensity and electrode placement on the efficacy and cognitive effects of electroconvulsive therapy. N Engl J Med 1993; 328:839–846 [A]

214. Krystal AD, Weiner RD: ECT seizure therapeutic adequacy. Convuls Ther 1994; 10:153–164 [F]

215. Weiner RD, Coffey CE, Krystal AD: The monitoring and management of electrically induced seizures. Psychiatr Clin North Am 1991; 14:845–869 [F]

216. Hales RE, Yudofsky SC, Talbott JA (eds): The American Psychiatric Press Textbook of Psychiatry, 3rd ed. Washington, DC, American Psychiatric Press, 1999 [G]

217. Lerer B, Shapira B, Calev A, Tubi N, Drexler H, Kindler S, Lidsky D, Schwartz JE: Antidepressant and cognitive effects of twice- versus three-times-weekly ECT. Am J Psychiatry 1995; 152:564–570 [A]

218. Shapira B, Gorfine M, Lerer B: A prospective study of lithium continuation therapy in depressed patients who have responded to electroconvulsive therapy. Convuls Ther 1995; 11:80–85 [B]

219. Schwarz T, Loewenstein J, Isenberg KE: Maintenance ECT: indications and outcome. Convuls Ther 1995; 11:14–23 [B]

220. Terman M, Terman JS, Quitkin FM, McGrath PJ, Stewart JW, Rafferty B: Light therapy for seasonal affective disorder: a review of efficacy. Neuropsychopharmacology 1989; 2:1–22 [B]

221. Eastman CI, Young MA, Fogg LF, Liu L, Meaden PM: Bright light treatment of winter depression: a placebo-controlled trial. Arch Gen Psychiatry 1998; 55:883–889 [B]

222. Terman M, Terman JS, Ross DC: A controlled trial of timed bright light and negative air ionization for treatment of winter depression. Arch Gen Psychiatry 1998; 55:875–882 [B]

223. Lewy AJ, Bauer VK, Cutler NL, Sack RL, Ahmed S, Thomas KH, Blood ML, Jackson JM: Morning versus evening light treatment of patients with winter depression. Arch Gen Psychiatry 1998; 55:890–896 [B]

224. Beck AT, Rush AJ, Shaw BF, Emery G: Cognitive Therapy of Depression. New York, Guilford, 1979 [G]

225. Gloaguen V, Cottraux J, Cucherat M, Blackburn IM: A meta-analysis of the effects of cognitive therapy in depressed patients. J Affect Disord 1998; 49:59–72 [E]

226. Dobson KS: A meta-analysis of the efficacy of cognitive therapy for depression. J Consult Clin Psychol 1989; 57:414–419 [E]

227. Gaffan EA, Tsaousis I, Kemp-Wheeler SM: Researcher allegiance and meta-analysis: the case of cognitive therapy for depression. J Consult Clin Psychol 1995; 63:966–980 [E]

228. Blackburn IM, Moore RG: Controlled acute and follow-up trial of cognitive therapy and pharmacotherapy in out-patients with recurrent depression. Br J Psychiatry 1997; 171:328–334 [B]

229. DeRubeis RJ, Gelfand LA, Tang TZ, Simons AD: Medications versus cognitive behavior therapy for severely depressed outpatients: mega-analysis of four randomized comparisons. Am J Psychiatry 1999; 156:1007–1013 [E]

230. Hollon SD, DeRubeis RJ, Evans MD, Wierner MJ, Garvey MJ, Grove WM, Tuason VB: Cognitive therapy and pharmacotherapy for depression. Arch Gen Psychiatry 1992; 49:774–781 [B]

231. Jarrett RB, Rush AJ: Short-term psychotherapy of depressive disorders: current status and future directions. Psychiatry 1994; 57:115–132 [F]

232. Clark DM, Salkovskis PM, Hackmann A, Middleton H, Anastasiades P, Gelder M: A comparison of cognitive therapy, applied relaxation and imipramine in the treatment of panic disorder. Br J Psychiatry 1994; 164:759–769 [B]

233. Elkin I, Shea Mt, Watkins JT, Imber SD, Sotsky SM, Collins JF, Glass DR, Pilkonis PA, Leber WR, Docherty JP: National Institute of Mental Health Treatment of Depression Collaborative Research Program: general effectiveness of treatments. Arch Gen Psychiatry 1989; 46:971–982 [F]

234. Evans MD, Hollong SD, Garvey MJ, Piasecki JM, Grove WM, Garvey MJ, Tuason VB: Differential relapse following cognitive therapy and pharmacotherapy for depression. Arch Gen Psychiatry 1992; 49:802–808 [B]

235. Joffe R, Segal Z, Singer W: Change in thyroid hormone levels following response to cognitive therapy for major depression. Am J Psychiatry 1996; 153:411–413 [B]

236. Thase ME, Dubé S, Bowler K, Howland RH, Myers JE, Friedman E, Jarrett DB: Hypothalamic-pituitary-adrenocortical activity and response to cognitive behavior therapy in unmedicated, hospitalized depressed patients. Am J Psychiatry 1996; 153:886–891 [B]

237. Thase ME, Simons AD, Reynolds CF: Abnormal electroencephalographic sleep profiles in major depression: association with response to cognitive behavior therapy. Arch Gen Psychiatry 1996; 53:99–108 [B]

238. Blatt SJ, Quinlan DM, Zuroff DC, Pilkonis PA: Interpersonal factors in brief treatment of depression: further analyses of the National Institute of Mental Health Treatment of Depression Collaborative Research Program. J Consult Clin Psychol 1996; 64:162–171 [F]

239. Patience DA, McGuire RJ, Scott AI, Freeman CP: The Edinburgh Primary Care Depression Study: personality disorders and outcome. Br J Psychiatry 1995; 167:324–330

240. Ferster CB: A functional analysis of depression. Am Psychol 1973; 10:857–870 [F]

241. Bandura A: Social Learning Theory. Englewood Cliffs, NJ, Prentice-Hall, 1977 [F]

242. Lewinsohn PM, Clarke G: Group treatment of depressed individuals: the Coping With Depression Course. Advances in Behavioral Research and Therapy 1984; 6:99–114 [F]

243. Rehm LP: Behavior Therapy for Depression. New York, Academic Press, 1979 [F]

244. Bellack AS, Hersen M: A comparison of social-skills training, pharmacotherapy and psychotherapy for depression. Behav Res Ther 1983; 21:101–107 [A]

245. Nezu AM: Efficacy of a social problem-solving therapy for unipolar depression. J Consult Clin Psychol 1986; 54:196–202 [A]

246. McLean PD, Hakstian AR: Clinical depression: comparative efficacies of outpatient treatments. J Consult Clin Psychol 1979; 47:818–836 [F]

247. Steuer JL, Mintz J, Hammen CL, Hill MA, Jarvik LF, McCarley T, Motoike P, Rosen R: Cognitive-behavioral and psychodynamic group psychotherapy in treatment of geriatric depression. J Consult Clin Psychol 1984; 52:180–189 [B]

248. Beach SR, O'Leary KD: Extramarital sex: impact on depression and commitment in couples seeking marital therapy. J Sex Marital Ther 1985; 11:99–108 [D]

249. Jacobson NS, Dobson K, Fruzetti AE, Schmaling KB, Salusky S: Marital therapy as a treatment for depression. J Consult Clin Psychol 1991; 59:547–557 [G]

250. Rabin AS, Kaslow NJ, Rehm LP: Factors influencing continuation in a behavioral therapy. Behav Res Ther 1985; 23:695–698 [C]

251. Thompson JK, Williams DE: An interpersonally based cognitive-behavioral psychotherapy. Prog Behav Modif 1987; 21:230–258 [G]

252. Miller IW, Norman WH, Keitner GI, Bishop SB: Cognitive-behavioral treatment of depressed inpatients. Behavior Therapy 1989; 20:25–47 [B]

253. Taylor S, McLean P: Outcome profiles in the treatment of unipolar depression. Behav Res Ther 1993; 31:325–330 [B]

254. McLean P, Taylor S: Severity of unipolar depression and choice of treatment. Behav Res Ther 1992; 30:443–451 [A]

255. Rohde P, Lewinsohn PM, Seeley JR: Response of depressed adolescents to cognitive-behavioral treatment: do differences in initial severity clarify the comparison of treatments? J Consult Clin Psychol 1994; 62:851–854 [B]

256. Thase ME, Simons AD, Cahalane J, McGeary J, Harden T: Severity of depression and response to cognitive behavior therapy. Am J Psychiatry 1991; 148:784–789 [B]

257. Kendall PC, Morris RJ: Child therapy: issues and recommendations. J Consult Clin Psychol 1991; 59:777–784 [F]

258. Klerman GL, Weissman MM, Rounsaville BJ, Chevron ES: Interpersonal Psychotherapy of Depression. New York, Basic Books, 1984 [G]

259. Elkin I, Shea MT, Watkins JT, Imber SD, Sotsky SM, Collins JF, Glass DR, Pilkonis PA, Leber WR, Docherty JP, Fiester SJ, Parloff MB: National Institute of Mental Health Treatment of Depression Collaborative Research Program: general effectiveness of treatments. Arch Gen Psychiatry 1989; 46:971–982 [A]

260. Schulberg HC, Block MR, Madonia MJ, Scott CP, Rodriguez E, Imber SD, Perel J, Lave J, Houck PR, Coulehan JL: Treating major depression in primary care practice: eight-month clinical outcomes. Arch Gen Psychiatry 1996; 53:913–919 [A]

261. Markowitz JC, Klerman GL, Clougherty KF, Spielman LA, Jacobsberg LB, Fishman B, Frances AJ, Kocsis JH, Perry SW III: Individual psychotherapies for depressed HIV-positive patients. Am J Psychiatry 1995; 152:1504–1509 [B]

262. Markowitz JC, Kocsis J, Fishman B, Spielman LA, Jacobsberg LB, Frances AJ, Klerman GL, Perry SW: Treatment of depressive symptoms in human immunodeficiency virus-positive patients. Arch Gen Psychiatry 1998; 55:452–457 [B]

263. Hardy GE, Barkham M, Shapiro DA, Reynolds S, Rees A, Stiles WB: Credibility and outcome of cognitive-behavioural and psychodynamic-interpersonal psychotherapy. Br J Clin Psychol 1995; 34:555–569 [F]

264. Barber JP, Muenz LR: The role of avoidance and obsessiveness in matching patients to cognitive and interpersonal psychotherapy: empirical findings from the Treatment for Depression Collaborative Research Program. J Consult Clin Psychol 1996; 64:951–958 [B]

265. Bash M: Understanding Psychotherapy: The Science Behind the Art. New York, Basic Books, 1988 [G]

266. Bibring E: Psychoanalysis and the dynamic psychotherapies. J Am Psychoanal Assoc 1954; 2:745–770 [F]

267. Gray SH: Quality assurance and utilization review of individual medical psychotherapies, in Manual of Quality Assurance Review. Edited by Mattson MR. Washington, DC, American Psychiatric Press, 1992, pp 159–166 [F]

268. Blatt SJ: Contributions of psychoanalysis to the understanding and treatment of depression. J Am Psychoanal Assoc 1998; 46:722–752 [F]

269. Brenner C: Depression, anxiety and affect theory. J Psychoanal 1974; 55:25–32 [F]

270. Freud S: Mourning and melancholia (1917 [1915]), in Complete Psychological Works, standard ed, vol 14. London, Hogarth Press, 1957, pp 243–258 [G]

271. Kohut H: Thoughts on narcissism and narcissistic rage. Psychoanal Study Child 1972; 27:360–400 [G]

272. Zetzel ER: On the incapacity to bear depression (1965), in The Capacity for Emotional Growth. New York, International Universities Press, 1970, pp 82–224 [G]

273. Loewald HW: Perspectives on memory (1972), in Papers on Psychoanalysis. New Haven, Conn, Yale University Press, 1980, pp 148–173 [G]

274. Tasman A, Kay J, Lieberman JA: Psychiatry. Philadelphia, WB Saunders, 1996 [G]

275. Brenner C: Psychoanalytic Technique and Psychic Conflict. New York, International Universities Press, 1976 [F]

276. Rado S: The problem of melancholia (1927), in Psychoanalysis of Behavior: Collected Papers. New York, Grune & Stratton, 1956 [G]

277. Karasu TB: Developmentalist metatheory of depression and psychotherapy. Am J Psychother 1992; 46:37–49 [G]

278. Covi L, Lipman RS, Derogatis LR, Smith JE III, Pattison JH: Drugs and group psychotherapy in neurotic depression. Am J Psychiatry 1974; 131:191–198 [A]

279. Daneman EA: Imipramine in office management of depressive reactions (a double-blind study). Dis Nerv Syst 1961; 22:213–217 [A]

280. Beach SRH, Sandeen EE, O'Leary KD: Depression in Marriage. New York, Guilford, 1990 [G]

281. Yager J: Mood disorders and marital and family problems, in American Psychiatric Press Review of Psychiatry, vol 11. Edited by Tasman A, Riba MB. Washington, DC, American Psychiatric Press, 1992, pp 477–493 [G]

282. Coyne JC, Kessler RC, Tal M, Turnball J, Wortman CB, Greden JF: Living with a depressed person. J Consult Clin Psychol 1987; 55:347–352 [F]

283. Hahlweg K, Markman HJ: Effectiveness of behavioral marital therapy: empirical status of behavioral techniques in preventing and alleviating marital distress. J Consult Clin Psychol 1988; 56:440–447 [F]

284. Jacobson NS, Martin B: Behavioral marriage therapy: current status. Psychol Bull 1976; 83:540–556 [F]

285. Jacobson N, Addis M: Research on couples and couple therapy: what do we know? where are we going? J Consult Clin Psychol 1993; 61:85–93 [F]

286. O'Leary KD, Beach SR: Marital therapy: a viable treatment for depression and marital discord. Am J Psychiatry 1990; 147:183–186 [G]

287. Bright JI, Baker KD, Neimeyer RA: Professional and paraprofessional group treatments for depression: a comparison of cognitive-behavioral and mutual support interventions. J Consult Clin Psychol 1999; 67:491–501 [A]

288. Neimeyer RA, Baker KD, Haykal RF, Akiskal HS: Patterns of symptomatic change in depressed patients in a private inpatient mood disorders program. Bull Menninger Clin 1995; 59:460–471 [C]

289. Neimeyer RA, Feixas G: The role of homework and skill acquisition in the outcome of group cognitive therapy for depression. Behavior Therapy 1990; 21:281–292 [B]

290. MacKenzie RR: Anti-depression interpersonal psychotherapy groups (IPT-G): preliminary effectiveness data. Society for Psychotherapy Research Conference, 1999 [B]

291. Yalom ID: The Theory and Practice of Group Psychotherapy, 4th ed. New York, Basic Books, 1995 [G]

292. Smith ML, Glass GV, Miller TI: The Benefits of Psychotherapy. Baltimore, Johns Hopkins Press, 1980 [G]

293. Toseland RW, Siporin M: When to recommend group treatment: a review of the clinical and group literature. Int J Group Psychother 1986; 36:171–201 [F]

294. Piper WE, Joyce AS: A consideration of factors influencing utilization of time-limited short-term group therapy. Int J Group Psychother 1996; 46:311–328 [F]

295. McRoberts C, Burlingame GM, Hoag MJ: Comparative efficacy of individual and group psychotherapy: a meta-analytic perspective. Group Dynamics: Theory, Research, and Practice 1998; 2:101–117 [E]

296. Targ EF, Karasic DH, Diefenbach PN, Anderson DA, Bystritsky A, Fawzy FI: Structured group therapy and fluoxetine to treat depression in HIV-positive persons. Psychosomatics 1994; 35:132–137 [B]

297. Lieberman MA, Borman LD: Self-Help Groups for Coping With Crisis. San Francisco, Jossey-Bass, 1979 [G]

298. Shapiro DA, Barkham M, Rees A, Hardy GE, Reynolds S, Startup M: Effects of treatment duration and severity of depression on the effectiveness of cognitive-behavioral and psychodynamic-interpersonal psychotherapy. J Consult Clin Psychol 1994; 62:522–534 [B]

299. Wexler BE, Cicchetti DV: The outpatient treatment of depression: implications of outcome research for clinical practice. J Nerv Ment Dis 1992; 180:277–286 [F]

300. Beck AT, Jallon SD, Young JE: Treatment of depression with cognitive therapy and amitriptyline. Arch Gen Psychiatry 1985; 42:142–148 [D]

301. Blackburn IM, Bishop S, Glen AI, Whalley LJ, Christie JE: The efficacy of cognitive therapy in depression: a treatment trial using cognitive therapy and pharmacotherapy, each alone and in combination. Br J Psychiatry 1981; 139:181–189 [A]

302. Chaudhry HR, Najam N, Naqvi A: The value of amineptine in depressed patients treated with cognitive behavioural psychotherapy. Hum Psychopharmacol 1998; 13:419–424 [A]

303. Hersen M, Bellack AS, Himmelhoch JM, Thase ME: Effects of social skill training, amitriptyline, and psychotherapy in unipolar depressed women. Behavior Therapy 1984; 15:21–40 [B]

304. Murphy GE, Simons AD, Wetzel RD, Lustman PJ: Cognitive therapy and pharmacotherapy: singly and together in the treatment of depression. Arch Gen Psychiatry 1984; 41:33–41 [A]

305. Thase ME, Greenhouse JB, Frank E, Reynolds CF, Pilkonis PA, Hurley K, Grochocinski VJ, Kupfer DJ: Treatment of major depression with psychotherapy or psychotherapy-pharmacotherapy combinations. Arch Gen Psychiatry 1997; 54:1009–1015 [E]

306. Fava GA, Grandi S, Zielezny M, Canestrari R, Morphy MA: Cognitive behavioral treatment of residual symptoms in primary major depressive disorder. Am J Psychiatry 1994; 151:1295–1299 [B]

307. Fava M, Kaji J: Continuation and maintenance treatments of major depressive disorder. Psychiatr Annals 1994; 24:281–290 [F]

308. Fava M, Davidson KG: Definition and epidemiology of treatment-resistant depression. Psychiatr Clin North Am 1996; 19:179–200 [F]

309. Fava GA, Rafanelli C, Grandi S, Conti S, Belluardo P: Prevention of recurrent depression with cognitive behavioral therapy: preliminary findings. Arch Gen Psychiatry 1998; 55:816–820 [G]

310. Consensus Development Panel: NIMH/NIH Consensus Development Conference Statement: mood disorders: pharmacologic prevention of recurrences. Am J Psychiatry 1985; 142:469–476 [F]

311. Maj M, Veltro F, Pirozzi R, Lobrace S, Magliano L: Pattern of recurrence of illness after recovery from an episode of major depression: a prospective study. Am J Psychiatry 1992; 149:795–800 [B]

312. Thase ME, Simons AD, McGeary J, Cahalane JF, Hughes C, Harden T, Friedman E: Relapse after cognitive behavior therapy of depression: potential implications for longer courses of treatment. Am J Psychiatry 1992; 149:1046–1052 [C]

313. Keller MD, Gelenberg AJ, Hirschfeld RM, Rush AJ, Thase ME, Kocsis JH, Markowitz JC, Fawcett JA, Koran LM, Klein DN, Russell JM, Kornstein SG, McCullough JP, Davis SM, Harrison WM: The treatment of chronic depression, part 2: a double-blind, randomized trial of sertraline and imipramine. J Clin Psychiatry 1998; 59:598–607 [A]

314. Prien RF, Kupfer DJ: Continuation drug therapy for major depressive episodes: how long should it be maintained? Am J Psychiatry 1986; 143:18–23 [B]

315. Jarrett DB, Basco MR, Riser R, Ramanan J, Marwill M, Rush AJ: Is there a role for continuation phase cognitive therapy for depressed outpatients? J Consult Clin Psychol 1998; 66:1036–1040 [B]

316. Fava GA, Grandi S, Zielezny M, Rafanelli C, Canestrari R: Four-year outcome for cognitive behavioral treatment of residual symptoms in major depression. Am J Psychiatry 1996; 153:945–947 [B]

317. Solomon DA, Bauer MS: Continuation and maintenance pharmacotherapy for unipolar and bipolar mood disorders. Psychiatr Clin North Am 1993; 16:515–540 [F]

318. Frank E, Kupfer DJ, Perel JM, Cornes C, Jarrett DB, Mallinger AG, Thase ME, McEachran AB, Grochocinski VJ: Three-year outcomes for maintenance therapies in recurrent depression. Arch Gen Psychiatry 1990; 47:1093–1099 [A]

319. Kupfer DJ, Frank E, Perel JM, Cornes C, Mallinger AG, Thase ME, McEachran AB, Grochocinski VJ: Five-year outcome for maintenance therapies in recurrent depression. Arch Gen Psychiatry 1992; 49:769–773 [A]

320. Frank E, Kupfer DJ, Perel JM, Cornes C, Mallinger AG, Thase ME, McEachran AB, Grochocinski VJ: Comparison of full-dose versus half-dose pharmacotherapy in the maintenance treatment of recurrent depression. J Affect Disord 1993; 27:139–145 [A]

321. Scott J: Chronic depression: can cognitive therapy succeed when other treatments fail? Behavioural Psychotherapy 1992; 20:25–36 [B]

322. Belsher G, Costello CB: Relapse after recovery from unipolar depression: a critical review. Psychol Bull 1988; 104:84–96 [F]

323. Petrides G, Dhossche D, Fink M, Francis A: Continuation ECT: relapse prevention in affective disorders. Convuls Ther 1994; 10:189–194 [B]

324. Vanelle JM, Loo H, Galinowski A, de Carvalho W, Bourdel MC, Brochier P, Bouvet O, Brochier T, Olie JP: Maintenance ECT in intractable manic-depressive disorders. Convuls Ther 1994; 10:195–205 [C]

325. Dilsaver SC, Kronfol Z, Sackellares JC, Greden JF: Antidepressant withdrawal syndromes: evidence supporting the cholinergic overdrive hypothesis. J Clin Psychopharmacol 1983; 3:157–164 [F]

PRACTICE GUIDELINE FOR THE
Treatment of Patients With Bipolar Disorder

WORK GROUP ON BIPOLAR DISORDER

Robert M.A. Hirschfeld, M.D., Chair

Paula J. Clayton, M.D.
Irvin Cohen, M.D.
Jan Fawcett, M.D.
Paul Keck, M.D.
Jon McClellan, M.D.
Susan McElroy, M.D.
Robert Post, M.D.
Aaron Satloff, M.D.

▶ NOTE TO THE READER

In this practice guideline, treatment recommendations are discussed in section II.E and II.F, and are summarized in Section III. Data regarding the safety and efficacy of available treatments are reviewed in Sections II.A, II.B, II.C, and II.D.

This practice guideline was published in *The American Journal of Psychiatry* in December 1994.

CONTENTS

DEVELOPMENT PROCESS

This practice guideline was developed under the auspices of the Steering Committee on Practice Guidelines. The development process is detailed in the Appendix to this volume. Key features of the process included: 1) initial drafting by a work group consisting of psychiatrists with clinical and research expertise in bipolar disorder; 2) a comprehensive literature review; 3) the production of multiple drafts, each of which received widespread review, with over 120 individuals and 40 organizations submitting comments (see sections V and VI); 4) approval by the APA Assembly and Board of Trustees; and 5) planned revisions at 3- to 5-year intervals.

Computerized searches of the relevant literature were conducted using MEDLINE. The key words used were "bipolar disorder–treatment" for the period January 1987 through October 1993; "bipolar disorder–psychological treatments" for the period January 1981 through December 1986 and "psychotic depression–treatment" for the period January 1987 through November 1993.

Papers selected from these searches for further review included those published in English in peer-reviewed journals. Preference was given to those articles based on randomized, placebo-controlled clinical trials. Clinical reports involving descriptions of patients or groups of patients were reviewed when data from controlled trials were not available. Review articles, especially those published in well-regarded peer-reviewed journals, and book chapters were reviewed.

INTRODUCTION

This guideline seeks to provide guidance to psychiatrists who treat patients with bipolar I disorder (manic-depressive illness). The pharmacologic, other somatic, and psychotherapeutic treatments that are used for patients with bipolar I disorder are summarized. Although many of the treatments discussed in this guideline may be effective for patients with bipolar II disorder or for patients with schizoaffective disorder, bipolar type, the focus is to guide the treatment of patients with bipolar I disorder. It should be assumed that the use of the term "bipolar disorder" in this document refers to bipolar I disorder, as defined in DSM-IV, unless a broader meaning is specified (e.g., "to include bipolar II disorder"). The guideline begins at the point where the psychiatrist has established the diagnosis of bipolar I disorder and has evaluated the patient for the presence of comorbid psychiatric conditions (e.g., alcohol and/or substance abuse or dependence disorder, personality disorders) as well as general medical conditions (e.g., thyroid disease, Cushing's disease, cerebral neoplasms) that could mimic bipolar disorder or be important to its treatment.

The purpose of this guideline is to assist the physician faced with the task of managing patients with bipolar disorder. This may involve different treatment strategies at different points in time. Because the needs of individual patients vary substantially during the course of this long-term disorder and because patients may have comorbid disorders, the psychiatrist should consider, but not be limited to, the recommendations in this treatment guideline.

I. DISEASE DEFINITION, EPIDEMIOLOGY, AND NATURAL HISTORY

▶ ## A. DIAGNOSIS OF BIPOLAR DISORDER

By DSM-IV definition, patients with bipolar I disorder have had at least one episode of mania. Some patients have had previous depressive episodes, and most patients will have subsequent episodes that can be either manic or depressive. In addition, hypomanic and mixed episodes can occur, as well as significant subthreshold mood lability between episodes.

▶ ## B. SPECIFIC FEATURES OF DIAGNOSIS

The assessment of a patient with bipolar disorder includes both cross-sectional (i.e., current or recent features of the patient's condition) and longitudinal (i.e., past and ongoing course of the disorder) issues.

1. Cross-sectional issues

There are a number of important clinical and psychosocial issues to consider in the cross-sectional evaluation of a patient with bipolar disorder. First, the psychiatrist should determine whether the patient meets DSM-IV criteria for a manic, hypomanic, depressive, or mixed episode.

Cross-sectional issues include assessment for the presence of psychotic features, cognitive impairment, risk of suicide, risk of violence to persons or property, risk-taking behavior (including financial extravagance), sexually inappropriate behavior, and substance abuse, as well as the DSM-IV specifiers for current or most recent episode. Assessment of the individual's ability to care for himself or herself, childbearing status or plans, and supports, including family and friends, housing, and financial resources, is important. The degree of distress and disability is also important. Careful attention to these factors will enable the psychiatrist to make a recommendation as to the site of treatment (e.g., inpatient, outpatient, partial hospitalization) and to formulate well-reasoned and appropriate clinical approaches to the patient and family.

2. Longitudinal issues

Bipolar disorder is an episodic, long-term illness with a variable course. In evaluating the individual patient in order to make immediate clinical recommendations and decisions, as well as in beginning to formulate a long-term treatment plan, a number of longitudinal issues must be considered. These include the number of prior episodes, the average length of episodes and average interepisode duration, the interval since the last episode of mania or depression, the level of psychosocial and symptomatic functioning between episodes of illness, and the response to prior treatment.

Bipolar disorder should always be considered in the differential diagnosis of patients with depression. Very often patients do not report prior episodes of mania and hypomania. Therefore, the psychiatrist needs to ask explicitly about such prior manic episodes because knowledge of their presence can influence treatment recommendations and decisions. The psychiatrist should also ask about a family history of mood disorders, including mania and hypomania. Consultation with family members and significant others may be extremely useful in establishing family history. DSM-IV specifiers describing the course of recurrent episodes include rapid cycling, seasonal pattern, and longitudinal course (with or without full interepisode recovery). Some patients switch rapidly and frequently between manic and depressive symptoms without experiencing an intervening period of euthymia. Although these patients are sometimes referred to as rapid cyclers, in this guideline we will refer to these patients as ultrarapid cyclers and reserve the term "rapid cycling" for those patients who have four or more episodes per year (i.e., the DSM-IV definition).

C. NATURAL HISTORY AND COURSE

The first episode of bipolar disorder may be manic, hypomanic, mixed, or depressive and may be followed by several years during which the patient is symptom-free. Because the illness may be associated with substance-related disorders, recklessness, impulsivity, truancy, and other antisocial behavior, the diagnosis of bipolar disorder must be carefully differentiated from substance-related disorders, antisocial behavior, or personality disorders. In children and adolescents, the diagnoses of attention deficit hyperactivity disorder and conduct disorder must also be considered.

Untreated patients with bipolar disorder may have more than 10 total episodes of mania and depression during their lifetime, with the duration of episodes and interepisode periods stabilizing after the fourth or fifth episode (1). Often 5 years or more may elapse between the first and second episode, but the time periods between subsequent episodes usually narrow. However, it must be emphasized that variability is the hallmark of this illness.

Bipolar disorder causes substantial psychosocial morbidity that frequently affects the patient's marriage, children, occupation, and other aspects of the patient's life. Divorce rates are substantially higher in patients with bipolar disorder, approaching two to three times the rate of normal comparison subjects (2). The occupational status of patients with bipolar disorder is twice as likely to deteriorate as that of comparison subjects (2).

In a review of studies of depressive and manic-depressive illnesses conducted between 1937 and 1988 involving over 9,000 patients, the mean suicide completion rate was 19% (1). The rate for bipolar disorder alone was not reported. Suicide occurs more often among males than females and is most likely during a depressive episode. Comorbid substance abuse and anxiety disorders substantially increase the risk of suicide.

Pharmacotherapy may substantially reduce the risk of suicide (3). For example, in an 11-year follow-up of 103 bipolar patients taking lithium, death rates were well below that expected for this group based on age and sex (4). Mortality in general is higher in those with mania in late life compared to those with depression alone (5).

D. EPIDEMIOLOGY

Bipolar I disorder affects approximately 0.8% of the adult population (estimates from community samples range between 0.4% and 1.6%) and bipolar II disorder affects approximately 0.5% over the course of a lifetime (6). Bipolar I disorder affects men and women fairly equally, although bipolar II disorder is more common in women. There are no known significant differences among racial groups in the prevalence of either bipolar I or bipolar II disorder.

The Epidemiologic Catchment Area study reported a mean age at onset of 21 years for bipolar disorder (7). When studies examining age at onset are stratified into 5-year intervals, the peak age at onset of first symptoms falls between ages 15–19, followed closely by ages 20–24. There is often a 5- to 10-year interval, however, between age at onset of illness and age at first treatment or first hospitalization. Onset of mania before age 15 has been less well studied. Clinical experience suggests that onset of bipolar disorder prior to age 12 is uncommon (8).

The first episode in males is more likely to be a manic episode. The first episode in females is more likely to be depressive episode. Frequently, a patient will experience several episodes of depression before a manic episode occurs (9–15).

Onset of mania after age 60 is less likely to be associated with a positive family history of bipolar disorder and is more likely to be associated with identifiable general medical factors, including cerebral vascular problems. Morbidity and mortality rates are especially high in patients over age 60 (5, 16).

Evidence from epidemiologic and twin studies strongly suggests that bipolar disorder is a heritable illness (17, 18). First-degree relatives of patients with bipolar disorder have significantly higher rates of mood disorder compared with relatives of nonpsychiatrically ill control populations. However, the mode of inheritance remains unknown, and the magnitude of the role played by environmental stressors, particularly early in the course of the illness, also remains uncertain. In clinical practice, a family history of mood disorder, especially of bipolar disorder, provides strong corroborative evidence of the existence of a mood disorder in a patient with otherwise predominantly psychotic features.

II. TREATMENT PRINCIPLES AND ALTERNATIVES

The development of a treatment plan for patients with bipolar disorder requires the consideration of many issues. The cross-sectional (e.g., current clinical status) and longitudinal (e.g., frequency, severity, and consequences of past episodes) context of the treatment decision should guide the psychiatrist and patient in choosing from among various possible treatments and treatment settings. These decisions must be based on knowledge of the beneficial and adverse effects of available options, along with information about patient preferences. In addition, treatment decisions should be continually reassessed as new information becomes available and/or the patient's clinical status changes. It should also be kept in mind that denial is often a prominent part of this disorder and may at times interfere with the patient's ability to make reasoned treatment decisions.

At this time there is no cure for bipolar disorder; however, treatment can decrease the associated morbidity and mortality. The specific goals of treatment are to decrease the frequency, severity, and psychosocial consequences of episodes and to improve psychosocial functioning between episodes. Some patients with severe and chronic impairments will need specific rehabilitative services.

This section is organized as follows. First, treatment options for patients with bipolar disorder, including psychiatric management, pharmacologic treatments, electroconvulsive therapy, and psychotherapeutic treatments are reviewed along with the evidence for their efficacy. Second, issues to be considered in choosing and implementing these treatment options (including the factors that underlie the choice of treatment setting) are discussed in the context of specific phases of the illness. Finally, the ways in which particular clinical features of the patient's illness alter the general treatment recommendations are elucidated.

A. PSYCHIATRIC MANAGEMENT

Psychiatric management includes a specific set of interventions, some of which have been included in the concept of "supportive psychotherapy" and/or "insight-oriented psychotherapy" and others in the concept of "clinical management." The general goals are to assess and treat acute exacerbations, prevent recurrences, improve interepisode functioning, and provide assistance, insight, and support to the patient and family.

Specific goals of psychiatric management include establishing and maintaining a therapeutic alliance, monitoring the patient's psychiatric status, providing education regarding bipolar disorder, enhancing treatment compliance, promoting regular patterns of activity and wakefulness, promoting understanding of and adaptation to the psychosocial effects of bipolar disorder, identifying new episodes early, and reducing the morbidity and sequelae of bipolar disorder (19).

1. Establishing and maintaining a therapeutic alliance

Bipolar disorder is a long-term illness that manifests itself in different ways at different points during its course. Establishing and maintaining a supportive therapeutic relationship is critical to the proper understanding and management of an individual patient. A crucial element of this alliance is the knowledge gained about the course of the patient's illness that allows new episodes to be identified as early as possible.

2. Monitoring the patient's psychiatric status

The psychiatrist should remain vigilant for changes in psychiatric status. While this is true for all mental disorders, it is especially important in bipolar disorder because lack of insight on the part of the patient is so frequent, especially during manic episodes, and because small changes in mood or behavior may herald the onset of an episode with potentially devastating consequences. Such monitoring may be enhanced by knowledge gained over time about particular characteristics of the patient's illness, including typical sequence (e.g., mania is usually followed by depression) and typical duration and severity of episodes (e.g., depressions are mild and often self-limiting).

3. Providing education regarding bipolar disorder

Patients with bipolar disorder often benefit from education and feedback regarding their illness, prognosis, and treatment. Frequently, their ability to understand and retain this information will vary over time and may be impeded by a tendency to deny the existence and consequences of the illness. Education should therefore be an ongoing process in which the psychiatrist gradually but persistently introduces facts about the illness, with adequate therapeutic attention to the psychological forces promoting denial and to the patient's stage of adaptation to the chronic illness. Importantly, patient education over an extended period of time will assist in reinforcing the patient's role as collaborator in the treatment of this persistent illness. In this capacity, the patient will know when to report subsyndromal symptoms and gradually learn to increase or decrease medications with the waxing and waning of the illness. Printed material on cross-sectional and longitudinal aspects of bipolar illness and its treatment can be helpful (20–23). Family members may also deny the illness and its consequences, and similar educational approaches by the psychiatrist may be important with family members.

4. Enhancing treatment compliance

Bipolar disorder is a long-term illness in which adherence to carefully designed treatment plans can improve the patient's health status. However, patients with this disorder are frequently ambivalent about treatment. This ambivalence often takes the form of noncompliance with medication and other treatments (24, 25). Noncompliance with mood-stabilizing medications is a major cause of relapse (26, 27).

Ambivalence about treatment stems from many factors. One is denial. Patients who do not believe that they have a serious illness are not likely to be willing to adhere to long-term treatment regimens. Patients with this disorder may minimize or deny the reality of a prior episode, their own behavior, and often the consequences of their behavior. Denial may be especially pronounced during a manic episode.

Another important factor for some patients is their reluctance to give up the experience of mania (24). The increased energy, euphoria, heightened self-esteem, and ability to focus may be very desirable and enjoyable. Patients often recall this experience and minimize or deny entirely the subsequent devastating features of full-blown mania or the extended demoralization of a depressive episode. They are therefore often reluctant to take medication that prevents mania.

Medication side effects and other demands of long-term treatment may be burdensome and need to be discussed realistically with the patient and family members. Many side effects can be corrected with careful attention to dosing, scheduling, and preparation. Troublesome side effects that remain must be discussed in the context of an informed assessment of the risks and benefits of the current treatment and its potential alternatives.

5. Promoting regular patterns of activity and wakefulness

Patients with bipolar disorder may benefit from regular patterns of daily activities, including sleeping, eating, physical activity, and social and/or emotional stimulation. The psychiatrist should help the patient determine the degree to which these factors affect mood states and to develop methods to monitor and modulate daily activities. Many patients find that if they establish regular patterns of sleeping, other important aspects of life fall into regular patterns as well.

6. Promoting understanding of and adaption to the psychosocial effects of bipolar disorder

All patients with bipolar disorder have had at least one manic episode. Many patients have had several episodes of mania and depression. Typically, such a history leaves patients with emotional, social, family, academic, occupational, and financial issues that require therapeutic help to address and deal with effectively.

During the episode itself, the psychiatrist should assist the patient with issues related to his or her environment, including interpersonal relationships, work and living conditions, and other medical or health-related needs. Examples of this assistance include helping the patient to avoid engaging in embarrassing behavior during manic episodes, assisting the patient in scheduling absences from work or other responsibilities as required, discouraging the patient from instituting major life changes that might be predicated on the depressed or manic state, helping to bolster the patient's morale by strengthening expectations of help and hope for the future, enlisting the support of others in the patient's social network and supporting them as necessary, and setting realistic, attainable, and tangible goals. Patients who have children may need help assessing their children's needs, both during and in the wake of the parent's episodes, and making appropriate plans to meet those needs. At times, it may be important to help the parent with bipolar disorder obtain a psychiatric evaluation for the child (e.g., if the parent reports that the child or adolescent is showing early signs of mood instability). Bipolar patients who are considering having children may benefit from genetic counseling (27).

7. Identifying new episodes early

The psychiatrist should help the patient and family members to identify early signs and symptoms of manic or depressive episodes. Such identification can help the patient to enhance mastery over his or her illness and can help ensure that adequate treatment is instituted as early as possible in the course of an episode. Early markers of episode onset vary from patient to patient. Many patients experience changes in sleep patterns early in the development of an episode. Other symptoms may be quite subtle and specific to the individual (e.g., participating in religious activities more or less often than usual). The identification of these early, prodromal signs or symptoms is facilitated by the presence of a consistent relationship between the psychiatrist and the patient, as well as the patient's family. The use of a graphic display of life events and mood can be very helpful in this process (28). First conceived by Kraepelin (29) and Meyer (30) and refined and advanced by Post et al. (28), a life chart provides a valuable display of illness course and episode sequence, polarity, severity, frequency, and relationship, if any, to environmental stressors, as well as response to treatment. A graphic display of sleep patterns may be sufficient for some patients to identify early signs of episodes.

8. Reducing the morbidity and sequelae of bipolar disorder

Through many of the activities already described, psychiatric management helps minimize the sequelae of abnormal mood states by helping the patient respond adaptively on an interpersonal, academic, occupational, social, and financial level.

Psychiatric management should be an ongoing process. Different interventions will be needed at different times as the patient experiences episodes of the illness and as the patient and family develop and grow in their ability to respond adaptively to the demands of the illness.

B. PHARMACOLOGIC TREATMENTS

Pharmacologic treatments are a critical component in the treatment of patients with bipolar disorder. Medications have been shown to be effective in the treatment of acute episodes, as well as in the prevention of future episodes. In addition, many patients benefit between episodes from the mood-stabilizing effects of some medications. The review of efficacy data for bipolar disorder is hampered somewhat by inconsistencies in the measurement and description of patient outcomes, as well as in the terms used to describe changes in the course of the illness.

Medications for patients with bipolar disorder include those that decrease symptoms of mania or depression, those that prevent episodes, and those that may not act primarily on mood but that are helpful at various times during the course of the disorder. These medications have been categorized in a variety of ways. In this guideline, we use the following categories: mood stabilizers (medications with both antimanic and antidepressive actions); antimanic agents; antidepressants; adjunctive medications; and new or atypical medications that have not been fully assessed.

The three mood stabilizers currently available—lithium, valproate, and carbamazepine—have been studied and used in the treatment of all phases of bipolar disorder. The following review of efficacy data for each medication is organized according to phase of disorder and goal of the treatment (e.g., during the manic phase, the goal is to reduce manic symptoms and shorten the episode).

Traditionally, lithium has been the primary pharmacologic treatment for patients with bipolar disorder. It was first reported to have antimanic effects in 1949 (31) and has been in widespread use in this country for the acute and preventive treatment of bipolar disorder since the mid 1960s (32). Valproate and carbamazepine, on the other hand, have only been reported useful for this disorder since the late 1970s. The total number of patients studied in lithium trials as well as the breadth of clinical experience with lithium far exceeds that for the two newer agents. However, the quality of study design and outcome measures have improved over time, so that some of the soundest studies include the newer agents.

1. Lithium

Lithium is effective in the acute treatment of manic and depressive episodes and in the prevention of recurrent manic and depressive episodes (1). In addition, lithium has been reported to decrease the mood instability that plagues many patients between episodes (1).

a) Acute mania

Considerable research supports the efficacy of lithium in the treatment of manic episodes. In a review of 10 early uncontrolled trials of 413 patients with bipolar disorder, 81% displayed reduced manic symptoms during acute lithium treatment (33). The overall response rate to lithium in four placebo-controlled studies of 116 patients with acute mania was 78% (34–38). These studies also demonstrated that up to 2 weeks of treatment with lithium may be necessary to reach maximal effectiveness for manic patients. In a recent randomized, double-blind, controlled study of lithium, divalproex, and placebo (39), 49% of the patients taking lithium had at least a 50% reduction in their mania rating scale score at 3 weeks, despite the fact that over half of the patients reported that lithium had not been effective for their most recent prior episode. Lithium was significantly more effective than placebo and was not statistically more or less effective than divalproex. Preliminary, unpublished data from this study suggest that lithium is more effective than divalproex in the treatment of "classic mania" and less effective than divalproex in the treatment of "mixed mania." These hypotheses need further study.

Lithium has also been compared with neuroleptics. While most studies are confounded by having included a wide diagnostic mix of patients, Janicak et al. (40) recently reviewed the available studies that included only patients with acute mania. They found that in these well-designed studies lithium was superior to neuroleptics in the acute treatment of mania.

b) Acute bipolar depression

A review of nine controlled studies comparing lithium with placebo in the treatment of the depressive phase of bipolar disorder (41) showed that 63 (79%) of 80 patients displayed an antidepressant response to lithium (41). Despite controversy over the methodology of some of these studies, it seems clear that many patients in the depressive phase of bipolar disorder can expect a clinically significant response to lithium. The time frame for response for depression is longer than that for mania, however. Many patients require lithium treatment for 6 to 8 weeks before a full response becomes evident. When the patient's clinical status prohibits such a long lag between the onset of treatment and a full response, the addition of psychotherapy, an antidepressant, or other medication may be warranted. These options are discussed in later sections.

c) Maintenance treatment

Open studies in the 1960s and 1970s of the prophylactic efficacy of lithium showed that the use of this drug reduces the frequency, duration, and severity of manic and depressive episodes (1). Many of these studies included patients with high rates of recurrence prior to treatment with lithium. In such patients the results were often dramatic. For example, in one study the average time ill during a 12-month period dropped from 13 weeks to 2 weeks (42).

These results have since been confirmed by 10 double-blind, placebo-controlled studies. A review of these studies found that patients taking lithium had a significantly lower probability of having an episode than those taking placebo (1). Overall, 34% of the patients taking lithium had an episode compared to 81% of those taking placebo, although these summary statistics are confounded by variations in entry criteria, definitions of relapse, and length of follow up.

Lithium appears to be equally effective in preventing episodes of mania and major episodes of depression. Many investigators have found that patients taking lithium prophylactically continue to have minor episodes of depression, however. This asymmetry of response between minor depressive and minor manic episodes may be based, in part, on the fact that patients are more likely to report mild depression than mild hypomania. Many investigators have also reported that lithium decreases the intensity of episodes that do occur and that lithium reduces subsyndromal mood variations between episodes. These two effects are often very valuable to patients and are frequently omitted from summary statistics of lithium's efficacy (1).

Discontinuation of long-term lithium therapy in patients with bipolar disorder has been associated with a significant short-term increase in risk of recurrence. In one study, over 50% of patients with bipolar disorder experienced recurrent mood episodes within 6 months of lithium discontinuation (43). Whether this represents a "lithium withdrawal syndrome" or simply a reemergence of the disorder is not clear (1, 44, 45). It is also possible that in some patients who choose to stop taking lithium, discontinuation itself may be an early manifestation of recurrence. If the decision is made to discontinue previously effective lithium therapy, slow tapering has been reported to reduce the risk of early recurrence (43). Some patients develop a more severe and relatively nonresponsive form of the illness following the discontinuation of effective prophylactic lithium (46). In this instance, switching to a medication with a novel mechanism of action, providing ECT, or discontinuing that medication for a period of time followed by a renewed trial may be successful, at least temporarily, in reinitiating a treatment response (47).

d) Pharmacokinetics and drug–drug interactions

Lithium is available in tablets or capsules as the carbonate salt or as lithium citrate in syrup form. A 300 mg tablet of lithium carbonate contains 8 meq (or mmol); 5 cc of the citrate syrup also contains 8 meq. Lithium is readily absorbed after oral administration; no parenteral forms are available. Standard preparations lead to peak serum levels in 1.5 to 2 hours; slow release forms lead to peak serum levels in 4 to 4.5 hours.

Lithium is excreted almost entirely by the kidneys, with a half-life between 14 and 30 hours. (Normally the lithium clearance is about one-fourth of the creatinine clearance.) The rate of lithium clearance is faster in younger persons and decreases in association with diminished glomerular function and age.

Therapeutic and toxic effects of lithium are correlated with serum levels, which are correlated, to a lesser extent, with oral dose. Therefore, safe and effective administration of lithium requires that serum levels be monitored. The relatively long half-life of lithium means that steady-state levels after a dosage change will not occur for 5 to 7 days. Trough levels are typically reported, and these are traditionally sampled 12 hours after the last dose. If this procedure is not followed, the results are likely to be unreliable and misleading. The availability of a slow-release form and the practice of switching from a multiple-dose regimen to a once-daily regimen may confuse the interpretation of serum levels. In general, a patient whose lithium regimen changes from twice a day to once a day can expect a 10% to 26% increase in 12-hour lithium levels (32).

Lithium is distributed in total body water, is not protein bound, and is not metabolized. Changes in hydration will affect lithium levels, with episodes of dehydration leading to higher levels. Lithium excretion, and therefore serum levels, can be affected by changes in renal function. Decreases in glomerular filtration rates, either due to age or disease, will decrease lithium clearance. In addition, sodium deficiency (secondary to diet, medication, or other causes) will increase lithium reabsorption and increase lithium levels. Thiazide diuretics increase lithium levels by 30% to 50%. Furosemide appears to have no direct effect on lithium levels, although lithium levels should be monitored in any patient beginning treatment with a diuretic because of potential changes in total body fluid. Many types of medications have been reported to increase lithium levels, including some nonsteroidal anti-inflammatory agents and angiotensin converting enzyme-inhibiting antihypertensive agents (1). Although there have been reports of enhanced neurotoxicity, including the development of neuroleptic malignant syndrome, when lithium was administered in conjunction with a neuroleptic (especially haloperidol), most investigators have found that these medications can be safely combined at standard doses, and are, in fact, used together quite commonly without severe adverse effects (32).

e) Side effects and toxicity

Up to 75% of patients treated with lithium experience some side effects (1, 32). These side effects vary in clinical significance; most are either minor or can be reduced or eliminated by lowering the lithium dose or changing the dosage schedule. For example, Schou (48) has reported a 30% reduction in side effects among patients treated with an average lithium level of 0.68 meq/liter compared to those with an average level of 0.85 meq/liter. Side effects that appear to be related to peak serum levels (e.g., tremor that peaks within 1 to 2 hours of a dose) may be reduced or eliminated by using a slow-release preparation or changing to a single bedtime dose.

(1) Dose-related side effects
Side effects of lithium include polyuria, polydypsia, weight gain, cognitive problems (e.g., dulling, impaired memory, poor concentration, confusion, mental slowness), tremor, sedation or lethargy, impaired coordination, gastrointestinal distress (e.g., nausea, vomiting, dyspepsia, diarrhea), hair loss, benign leukocytosis, acne, and edema. Side effects persisting despite dosage adjustment may be managed with other medications (e.g., β-blockers for tremor; diuretics for polyuria, polydipsia or edema; topical antibiotics or retinoic acid for acne). Gastrointestinal disturbances can be man-

aged by administering lithium with meals or switching lithium preparations (especially to lithium citrate).

Lithium may cause benign ECG changes associated with repolarization. Less commonly, cardiac conduction abnormalities have been associated with lithium treatment. Anecdotal reports have linked lithium with other ECG changes, including the exacerbation of existing arrhythmias and, less commonly, the development of new arrhythmias (32).

The most common renal effect of lithium is impaired concentrating capacity due to reduced renal response to ADH, manifested as polyuria and/or polydipsia. Although the polyuria associated with early lithium treatment may resolve, persistent polyuria (ranging from mild and well tolerated to severe nephrogenic diabetes insipidus) may occur. Polyuria can frequently be managed by changing to a once-daily bedtime dose. If the polyuria persists, management includes ensuring that fluid intake is adequate and that the lithium dose is as low as possible. Some clinicians have found that decreasing the total daily protein intake, in conjunction with a nutritional assessment, is helpful. If these measures do not ameliorate the problem, then concurrent administration of a thiazide diuretic (e.g., hydrochlorothiazide at a dose of 50 mg/day) may be helpful. The dosage of lithium will usually need to be decreased (typically by 50%) to account for the increased reabsorption induced by thiazides (32). In addition, potassium levels will need to be monitored, and potassium replacement may be necessary. Amiloride, a potassium-sparing diuretic, is reported to be effective in treating lithium-induced polyuria and polydipsia; its advantages are that it does not alter lithium levels and does not cause potassium depletion. Amiloride may be started at 5 mg b.i.d. and may be increased to 10 mg b.i.d., as needed (49).

Hypothyroidism occurs in 5% to 35% of patients treated with lithium, is more frequent in women, tends to appear after 6 to 18 months of lithium treatment, and may be associated with rapid cycling (1, 32, 50). Lithium-induced hypothyroidism is generally reversible when lithium is discontinued. However, lithium-induced hypothyroidism is not a contraindication to continuing lithium treatment. When lithium is continued, the associated hypothyroidism is easily treated by administration of levothyroxine (32). In addition to the classic signs and symptoms of hypothyroidism, patients with bipolar disorder are at risk of developing depression and/or rapid cycling as a consequence of suboptimal thyroid functioning. If these symptoms occur in the presence of laboratory evidence of suboptimal thyroid functioning, then thyroid supplementation and/or discontinuation of lithium should be considered (51, 52).

(2) Idiosyncratic side effects

A small number of case reports describe exacerbation or first occurrences of psoriasis associated with lithium treatment. Some of these patients improved with appropriate dermatologic treatment and/or when the lithium dose was lowered. In some cases, however, lithium seemed to block the effects of dermatologic treatment, and the condition cleared only after lithium was discontinued. In addition, occasionally patients experience severe pustular acne that does not respond well to standard dermatologic treatments and only resolves once the lithium has been discontinued. (This is in contrast to the more common mild to moderate acne that can occur with lithium treatment and that is usually responsive to standard treatments [32].)

Much concern has been raised about whether long-term lithium exposure may cause irreversible kidney damage. Approximately 10% to 20% of patients receiving long-term lithium treatment (more than 10 years) display morphological kidney changes—usually interstitial fibrosis, tubular atrophy, and sometimes glomerular sclerosis. These changes may be associated with impairment of water reabsorption, but not with reduction in glomerular filtration rate or development of renal insufficiency (1, 32, 53–55). Although irreversible renal failure due to lithium has not been unequivocally established, there are two case reports of probable lithium-induced renal insufficiency (55, 56). Additionally, several studies show that a small percentage of patients treated with lithium may develop rising serum creatinine concentrations after 10 years or more of treatment (55).

(3) Toxicity/overdose

Toxic effects of lithium become more likely as the serum level rises. Most patients will experience some toxic effects with levels above 1.5 meq/liter; levels above 2.0 meq/liter are commonly associated with life-threatening side effects. For many patients, the therapeutic range within which beneficial effects outweigh toxic effects is quite narrow, so that small changes in serum level may lead to clinically significant alterations in the beneficial and harmful effects of lithium. Elderly patients may experience toxic effects at lower levels and have a correspondingly narrower therapeutic window.

Signs and symptoms of early intoxication (with levels above 1.5 meq/liter) include marked tremor, nausea and diarrhea, blurred vision, vertigo, confusion, and increased deep tendon reflexes. With levels above 2.5 meq/liter, patients may experience more severe neurological complications and eventually experience seizures, coma, cardiac dysrhythmia, and permanent neurological impairment. The magnitude of the serum level and the duration of exposure to a high level of lithium are both correlated with risk of adverse effects. Therefore, rapid steps to reduce the serum level are essential. In addition, during treatment for severe intoxication, patients may experience "secondary peaks," during which the serum level rises after a period of relative decline; the clinician must therefore continue to monitor serum levels during treatment for severe intoxication. The patient with lithium intoxication should be treated with supportive care (e.g., maintenance of fluid and electrolyte balance), and steps should be taken to prevent further absorption of the medication (e.g., induction of emesis in the alert patient, gastric lavage). Hemodialysis is the only reliable method of rapidly removing excess lithium from the body and is more effective than peritoneal dialysis for this purpose. Criteria for use of hemodialysis in lithium intoxication are not firmly established, and the decision to dialyze must take into account both the patient's clinical status and the serum lithium level. While most authorities agree that dialysis should be used in instances when clinical signs of intoxication are severe, it is not clear that a clinically tolerated high lithium level is, by itself, an indication for dialysis.

f) Implementing lithium treatment

Prior to beginning lithium treatment, the patient's general medical history should be reviewed, with special reference to those systems that might affect, or be affected by, lithium therapy (i.e., renal, thyroid, and cardiac functioning). In addition, pregnancy or the presence of a dermatologic disorder must be ascertained.

In general, laboratory measures and other diagnostic tests are recommended based on knowledge of pathophysiology and anticipated clinical decisions, rather than on evidence from experimental studies that indicate their clinical utility. The decision to recommend a test is based on the probability of detecting a finding that would alter treatment and the expected benefit of the resulting alteration in treatment. Recommended tests fall into three categories: 1) baseline measures that are used to facilitate the later interpretation of laboratory tests (e.g., ECG, CBC); 2) tests to determine whether different or additional treatments are needed (e.g., pregnancy, thyroid-stimulating hormone level); and 3) tests to determine whether the standard dosage regimen of lithium needs to be altered (e.g., creatinine level).

Based on these considerations, the following are generally recommended prior to beginning lithium therapy: general medical history and physical examination; BUN and creatinine levels; pregnancy test; tests of thyroid function; ECG with rhythm strip for patients over age 40; and some authorities suggest a CBC.

There are two methods to initiate lithium treatment and achieve therapeutic serum levels. The first involves administering a single test dose of lithium, obtaining a serum level 24 hours later, and using a nomogram to predict the appropriate daily dose (57). Alternatively, lithium may be started in low divided doses to minimize side effects (e.g., 300 mg t.i.d. or less, depending on the patient's weight and age) and the dose titrated upward (generally to serum concentrations of 0.5 to 1.2 meq/liter) according to response and side effects (58). Lithium levels should be checked after each dosage increase (and prior to the next); steady-state levels are likely to be reached approximately 5 days after a dosage adjustment, but levels may need to be checked sooner if a rapid increase is necessary (e.g., in the treatment of acute mania) or if toxicity is suspected. As levels approach the upper limits of the therapeutic range (i.e., ≥ 1.0 meq/liter), levels should be checked at shorter intervals after each dosage increase to minimize the risk of toxicity.

Serum concentrations required for prophylaxis may be, in some cases, as high as those required for treatment of the acute episode. A controlled study by Gelenberg et al. (58) found that patients randomly assigned to a "low" lithium level (0.4–0.6 meq/liter) had fewer side effects but more episodes than patients in the "standard" lithium group (0.8–1.0 meq/liter). However, the lithium levels of some of the patients in the "low" group decreased relatively rapidly from their previous treatment levels, which could have increased their risk of relapse. Although the prophylactic efficacy of lithium levels between 0.6–0.8 meq/liter has not been formally studied, this range is commonly chosen by patients and their psychiatrists. Despite the lack of formal study, it is likely that for many patients increases in maintenance lithium levels will result in a trade off between greater protection from episodes at the cost of increased side effects. The "optimal" maintenance level may therefore vary somewhat from patient to patient. Some patients find that a single daily dose facilitates treatment compliance and reduces or does not change side effects.

The clinical status of patients on lithium needs to be monitored especially closely, with the frequency of monitoring dependent on the individual patient's clinical situation, but generally no less than every 6 months in stable patients. The optimal frequency of serum level monitoring in an individual patient will depend on the following features: the range of therapeutic lithium levels; the stability of lithium levels during the average course of events for that patient; and the degree to which the patient can be relied upon to notice and report symptoms. These features will vary with the phase of the illness.

In general, renal function should be tested every 2 to 3 months during the first 6 months of treatment, and thyroid function should be tested once or twice during the first 6 months of lithium treatment. Subsequently, renal and thyroid function may be checked every 6 months to 1 year in stable patients or whenever clinically indicated (e.g., in the presence of breakthrough affective symptoms, changes in side effects, or new general medical or psychiatric signs or symptoms) (32, 54).

2. Valproate

Valproate has been studied alone and in combination with other mood stabilizers in all phases of bipolar disorder.

a) Acute mania

Janicak et al. (40) reviewed the available data on the use of valproate in the treatment of acute mania. They found that numerous studies, comprising 297 patients, demonstrate an overall "moderate to marked" response rate of 56%. However, these studies had many methodologic problems, including a lack of standard diagnostic information about the patients, nonblind conditions, and the use of valproate in conjunction with other active medications.

Two double-blind, placebo-controlled trials of valproate in the acute treatment of mania have been reported, with a total of 36 patients in one study (59) and 179 patients in the other (39). These studies used careful diagnostic criteria, limited supplemental medications, and employed double-blind conditions. The study by Bowden et al. (39) included three treatment groups: placebo, lithium, and valproate. Taken together, these two studies demonstrate that over a 3-week period, valproate is superior to placebo and is as effective as lithium for patients with acute mania. In addition, as mentioned earlier, preliminary unpublished data suggest that divalproex may be more effective than lithium for patients with mixed mania and less effective than lithium for patients with classic mania. These hypotheses need to be tested in further studies.

Improvement in manic symptoms has been observed within 3 days using oral loading (60, 61) and within 5 days with standard dosing regimens (39). Other studies have demonstrated that certain patients who are resistant to the antimanic effects of a single mood stabilizer may benefit from the combination of valproate with lithium, valproate with carbamazepine, and valproate with neuroleptics, including clozapine (62–64).

b) Acute bipolar depression

There are no controlled studies examining the efficacy of valproate in acute bipolar depression. Open studies have had response rates that are in the range consistent with a placebo mechanism of action; 30% of depressed bipolar patients had "some response" and significantly fewer had a "marked response" to valproate (65–69).

There may be a role for valproate in the treatment of depressed bipolar patients who require an antidepressant but need to be protected from the induction of mania (68).

c) Maintenance treatment

There are no controlled studies of valproate in the maintenance phase of bipolar disorder. Open studies indicate that valproate may reduce the frequency and/or intensity of recurrent episodes over extended periods of time in some patients with bipolar disorder, including those with rapid cycling (65, 67, 69, 70).

d) Pharmacokinetics and drug–drug interactions

Valproate is commercially available in the United States in a wide variety of preparations: valproate (available in capsules and syrup), divalproex sodium (an enteric-coated, stable coordination compound containing equal proportions of valproic acid and sodium valproate), and divalproex sodium sprinkle capsules (containing coated particles of divalproex sodium that can be ingested intact or pulled apart and sprinkled on food). There are only minor differences in the pharmacokinetic properties of these different preparations (71–74), and valproate is the common compound in plasma. Valproate, in both capsules and syrup, is rapidly absorbed after ingestion; peak serum concentrations are reached within 2 hours. Peak serum concentrations of divalproex sodium are attained within 3 to 8 hours. The plasma half-life of both valproate and divalproex sodium ranges from 6 to 16 hours.

The relationship between valproate serum concentrations and mood-stabilizing effects is not fully defined. The range considered therapeutic for epilepsy is 50–100 μg/ml (75). A recent study of the use of valproate in patients with acute mania found that the beneficial effects increased markedly with levels above 45 μg/ml and certain adverse effects increased markedly with levels above 125 μg/ml (unpublished 1994 study of Bowden et al.).

Because valproate is extensively metabolized by the liver and highly protein bound, interactions may occur with other metabolized or protein-bound drugs (71, 72). In addition, valproate weakly inhibits drug oxidation, so serum concentrations of drugs that undergo oxidative metabolization (e.g., phenobarbital, phenytoin, and tricyclics) can be increased when coadministered with valproate. Conversely, valproate serum concentrations can be decreased by coadministration of microsomal enzyme-inducing drugs (e.g., carbamazepine) or increased by drugs that inhibit metabolism (e.g., fluoxetine) (76). Also, serum valproate free fraction concentrations can be increased and valproate toxicity precipitated by coadministration of other highly protein-bound drugs (e.g., aspirin), which can displace valproate from its protein binding sites.

e) Side effects and toxicity

Minor side effects of valproate, such as sedation or gastrointestinal distress, are common initially and typically resolve with continued treatment or dosage adjustment. In addition, the medication has a wide therapeutic window. Inadvertent overdose is uncommon, and purposeful overdose less likely to be lethal than with lithium. However, the medication can rarely cause life-threatening reactions, and patients must be relied upon to report the often quite subtle symptoms of these reactions promptly.

(1) Dose-related side effects

Common dose-related side effects of valproate include gastrointestinal distress (e.g., anorexia, nausea, dyspepsia, vomiting, diarrhea), benign hepatic transaminase elevations, tremor, and sedation. Patients with past or current hepatic disease may be at increased risk for hepatotoxicity. Mild, asymptomatic leukopenia and thrombocytopenia (reversible upon drug discontinuation) occur less frequently. Other side effects often bothersome to the patient include hair loss (usually transient), increased appetite, and weight gain. Persistent gastrointestinal distress associated with valproate can be alleviated by dosage reduction, change of preparation (use of the divalproex sodium formulation rather than valproic acid), or by administration of a histamine-2-antagonist (e.g., famotidine or cimetidine) (77). Tremor can be managed with dosage reduction or coadministration of β-blockers. If mild, asymptomatic thrombocytopenia occurs, a decrease in valproate dosage will usually restore the platelet count to normal. Similarly, cases of mild, asymptomatic leukopenia (total WBC count above 3000 and polymorphonuclear leukocyte count above 1500) is usually reversible upon dosage reduction or discontinuation.

(2) Idiosyncratic side effects

One recent uncontrolled report indicated that 80% of women receiving long-term valproate treatment for epilepsy before the age of 20 had polycystic ovaries or hyperandrogenism (78). The implications of this for women who take valproate for bipolar disorder (both for acute and perhaps maintenance treatment) need to be assessed. Rare, idiosyncratic, but potentially fatal adverse events include irreversible hepatic failure, pancreatitis, and agranulocytosis. Patients taking valproate need to be instructed to contact their psychiatrist immediately if they develop symptoms of these conditions.

(3) Toxicity/overdose

Valproate has a wide therapeutic window, and unintentional overdose is therefore uncommon. Signs of overdose include somnolence, heart block, and eventually coma. Deaths have been reported. Overdose can be treated with hemodialysis and/or naloxone (40, 75).

f) Implementing valproate treatment

Before initiating valproate treatment, a general medical history should be taken, with special attention to hepatic, hematologic, and bleeding abnormalities. Ideally, liver function and hematologic measures should be obtained at baseline prior to drug administration to evaluate general medical health.

Valproate may be initiated in low, divided doses to minimize gastrointestinal and neurologic toxicity. Dosage should generally be started at 250 mg t.i.d., with the dose increased every few days as side effects allow (49). The dose is then titrated upward by 250–500 mg/day every several days according to response and side effects, generally to a serum concentration between 50–100 μg/ml (with a maximum adult daily dose of 60 mg/kg per day) (75). Patients with acute mania may tolerate larger initial doses of up to 20 mg/kg per day (valproate loading) and more rapid dosage increments than elderly patients and patients who are hypomanic, euthymic, or depressed (60, 61). Once the patient is stable, valproate dosage regimens can be simplified to enhance convenience and compliance.

Asymptomatic hepatic enzyme elevations, leukopenia, and thrombocytopenia do not reliably predict life-threatening hepatic or bone marrow failure. In conjunction with careful monitoring of clinical status, educating patients about the signs and symptoms of hepatic and hematologic dysfunction and instructing them to report these symptoms if they occur is essential. Some investigators believe that routine monitoring of hematologic and hepatic function in otherwise healthy patients with epilepsy receiving long-term valproate treatment is not necessary (79). Nevertheless, most psychiatrists perform clinical assessments, including tests of hematologic and hepatic function, at a minimum of every 6 months for stable patients who are taking valproate (61, 80, 81). Patients who cannot reliably report signs or symptoms of toxicity need to be monitored more frequently.

3. Carbamazepine

Carbamazepine has been studied alone and in combination with other mood stabilizers in the treatment of all phases of bipolar disorder (63, 80–84).

a) Acute mania

Janicak et al. (40) reviewed 16 studies of carbamazepine that included patients with acute mania. The data generally support the conclusion that carbamazepine is effective in the acute treatment of manic episodes. However, precise interpretation of the data is difficult because of inadequate study design, frequent concomitant use of other active medications, and the use of patient samples that are likely to be atypical.

The results of studies comparing carbamazepine to lithium are mixed, with one investigator finding lithium to be superior (85) and one finding the two drugs to be statistically equivalent, with a trend toward greater efficacy of lithium (86). Studies comparing carbamazepine to neuroleptics have generally found the two medications to be equivalent in efficacy (87–89).

b) Acute bipolar depression

There are two double-blind comparisons of carbamazepine with placebo in the treatment of bipolar depression (90, 91). These studies included patients with bipolar I and bipolar II disorder. In total, 10 of 17 patients had a good or partial response. Another double-blind, controlled study of 13 patients with bipolar I disorder who had not responded to carbamazepine alone found that six responded to lithium augmentation (92).

c) Maintenance treatment

Reviews of the data on carbamazepine in the maintenance phase of bipolar disorder have concluded that carbamazepine may effectively reduce the frequency and severity of episodes for some patients (40, 93). However, the data are limited by such methodologic flaws as lack of a randomized, double-blind, placebo-controlled design; concomitant administration of other active medications; and insufficient doses (40, 94–98).

d) Pharmacokinetics and drug–drug interactions

Carbamazepine is available in a wide variety of preparations, including solutions, suspensions, syrups, and newly developed chewable and slow-release formulations. All of these preparations appear to have similar bioavailability. Peak plasma carbamazepine concentrations are generally obtained between 4 and 8 hours after ingestion, but peaks as late as 26 hours have been reported. The elimination half-life of carbamazepine ranges from 18 to 55 hours. With maintenance treatment, carbamazepine induces its own metabolism, and its half-life may be decreased to 5 to 26 hours.

Because carbamazepine also induces the metabolism of other drugs metabolized by the liver and is highly protein bound, it can have clinically important interactions with other drugs stemming from changes in protein binding and hepatic metabolism (71, 72, 99, 100). Carbamazepine decreases the plasma levels of many medications metabolized by the liver, including neuroleptics, benzodiazepines (except clonazepam), tricyclic antidepressants, anticonvulsants, sex steroids and hormonal contraceptives, and thyroid hormones. Conversely, carbamazepine serum concentrations can be increased by drugs that inhibit carbamazepine metabolism, including erythromycin, the calcium channel blockers diltiazem and verapamil (but not nifedipine or nimodipine), and serotonin reuptake inhibitors (40, 75).

e) Side effects and toxicity

Up to 50% of patients receiving carbamazepine experience side effects, and the drug is associated with potentially serious adverse reactions (72, 79, 101).

(1) Dose-related side effects

The most common side effects of carbamazepine include neurological symptoms, such as diplopia, blurred vision, fatigue, nausea, and ataxia. These effects are usually dose related, transient, and often reversible with dosage reduction. Elderly patients, however, may be more sensitive to the side effects. Less frequent side effects include skin rashes, mild leukopenia, mild thrombocytopenia, hyponatremia and (less commonly) hyposmolality, and mild liver enzyme elevations (occurring in 5%–15% of patients). Mild asymptomatic leukopenia is not related to serious idiopathic dyscrasia and usually resolves with dosage reduction or spontaneously with continuation of carbamazepine treatment. In the event of asymptomatic leukopenia, thrombocytopenia, or elevated liver enzymes, the carbamazepine dosage can be reduced or, with severe changes, the drug discontinued. Hyponatremia may be related to water retention due to carbamazepine's antidiuretic effect. Hyponatremia occurs in 6% to 31% of patients, is rare in children but probably more common in the elderly, occasionally develops many months after the initiation of carbamazepine treatment, and sometimes necessitates carbamazepine discontinuation. In addition, carbamazepine may decrease total and free thyroxine levels and increase free cortisol levels, but these effects are rarely clinically significant.

(2) Idiosyncratic side effects

Rare, idiosyncratic, but serious and potentially fatal side effects of carbamazepine include agranulocytosis, aplastic anemia, hepatic failure, exfoliative dermatitis (e.g., Stevens-Johnson Syndrome), and pancreatitis (79, 102). Although these side effects usually occur within the first 3 to 6 months of carbamazepine treatment, in some cases they occurred after more extended periods of treatment. Routine blood monitoring does not reliably predict blood dyscrasias, hepatic failure, or exfoliative dermatitis. Thus, in addition to careful monitoring of clinical status, it is essential to educate patients about the signs and symptoms of hepatic, hematologic, or dermatologic reactions and instruct them to report symptoms if they occur. Other rare side effects include systemic hypersensitivity reactions; cardiac conduction disturbances; psychiatric symptoms, including sporadic cases of mania and psychosis; and, very rarely, renal effects, including renal failure, oliguria, hematuria, and proteinuria.

(3) Toxicity/overdose

Carbamazepine may be fatal in overdose (deaths have been reported with ingestions of more than 6 g). Signs of impending carbamazepine toxicity include dizziness, ataxia, sedation, and diplopia. Acute intoxication can result in hyperirritability, stupor, or coma. The most common symptoms of carbamazepine overdose are nystagmus, ophthalmoplegia, cerebellar and extrapyramidal signs, impairment of consciousness, convulsions, and respiratory dysfunction. Cardiac symptoms may include tachycardia, arrhythmia, conduction disturbances, and hypotension. Gastrointestinal and anticholinergic symptoms may also occur. Management of carbamazepine intoxication includes symptomatic treatment, gastrolavage, and hemoperfusion.

f)   Implementing carbamazepine treatment

The pretreatment evaluation for carbamazepine should include a general medical history and physical examination, with special emphasis on prior history of blood dyscrasias or liver disease. Most authorities recommend that the minimum baseline evaluation include a CBC with differential and platelet count, a liver profile (LDH, SGOT, SGPT, bilirubin, alkaline phosphatase), and renal function tests (49). Serum electrolytes may also be obtained, especially in the elderly, who may be at higher risk for hyponatremia.

Although dosages can range from 200–1800 mg/day, the relationships among dose, serum concentration, response, and side effects are variable. Therefore, the dose should be titrated upward according to response and side effects. In patients over the age of 12, carbamazepine is usually begun at a total daily dosage of 200–600 mg, in three to four divided doses. In hospitalized patients with acute mania, the dosage may be increased in increments of 200 mg/day up to 800–1000 mg/day (unless side effects develop), with slower increases thereafter as indicated. In less acutely ill outpatients, dosage adjustments should be slower, as rapid increases may cause patients to develop nausea and vomiting or mild neurologic symptoms such as drowsiness, dizziness, ataxia, clumsiness, or diplopia. Should such side effects occur, the dose can be decreased temporarily and then increased again more slowly once these side effects have passed.

While therapeutic serum levels for bipolar disorder have not been established, levels established for treatment of seizure disorders (serum concentration between 4–15 $\mu g/ml$) are generally applied to patients with bipolar disorder. Trough levels are most meaningful for establishing an effective level for a given patient and are conveniently drawn prior to the first morning dose and then 5 days after a dosage change, or sooner if toxicity is suspected. Maintenance doses average about 1000 mg/day, but may range from 200–1600 mg/day in routine clinical practice (49). Doses higher than 1600 mg/day are not recommended. CBC, platelets, and liver function tests should be performed every 2 weeks during the first 2 months of carbamazepine treatment. Thereafter, if laboratory tests remain normal and no symptoms of bone marrow suppression or hepatitis appear, blood counts and liver function tests should be obtained at least every 3 months (49). More frequent monitoring is necessary in patients with laboratory findings, signs, or symptoms consistent with hematologic or hepatic abnormalities. Life-threatening reactions, however, are not always detected by routine monitoring. The psychiatrist should educate patients about signs and symptoms of hepatic, hematologic, or dermatologic reactions and instruct patients to report these symptoms if they occur. More frequent clinical and laboratory assessment is needed for those patients who cannot reliably report symptoms.

The combination of carbamazepine and lithium may be particularly effective for some patients, although it appears to increase their risk of developing an acute confusional state. If this combination is used, it is prudent to attempt to taper one of the medications once the patient is stable. While the majority of patients will not require the continued use of lithium and carbamazepine, the condition of some patients who discontinue combined treatment will worsen and require resumption of both mood stabilizers. During combined treatment, it is important to minimize the use or dose of other medications (e.g., neuroleptics, anticholinergics, benzodiazepines) that may contribute to the development of a confusional state. If the patient's mental status worsens, the possibility of drug toxicity should be considered (49).

4. Neuroleptics

Controlled studies have shown that neuroleptics are superior to placebo in the treatment of acute mania (1) (see section II.B.1.). Studies comparing lithium with neuroleptics (usually chlorpromazine) further suggest that while lithium may be superior to neuroleptics for the specific normalization of mood, neuroleptics may have a quicker onset of action and therefore may be useful, at least initially, in the highly agitated or psychotic patient (103). Neuroleptics may be used in the treatment of mania before a mood stabilizer is started to enhance compliance or in conjunction with a mood stabilizer to reduce symptoms while waiting for the effects of the mood stabilizer to become apparent. However, the use of benzodiazepines should be considered as an alternative to neuroleptics in the adjunctive treatment of mania. Benzodiazepines are frequently as effective as neuroleptics for adjunctive treatment of mania, yet do not pose a risk of extrapyramidal symptoms or tardive dyskinesia (1, 104–108).

Neuroleptics have been shown to be effective in conjunction with antidepressants in the treatment of unipolar and bipolar patients with psychotic depression (109, 110). However, clinical experience suggests that some patients with psychotic depression in the context of bipolar disorder may respond to the combination of a mood stabilizer and an antidepressant alone and therefore may not inevitably require a neuroleptic.

Little research supports the routine use of neuroleptics alone as a maintenance treatment for bipolar disorder. Some investigators believe that neuroleptics may exacerbate postmanic major depressive episodes and induce rapid cycling in some bipolar patients (111). However, use of neuroleptics, either intermittently or long term in conjunction with other mood-stabilizing agents, may be necessary in those patients whose psychotic symptoms have inadequately responded to standard mood-stabilizing agents (112).

Depot neuroleptics may be the only treatment option in those patients with seriously disruptive manic and/or psychotic symptoms who are noncompliant with oral medication regimens. In such cases, the risk of tardive dyskinesia should be balanced against the consequences of repeated manic episodes or chronic manic symptoms.

It is possible that clozapine and other newer antipsychotic agents will be effective alternatives for some patients with bipolar disorder (see section II.B.7.).

5. Benzodiazepines

Clonazepam and lorazepam have been studied alone and in combination with lithium in the treatment of acute mania. The interpretation of many of these studies is confounded by small sample sizes, short durations of treatment, concomitant use of neuroleptics, and difficulties in distinguishing putative specific antimanic effects from nonspecific sedative effects (104, 113–117). Taken together, these studies suggest that benzodiazepines are effective, in place of or in conjunction with a neuroleptic, in sedating the acutely agitated manic patient while waiting for the effects of other primary mood-stabilizing agents to become evident. The fact that lorazepam is well absorbed after intramuscular injection (unlike other benzodiazepines) has made it particularly useful for some very agitated patients.

Benzodiazepines are not effective antidepressants and may, in fact, exacerbate depressive symptoms in some patients. However, many depressed patients have anxiety and/or insomnia (either as a consequence of the depression or as a side effect of another medication) and may benefit from a benzodiazepine in addition to their specific antidepressant or mood-stabilizing medication.

Two studies have examined the prophylactic efficacy of benzodiazepines in bipolar disorder. One study demonstrated that clonazepam could successfully replace haloperidol in patients who required an adjunct to their maintenance lithium therapy (118). However, the other study demonstrated that patients who were relatively treatment refractory to the combination of neuroleptics and mood stabilizers could not successfully be treated with the combination of clonazepam and a mood stabilizer (119). Patients with anxiety and/or insomnia may benefit from the adjunctive use of a benzodiazepine. This is especially important for those patients who seem to be particularly vulnerable to the precipitation of an episode during periods of relative sleep deprivation. During these periods, the prompt institution of a benzodiazepine at bedtime may effectively decrease the risk of a relapse.

Although benzodiazepines may be helpful for many patients with bipolar disorder, two cautions are necessary. 1) Benzodiazepines have the potential to cause either dysphoria or disinhibition (with increased agitation) in some patients. 2) Benzodiazepines can produce dependency and in patients with comorbid substance use disorder can induce a relapse of another substance use disorder (120, 121). Patients with comorbid substance-related disorders who are taking benzodiazepines must be monitored particularly closely.

6. Antidepressants

Although antidepressant medications have been extensively studied in patients with unipolar depression (122) and in mixed groups of patients with unipolar and bipolar disorder, there are few sources of controlled data on their use in the depressive phase of bipolar disorder. In addition, all of these studies have methodologic limitations (41).

Zornberg and Pope reviewed seven controlled studies that examined the efficacy of tricyclic antidepressants in the treatment of bipolar depression (41). In general, the data indicate that tricyclic antidepressants are more effective than placebo for patients with bipolar depression. Their efficacy relative to lithium and other antidepressants is less certain. In addition, their utility when combined with lithium, or an alternative mood stabilizer, has not been systematically studied (although this is the manner in which they are frequently used).

Two controlled studies have tested monoamine oxidase inhibitors (MAOI) in patients with bipolar depression. One study found moclobemide (a reversible MAOI) to be equivalent to imipramine among a heterogeneous group of depressed patients, including 33 bipolar patients (123). The other study showed that tranylcypromine was significantly superior to imipramine (without concomitant lithium) in the treatment of the anergic subtype of bipolar depression in patients with bipolar I and bipolar II disorder (124). It is unclear to what extent these findings would apply to bipolar patients without atypical features.

Selective serotonin reuptake inhibitors have not been well studied in the treatment of acute bipolar depression. One controlled study found that fluoxetine was superior to imipramine and placebo in the treatment of acute bipolar depression (125); some of the patients were receiving lithium and some were not (41). Conclusions about the efficacy and risks associated with these medications must await further systematic studies.

Case reports and two clinical trials suggest that bupropion is effective in the prevention and treatment of episodes of bipolar disorder, especially depressive episodes (126–130). Some investigators report that bupropion is less likely than other antidepressants to induce mania and hypomania, but the evidence supporting this is weak.

Virtually every available antidepressant agent has been associated with the emergence of mania in bipolar patients (41, 131, 132). The study of this issue is complicated, however, by the fact that patients with depression have a baseline risk of switching to mania. This risk has been difficult to characterize because of variations in patient groups and treatment regimens across studies. Of further concern is the fact that some investigators have reported an association between the use of antidepressants and the development of rapid cycling (133) and mixed affective states (134). It has therefore been hypothesized that antidepressants may worsen the overall course of bipolar disorder (133). Unfortunately, the phenomenon of antidepressants inducing the switch to mania, hypomania, rapid cycling, or mixed affective states has not been systematically evaluated in most studies of antidepressants and bipolar depression. It is therefore unknown whether different antidepressants are more or less likely to induce the switch process, although recent preliminary data suggest that bupropion may be less likely than tricyclic antidepressants to induce a switch (126).

In general, psychiatrists should be cautious in prescribing antidepressants for patients with bipolar disorder. However, as some bipolar patients continue to develop depression despite optimal use of mood stabilizers, antidepressants are often necessary for acute and/or prophylactic treatment. Patients who require antidepressant treatment should receive the lowest effective dose for the shortest time necessary.

7. Novel and adjunctive pharmacologic treatments

A number of alternative treatments have been reported to be useful in the treatment of various phases of bipolar disorder (93, 135). These include calcium channel blockers, thyroid hormones, clozapine, psychostimulants, light therapy, and sleep manipulation. Some manic patients may respond to calcium channel blockers (136–146), although preliminary data suggest that these may be the same patients who respond to lithium, making these agents less useful in treatment-refractory patients.

Thyroid hormones thyroxine (T_4) and triiodothyronine (T_3), sometimes in "hyperthyroxinemic" (i.e., higher than physiologic) doses and regardless of baseline thyroid status, may have mood-stabilizing effects in patients with rapid-cycling bipolar disorder, usually when used adjunctively with other mood-stabilizing agents, such as lithium, carbamazepine, or valproate (50, 147, 148). Some investigative groups have recommended high initial doses of T_4 (150–400 µg/day), with an increase in dose to an end point of 50% above normal in the free thyroxine index (50, 147). The possibility of adverse cardiac effects, weight loss, depletion of bone mass, and anxiety must be considered (149–151); however, studies have not confirmed concerns about osteoporosis (152, and unpublished 1994 study of Gyulai et al.).

Retrospective and prospective open studies also suggest that the atypical antipsychotic agent clozapine may have mood-stabilizing as well as antipsychotic effects in bipolar patients with psychotic features, including those with rapid cycling and mixed episodes (62, 153, and unpublished 1992 study of Calabrese et al.). Although systematic studies in patients with bipolar disorder are lacking, clozapine appears to have a unique mechanism of action and side-effect profile compared with other neuroleptics. In particular, it does not appear to be associated with akathisia or acute extrapyramidal side effects or, more importantly, tardive dyskinesia. However, clozapine does cause serious side effects, such as seizures and potentially fatal leukopenia.

Psychostimulants, often in conjunction with an antidepressant medication, may be helpful in treatment-resistant depression, although the combination of psychostimulants and an MAOI may pose serious risks that require careful monitoring (122). Their use for the treatment of bipolar depression should be attempted very cautiously because they may precipitate mania.

Other drugs evaluated in the treatment of acute mania, including cholinergic drugs, β-blockers, serotonergic agents (such as fenfluramine, methysergide, and L-tryptophan), and the α-2 adrenergic agonist clonidine, have generally produced unpromising results.

Nonpharmacologic somatic treatments other than ECT, such as sleep deprivation and light therapy, have not yet been rigorously studied in patients with bipolar disorder. However, as noted in the *Practice Guideline for Major Depressive Disorder in Adults* (122; Second Edition included in this volume), light therapy is effective for some patients with seasonal patterns of depressive episodes and may be useful in promoting regular sleep/wake cycles (154). The specific role of light therapy for patients with bipolar disorder, and its potential to induce mania, needs further clarification. Sleep deprivation may be useful for bipolar depression, although it may induce mania.

▶ C. ELECTROCONVULSIVE THERAPY

ECT is efficacious in the treatment of both phases of bipolar disorder. Since the treatment data are specific to the phase of the disorder, they will be discussed separately.

1. Acute mania

ECT has been demonstrated to be rapidly effective as a treatment for acute mania (155). In a review of the studies in which ECT was used to treat acute manic episodes, 470 of 589 patients (80%) showed marked clinical improvement (155). Retrospective analyses of the efficacy and safety of ECT and lithium (with or without antipsychotic drugs) have found both to be roughly equivalent in efficacy (156–158). In controlled prospective studies, ECT was found to be equal to or more effective than pharmacotherapy (159–161).

Many manic patients will experience a relatively rapid response to ECT. For example, in one study with very strict clinical standards, complete remission occurred after six treatments (161). Recommended frequency is three treatments per week; no differences in response rate were found with more frequent treatments (161). The efficacy of frequent and/or prolonged ECT has not been supported by retrospective (156–158, 162) or prospective (160, 161) studies.

ECT is typically not considered a first-line treatment for manic episodes, given that a majority of patients will exhibit an acute response to a mood-stabilizing medication, which may then be continued for maintenance treatment. Consequently, the majority of manic patients treated with ECT are likely to be resistant to conventional antimanic pharmacological agents. One prospective study examined the efficacy of ECT in such medication-resistant patients and found that 13 of 24 (54%) responded to ECT (161). The role of ECT for patients who fail to respond to other mood stabilizers has not been systematically examined.

The rare syndrome of manic delirium that may be associated with severe hyperthermia represents a primary indication for the use of ECT, as ECT is rapidly effective and has a high margin of safety (163–166). ECT should also be considered as a first-line treatment in the presence of pregnancy, neuroleptic malignant syndrome, catatonia, and general medical conditions that preclude the use of standard pharmacological treatments.

2. Acute bipolar depression

ECT is generally considered the most effective antidepressant treatment available, although no study has focused exclusively on the use of ECT in bipolar depression (167–169).

The efficacy of ECT in the treatment of mixed groups of patients with unipolar and bipolar depression has been established in a series of double-blind studies comparing ECT with the administration of anesthesia alone and with antidepressant medications and in studies comparing different forms of ECT administration (170). Patients with psychotic depression may be particularly responsive to ECT. Several investigators have compared rates of response to ECT in patients with bipolar and unipolar depression (157, 171–173). In general, the unipolar/bipolar distinction does not have predictive value with regard to short-term ECT outcome. Consequently, ECT is considered an extremely effective treatment for the depressed phase of bipolar disorder. There is limited information on the efficacy of ECT in bipolar patients with established medication resistance. Recent studies suggest that approximately 50% of bipolar patients with acute depression who have failed at least one adequate trial of antidepressant medication show marked clinical improvement when treated with bilateral ECT (174).

ECT should be considered as a primary treatment in bipolar depression whenever a rapid response is necessary or when pharmacologic interventions are contraindicated (e.g., in pregnancy).

3. Implementing ECT treatment

ECT, like antidepressant medications, may provoke hypomania or mania. This phenomenon is relatively rare during the ECT course (175), and its management is uncertain. Some practitioners continue with ECT, while others discontinue ECT and start lithium treatment (169).

Patients receiving lithium during ECT may be at a higher risk for delirium and status epilepticus (176–182). However, adverse reactions to the combination of ECT and lithium are rare, and delirium associated with the combined treatment rapidly improves once lithium is discontinued. Benzodiazepines raise seizure threshold and reduce the duration of seizures and thus may impair the efficacy of ECT (177, 178, 183, 184). Antipsychotic drugs may be continued during the course of ECT for psychotic or highly agitated patients, but are generally discontinued after such symptoms remit. Like benzodiazepines, anticonvulsants may interfere with the production or duration of seizures and preferably should be discontinued. However, patients maintained on anticonvulsants to treat a concurrent seizure disorder may be safely treated with ECT, often with excellent clinical results.

ECT is extremely safe when administered using modern methods, which include current anesthesia practice, alterations in the delivery of the electrical stimulus, the selected use of unilateral treatment, and advanced cardiopulmonary monitoring. At this time no absolute contraindications to ECT are known. The reader is referred to the 1990 report of the APA Task Force on Electroconvulsive Therapy as the best available summary of indications, complications, side effects, and general implementation of ECT (169).

D. PSYCHOTHERAPEUTIC TREATMENTS

Psychiatric management and pharmacologic therapy are essential components of treatment for acute episodes and for prevention of future episodes in patients with bipolar disorder. In addition, other specific psychotherapeutic treatments may be critical components of the treatment plan for some patients. Patients with bipolar disorder suffer from the psychosocial consequences of past episodes, the ongoing vulnerability to future episodes, and the burdens of adhering to a long-term treatment plan that may involve some unpleasant side effects. In addition, many patients have clinically significant mood instability between episodes. The goals of psychotherapeutic treatments (including psychiatric management) are to reduce distress and improve the patient's functioning between episodes and to decrease the frequency of future episodes (185). Most patients with bipolar disorder will struggle with some of the following issues: 1) emotional consequences of periods of major mood disorder and diagnosis of a chronic mental illness; 2) developmental deviations and delays caused by past episodes; 3) problems associated with stigmatization; 4) problems regulating self-esteem; 5) fears of recurrence and consequent inhibition of normal psychosocial functioning; 6) interpersonal difficulties; 7) marriage, family, childbearing, and parenting issues; 8) academic and occupational problems; and 9) other legal, social, and emotional problems that arise from reckless, violent, withdrawn, or bizarre behavior that may occur during episodes. For some patients, a specific psychotherapy (in addition to psychiatric management) will be needed to address these issues, although the form, intensity, and focus of psychotherapeutic treatment are likely to vary over time for each patient.

In addition to psychiatric management (see section II.A.), there are a range of specific psychotherapeutic interventions that may be helpful for some patients. In general, judgments regarding the efficacy of these treatments are based on strong clinical consensus regarding their beneficial effects for selected patients, rather than on formal controlled trials. The individual treatment approaches include psychodynamic, interpersonal, behavioral, and cognitive. In addition, couples therapy, family therapy, and group therapy may be indicated for some patients. Formal studies are currently being conducted for many of these treatments in patients with bipolar disorder.

The available psychotherapeutic treatments are discussed as separate entities, even though in practice psychiatrists commonly use a combination or synthesis of different approaches depending on the patient's needs and preferences.

1. Specific psychosocial interventions

Research on the application of specific psychosocial interventions for patients with bipolar disorder is sparse. The research summarized here involves formal psychotherapies that have as their goals many of the features of psychiatric management.

Inpatient family intervention (186) has been applied both in schizophrenia and bipolar disorder. Family treatment is brief (approximately six sessions) and includes a psychoeducational component. Goals include accepting the reality of the illness, identifying precipitating stresses and likely future stresses inside and outside the family, elucidating family interactions that produce stress on the patient, planning strategies for managing and/or minimizing future stresses, and bringing about the patient's family's acceptance of the need for continued treatment after hospital discharge. Systematic study of this approach in patients with bipolar disorder is limited, although there is some evidence that it is helpful for some patients (187).

Behavioral family management is a treatment for patients who have recently been hospitalized for an episode of mania. Behavioral family management is based on a home-centered psychosocial treatment for schizophrenia developed by Falloon (188). The treatment includes psychoeducation, communication skills training, and problem-solving skills training. A behavioral family treatment intervention has also been outlined (189). Although definitive trials of behavioral family treatment have not been completed, preliminary evidence suggests that behavioral family management/behavioral family treatment in concert with adequate pharmacotherapy leads to a substantial decrease in relapse rates.

A pilot study of the impact of family therapy and psychoeducation (in addition to pharmacologic and milieu treatment) on patients with bipolar disorder has been reported (190). Patients who were randomly assigned to the family therapy group had lower rates of family separations, greater improvements in level of family functioning, higher rates of full recovery, and lower rates of rehospitalization for 2 years following family treatment.

A cognitive behavioral treatment package for patients with bipolar disorder has been developed by Basco and Rush (191). The goals of the program are to educate the patient regarding bipolar disorder and its treatment, teach cognitive behavioral skills for coping with psychosocial stressors and attendant problems, facilitate compliance with treatment, and monitor the occurrence and severity of symptoms.

The observation that many bipolar patients experience less mood lability when they maintain a regular pattern of daily activities (including sleeping, eating, physical activity, and emotional stimulation) has led to the development of a formalized psychotherapy called interpersonal and social rhythm therapy (192). This form of psychotherapy is currently being tested in combination with pharmacotherapy in a randomized clinical trial during the maintenance phase of bipolar disorder.

2. Specific psychotherapies for depressive episodes

There are a range of psychotherapeutic interventions that may be useful for patients with major depressive episodes. Some of these interventions have been studied in patients with bipolar depression as well as in those with unipolar depression. Others have only been studied in patients with unipolar depression. We did not identify any completed controlled studies of psychotherapeutic treatments in patients with bipolar (and not unipolar) depression, although some studies are underway. It is not clear to what extent patients with bipolar and unipolar depression are similar in their responsiveness to psychotherapy. However, it seems likely that the following treatments may benefit some patients with bipolar depressive disorders, especially when the depressive episodes seem to be precipitated or exacerbated by psychosocial issues or are the cause of significant psychosocial morbidity. This discussion is summarized from the APA *Practice Guideline for Major Depressive Disorder in Adults* (122; Second Edition included in this volume).

Psychodynamic psychotherapy and psychoanalytic treatments are based on observed beneficial effects of clarifying intrapsychic processes that may precipitate and/or perpetuate affective dysregulation in vulnerable patients. Once these forces are made conscious, difficulties can be anticipated and mastered or conflicts neutralized through the process of insight. Mastery and insight, experienced in the supportive or interpretive relationship with the therapist, permit the patient not only to overcome ongoing negative or disorganizing effects of illness but to ward off recurrent dysregulation. In vulnerable individuals who are excessively sensitive to loss and who use reaction formation and aggression turned inward as defense mechanisms to control the aggressive impulse, the detection and alteration of these psychodynamic mechanisms are of central importance in the treatment of depression (193). The supportive psychodynamic approach seeks to alleviate ongoing symptoms and help the patient adapt to life circumstances.

Interpersonal therapy seeks to recognize and explore depressive precipitants that involve interpersonal losses, role disputes and transitions, social isolation, or deficits in social skills (194). There is some evidence in controlled studies that interpersonal therapy without pharmacotherapy is effective in reducing depressive symptoms in the acute phase of less severe unipolar depressive episodes (195, 196) and that it is especially effective in ameliorating occupational and social aspects of the patient's dysfunction (197). There is evidence that monthly interpersonal therapy also has a prophylactic effect during the maintenance phase of unipolar depression (198). The role of interpersonal therapy in the maintenance phase of bipolar disorder is not known.

Behavior therapy of depression is based on a functional analysis of behavior theory (199) and/or social learning theory (200). The techniques involve activity scheduling (201, 202), self-control therapy (203), social skills training (204), and problem solving (205). Behavior therapy has been reported to be effective in the acute treatment of patients with mild to moderately severe unipolar depression, especially when combined with pharmacotherapy (206–209). Studies of the prophylactic value of behavior therapy in the acute phase of depression, once therapy is discontinued, have been inconclusive (210, 211). The utility of behavior therapy in continuation- and maintenance-phase treatment of patients with bipolar depression has not been subjected to controlled studies.

Cognitive therapy maintains that irrational beliefs and distorted attitudes toward the self, the environment, and the future perpetuate depressive affects and that these beliefs may be reversed through cognitive behavior therapy (212). There is some evidence that cognitive therapy reduces depressive symptoms during the acute phase of less severe, nonmelancholic forms of unipolar depression (196, 213). Studies of the prophylactic effect of acute-phase cognitive behavior therapy in unipolar patients, once therapy is discontinued, have had mixed results. No randomized, controlled studies are available on the role of cognitive therapy for bipolar patients in either the acute or maintenance phase of treatment (211, 214–217).

The effects of protracted depression can lead to severe strains in marital and family relationships. Comprehensive treatment includes an assessment of and efforts to address these problems. Marital and family problems may be a consequence of depression, but may also increase vulnerability to depression and in some instances retard recovery (218, 219). Techniques for using marital and family approaches for the treatment of depression include behavioral approaches (218), a psychoeducational approach, and a "strategic marital therapy" approach (220). In addition, family therapy in the inpatient treatment of depressed patients has been studied (221). Research suggests that marital and family therapy may reduce depressive symptoms and the risk of relapse in patients with unipolar depression who have marital and family problems (217, 222). The role of these treatments for patients with bipolar disorder has not been formally studied.

The role of group therapy in the treatment of patients with depression is based on clinical experience, rather than on systematic controlled studies. Group therapy may be particularly useful in the treatment of depression in the context of bereavement or such common stressors as chronic illness. Individuals in such circumstances may benefit from the example of others who have successfully dealt with the same or similar challenges. The role of group therapy in patients with bipolar depression has not been formally studied.

3. Specific psychotherapies for manic episodes

Management of severe manic episodes poses one of the greatest challenges in psychiatry. While it is generally not beneficial to implement a specific psychotherapy during a manic episode, there are important psychosocial and environmental approaches that may be applied. A plan that sets and enforces clear limits in a firm and unprovocative manner is generally recommended, but may be difficult to implement. Isolation of the patient from other individuals may sometimes be required to protect both the patient and others. Clinical consensus seems to indicate that reducing external stimulation may help calm the manic patient. Thus, a quiet room with few distractions may be desirable. A regular schedule of meetings with the patient may be helpful.

4. Specific psychotherapies for associated comorbidity and complications

Patients in remission from bipolar disorder suffer from the psychosocial consequences of past episodes and ongoing vulnerability to future episodes. In addition, patients with this disorder remain vulnerable to other psychiatric disorders, including, most commonly, substance use disorders (223) and personality disorders (224, 225). Each of these comorbid disorders has particular consequences and increases the overall psychosocial vulnerability of the bipolar patient. Psychosocial treatments should address comorbidities and complications that are present.

Clinical experience and preliminary research suggests that group psychotherapy, in conjunction with appropriate medication, may help certain patients to address such issues as adherence to a treatment plan, adaptation to a chronic illness, regulation of self-esteem, and management of marital as well as other psychosocial issues (226–232).

5. Support groups

Many support groups provide useful information about bipolar disorder and its treatment. Patients in these groups often benefit from hearing the experiences of others who are struggling with such issues as denial versus acceptance of the need for medication, problems with side effects, and how to shoulder other burdens associated with the illness and its treatment. Advocacy groups such as the National Depressive and Manic-Depressive Association and the National Alliance for the Mentally Ill have many local chapters that provide both support and educational material to patients and their families.

E. FORMULATION AND IMPLEMENTATION OF A TREATMENT PLAN

The psychiatrist should use the information presented in this guideline to arrive at treatment recommendations. Treatment decisions will of course depend on cross-sectional and longitudinal features of the patient's illness. Considerations involved in these decisions are discussed in this section.

1. Choosing the site of treatment

One of the first decisions the psychiatrist must make is the overall level of care that the patient requires. Such a decision will, in part, be determined by the particular options of hospital, partial hospital, and outpatient services that are available in a given community. Many of the factors that underlie the choice of treatment setting discussed here are broadly applicable.

Acute episodes of bipolar disorder are frequently of such severity that patients will require treatment in either a full or partial hospital setting. The decision about the appropriate site of treatment should be based on the same considerations that guide the care of all patients with a severe mental disorder. In general, the least restrictive setting that is likely to allow for safe and effective treatment should be chosen.

Abnormal mood states (either manic or depressed) are characteristically accompanied by impaired judgment, and a substantial number of patients with a full mood episode will have psychotic symptoms (1). Patients may engage in risky behaviors that are explicitly designed to cause harm (e.g., suicidal or homicidal behavior) or have unanticipated consequences that are nonetheless harmful (e.g., promiscuous sexual activity, substance abuse, reckless driving). Some patients with a major mood disorder may not be judged to be at imminent risk, but nevertheless may require inpatient or partial hospital treatment to facilitate adequate treatment.

Unfortunately, the impaired judgment associated with acute episodes may interfere with the patient's ability to make reasonable treatment decisions. As a result, considerable effort should be put into working with patients and their families to help them appreciate the clinical situation and the reasons for the treatment recommendations. Anticipation of such situations during periods of mood stability, and the development of a treatment plan in case of a major mood episode, is frequently helpful. A long-term relationship between the psychiatrist and the patient (and family) can facilitate these discussions. Despite all efforts, however, some patients with acute episodes of bipolar disorder will need to be hospitalized involuntarily in order to receive necessary treatment. Guidelines for instituting such action are determined by specific state laws regarding involuntary commitment. Some patients during manic episodes seem to be capable of presenting different clinical pictures to different parties (e.g., judges, family members, treating psychiatrist), which may lead to profound disagreements among those involved over the best course of action. One of the psychiatrist's tasks in such a case is to educate the other concerned parties about the nature of mania and the risks to the patient despite the patient's apparent ability to appear relatively healthy at times.

a) The patient lacking the capacity to cooperate with treatment

Patients who, along with any available social supports, are unable to care for themselves adequately, cooperate with outpatient treatment of their mood disorder, or provide reliable feedback to their psychiatrist regarding their clinical status are candidates for full or partial hospitalization, even in the absence of a tendency toward intentional self-harm.

b) The patient at risk for suicide or homicide

Patients with suicidal or homicidal ideation, intention, or plan require close monitoring. Patients at particularly high risk may benefit from hospitalization, during which close observation, restricted access to violent means, and more intensive treatment are possible. Some patients with bipolar disorder are prone to rapid mood fluctuations, especially in the context of substance use, making the assessment of suicide risk particularly difficult and highlighting the need to attempt to understand, for each individual patient, the potential precipitants to suicidal thoughts and actions.

c) The patient lacking psychosocial supports

Recovery from acute bipolar episodes is aided by an environment that encourages safety, constructive activity, positive interpersonal interactions, and compliance with treatment. If the home environment lacks these features or exposes the patient to undesirable or dangerous activities, such as alcohol or drug abuse, admission to a hospital or an intensive day program may be necessary.

d) Other factors influencing the need for hospitalization

Hospitalization may be necessary for patients with complicating psychiatric or general medical conditions that make outpatient treatment unsafe. Detoxification or withdrawal from psychoactive substances may necessitate hospitalization. Patients with bipolar disorder, especially those with psychotic symptoms, may engage in bizarre or imprudent behavior that may endanger their important relationships, reputation, or assets; hospitalization may be necessary to protect the patient and others. The presence of severe psychotic features, catatonia, severe depression, or severe mixed states and the risk of ultrarapid cycling are often factors to be considered. Patients who have not responded to outpatient treatment may need to be hospitalized in order to receive the type or intensity of treatment deemed necessary. Hospitalization may also be necessary for patients who cannot receive the type or intensity of outpatient treatment required because of the local community lacks appropriate resources.

2. Development of a treatment plan

Before starting treatment with a patient with bipolar disorder, a comprehensive general medical and psychiatric evaluation should be conducted. Examination of an acutely ill patient is sometimes impossible, in which case the psychiatrist must rely on his or her best judgment about the patient's safety. The psychiatrist should consider potential general medical and substance-induced causes of manic or depressive symptoms, especially when dealing with a patient's first episode. Laboratory and other diagnostic studies should be guided by the psychiatrist's evaluation of the patient's condition and by the choice of treatment, as outlined in section II.B. Attention should be given to the patient's psychosocial stressors, social supports, and general living situation.

Bipolar disorder is a chronic condition that has potentially devastating effects on many aspects of the patient's life and that carries with it a high risk of suicide. Care of the patient involves multiple efforts to reduce the frequency and severity of episodes and to reduce the overall morbidity and mortality of the disorder.

3. Psychiatric management

Patients with bipolar disorder need different types and intensities of care at different times. The psychiatrist should have a relationship with the patient (and family, if appropriate) that allows him or her to monitor the patient's status and adjust the treatment recommendations accordingly. Psychiatric management (see section II.A.) is the foundation for all of the treatments for bipolar disorder. The specific nature and focus of psychiatric management will change as the patient's psychiatric status fluctuates and ability to respond adaptively to the demands of the illness expands.

4. Choice of a mood-stabilizing medication and/or ECT

Lithium, valproate, carbamazepine, and ECT are all used as primary agents in the treatment of patients with bipolar disorder. ECT is generally reserved for those patients who are unable to safely wait until a medication becomes effective, who are unable to safely tolerate one of the effective medications, who have been unresponsive to the available medications, or who prefer ECT.

Although the pharmacologic treatment of patients with bipolar disorder varies with the phase of the illness, almost all patients will require the use of a mood stabilizer for individual episodes, and many will require a mood stabilizer for maintenance treatment as well. Therefore, one of the first decisions a psychiatrist must make is which mood stabilizer to use to initiate treatment (even though many patients will require additional pharmacologic treatments as well).

The choice of medication depends on an individualized assessment of the risks and benefits of, and preferences for, each of the three mood stabilizers. This decision may be informed by prior response to a given medication. In addition, the potential need for maintenance treatment is frequently relevant to the decision.

a) Benefits

Four placebo-controlled trials of lithium have all demonstrated its efficacy in patients with acute mania (34–38). On the whole, about 50% to 80% of patients are expected to have some response to lithium, although the percentage varies with the study and the definition of "response." Fewer studies have been conducted using valproate, but in one recent double-blind trial in acute mania valproate was shown to be significantly more effective than placebo, with 48% of the patients having at least a 50% reduction in mania rating scale scores at 3 weeks (39). This study showed valproate and lithium to be similarly efficacious; other studies specifically designed to address the comparative efficacy of these two medications are needed. The effect of carbamazepine in acute mania is more difficult to evaluate because of the methodologic limitations of available studies. The available data, however, are supportive of the efficacy of carbamazepine in mania, though its efficacy relative to lithium and valproate is not known.

Studies of bipolar depression are generally difficult to interpret because of methodologic flaws involving the inclusion of patients with different diagnoses (i.e., bipolar I, bipolar II, unipolar depression), the use of concomitant medication, and other design problems. The data are strongest for lithium, which has been shown to be effective for depressed patients with bipolar I disorder. In addition, all three mood stabilizers have been used successfully in conjunction with antidepressants for these patients.

Only lithium has been proven to decrease the frequency and severity of episodes during maintenance treatment. Both valproate and carbamazepine have demonstrated prophylactic effect as well, although the evidence base is smaller than that for lithium and the available studies have significant methodologic flaws.

b) Risks

All three mood stabilizers are associated with potentially unpleasant dose-related side effects, most of which can be better tolerated over time or ameliorated by alterations in preparation, dose, or schedule. All of the mood stabilizers can interact with other medications, and care should be taken to avoid certain drug combinations or adjust doses accordingly.

Lithium has been extensively studied in the short- and long-term treatment of bipolar disorder. Lithium induces dose-related side effects that can be effectively controlled by dosage adjustment. However, its relatively narrow therapeutic window means that for some patients lower rates of side effects will be traded off against slightly lower efficacy. Some patients may have toxic reactions to lithium after substantial shifts in total body fluid levels brought on by general medical illness, changes in medications, or alcohol binges; unreliable patients may attain toxic lithium levels after unauthorized dosage increases (e.g., "as needed" use of extra lithium for "nerves"). In addition, lithium is dangerous in overdose. Potentially serious side effects at therapeutic doses are rare, but include the induction of serious dermatologic conditions (that resolve with cessation of medication) and the possibility of long-term renal effects (manifested by rising creatinine levels) after 10 or more years of treatment.

During short-term treatment with valproate, dose-related side effects may occur, most of which are relieved over time or by dosage adjustment. Valproate can cause potentially life-threatening effects on bone marrow, liver, and pancreas. These rare reactions cannot be reliably predicted by routine laboratory monitoring. It is essential that patients taking valproate be made aware of the early symptoms of these conditions and instructed to report their occurrence promptly. The therapeutic window for valproate is wider than that for lithium, making the occurrence of unintentional toxic levels less likely.

Carbamazepine produces dose-related side effects, many of which can be relieved over time or by alterations in dosage. Potentially life-threatening reactions that are not dose related include blood dyscrasias, hepatic failure, exfoliative dermatitis, and pancreatitis. These rare reactions cannot be reliably predicted by routine laboratory monitoring. It is essential that patients taking carbamazepine be made aware of the early symptoms of these conditions and instructed to report their occurrence promptly.

c) Patient preferences

In choosing a medication, informed patients should consider many factors in addition to evidence about efficacy, including the specific side-effect profile (which may be informed by prior use of a particular medication), other burdens of taking the medication, and costs. These considerations may be particularly important in the choice of a maintenance medication.

For the three mood stabilizers, these considerations may be summarized as follows. Lithium requires more frequent blood monitoring, but if recommendations are followed, does not carry a significant risk of life-threatening reactions. The specific side effects of valproate and carbamazepine may be preferable to some patients, but both carry a very small, though not negligible, risk of life-threatening reactions. The costs of the three medications may vary, depending, in part, on the availability of generic preparations. In most situations, lithium will likely be the least expensive agent.

5. Manic episodes

In addition to intensified psychiatric management, the primary treatment of a manic episode involves the use of a mood-stabilizing medication or ECT. The choice of ECT is governed by the same factors discussed earlier (i.e., safety, efficacy, and patient preference). ECT would be appropriate in those situations in which a rapid response is necessary, medications are contraindicated or have not been effective in the past, or the patient is known to prefer ECT as a first-line treatment. If the patient refuses blood testing, treatment with a mood stabilizer may be initiated and laboratory tests obtained once the patient has begun to respond and is more cooperative. The choice of a medication should be determined by the factors discussed earlier. If a new medication is to be started or if the patient is already on a mood stabilizer, the first step is to ensure adequate serum levels, as defined previously. It must be kept in mind, however, that within the documented therapeutic ranges for each of these medications, there is likely to be a dose-response curve for each patient. Therefore, within the target range, the precise choice of serum level will need to be guided by the patient's beneficial and adverse responses to the medication. Simultaneously, the patient's general medical condition, including thyroid status, should be checked and any abnormalities treated. Any antidepressant medications should be discontinued unless the addition of a mood stabilizer brings prompt cessation of the manic symptoms and the patient is thought to require continued use of the antidepressant to control depressive symptoms (e.g., the patient has a prior history of positive response to antidepressants).

Since mood stabilizers may take up to 2 to 3 weeks to become fully effective, many patients will require adjunctive medication in the interim to control agitated, psychotic, or otherwise dangerous behavior. Both benzodiazepines and neuroleptics have been shown to be helpful and often necessary for extremely agitated or psychotic patients. Benzodiazepines are safer; however, neuroleptics have been more widely used and studied. Some patients will not be able to safely tolerate the side effects of the mood stabilizer, in which case the initial medication should be replaced by one of the other available agents.

If after 2 to 3 weeks on a mood stabilizer at therapeutic levels the patient has not substantially improved, a second mood stabilizer or ECT may be added to the treatment regimen. These interventions may need to be instituted earlier in patients with severe forms of mania. It is usually considered preferable to add another mood stabilizer rather than substitute a second agent for the first to avoid the possibility of exacerbating the patient's condition as a result of the cessation of the first medication.

If the decision is made to use carbamazepine and valproate simultaneously, the dose of carbamazepine may need to be decreased and the dose of valproate increased because of their pharmacokinetic interactions. In addition, there is some concern about increased neurotoxicity from this combination, so careful monitoring is essential.

Patients with manic episodes may require the use of adjunctive agents (e.g., benzodiazepines, neuroleptics) beyond the initial phase of treatment and/or other medications to treat side effects from the mood stabilizer(s) or to treat comorbid conditions.

6. Depressive episodes

The treatment options for bipolar patients with depressive episodes include psychiatric management, mood-stabilizing medication, specific psychotherapy, antidepressant medication, and ECT.

Psychiatric management may need to be intensified to allow for: assessment of the patient's condition, with particular attention to the use of (or adequate dosage of) mood-stabilizing medication; the possible role of psychosocial factors (e.g., the loss of an important relationship) or general medical factors (e.g., abnormal thyroid functioning) that may be contributing to the depression and initiation of any specific intervention designed to address these factors; assessment and monitoring of the patient's psychiatric status, with particular vigilance for suicidality, changes in severity of depression, or signs of a switch to mania; and efforts to reduce the psychosocial morbidity associated with the depressive episode.

For patients who are already taking an adequate dose of a mood stabilizer when they become depressed, the continued use of the mood stabilizer and intensified psychiatric management may be combined with one or more of the following interventions: 1) a specific psychotherapy, 2) an antidepressant medication, and 3) ECT (although this may require temporary discontinuation of the mood stabilizer).

For patients who are not taking a mood stabilizer when they become depressed (or are not taking an adequate dosage), a mood-stabilizing medication should be initiated (or an adequate dosage achieved). Data show lithium to be the most efficacious mood stabilizer for depression in bipolar patients, so this agent would most often be the logical initial choice. Since clinical experience suggests that the antidepressant efficacy of lithium may not be evident for 4 to 6 weeks after adequate serum levels have been achieved (with the full effect taking somewhat longer), other treatments noted above should also be considered.

The decision to initiate a specific psychotherapy, and the particular choice of psychotherapy, depends on the factors discussed earlier, including knowledge of the patient's response to treatment of earlier episodes, as well as an assessment of the factors that may play a role in the precipitation, exacerbation, perpetuation, or psychosocial consequences of the episode. Further considerations are discussed in the *Practice Guideline for Major Depressive Disorder in Adults* (122; Second Edition included in this volume).

Decisions regarding the use of antidepressant medication require an assessment of the benefits (e.g., the likelihood of relatively rapid relief of symptoms) and burdens (e.g., potential side effects of the medication, increased risk of developing a manic episode). The decision will therefore depend on the patient's specific clinical features (e.g., severity of depression, previous course of depressive episodes) and preferences (e.g., concerns about side effects, availability of supports in the event of a manic episode).

For some patients with mild depression or a history of self-limited depressive episodes that are not unduly disruptive, the combination of psychiatric management, with or without a specific psychotherapy, and use of a mood stabilizer may be sufficient.

The addition of an antidepressant medication to the mood-stabilizing regimen is likely to be beneficial for the following groups of patients: patients who cannot safely tolerate or are unwilling to tolerate a 4- to 6-week delay before response to the initiation (or dosage adjustment) of a mood-stabilizing medication; patients who have a history of beneficial response to previous treatment with an antidepressant medication; or patients who have not responded to the combination of psychiatric management, a mood stabilizer, and, if indicated, a specific psychotherapy.

All antidepressant medications that have been shown to be effective for patients with major depressive disorder are also probably effective for patients in the depressed phase of bipolar disorder. However, these medications are likely to increase the bipolar patient's baseline risk of developing a manic episode. The simultaneous use of a mood-stabilizing medication is recommended to decrease this risk. Patients who take antidepressant medications should be informed of the risks of developing a manic episode and should be educated about the early warning signs of such a switch. A plan should be made for immediate intervention should a switch to mania occur; it is frequently helpful to involve the patient's family in such a plan. Patients who refuse treatment with a mood stabilizer and prefer treatment with an antidepressant alone may be at particular risk of switching to mania and should be so informed.

Available data indicate that the choice of antidepressant agents for bipolar patients is governed by the same factors that guide the choice in unipolar patients. Thus, the prior response of the patient, the side effect profile, the presence of atypical features (which would favor the use of an MAOI or a selective serotonin reuptake inhibitor), and patient preference are relevant to the decision. As in all depressed patients, the presence of suicidality should be continually assessed. Suicidal patients may be most safely treated with agents that are less toxic in overdose (e.g., selective serotonin reuptake inhibitors).

ECT is another alternative for depressed patients. The use of ECT is governed by the same factors discussed previously, including the need for a rapid response, the presence of contraindications to the use of medication, the history of nonresponse to medication, or patient preference.

Treatment decisions for psychotically depressed patients are similar to those for all severely depressed patients. Although some patients with psychotic depression may respond to the combination of a mood stabilizer and an antidepressant, others will require the additional use of a neuroleptic. ECT is also an appropriate first-line treatment for these patients.

Patients with a major depressive episode may at times require other adjunctive agents, which are discussed in the *Practice Guideline for Major Depressive Disorder in Adults* (122; Second Edition included in this volume).

7. Mixed episodes and ultrarapid cycling

The treatment principles for patients with mixed episodes are the same as those for patients with pure mania. Antidepressants may exacerbate mixed states and should be avoided, if possible. Preliminary data from one controlled study suggests that valproate may be more effective than lithium for patients with mixed episodes (C Bowden, personal communication); however, this finding needs to be tested in further studies.

Patients who experience rapid changes in mood state between depression and mania share many features with patients who have mixed states. A general medical evaluation should be conducted, with particular attention to thyroid status. If there are indications of decreased thyroid function, thyroxine or T_3 should be added and the measures of thyroid function brought into the upper range of normal distribution. Other general medical conditions, as well as comorbid alcohol or substance abuse, could be exacerbating the ongoing mood abnormality and should be treated. Some investigators believe that the use of antidepressants should be discontinued or avoided, if possible, and the subsequent course of illness reevaluated.

If these interventions are not sufficient to halt the ultrarapid cycling, treatment with a second mood stabilizer should be initiated and response over time (preferably after at least two cycles) carefully evaluated. If hypomanic and manic symptoms are relieved but depression persists, thyroid hormone or an antidepressant may be added. Occasionally, a third mood stabilizer may be necessary.

A small series of studies suggest the utility of very high doses of thyroid hormone, used concomitantly with mood-stabilizing agents, in the treatment of rapid-cycling patients (50, 147, 148). This is discussed in more detail in section II.B.7.

8. Maintenance phase

Bipolar disorder is a recurrent and sometimes chronic disorder. Therefore, the psychiatrist should address maintenance and other long-term issues with the patient and the family as early in treatment as is feasible. The decision to implement maintenance pharmacotherapy should involve the participation of the psychiatrist, the patient, and, at times, family members. A decision to initiate maintenance treatment depends on 1) the probability of a recurrence with or without a mood-stabilizing agent, 2) the likely consequences of a recurrence, and 3) the benefits and burdens of taking a mood-stabilizing agent (233). Information about past episodes is essential in making these judgments.

Many psychiatrists recommend maintenance medication following a single manic episode, particularly if there are no contraindications to the use of a mood-stabilizing medication. Although this option should be made available to all patients after their first manic episode, clearly different patients may rationally make different decisions regarding the initiation and continuation of maintenance treatment depending on their individual circumstances and attitudes. Decisions regarding maintenance treatment should be reassessed whenever the patient's clinical status changes, or approximately annually in stable patients. It is likely that after two manic episodes, the benefits of prophylaxis would outweigh the burdens for most patients.

The choice of a maintenance medication should be guided by the factors discussed earlier. Data are strongest for the efficacy and safety of lithium in this phase. However, patients who are nonresponsive or acutely intolerant to lithium, may benefit from an alternative mood stabilizer for maintenance. Additionally, some patients achieve better prophylaxis with a combination of mood stabilizers.

The choice of a target serum level should also be guided by the factors discussed previously. The narrow therapeutic window for lithium means that some patients will need to determine their preferred balance between side effects and efficacy. Other patients will be able to tolerate the higher range of therapeutic levels with easily remediable or only insignificant side effects. Many psychiatrists and their patients find that lithium levels between 0.6 and 0.8 meq/liter are optimal; others will prefer higher or lower doses.

During this phase, patients must deal with the psychological consequences of past episodes, the ongoing vulnerability to future episodes, and, for some patients, a significant degree of mood lability that falls short of a full mood episode. In addition to psychiatric management, some patients appear likely to benefit from a specific psychotherapeutic treatment. The range of available treatments and the factors guiding treatment choice and implementation are discussed in section II.D.

Even with optimal serum levels of a mood stabilizer and the appropriate use of psychotherapy, many patients will have occasional episodes of mania or depression. A critical role of psychiatric management is to help patients identify precipitants to, or early manifestations of, such episodes, so that treatment can be initiated promptly. Patients can benefit from anticipating and planning for such an event, so that critical treatment and other decisions can be made while the patient is still relatively euthymic.

The first step in treating early symptoms of a major mood episode is to ensure that the serum level of the mood stabilizer is adequate. In addition, the presence of a general medical condition (e.g., alteration in thyroid status or addition of a medication that may alter the bioavailability of the mood stabilizer) or a psychological factor (e.g., loss of a valued relationship) that could be contributing to the episode should be determined and addressed. Insomnia may be a precipitant or an early indicator of mania. Education about the importance of regular sleep habits and the occasional use of a benzodiazepine to promote regular sleep patterns are felt to be important for some patients in the prevention of full-blown manic episodes (234). Other subtle or early signs of mania can sometimes be managed with short-term use of a benzodiazepine or a neuroleptic.

Some patients will require additional treatments for a major mood episode, as described in sections II. A., B., C., and D.

9. Discontinuation of maintenance medication

Discontinuation of effective lithium prophylaxis is associated with an increased risk of early relapse. Such risk may be minimized by gradual, rather than rapid, discontinuation. In addition, there have been reports of patients who seem to develop a more severe and relatively nonresponsive form of the illness following discontinuation of effective prophylactic lithium. The risks associated with the discontinuation of maintenance valproate or carbamazepine are not clear.

The development of an episode during maintenance treatment does not necessarily imply treatment failure. Rather, the efficacy of a maintenance medication regimen should be assessed by comparing the actual course of the illness with the predicted course without medication. Although in practice such determinations may be difficult, it is important that an effective treatment not be abandoned in search of a regimen that will confer 100% protection against all future episodes. Severe or repeated breakthrough episodes should trigger a reassessment of the treatment plan. The use of life charts before and after the institution of maintenance treatment may be helpful. It is possible for patients to show a gradual decrease in responsiveness to a previously effective mood stabilizer. In this instance, switching to a medication with a novel mechanism of action, providing ECT, or discontinuing the new medication for a period of time followed by a renewed trial may be successful, at least temporarily, in reinitiating a treatment response.

F. CLINICAL FEATURES INFLUENCING TREATMENT

This section summarizes considerations pertaining to clinical features influencing treatment. The reader is referred to pertinent sections of the guideline that cover in greater detail subjects touched upon here.

1. Psychiatric factors

a) Psychotic or catatonic features

Patients may experience delusions and/or hallucinations during episodes of mania or depression. These symptoms can be treated with mood stabilizers alone or with the addition of an antipsychotic agent. In addition, ECT may be used.

Occasionally, catatonic features may develop in patients during a manic episode. A careful assessment is indicated to rule out a general medical etiology and to clarify the psychiatric diagnosis. If the diagnosis of mania is confirmed, treatment should be directed accordingly. ECT has been successfully used for patients with catatonic features and is probably the treatment of choice (235). Neuroleptics and benzodiazepines have also been used.

b) Risk of suicide, homicide, and violence

Among patients with psychiatric disorders, bipolar patients are among those at highest risk for suicide (236, 237). While patients with bipolar disorder have a mortality rate that is two to three times higher than that of the general population, the mortality rate of patients in long-term lithium treatment does not appear to differ significantly from that of the general population (238). Lithium maintenance treatment is associated with lowering the frequency of suicide attempts and completions (3).

Numerous risk factors for suicide among bipolar patients have been determined. In addition to general risk factors for suicide (e.g., previous suicide attempt, suicidal ideation, substance use in conjunction with another psychiatric disorder), patients with bipolar disorder have been shown to have other risk factors, including mood cycling within an episode and depressive turmoil, or rapid shifting from one mood state to another (e.g., from euphoria to anger to depression) (237). In these patients, absence of general risk factors should not be taken as reassurance that the patient is not at high risk for suicide (237). In general, a detailed evaluation of the individual patient is necessary to assess suicidal risk. Decisions must be made with the understanding that judgments of suicidality cannot be perfect, and it is prudent to err on the side of caution.

The potential for violence in patients with bipolar disorder is less well studied than is risk for suicide. Clinical experience attests to the presence of violent behavior in some of these patients, and violence may be an indication for hospitalization. In some instances, the threat is explicit through the patient's verbalizations and expressed intent. In other instances, the risk can only be inferred from the patient's agitation and dysphoric mood states combined with paranoid delusional thinking. When these features are associated with very rapid mood cycling, the risk of violence may be high.

c) Substance-related disorders

The rate of comorbidity between bipolar disorder and substance-related disorders is high. Substance abuse and its associated behaviors may lead psychiatrists and family members to fail to diagnose bipolar disorder. Conversely, the diagnosis of substance-related disorders may be overlooked in patients with bipolar disorder. In addition, substance abuse may worsen the course of bipolar disorder, perhaps by decreasing compliance with the treatment regimen (1).

Treatment for the substance use disorder and mood disorder should proceed concurrently, to the extent possible. The treatment of one disorder may have effects on the treatment of the other. For example, increased thirst secondary to lithium treatment may lead to increased alcohol consumption, and dehydration associated with alcohol abuse may increase serum lithium levels. Also, lithium may decrease the psychological effects of alcohol, thus stimulating greater alcohol consumption. As suicide risk often increases during alcohol detoxification, inpatient hospitalization may be required.

d) Other psychiatric comorbidities

Patients with comorbid personality disorders pose complicated diagnostic pictures. They are clearly at greater risk for experiencing intrapsychic and psychosocial stress that can precipitate or exacerbate major mood episodes. In addition, these patients may have particular difficulty adhering to long-term treatment regimens. The choice of a psychotherapeutic treatment should be guided by patient needs and preferences, but should include as an important focus the psychiatric management tasks required for adequate treatment of bipolar disorder.

The presence of a comorbid anxiety disorder may complicate the assessment of mood states in patients with bipolar disorder. The anxiety disorder should be assessed and treated concurrently with bipolar disorder.

The presence of attention deficit hyperactivity disorder, especially in children and adolescents, complicates the assessment of changes in mood states in patients with bipolar disorder. Early manifestations of mania and hypomania can be particularly difficult to distinguish from the ongoing symptoms of attention deficit hyperactivity disorder. Careful tracking of symptoms and behaviors is helpful. In addition, psychiatrists should consider the implications of pharmacologic treatments for attention deficit hyperactivity disorder on the course of the bipolar disorder (e.g., the use of tricyclic antidepressants or psychostimulants may exacerbate the course of bipolar illness).

The presence of comorbid conduct disorder in children and adolescents with bipolar disorder is likely to interfere with the development of a treatment alliance, decrease the likelihood of adherence to a long-term treatment regimen, increase the risk of substance use and other forms of risk-taking behavior, and increase the exposure of the patient to psychosocial stress, which could precipitate or exacerbate major mood episodes. Such patients may require intensive approaches to maximize potential treatment benefit and minimize risks from imprudent behavior.

2. Concurrent general medical conditions

The presence of a general medical condition may affect the treatment of a patient with bipolar disorder by exacerbating the course or severity of the disorder or by complicating treatment.

For example, the course of bipolar disorder may be exacerbated any condition that requires intermittent or regular use of steroids (e.g., asthma, inflammatory bowel disease) or that leads to abnormal thyroid functioning. Psychiatrists who treat HIV-infected patients often find that lower doses of mood stabilizers are indicated because of the patient's increased sensitivity to side effects.

The treatment of patients with bipolar disorder may be complicated by conditions that affect renal or hepatic function, which may restrict the choice or dosage of mood-stabilizing agents; require the use of diuretics that affect lithium excretion (e.g., edema); or are associated with abnormal cardiac conduction or rhythm, which may limit the choice of mood-stabilizing medications.

The possibility of adverse drug–drug interactions should always be considered whenever patients are taking more than one medication. Patients should be educated about the importance of informing their psychiatrist and other physicians about their current medications whenever new medications are prescribed.

3. Family history

The treatment of patients with bipolar disorder is not dependent on family history, although a positive family history may increase the chance that a patient with a major depressive episode may develop bipolar disorder. Thus, a careful history for prior episodes of mania or hypomania and adequate patient education about the risk of developing mania while taking an antidepressant medication are recommended.

4. Demographic and psychosocial variables

a) Children and adolescents

The treatment of bipolar disorder in children and adolescents, based on numerous case reports and open trials, is similar to that for adults. Lithium has traditionally been used as a first-line mood stabilizer (239). However, overall response to lithium may be lower in younger patients with bipolar disorder than adults because children, and especially adolescents, with mania often have either mixed episodes or a predominance of psychotic symptoms, both of which are generally more refractory to treatment.

Several studies have documented the effectiveness of lithium for adolescents with bipolar disorder (240–243). The prophylactic effectiveness of lithium in preventing and reducing the rate of relapses in children and adolescents was demonstrated by Strober et al. (14). In this study, 37.5% of patients who completed an 18-month trial of lithium experienced at least one relapse compared to 92.3% of those who did not complete the trial. Further, those patients who completed the trial and who had at least one relapse had a decreased frequency of episodes during lithium treatment compared to baseline.

While the spectrum of lithium side effects seen in children and adolescents is similar to that seen in adults, the long-term effects of lithium in children and adolescents have not been studied. In particular, potential interactions with the developmental maturation of a child (e.g., with skeletal growth given lithium's interaction with calcium metabolism) need further research.

Children generally excrete lithium more rapidly than do adults (1); this reduced half-life means that dosage can frequently be adjusted after shorter intervals (244). Therapeutic levels are the same as for adults, with dosage adjustment recommended according to individual response.

The frequency of lithium monitoring in children and adolescents may be determined by the same considerations that apply to adult patients. While either serum or saliva sampling may be used to monitor lithium levels, serum sampling is recommended. Saliva sampling should be used only in extreme situations because saliva lithium levels are more variable, and therefore less reliable, than serum levels and children would need to avoid eating or drinking for 12 hours prior to saliva samples being obtained (245).

As in adults, adjunctive agents such as benzodiazepines, neuroleptics, and antidepressants are often used in combination with lithium. The specific risks of each of these agents should be carefully considered (e.g., tardive dyskinesia with neuroleptics, cardiac effects of tricyclic antidepressants, development or exacerbation of a substance-related disorder with benzodiazepines). Carbamazepine and valproate are also used either as adjuncts to lithium or alone. The use of these agents is primarily based on studies of adults; the literature on their use with children and adolescents is quite limited.

Although there are case reports of ECT being used effectively in children and adolescents with bipolar disorder, systematic studies are not available (246).

Psychosocial treatments are necessary to address the morbidity and sequelae of bipolar disorder in children and adolescents (247). Psychiatric management of children and adolescents must be informed by an assessment of the individual's emotional, social, and academic capacities and skills, as chronic mood lability and major mood episodes may interfere with normal development in these areas. Comorbid conditions, such as substance-related disorders and learning problems, also need to be addressed.

Some children and adolescents will benefit from a specific, more intensive intervention. For example, individual and/or family psychotherapy may be indicated to address interpersonal, intrapsychic, and social conflicts; school consultation may be necessary to develop an appropriate educational environment for the child or adolescent.

b) The elderly

There are patients who have a first manic episode after age 60. The majority of these patients had previous depressive episodes in their 40s and 50s. Any patient who has an onset of mania after age 60 should be evaluated especially carefully for general medical (including neurological) causes. These patients more often have concurrent general medical conditions and thus need a thorough general medical as well as psychiatric evaluation.

Many elderly patients appear to be more sensitive to lithium, requiring lower serum levels than younger patients to achieve similar beneficial and adverse effects. For example, it is common for elderly patients to be intolerant of levels above 0.7 meq/liter and to have a beneficial response at even lower levels. In addition, certain side effects (e.g., lithium-induced tremor) may be more common in elderly patients.

c) Family history and current family functioning

A family history of bipolar disorder is common in patients with bipolar disorder. A positive family history may increase the likelihood that a patient with a major depressive episode will eventually have a manic episode and be diagnosed with bipolar I disorder. In addition, individuals with bipolar disorder who are considering having children may benefit from genetic counseling (27). Children of individuals with bipolar disorder have genetic as well as psychosocial risk factors for developing a psychiatric disorder (1). Patients may need help anticipating, assessing, and addressing their children's needs both during and between parental episodes.

Recognizing distress or dysfunction in the family of a patient with bipolar disorder is important because such ongoing stress may exacerbate the patient's condition or interfere with treatment. In addition, poor family functioning will increase the psychosocial risks for the patient's children and other family members, including siblings of children and adolescents with bipolar disorder. Even if dysfunction is not apparent, it is important to educate the family about bipolar disorder and enlist their support and cooperation.

d) Gender and pregnancy

A number of issues related to gender must be considered when treating patients with bipolar disorder. Hypothyroidism is more common in women, and women may be more susceptible to the antithyroid effects of lithium. Because of the increased risk of birth defects associated with many medications used to treat bipolar disorder, the psychiatrist should encourage careful contraceptive practices for all female patients of childbearing age who are receiving pharmacologic treatment (248). Further, the metabolism of birth control pills is increased by carbamazepine and dosages may need to be adjusted accordingly. This effect does not occur with other medications used to treat bipolar disorder.

Pregnancy and the postpartum state are major factors to be considered in the treatment of women with bipolar disorder. Women with bipolar disorder may exhibit significant affective symptoms while pregnant or during the postpartum period (249). However, first trimester exposure to any of the three mood stabilizers—lithium, carbamazepine, and valproate—is associated with increased risk of birth defects. The absolute risk of major congenital anomalies among children of women treated with lithium during early pregnancy is estimated at 4% to 12%, compared to 2% to 4% in untreated comparison groups (248). Carbamazepine may have teratogenic effects, especially with first trimester exposure, including neural tube defects (250, 251), craniofacial defects, fingernail hypoplasia, and developmental delay. Valproate has been associated with a 1% to 2% risk of neural tube defects (252). Exposure to fluoxetine and tricyclic antidepressants during the first trimester may increase the risk of miscarriage (253).

Because of the risks of pharmacologic treatment, psychotherapeutic treatment alone is an important alternative for female patients who are pregnant or trying to conceive. In pregnant women who are manic, depressed, or psychotically depressed, the safest and most effective treatment is usually ECT.

Decisions regarding treatment with mood stabilizers for women who are pregnant or trying to conceive require careful discussion of risks, benefits, and alternatives. In women with severe bipolar disorder for whom discontinuation of pharmacologic treatment poses a substantial risk of increased morbidity, treatment with mood stabilizers should be discontinued for a period coinciding as closely as possible with that of embryogenesis, and preferably throughout the first trimester. Nevertheless, for some women with severe bipolar disorder, brief discontinuation of mood stabilizers will pose an unacceptable risk of increased morbidity. Therefore, if mood stabilizers are to be taken during all or part of the first trimester, the patient should 1) receive reproductive risk counseling as early as possible during the pregnancy; and 2) be offered monitoring of fetal development, including a fetal echocardiography and high-resolution ultrasound examination at 16–18 weeks' gestation and tests of serum and amniotic fluid α-fetoprotein levels (248). Throughout pregnancy, dosages of mood stabilizers may need to be adjusted because of changes in renal clearance and increases in hepatic metabolism induced by maternal hormones. Accordingly, regular monitoring of serum concentrations of mood stabilizers is recommended throughout pregnancy.

It is advisable to discontinue mood stabilizers a few days before delivery to minimize toxic effects on the infant and to resume treatment a few days afterward to reduce the risk of a postpartum episode. If pharmacologic treatment is continued, however, it is important to be aware of the large changes in total body water expected at the time of delivery. Lithium levels need to be monitored very closely after delivery until a stable level is achieved to avoid the risks of toxicity with higher levels and untreated mania with lower levels (254). Because psychotropic medications are excreted in breast milk and their long-term effects on the developing child are unknown, most authorities recommend against breast feeding if psychotropic medications are being used.

e) Cross-cultural issues

Culture can influence the experience and communication of symptoms of depression and mania. Underdiagnosis or misdiagnosis, as well as delayed detection of early signs of recurrence, can be reduced by being alert to specific ethnic and cultural differences in reporting complaints of a major mood episode. Ethnic groups may differ in their response to antidepressant agents (255, 256).

f) Environment

During the manic phase of bipolar disorder, maintaining a routine and calm environment is optimal. Since the manic patient is stimulated by outside events, television, videos, music, animated conversations, and alcohol can heighten manic thought processes and activities. Manic patients may also need room to pace or exercise as a way to use energy and ensure sleep. Patients and their families should be advised that during manic episodes patients may engage in reckless driving and that, at times, steps should be taken to limit access to a car.

g) Stressors

An association between psychosocial stressors and the precipitation of mania in the first four episodes has been reported (257), although many episodes of mania have no identifiable precipitants (258). As the illness progresses, more episodes may seem to occur spontaneously. There have been occasional reports of an association between bereavement and the onset of mania, which may be mediated through poor sleep. Patients and their families should work with the psychiatrist to develop an understanding of the unique association for each individual patient between stressful events and the onset of symptoms; they should be encouraged to contact the psychiatrist during such times.

III. SUMMARY OF RECOMMENDATIONS

▶ A. CODING SYSTEM

Each recommendation is identified as falling into one of three categories of endorsement, by a bracketed Roman numeral following the statement. The three categories represent varying levels of clinical confidence in the recommendation.

[I] Indicates recommended with substantial clinical confidence.
[II] Indicates recommended with moderate clinical confidence.
[III] Indicates options that may be recommended on the basis of individual circumstances.

▶ B. GENERAL CONSIDERATIONS

Patients with bipolar disorder suffer from a severe long-term psychiatric illness. Without treatment, patients with bipolar disorder will face substantial and prolonged distress and impairment, as well as the risk of significant morbidity and mortality. While effective treatments exist, there is no cure and even with optimal treatment most patients need some level of longitudinal psychiatric care. A careful and thorough psychiatric and general medical evaluation is essential prior to initiating treatment and at times of significant clinical change throughout the illness [I]. The presence of a substance use disorder should be ascertained and treated [I]. A graphic display of the course of the patient's disorder (e.g., a life chart) is frequently helpful in detecting patterns in the development and amelioration of episodes and their sequelae. Such information may be helpful in guiding and assessing attempts to decrease the frequency, severity, and consequences of future episodes. Treatment decisions depend on both cross-sectional and longitudinal features of the patient's illness.

1. Choosing the site of treatment

The psychiatrist must determine the overall level of care that a patient with bipolar disorder needs; such a decision will depend, in part, on the availability of inpatient, partial hospital, and outpatient services in the community. In general, the least restrictive setting that is likely to allow for safe and effective treatment should be chosen. Factors guiding the choice of a treatment setting include [I]: the patient's ability to cooperate with treatment, the patient's risk for suicidal or homicidal behavior, the availability of psychosocial supports, and other clinical factors that make outpatient treatment unsafe or unlikely to be effective. Involuntary hospitalization may be necessary to protect and adequately treat the patient.

2. Development of a treatment plan

Treatment must be preceded by a careful general medical and psychiatric examination to determine precipitants of the episode, barriers to treatment, and the presence of other disorders or factors that may complicate treatment or that require specific interventions. Patients with full-blown manic episodes may require treatment prior to the completion of a full assessment. Laboratory and other diagnostic studies should be guided by the psychiatrist's evaluation of the patient's condition and by the choice of treatment, as outlined in section II.B.

3. Psychiatric management

Psychiatric management is the foundation for all of the treatments for bipolar disorder [I]. The intensity and focus of treatment may change as the patient's psychiatric status fluctuates and as the patient expands his or her ability to respond adaptively to the demands of the illness. The goals of psychiatric management include: establishing and maintaining a therapeutic alliance, monitoring the patient's psychiatric status, providing education regarding bipolar disorder, enhancing treatment compliance, promoting regular patterns of activity and wakefulness, promoting understanding of and adaptation to the psychosocial effects of bipolar disorder, identifying new episodes early, and reducing the morbidity and sequelae of the disorder. The patient's family and other social supports may be critical components of a treatment plan.

4. Choice of a mood-stabilizing medication and/or ECT

Lithium, valproate, carbamazepine, and ECT are all used as primary agents in the treatment of patients with bipolar disorder [I]. ECT is generally reserved for those patients who are unable to safely wait until a medication becomes effective, who are not responsive to or unable to safely tolerate one of the effective medications, or who prefer ECT [I]. Most patients will require the use of a mood-stabilizing medication for the treatment of acute episodes, and many will require a mood stabilizer for maintenance treatment as well [I].

The choice of medication depends on an individualized assessment of the benefits and risks of, and preferences for, each of the three mood stabilizers. A discussion of these issues is summarized in section II.E.4. The data regarding efficacy and safety, in both the acute and maintenance phases, are most favorable for lithium [I]. However, some patients and psychiatrists will choose either valproate or carbamazepine based on preferences for the specific side-effect profile or based on a history of nonresponse or intolerance to lithium [II]. The use of any of these medications requires laboratory monitoring both prior to and during treatment. In addition, all three agents have recommended therapeutic ranges that may serve as general guidelines, but the specific dosage must be individualized for each patient [II]. These issues are discussed in section II.B.

C. MANIC EPISODES

The primary treatment of a manic episode involves the use of a mood-stabilizing medication or ECT [I]. The first step is to ensure that the patient has an adequate serum level of the medication. The choice of a target serum level may involve a compromise between maximizing efficacy and minimizing side effects. Simultaneously, the patient's general medical condition, including thyroid function, should be checked and any abnormalities treated [I]. The use of antidepressant medications should be discontinued or avoided, unless continued use is necessary based on knowledge of the patient's prior course [II].

Adjunctive benzodiazepines or neuroleptics may be used to manage symptoms of agitation, psychosis, or other dangerous behavior while awaiting the full effects of a primary mood stabilizer, or to augment the effects of the mood stabilizer [I].

If the patient has not significantly improved within 2 to 3 weeks, a second mood stabilizer should be added to the treatment regimen [II]. Pharmacokinetic interactions among medications must be kept in mind to ensure safe and effective treatment. Alternatively, ECT may be considered based on judgments about safety, efficacy, and patient preference [I].

D. DEPRESSIVE EPISODES

The treatment of depressed bipolar patients who are on an adequate dose of a mood-stabilizing medication includes intensified psychiatric management and continued use of the mood-stabilizing medication [II]. In addition, some patients will need one or more of the following: specific psychotherapy, antidepressant medication, and ECT.

For patients who are not taking an adequate dose of a mood stabilizer when they become depressed, a mood-stabilizing medication should be initiated (or an adequate dosage achieved) [II]. The strongest efficacy data are for lithium, so this agent would most often be the logical initial choice of mood stabilizer. Other treatments noted above should also be considered.

The decision to initiate a specific psychotherapy, and the particular choice of psychotherapy, depends on the factors discussed earlier, including knowledge of the patient's response to earlier episodes of treatment, as well as an assessment of the factors that may play a role in the precipitation, exacerbation, perpetuation, or psychosocial consequences of the episode [II].

Decisions regarding the use of antidepressant medication require an assessment of the benefits (e.g., the likelihood of relatively rapid relief of symptoms) and burdens (e.g., potential side effects of the medication, increased risk of developing a manic episode). The decision will therefore depend on the patient's specific clinical features and preferences [II].

The choice of antidepressant medication for bipolar patients is governed by the prior response of the patient to antidepressants, the side-effect profile, the presence of atypical features, the risk of inducing a manic episode, and patient preference [II].

ECT is another alternative for depressed patients [I]; its use is governed by the same factors discussed previously.

Treatment decisions for psychotically depressed patients are similar to those for all severely depressed patients. Although some patients with psychotic depression may respond to the combination of a mood stabilizer and an antidepressant, others will require the additional use of a neuroleptic [II]. ECT is also a possible treatment for these patients.

Patients with a major depressive episode may, at times, require other adjunctive agents. Further considerations are discussed in the *Practice Guideline for Major Depressive Disorder in Adults* (122; Second Edition included in this volume).

▶ E. MIXED EPISODES AND ULTRARAPID CYCLING

The treatment of patients with mixed episodes is guided by the same principles underlying the treatment of manic patients [II]. The use of antidepressants should be avoided if possible [II]. Patients who switch rapidly between depressive and manic states share many features with patients who have mixed episodes. Treatment of general medical conditions, including optimization of thyroid functioning, may be effective. Some patients may respond to the elimination of antidepressants from their treatment regimen [III]. Preliminary data suggest that patients with mixed mania may be more likely to respond to valproate, and patients with classic mania may be more likely to respond to lithium (III). Augmentation with thyroid hormone has been suggested by some investigators [III].

▶ F. MAINTENANCE PHASE

All patients with bipolar disorder should be informed of the option of maintenance medication [I]. A decision to initiate maintenance medication treatment depends on a judgment regarding the probability of a recurrence with and without medication, the likely consequences of a recurrence, and the risks and other burdens associated with taking a maintenance medication. Such decisions should be made by the patient in conjunction with the psychiatrist and, if appropriate, family members [I]. Decisions regarding maintenance treatment should be reviewed at times of clinical change and approximately annually in stable patients [I].

Data are strongest for the efficacy and safety of lithium in the maintenance phase [I]. However, patients who are nonresponsive or intolerant to lithium, or for other reasons prefer an alternative medication, may benefit from either valproate or carbamazepine maintenance treatment [II]. The choice of a target serum level for each of these medications should be guided by the factors discussed previously and may need to be individualized according to the patient's response and preference.

In addition to psychiatric management, some patients will benefit from a specific psychotherapeutic treatment [II]. The range of available treatments and the factors guiding their choice and implementation are discussed in section II.D.

A critical role of psychiatric management is to help patients to identify precipitants or early manifestations of breakthrough episodes, so that treatment can be initiated promptly [I]. Patients can benefit from anticipating and planning for such events, so that critical decisions can be made during periods of relative mood stability.

Early signs of breakthrough episodes should be treated according to the guidelines for the treatment of acute episodes [II]. Insomnia may be either a precipitant or an early indicator of mania or depression. Education about the importance of regular sleep habits and the occasional use of benzodiazepines to promote normal sleep patterns may be useful in preventing the development of a manic episode [III]. Other early or subtle signs of mania may be treated with the short-term use of benzodiazepines or neuroleptics [II].

▶ G. DISCONTINUATION OF MAINTENANCE MEDICATION

Discontinuation of maintenance lithium should be gradual to minimize the risk of early relapse [II]. While it is not known what risks are associated with the discontinuation of maintenance valproate or carbamazepine, most clinicians recommend gradual reduction in dosage.

IV. RESEARCH DIRECTIONS

The relative effectiveness of various possible treatment regimens, including all three primary mood stabilizers, needs to be clarified in the full range of bipolar patients. The magnitude of the risks and benefits of these treatments should be clarified to enable patients and their psychiatrists to optimize individual treatment regimens. In addition, more data regarding the optimal treatment(s) for patients who have not responded to first- and second-line treatments are needed. Clinical decisions would be improved by better quantitative data on the course of this disorder with and without available treatments. A better understanding of the spectrum of patients' preferences for different treatments and outcomes would facilitate the development of general recommendations for treatment.

The treatment of bipolar depression is vastly understudied and is of substantial clinical importance given the number of bipolar patients who initially present with depression. The efficacy and safety of antidepressants in the acute and maintenance treatment of bipolar depression need further elucidation.

Psychosocial and biological research to elucidate factors leading to the initiation and exacerbation of episodes would pave the way for improved maintenance treatments. For example, research designed to clarify the role of emotional stress and sleep deprivation in the induction of episodes, and the efficacy of treatments aimed at reducing these factors, could lead to important new treatments for patients with this disorder.

Psychotherapeutic treatments for patients with bipolar disorder must be formalized to allow for careful study of their essential features and effectiveness in patients with bipolar disorder at specific phases.

The diagnosis and optimal treatment of bipolar disorder in children and adolescents requires further study. In addition, the development and testing of interventions to improve the outcome for children of parents with bipolar disorder is important.

Research into the genetic mechanisms of bipolar illness is a high priority. Ascertaining the gene(s) responsible for bipolar illness carries with it the probability of early and more accurate diagnosis, as well as the potential for more specific treatments derived from an understanding of the illness at its molecular level.

The treatment implications for bipolar II disorder or schizoaffective disorder—as opposed to bipolar I disorder—need to be clarified. The optimal treatment of patients with bipolar disorder and comorbid psychiatric disorders (e.g., substance use, personality disorders) needs further study. In addition, the need for modifications in the treatment plan based on such factors as age, gender, culture, ethnicity, family history, and other psychosocial factors must be assessed in order to better individualize treatment.

V. REVIEWERS AND CONSULTANTS

Hagop S. Akiskal, M.D.
Lori Altshuler, M.D.
James Ballenger, M.D.
Richard Balon, M.D.
Donald Banzhaf, M.D.
David J. Barry, M.D.
Monica Ramirez Basco, Ph.D.
Mark S. Bauer, M.D.
Lee H. Beecher, M.D.
Carl C. Bell, M.D.
Deborah Blacker, M.D., Sc.D.
Charles H. Blackinton, M.D.
Mary C. Blehar, Ph.D.
Carrie M. Borchardt, M.D.
Jonathan F. Borus, M.D.
Nashaat Boutros, M.D.
Charles L. Bowden, M.D.
R.C. Bowen, M.D., F.R.C.P.(C.)
Robert Paul Cabaj, M.D.
Joseph Calabrese, M.D.
Oliver G. Cameron, M.D., Ph.D.
James M. Campbell, M.D.
Gabrielle Carlson, Ph.D.
Brendan T. Carroll, M.D.
K. Himasiri De Silva, M.D.
Ronald J. Diamond, M.D.
David L. Dunner, M.D.
Jean Endicott, Ph.D.
Irl Extein, M.D.
Terry F. Fitzgerald, Ph.D.
Lois T. Flaherty, M.D.
David L. Fogelson, M.D.
Ellen Frank, Ph.D.
Alan J. Gelenberg, M.D.
Barbara Geller, M.D.
Samuel Gershon, M.D.
Mary Gillette, Ph.D.
Katharine Gillis, M.D.
Sheila Hafter Gray, M.D.
John Greden, M.D.

John Greist, M.D.
George T. Grossberg, M.D.
Ellen Haller, M.D.
Constance Hammen, Ph.D.
Sandra G. Hershberg, M.D.
Abram M. Hostetter, M.D.
Michael Hughes, M.D.
Steven Hyman, M.D.
William S. James, M.D.
Kay Jamison, Ph.D.
James W. Jefferson, M.D.
Kathleen Kannenberg, M.A., OTRLH
Roger G. Kathol, M.D.
David L. Keegan, M.D.
Marin B. Keller, M.D.
Lawrence L. Kennedy, M.D.
Howard D. Kibel, M.D.
Donald F. Klein, M.D.
David J. Kupfer, M.D.
Henry Lahmeyer, M.D.
Barry J. Landau, M.D.
William B. Lawson, M.D., Ph.D.
Ellen Liebenluft, M.D.
Alan B. Levy, M.D.
Francis Lu, M.D.
Stephan C. Mann, M.D.
Velandy Manohar, M.D.
Ronald L. Martin, M.D.
Marlin Mattson, M.D.
Jon McClellan, M.D.
J. Stephen Meredith, M.D.
Arnold E. Merriam, M.D.
Jerome A. Motto, M.D.
J. Craig Nelson, M.D.
Charles Nemeroff, M.D., Ph.D.
Arthur M. Nezu, Ph.D.
Andrei Novac, M.D.
John I. Nurnberger, Jr., M.D., Ph.D.
Joseph Parks, M.D.
Eugene Patterson, M.D.

Teri Pearlstein, M.D.
Glen N. Peterson, M.D.
Herbert Peyser, M.D.
Robert Prien, Ph.D.
John C. Racy, M.D.
Shahzad Rahman, M.D.
Lynn Rehm, Ph.D., ABPP
William H. Reid, M.D., M.P.H.
Ronald A. Remick, M.D., F.R.C.P.(C.)
Richard Ries, M.D.
A. John Rush, M.D.
Gary Sachs, M.D.
Harold A. Sackeim, Ph.D.
Alan Schatzberg, M.D.
Stephen Scheiber, M.D.
Jerome M. Schnitt, M.D.
Mogens Schou, M.D.
Aimee Schwartz, M.D.
Paul M. Schyve, M.D.
Steven S. Sharfstein, M.D.

Michael Silver, M.D.
Issac Slaughter, M.D.
Joyce G. Small, M.D.
David A. Solomon, M.D.
Harvey Sternbach, M.D.
Andrew L. Stoll, M.D.
Stephen M. Strakowski, M.D.
John Strauss, M.D.
Patricia Suppes, M.D.
Margery Sved, M.D.
Clifton R. Tennison, M.D.
Claudewell Thomas, M.D.
Mauricio Tohen, M.D., Dr.P.H.
Ming T. Tsuang, M.D., Ph.D.
Robert J. Ursano, M.D.
Richard Weiner, M.D.
Myrna Weissman, M.D.
Peter Whybrow, M.D.
Philip Woollcott, Jr., M.D.
Herbert F. Young, M.D.

VI. ORGANIZATIONS SUBMITTING COMMENTS

Academy of Psychosomatic Medicine
American Academy of Child and Adolescent Psychiatry
American Academy of Family Physicians
American Academy of Neurology
American Academy of Psychiatrists in Alcoholism and Addiction
American Academy of Psychoanalysis
American Association of Community Psychiatrists
American Association of Psychiatric Administrators
American Association of Psychiatrists from India
American Association of Suicidology
American Board of Psychiatry and Neurology
American College of Neuropsychopharmacology
American College of Occupational and Environmental Medicine
American Geriatrics Society
American Group Psychotherapy Association
American Occupational Therapy Association
American Psychiatric Electrophysiology Association
American Psychoanalytic Association
American Psychological Association
American Psychosomatic Society
American Society for Adolescent Psychiatry
American Society of Addiction Medicine
Association for Academic Psychiatry
Association for the Advancement of Behavior Therapy

Association of Gay and Lesbian Psychiatrists
Association of Women in Psychology
Baltimore-Washington Society for Psychoanalysis
Black Psychiatrists of America
Joint Commission on Accreditation of Health Care Organizations
National Alliance for the Mentally Ill
National Association of Psychiatric Health Systems
National Association of Social Workers
National Association of State Mental Health Program Directors
National Community Mental Healthcare Council
National Depressive and Manic Depressive Association
National Guild of Catholic Psychiatrists
National Institute of Mental Health
National Mental Health Association
Recovery, Inc.
Society of Biological Psychiatry

VII. REFERENCES

The bracketed letter following each reference indicates the nature of the supporting evidence, as follows:

[A]   *Randomized controlled clinical trial.* A study of an intervention in which subjects are prospectively followed over time; subjects are randomly assigned to treatment and control groups; both the subjects and the investigators are blind to the assignments.

[B]   *Clinical trial.* A prospective study in which an intervention is made and the results of that intervention are tracked longitudinally; study does not meet standards for a randomized clinical trial.

[C]   *Cohort or longitudinal study.* A study in which subjects are prospectively followed over time without any specific intervention.

[D]   *Case-control study.* A study in which a group of patients is identified and information about them is pursued retrospectively.

[E]   *Review with secondary data analysis.* A structured analytic review of existing data, e.g., a metanalysis or a decision analysis.

[F]   *Review.* A qualitative review and discussion of previously published literature without a quantitative synthesis of the data.

[G]   *Other.* Expert opinion, case reports, and other reports not included above.

1. Goodwin FK, Jamison KR: Manic-Depressive Illness. New York, Oxford University Press, 1990 [F]

2. Coryell W, Scheftner W, Keller, Endicott J, Maser J, Klerman GL: The enduring psychosocial consequences of mania and depression. Am J Psychiatry 1993; 150:720–727 [C]

3. Müller-Oerlinghausen B, Muser-Causemann B, Volk J: Suicides and parasuicides in a high risk patient group on and off lithium long-term medication. J Affect Disord 1992; 25:261–269 [C]

4. Coppen A, Standish-Barry H, Bailey J, Houston G, Silcocks P, Hermon C: Does lithium reduce the mortality of recurrent mood disorders? J Affect Disord 1991; 23:1–7 [C]

5. Shulman KI, Tohen M, Satlin A, Mallya G, Kalunian D: Mania compared with unipolar depression in old age. Am J Psychiatry 1992; 149:341–345 [C]

6. Weissman MM, Bruce ML, Leaf PJ, Florio LP, Holzer III CE: Affective disorders, in Psychiatric Disorders in America. Edited by Robins L, Regier DA. New York, Free Press, 1990 [C]

7. Weissman MM, Leaf PJ, Tischler GL, Blazer DG, Karno M, Bruce ML, Florio EF: Affective disorders in five United States communities. Psychol Med 1988; 18:141–153 [C]

8. Weller BW, Weller RA: Mood disorders, in Child and Adolescent Psychiatry: A Comprehensive Textbook. Edited by Lewis M. Baltimore, Williams & Wilkins, 1991 [F]

9. Carlson GA, Strober M: Manic depressive-illness in early adolescence: a study of clinical and diagnostic characteristics in six cases. J Am Acad Child Adolesc Psychiatry 1978; 17:138–153 [G]

10. Strober M, Carlson G: Bipolar illness in adolescents with major depression: clinical, genetic, and psychopharmacologic predictors in a three- to four-year prospective follow-up investigation. Arch Gen Psychiatry 1982; 39:549–555 [C]

11. Weller RA, Weller EB, Tucker SG, Fristad MA: Mania in prepubertal children: has it been underdiagnosed? J Affect Disord 1986; 11:151–154 [F]

12. DeLong GR, Aldershof AL: Long-term experience with lithium treatment in childhood: correlation with clinical diagnosis. J Am Acad Child Adolesc Psychiatry 1987; 26:389–394 [B]

13. Varanka TM, Weller RA, Weller EB, Fristad MA: Lithium treatment of manic episodes with psychotic features in prepubertal children. Am J Psychiatry 1988; 145:1557–1559 [B]

14. Strober M, Morrell W, Lampert C, Burroughs J: Relapse following discontinuation of lithium maintenance therapy in adolescents with bipolar I illness: a naturalistic study. Am J Psychiatry 1990; 147:457–461 [C]

15. Werry JS, McClellan JM, Chard L: Childhood and adolescent schizophrenic, bipolar, and schizoaffective disorders: a clinical and outcome study. J Am Acad Child Adolesc Psychiatry 1991; 30:457–465 [D]

16. Tohen M, Shulman KT, Satlin A: First-episode mania in late life. Am J Psychiatry 1994; 151:130–132 [C]

17. Gershon ES, Berrettini W, Nurnberger J, Goldin LR: Genetics of affective illness, in Psychopharmacology: The Third Generation of Progress. Edited by Meltzer HL. New York, Raven Press, 1987 [F]

18. Nurnberger JI, Gershon E: Genetics, in Handbook of Affective Disorders, 2nd ed. Edited by Paykel ES. New York, Churchill Livingstone, 1992 [E]

19. Akiskal HS: The clinical management of affective disorders, in Psychiatry, vol 1. Edited by Michels R, Cooper AM, Guze SB, Judd LL, Klerman GL, Solnit AJ. Philadelphia, JB Lippincott, 1985 [G]

20. Schou M: Lithium Treatment of Manic-Depressive Illness: A Practical Guide, 5th ed. New York, S Karger, 1993 [F]

21. Bohn J, Jefferson JW: Lithium and Manic Depression: A Guide, 2nd ed. Madison, Wis, Lithium Information Center, Dean Foundation, 1993 [G]

22. Jefferson JW, Greist JH: Valproate and Manic Depression: A Guide, 2nd ed. Madison, Wis, Lithium Information Center, Dean Foundation, 1993 [G]

23. Medenwald JR, Greist JH, Jefferson JW: Carbamazepine and Manic Depression: A Guide, 2nd ed. Madison, Wis, Lithium Information Center, Dean Foundation, 1993 [G]

24. Gutheil TG: The psychology of psychopharmacology. Bull Menninger Clin 1982; 46:321–330 [G]

25. Jamison KR: Manic-depressive illness: the overlooked need for psychotherapy, in Integrating Pharmacotherapy and Psychotherapy. Edited by Beitman BD, Klerman GL. Washington, DC, American Psychiatric Press, 1991 [F]

26. Jamison KR, Akiskal HS: Medication compliance in patients with bipolar disorder. Psychiatr Clin North Am 1983; 6:175–192 [F]

27. Pardes H, Kaufman CA, Pincus HA, West A: Genetics and psychiatry: past discoveries, current dilemmas, and future directions. Am J Psychiatry 1989; 146:435–443 [G]

28. Post RM, Roy-Byrne PP, Uhde TW: Graphic representation of the life course of illness in patients with affective disorder. Am J Psychiatry 1988; 145:844–848 [G]

29. Kraepelin E: Manic-Depressive Insanity and Paranoia (1921). Translated by Barclay RM; edited by Robertson GM. New York, Arno Press, 1976 [G]

30. Meyer A: The Collected Papers of Adolph Meyer. Edited by Winters EE. Baltimore, Johns Hopkins University Press, 1950–52 [G]

31. Cade JFJ: Lithium salts in the treatment of psychotic excitement. Med J Aust 1949; 36:349–352 [G]

32. Jefferson JW, Greist JH, Acherman DL, Carroll JA: Lithium Encyclopedia for Clinical Practice, 2nd ed. Washington, DC, American Psychiatric Press, 1987 [F]

33. Goodwin FK, Ebert M: Lithium in mania: clinical trials and controlled studies, in Lithium: Its Role in Psychiatric Research and Treatment. Edited by Gershon S, Shopsin B. New York, Plenum Press, 1973 [E]

34. Schou M, Juel-Nielson, Strömgren E, Voldby H: The treatment of manic psychoses by administration of lithium salts. J Neurol Neurosurg Psychiatry 1954; 17:250–260 [B]

35. Maggs R: Treatment of manic illness with lithium carbonate. Br J Psychiatry 1963; 109:56–65 [B]

36. Goodwin FK, Murphy DL, Bunney WF Jr: Lithium carbonate treatment in depression and mania: a longitudinal double-blind study. Arch Gen Psychiatry 1969; 21:486–496 [B]

37. Stokes PE, Shamoian CA, Stoll PM, Patton MJ: Efficacy of lithium as acute treatment of manic-depressive illness. Lancet 1971; 1:1319–1325 [B]

38. Goodwin FK, Zis AP: Lithium in the treatment if mania: comparisons with neuroleptics. Arch Gen Psychiatry 1979; 36:840–844 [F]

39. Bowden CL, Brugger AM, Swann AC, Calabrese JR, Janicak PG, Petty F, Dilsaver SC, Davis JM, Rush AJ, Small JG, Garza-Treviño ES, Risch SC, Goodnick PJ, Morris DD: Efficacy of divalproex vs lithium and placebo in the treatment of mania. The Depakote Mania Study Group. JAMA 1994; 271:918–924 [A]

40. Janicak PG, Davis JM, Preskorn SH, Ayd FJ: Principles and Practice of Psychopharmacotherapy. Baltimore, Williams & Wilkins, 1993 [F]

41. Zornberg GL, Pope HG Jr: Treatment of depression in bipolar disorder: new directions for research. J Clin Psychopharm 1993; 13:397–408 [E]

42. Baastrup PC, Schou M: Lithium as a prophylactic agent: its effect against recurrent depression and manic-depressive psychosis. Arch Gen Psychiatry 1967; 16:162–172 [B]

43. Faedda GL, Tondo L, Baldessarini RJ, Suppes T, Tohen M: Outcome after rapid vs. gradual discontinuation of lithium treatment in bipolar disorders. Arch Gen Psychiatry 1993; 50:448–455 [B]

44. Suppes T, Baldessarini RJ, Faedda GL, Tohen M: Risk of recurrence following discontinuation of lithium treatment in bipolar disorder. Arch Gen Psychiatry 1991; 48:1082–1088 [E]

45. Schou M: Is there a lithium withdrawal syndrome? an examination of the evidence. Br J Psychiatry 1993; 163:514–518 [F]

46. Post RM, Leverich GS, Altshuler L, Mikalauskas K: Lithium-discontinuation-induced refractoriness: preliminary observations. Am J Psychiatry 1992; 149:1727–1729 [G]

47. Pazzaglia PJ, Post RM: Contingent tolerance and reresponse to carbamazepine: a case study in a patient with trigeminal neuralgia and bipolar disorder. J Neuropsychiatry Clin Neurosci 1992; 4:76–81 [G]

48. Schou M: Lithium prophylaxis: myths and realities. Am J Psychiatry 1989; 146:573–576 [F]

49. Arana GW, Hyman SE: Handbook of Psychiatric Drug Therapy, 2nd ed. Boston, Little, Brown, 1991 [F]

50. Bauer MS, Whybrow PC: Rapid cycling bipolar affective disorder. II. Treatment of refractory rapid cycling with high-dose levothyroxine: a preliminary study. Arch Gen Psychiatry 1990; 47:435–440 [G]

51. Smigan L, Wahlin A, Jacobsson L, von Knorring L: Lithium therapy and thyroid function tests: a prospective study. Neuropsychobiology 1984; 17:39–43 [B]

52. Bocchetta A, Bernardi F, Burrai C, Pedditzi M, Loviselli A, Velluzzi F, Martino E, Del Zompo M: The course of thyroid abnormalities during lithium treatment: a two year follow-up study. Acta Psychiatr Scand 1992; 86:38–41 [C]

53. Vestergaard P, Schou M, Thomsen K: Monitoring of patients in prophylactic lithium treatment: an assessment based on recent kidney studies. Br J Psychiatry 1982; 140:185–187 [C]

54. Schou M: Effects of long-term lithium treatment on kidney function: an overview. J Psychiatry Res 1988; 22:287–296 [F]

55. Gitlin MJ: Lithium-induced renal insufficiency. J Clin Psychopharmacol 1993; 13:276–279 [C]

56. von Knorring L, Wahlin A, Nystrom K, Bohman SO: Uraemia induced by long-term lithium treatment. Lithium 1990; 1:251–253 [G]

57. Cooper TB, Bergner PE, Simpson GM: The 24-hour serum lithium level as a prognosticator of dosage requirements. Am J Psychiatry 1973; 130:601–603 [C]

58. Gelenberg AJ, Kane JM, Keller MB, Lavori P, Rosenbaum JF, Cole K, Lavelle J: Comparison of standard and low serum levels of lithium for maintenance treatment of bipolar disorder. N Engl J Med 1989; 321:1489–1493 [A]

59. Pope HG Jr, McElroy SL, Keck PE Jr, Hudson JI: Valproate in the treatment of acute mania: a placebo controlled study. Arch Gen Psychiatry 1991; 48:62–68 [A]

60. Keck PE Jr, McElroy SL, Tugrul KC, Bennett JA: Valproate oral loading in the treatment of acute mania. J Clin Psychiatry 1993; 54:305–308 [B]

61. McElroy SL, Keck PE, Jr: Treatment guidelines for valproate in bipolar and schizoaffective disorders. Can J Psychiatry 1993; 38(3 suppl 2):S62–S66 [F]

62. McElroy SL, Dessain EC, Pope HG Jr, Cole JO, Keck PE Jr, Frankenberg FR, Aizley HG, O'Brien S: Clozapine in the treatment of psychotic mood disorders, schizoaffective disorder, and schizophrenia. J Clin Psychiatry 1991; 52:411–414 [G]

63. Keck PE Jr, McElroy SL, Nemeroff CB: Anticonvulsants in the treatment of bipolar disorder. J Neuropsychiatry Clin Neurosci 1992; 4:395–405 [F]

64. Ketter TA, Pazzaglia PJ, Post RM: Synergy of carbamazepine and valproic acid in affective illness: case report and review of literature. J Clin Psychopharmacol 1992; 12:276–281 [F]

65. Puzynski S, Kosiewicz L: Valproic acid amide as a prophylactic agent in affective and schizoaffective disorders. Psychopharmacol Bull 1984; 20:151–159 [B]

66. Hayes SG: The long-term use of valproate in primary psychiatric disorders. J Clin Psychiatry 1989; 50(3 suppl):35–39 [D]

67. Calabrese JR, Delucchi GA: Spectrum of efficacy of valproate in 55 patients with rapid-cycling bipolar disorder. Am J Psychiatry 1990; 147:431–434 [B]

68. Calabrese JR, Markovitz PJ, Kimmel SE, Wagner SC: Spectrum of efficacy of valproate in 78 rapid-cycling bipolar patients. J Clin Psychopharmacol 1992; 12(1 suppl):53S–56S [B]

69. McElroy SL, Keck PE Jr, Pope HG Jr, Hudson JI: The use of valproate in psychiatric disorders: literature review and clinical guidelines. J Clin Psychiatry 1989; 50(Mar suppl):23–29 [F]

70. Jacobsen FM: Low-dose valproate: a new treatment for cyclothymia, mild rapid cycling disorders, and premenstrual syndrome. J Clin Psychiatry 1993; 54:229–234 [B]

71. Rall TW, Schleifer LS: Drugs effective in the therapy of the epilepsies, in Goodman and Gilman's: The Pharmacological Basis of Therapeutics, 8th ed. Edited by Gilman LS, Goodman AG, Rall TW. New York, Macmillan, 1991 [F]

72. Rimmer EM, Richens A: An update on sodium valproate. Pharmacotherapy 1985; 5:171–184 [F]

73. Penry JK, Dean JC: The scope and use of valproate in epilepsy. J Clin Psychiatry 1989; 50(Mar suppl):17–22 [F]

74. Wilder BJ, Karas BJ, Penry JK, Asconape J: Gastrointestinal tolerance of divalproex sodium. Neurology 1983; 33:808–811 [B]

75. Goodman AG, Zall TW, Nies AS, Taylor P: Goodman and Gilman's: The Pharmacological Basis of Therapeutics, 8th ed. New York, Macmillan, 1991 [G]

76. Sovner R, Davis JM: A potential drug interaction between fluoxetine and valproic acid (letter). J Clin Psychopharmacol 1991; 11: 389 [G]

77. Stoll AL, Vuckovic A, McElroy SL: Histamine-2-receptor antagonists for the treatment of valproate-induced gastrointestinal distress. Ann Clin Psychiatry 1991; 3:301–304 [G]

78. Isojarvi JI, Laatikainen TJ, Pakarinen AJ, Juntunen KT, Myllyla VV: Polycystic ovaries and hyperandrogenism in women taking valproate for epilepsy. N Engl J Med 1993; 329:1383–1388 [G]

79. Pellock JM, Willmore LJ: A rational guide to routine blood monitoring in patients receiving antiepileptic drugs. Neurology 1991; 41:961–964 [G]

80. McElroy SL, Keck PE Jr, Pope HG Jr, Hudson JI: Valproate in the treatment of bipolar disorder: literature review and clinical guidelines. J Clin Psychopharmacol 1992; 12(1 suppl):42S–52S [F]

81. McElroy SL, Keck PE Jr, Pope HG Jr, Hudson JI, Faedda GL, Swann AC: Clinical and research implications of the diagnosis of dysphoric or mixed mania or hypomania. Am J Psychiatry 1992; 149:1633–1644 [F]

82. Post RM, Leverich GS, Rosoff AS, Altshuler LL: Carbamazepine prophylaxis in refractory affective disorders: a focus on long-term follow-up. J Clin Psychopharmacol 1990; 10:318–327 [C]

83. Lipinski JF Jr, Pope HG Jr: Possible synergistic action between carbamazepine and lithium carbonate: a report of three cases. Am J Psychiatry 1982; 139:938–939 [B]

84. Keck PE Jr, McElroy SL, Vuckovic A, Friedman LM: Combined valproate and carbamazepine treatment of bipolar disorder. J Neuropsychiatry Clin Neurosci 1992; 4:319–322 [B]

85. Lerer B, Moore M, Meyendorff E, Cho SR, Gershon S: Carbamazepine versus lithium in mania: a double-blind study. J Clin Psychiatry 1987; 48:89–93 [A]

86. Small JG, Klapper MH, Milstein V, Kellams JJ, Miller MJ, Marhenke JD, Small IF: Carbamazepine compared with lithium in the treatment of mania. Arch Gen Psychiatry 1991; 48:915–921 [A]

87. Colgate R: The ranking of therapeutic and toxic side effects of lithium carbonate. Psychiatr Bull 1992; 16:473–475 [G]

88. Ayd FJ: Acute self-poisoning with lithium. Int Drug Therapy Newsletter 1988; 23:1–2 [G]

89. Ragheb M: The clinical significance of lithium-nonsteroidal anti-inflammatory drug interactions. J Clin Psychopharmacol 1990; 10:350–354 [G]

90. Ballenger JC, Post RM: Carbamazepine in manic-depressive illness: a new treatment. Am J Psychiatry 1980; 137:782–790 [A]

91. Post RM, Uhde TW, Ballenger JC, Squillace KM: Prophylactic efficacy of carbamazepine in manic-depressive illness. Am J Psychiatry 1983; 140:1602–1604 [G]

92. Kramlinger KG, Post RM: The addition of lithium to carbamazepine: antidepressant efficacy in treatment-resistant depression. Arch Gen Psychiatry 1989; 46:794–800 [B]

93. Prien RF, Gelenberg AJ: Alternatives to lithium for preventive treatment of bipolar disorder. Am J Psychiatry 1989; 146:840–848 [F]

94. Lusznat RM, Murphy DP, Nunn CMH: Carbamazepine vs lithium in the treatment and prophylaxis of mania. Br J Psychiatry 1988; 153:198–204 [A]

95. Okuma T, Inanaga K, Otsuki S, Sarai K, Takahashi R, Hazama H, Mori A, Watanabe S: A preliminary double-blind study on the efficacy of carbamazepine in prophylaxis of manic-depressive illness. Psychopharmacology (Berl) 1981; 73:95–96 [A]

96. Placidi GF, Lenzi A, Lazzerini F, Cassano GB, Akiskal HS: The comparative efficacy and safety of carbamazepine versus lithium: a randomized, double-blind, 3 year trial in 83 patients. J Clin Psychiatry 1986; 47:490–494 [A]

97. Watkins SE, Callender K, Thomas DR, Tidmarsh SF, Shaw DM: The effect of carbamazepine and lithium on remission from affective illness. Br J Psychiatry 1987; 150:180–182 [A]

98. Murphy DJ, Gannon MA, McGennis A: Carbamazepine in bipolar affective disorder (letter). Lancet 1989; 2:1151–1152 [G]

99. Ketter TA, Post RM, Worthington K: Principles of clinically important drug interactions with carbamazepine. Part I. J Clin Psychopharmacology 1991; 11:198–203 [F]

100. Ketter TA, Post RM, Worthington K: Principles of clinically important drug interactions with carbamazepine. Part II. J Clin Psychopharmacology 1991; 11:306–313 [F]

101. Smith MC, Bleck TP: Convulsive disorders: toxicity of anti-convulsants. Clin Neuropharmacol 1991; 14:97–115 [F]

102. Seetharam MN, Pellock JM: Risk-benefit assessment of carbamazepine in children. Drug Safety 1991; 6:148–158 [F]

103. Prien RF, Caffey EM, Klett CJ: Comparison of lithium carbonate and chlorpromazine in the treatment of mania. Report of the Veterans Administration and National Institute of Mental Health Collaborative Study Group. Arch Gen Psychiatry 1972; 26:146–153 [A]

104. Lenox RH, Newhouse PA, Creelman WL, Whitaker TM: Adjunctive treatment of manic agitation with lorazepam versus haloperidol: a double-blind study. J Clin Psychiatry 1992; 53: 47–52 [A]

105. Shopsin B, Gershon S, Thompson H, Collins P: Psychoactive drugs in mania. A controlled comparison of lithium carbonate, chlorpromazine, and haloperidol. Arch Gen Psychiatry 1975; 32:34–42 [A]

106. Davis JM: Overview: maintenance therapy in psychiatry: II. Affective disorders. Am J Psychiatry 1976; 133:1–13 [E]

107. Mukherjee S, Rosen AM, Caracci G, Shukla S: Persistent tardive dyskinesia in bipolar patients. Arch Gen Psychiatry 1986; 43: 342–346 [C]

108. Tardive Dyskinesia: A Task Force Report of the American Psychiatric Association. Washington, DC, APA, 1991 [F]

109. Parker G, Roy K, Hadzi-Pavlovic D, Pedic F: Psychotic (delusional) depression: a meta-analysis of physical treatments. J Affect Disord 1992; 24:17–24 [E]

110. Spiker DG, Weiss JC, Dealy RS, Griffin SJ, Hanin I, Neil JF, Perel JM, Rossi AJ, Soloff PH: The pharmacological treatment of delusional depression. Am J Psychiatry 1985; 142:430–436 [A]

111. Kukopulos A, Reginaldi D, Laddomada P, Floris G, Serra G, Tondo L: Course of the manic-depressive cycle and changes caused by treatment. Pharmakopsychiatrie-Neuropsychopharmakol 1980; 13:156–167 [C]

112. Sernyak MJ, Woods SW: Chronic neuroleptic use in manic-depressive illness. Psychopharmacol Bull 1993; 29:375–381 [B]

113. Edwards R, Stephenson U, Flewett T: Clonazepam in acute mania: a double-blind trial. Aust N Z J Psychiatry 1991; 25:238–242 [A]

114. Chouinard G, Young SN, Annable L: Antimanic effect of clonazepam. Biol Psychiatry 1983; 18:451–466 [F]

115. Chouinard G: Clonazepam in acute and maintenance treatment of bipolar disorder. J Clin Psychiatry 1987; 48(Oct suppl):29–37 [F]

116. Bradwejn J, Shriqui C, Koszycki D, Meterissian G: Double-blind comparison of the effects of clonazepam and lorazepam in acute mania. J Clin Psychopharmacol 1990; 10:403–408 [A]

117. Chouinard G, Annable L, Turnier L, Holobow N, Szkrumelak N: A double-blind randomized clinical trial of rapid tranquilization with I.M. clonazepam and I.M. haloperidol in agitated psychotic patients with manic symptoms. Can J Psychiatry 1993; 38(suppl 4):S114–S121 [A]

118. Sachs GS, Weilburg JB, Rosenbaum JF: Clonazepam vs neuroleptics as adjuncts to lithium maintenance. Psychopharmacol Bull 1990; 26:137–143 [F]

119. Aronson TA, Shukla S, Hirschowitz J: Clonazepam treatment of five lithium-refractory patients with bipolar disorder. Am J Psychiatry 1989; 146:77–80 [G]

120. Miller NS, Gold MS: Abuse, addiction, tolerance, and dependence to benzodiazepines in medical and nonmedical populations. Am J Drug Alcohol Abuse 1991; 17:27–37 [F]

121. Busto V, Sellers EM, Naranjo CA, Cappell HD, Sanchez-Craig M, Simpkins J: Patterns of benzodiazepine abuse and dependence. Br J Addiction 1986; 81:87–94 [C]

122. American Psychiatric Association: Practice Guideline for Major Depressive Disorder in Adults. Am J Psychiatry 1993; 150(Apr suppl) [F]

123. Baumhackl U, Biziere K, Fischbach R, Geretsegger CH, Hebenstreit G, Radmayr E, Stabl M: Efficacy and tolerability of moclobemide compared with imipramine in depressive disorder (DSM-III): an Austrian double-blind, multicentre study. Br J Psychiatry 1989; 155(Oct suppl):78–83 [A]

124. Himmelhoch JM, Thase ME, Mallinger AG, Houck P: Tranylcypromine versus imipramine in anergic bipolar depression. Am J Psychiatry 1991; 148:910–916 [A]

125. Cohn JB, Collins G, Ashbrook E, Wernicke JF: A comparison of fluoxetine imipramine and placebo in patients with bipolar depressive disorder. Int Clin Psychopharmacology 1989; 4:313–322 [A]

126. Sachs GS, Lafer B, Stoll AL, Banov M, Thibault AB, Tohen M, Rosenbaum JF: A double-blind trial of bupropion versus desipramine for bipolar depression. J Clin Psychiatry 1994; 55:391–393 [A]

127. Fogelson DL, Bystritsky A, Pasnau R: Bupropion in the treatment of bipolar disorders: the same old story? J Clin Psychiatry 1992; 53:443–446 [G]

128. Shopsin B. Bupropion's prophylactic efficacy in bipolar affective illness. J Clin Psychiatry 1983; 44(5, sec 2):163–169 [B]

129. Haykal RF, Akiskal HS: Bupropion as a promising approach to rapid cycling bipolar II patients. J Clin Psychiatry 1990; 51:450–455 [G]

130. Wright G, Galloway L, Kim J, Dalton M, Miller L Stern W: Bupropion in the long-term treatment of cyclic mood disorders: mood stabilizing effects. J Clin Psychiatry 1985; 46:22–25 [F]

131. Wehr TA, Goodwin FK: Do antidepressants cause mania? Psychopharmacol Bull 1987; 23:61–65 [G]

132. Peet M: Induction of mania with selective serotonin re-uptake inhibitors and tricyclic antidepressants. Br J Psychiatry 1994; 164:549–550 [E]

133. Wehr TA, Goodwin FK: Rapid cycling in manic-depressives induced by tricyclic antidepressants. Arch Gen Psychiatry 1979; 36:555–559 [B]

134. Akiskal HS, Mallya G: Criteria for the "soft" bipolar spectrum: treatment implications. Psychopharmacol Bull 1987; 23:68–73 [G]

135. Prien RF, Potter WZ: NIMH workshop report on treatment of bipolar disorder. Psychopharmacol Bull 1990; 26:409–427 [F]

136. Dubovsky SL, Franks RD, Lifschitz M, Coen P: Effectiveness of verapamil in the treatment of a manic patient. Am J Psychiatry 1982; 139:502–504 [G]

137. Dubovsky S, Franks RD, Schrier D: Phenelzine-induced hypomania: effect of verapamil. Biol Psychiatry 1985; 20:1009–1014 [G]

138. Dubovsky SL, Franks RD, Allen S, Murphy J: Calcium antagonists in mania: a double-blind study of verapamil. Psychiatry Res 1986; 18:309–320 [A]

139. Dubovsky SL, Franks RD, Allen S: Verapamil: a new antimanic drug with potential interactions with lithium. J Clin Psychiatry 1987; 48:371–372 [G]

140. Dubovsky SL, Franks RD: Intracellular calcium ions in affective disorders: a review and an hypothesis. Biol Psychiatry 1983; 18:781–797 [F]

141. Hoschl C: Verapamil for depression? (letter). Am J Psychiatry 1983; 140:1100 [G]

142. Giannini AJ, Houser WL Jr, Loiselle RH, Giannini MC, Price WA: Antimanic effects of verapamil. Am J Psychiatry 1984; 141:1602–1603 [B]

143. Giannini AJ, Taraszewski R, Loiselle RH: Verapamil and lithium in maintenance therapy of manic patients. J Clin Pharmacol 1987; 27:980–982 [A]

144. Dose M, Emrich HM, Cording-Tommel C, Von Zerssen D: Use of calcium antagonists in mania. Psychoneuroendocrinology 1986; 11:241–243 [F]

145. Hoschl C, Kozeny J: Verapamil in affective disorders: a controlled, double-blind study. Biol Psychiatry 1989; 25:128–140 [B]

146. Garza-Treviño ES, Overall JE, Hollister LE: Verapamil versus lithium in acute mania. Am J Psychiatry 1992; 149:121–122 [A]

147. Stancer HC, Persad E: Treatment of intractable rapid-cycling manic-depressive disorder with levothyroxine: clinical observations. Arch Gen Psychiatry 1982: 39:311–312 [G]

148. Stein D, Avni J: Thyroid hormones in the treatment of affective disorders. Acta Psychiatr Scand 1988; 77:623–636 [F]

149. Banovac K, Papic M, Bilsker MS, Zakarija M, McKensie JM: Evidence of hyperthyroidism in apparently euthyroid patients treated with levothyroxine. Arch Intern Med 1989; 149:809–812 [C]

150. Stall GM, Harris S, Sokoll LJ, Dawson-Hughes B: Accelerated bone loss in hypothyroid patients overtreated with L-thyroxine. Ann Intern Med 1990; 113:265–269 [C]

151. Coindre JM, David JP, Riviere L, Goussot JF, Roger P, de Mascarel A, Meunier PJ: Bone loss in hypothyroidism with hormone replacement: a histomorphic study. Arch Intern Med 1986; 146: 48–53 [G]

152. Gyulai L, Lew PY, Bauer MS, Rubin L, Rounkin S, Jaggi J, Whybrow P: High dose thyroxine does not decrease bone density, in CME Syllabus and Scientific Proceedings in Summary Form, 146th Annual Meeting of the American Psychiatric Association. Washington, DC, APA, 1993 [F]

153. Suppes T, McElroy SL, Gilbert J, Dessain EC, Cole JO: Clozapine in the treatment of dysphoric mania. Biol Psychiatry 1992; 32:270–280 [B]

154. Deltito JA, Moline M, Pollak C, Martin LY, Maremmani I: Effects of phototherapy on nonseason unipolar and bipolar depressive spectrum disorders. J Affect Disord 1991 23:231–237 [B]

155. Mukherjee S, Sackeim HA, Schnurr DB: Electroconvulsive therapy of acute manic episodes: a review. Am J Psychiatry 1994; 151:169–176 [F]

156. Thomas J, Reddy B: The treatment of mania: a retrospective evaluation of the effects of ECT, chlorpromazine, and lithium. J Affect Disord 1982; 4:85–92 [D]

157. Black DW, Winokur G, Nasrallah A: Treatment of mania: a naturalistic study of electroconvulsive therapy versus lithium in 438 patients. J Clin Psychiatry 1987; 48:132–139 [C]

158. Alexander RC, Salomon M, Ionescu-Pioggia M, Cole JO: Convulsive therapy in the treatment of mania. Convulsive Therapy 1988; 4:115–125 [D]

159. Milstein V, Small JG, Klapper MH, Small IF, Miller MJ, Kellams JJ: Uni- versus bilateral ECT in the treatment of mania. Convulsive Therapy 1987; 3:1–9 [B]

160. Small JG, Klapper MH, Kellams JJ, Miller MJ, Milstein V, Sharpley PH, Small IF: Electroconvulsive treatment compared with lithium in the management of manic states. Arch Gen Psychiatry 1988; 45:727–732 [B]

161. Mukherjee S, Sackeim HA, Lee C: Unilateral ECT in the treatment of manic episodes. Convulsive Therapy 1988; 4:74–80 [B]

162. Strömgren LS: Electroconvulsive therapy in Aarhus, Denmark, in 1984: its application in nondepressive disorders. Convulsive Therapy 1988; 4:306–313 [D]

163. Heshe J, Roeder E: [Electroconvulsive therapy in Denmark. Review of the technique, employment, indications and complications.] Ugeskrift for Laeger 1975; 137:939–944 [G]

164. Kramp P, Bolwig TG: Electroconvulsive therapy in acute delirious states. Compr Psychiatry 1981; 22:368–371 [F]

165. Mann SC, Caroff SN, Bleier HR, Welz WK, Kling MA, Hayashida M: Lethal catatonia. Am J Psychiatry 1986; 143:1374–1381 [F]

166. Mann SC, Caroff SN, Bleier HR, Anttelo RE, Un H: Electroconvulsive therapy of the lethal catatonia syndrome. Convulsive Therapy 1990; 6:239–247 [F]

167. Janicak PG, Davis JM, Gibbons RD, Ericksen S, Chang S, Gallagher P: Efficacy of ECT: a meta-analysis. Am J Psychiatry 1985; 142:297–302 [E]

168. Hamilton M: Electroconvulsive therapy: indications and contraindications. Ann NY Acad Sci 1986; 462:5–11 [F]

169. The Practice of Electroconvulsive Therapy: Recommendations for Treatment, Training, and Privileging: A Task Force Report of the American Psychiatric Association. Washington, DC, American Psychiatric Press, 1990 [F]

170. Sackheim HA: The efficacy of electroconvulsive therapy in the treatment of major depressive disorder, in The Limits of Biological Treatments for Psychological Distress. Edited by Fisher S, Greenberg RP. Hillsdale, NJ, Erlbaum Publishing, 1989 [F]

171. Perris C, d'Elia G: A study of bipolar (manic-depressive) and unipolar recurrent depressive psychoses. IX. Therapy and prognosis. Acta Psychiatr Scand Suppl 1966; 194:153–171 [B]

172. Strömgren LS: Unilateral versus bilateral electroconvulsive therapy. Investigations into the therapeutic effect in endogenous depression. Acta Psychiatr Scand Suppl 1973; 240:8–65 [B]

173. Abrams R, Taylor MA: Unipolar and bipolar depressive illness. Phenomenology and response to electroconvulsive therapy. Arch Gen Psychiatry 1974; 30:320–321 [B]

174. Prudic J, Sackeim HA, Devanand DP: Medication resistance and clinical response to electroconvulsive therapy. Psychiatry Res 1990; 31:287–296 [B]

175. Devanand DP, Sackeim HA, Decina P, Prudic J: The development of mania and organic euphoria during ECT. J Clin Psychiatry 1988; 49:69–71 [G]

176. Small JG, Kellams JJ, Milstein V, Small IF: Complications with electroconvulsive treatment combined with lithium. Biol Psychiatry 1985; 20:125–134 [D]

177. Strömgren LS, Dahl J, Fjeldborg N, Thomsen A: Factors influencing seizure duration and number of seizures applied in unilateral electroconvulsive therapy: anaesthetics and benzodiazepines. Acta Psychiatr Scand 1980; 62;158–165 [A]

178. Standish-Barry HMAS, Bouras N, Hale AS, Bridges PK, Bartlett JR: Ventricular size and CSF transmitter metabolite concentrations in severe endogenous depression. Br J Psychiatry 1986; 148:386–392 [C]

179. Rudorfer MV, Linnoila M, Potter WZ: Combined lithium and electroconvulsive therapy: pharmacokinetic and pharmacodynamic interactions. Convulsive Therapy 1987; 3:40–45 [F]

180. El-Mallakh RS: Complications of concurrent lithium and electroconvulsive therapy: a review of clinical material and theoretical considerations. Psychopharmacol Bull 1987; 23:595–601 [F]

181. Ahmed SK, Stein GS: Negative interaction between lithium and ECT (letter). Br J Psychiatry 1987; 151:419–420 [G]

182. Small JG, Milstein V, Miller MJ, Sharpley PH, Small IF, Malloy FW, Klapper MH: Clinical, neuropsychological, and EEG evidence for mechanisms of action of ECT. Convulsive Therapy 1988; 4:280–291 [F]

183. Pettinati HM, Willis KW, Nilsen SM, Robin SE: Benzodiazepines reduce ECT's therapeutic effect, in New Research Program and Abstracts, 140th Annual Meeting of the American Psychiatric Association. Washington, DC, APA, 1987

184. Nettleblatt P: Factors influencing number of treatments and seizure duration in ECT: drug treatment, social class. Convulsive Therapy 1988; 4:160–168 [C]

185. Kahn DA: The use of psychodynamic psychotherapy in manic-depressive illness. J Am Acad Psychoanal 1993; 21:441–455 [F]

186. Haas GL, Glick ID, Clarkin JF, Spencer JH, Lewis AB, Peyser J, DeMane N, Good-Ellis M, Harris E, Lestelle V: Inpatient family intervention: a randomized clinical trial. II. Results at hospital discharge. Arch Gen Psychiatry 1988; 45:217–224 [B]

187. Clarkin JF, Glick ID, Haas GL, Spencer JH, Lewis AB, Peyser J, DeMane N, Good-Ellis M, Harris E, Lestelle V: A randomized clinical trial of inpatient family intervention. V. Results for affective disorders. J Affect Disord 1990; 18:17–28 [A]

188. Falloon IRH, Boyd JL, McGill CW: Family Care for Schizophrenia: A Problem-Solving Approach to Mental Illness. New York, Guilford Press, 1984 [G]

189. Miklowitz DJ, Goldstein MJ: Behavioral family treatment for patients with bipolar affective disorder. Behavior Modification 1990; 14:457–489 [G]

190. Miller IW, Keitner GI, Epstein NB, Bishop DS, Ryan CE: Families of bipolar patients: dysfunction, course of illness, and pilot treatment study, in Proceedings of the 22nd Meeting of the Society for Psychotherapy Research. Pittsburgh, Society for Psychotherapy Research, 1991 [B]

191. Basco MR, Rush AJ: Cognitive-behavioral therapy for bipolar disorder, in Cognitive Behavioral Treatment of Manic Depressive Disorder. New York, Guilford Press (in press) [F]

192. Frank E: Interpersonal and social rhythm therapy for bipolar disorder: integrating interpersonal and behavioral approaches. Behavior Therapist (in press) [F]

193. Karasu TB: Developmentalist metatheory of depression and psychotherapy. Am J Psychother 1992; 46:37–49 [G]

194. Klerman GL, Weissman MM, Rounsaville BJ, Chevron ES: Interpersonal Psychotherapy of Depression. New York, Basic Books, 1984 [G]

195. DiMascio A, Weissman MM, Prusoff BA, Neu C, Zwilling M, Klerman GL: Differential symptom reduction by drugs and psychotherapy in acute depression. Arch Gen Psychiatry 1979; 36: 1450–1456 [A]

196. Elkin I, Shea MT, Watkins JT, Imber SD, Sotsky SM, Collins JF, Glass DR, Pilkonis PA, Leber WR, Docherty JP, Fiester SJ, Parloff MB: National Institute of Mental Health Treatment of Depression Collaborative Research Program: general effectiveness of treatments. Arch Gen Psychiatry 1989; 46:971–982 [A]

197. Klerman GL, DiMascio A, Weissman M, Prusoff B, Paykel ES: Treatment of depression by drugs and psychotherapy. Am J Psychiatry 1974; 131:186–191 [A]

198. Frank E, Kupfer DJ, Perel JM, Cornes C, Jarrett DB, Mallinger AG, Thase ME, McEachran AB, Grochocinski VJ: Three-year outcomes for maintenance therapies in recurrent depression. Arch Gen Psychiatry 1990; 47:1093–1099 [B]

199. Ferster CB: A functional analysis of depression. Am Psychol 1973; 28:857–870 [F]

200. Bandura A: Social Learning Theory. Englewood Cliffs, NJ, Prentice-Hall, 1977 [F]

201. Lewinsohn PM, Antonuccio DA, Steinmetz-Breckinridge J, Teri L: The Coping with Depression Course: A Psychoeducational Intervention for Unipolar Depression. Eugene, Ore, Castalia Publishing, 1984 [F]

202. Lewinsohn P, Clarke G: Group treatment of depressed individuals: the "Coping with Depression" course. Advances in Behaviour Research Therapy 1984; 6:99–114 [F]

203. Rehm LP: Behavior Therapy for Depression: Present Status and Future Directions. New York, Academic Press, 1980 [F]

204. Bellack AS, Hersen M, Himmelhoch JM: A comparison of social-skills training, pharmacotherapy and psychotherapy for depression. Behav Res Ther 1983; 21:101–107 [A]

205. Nezu AM: Efficacy of a social problem-solving therapy for unipolar depression. J Consult Clin Psychol 1986; 54:196–202 [B]

206. Thompson LW, Gallagher D, Breckenridge JS: Comparative effectiveness of psychotherapies for depressed elders. J Consult Clin Psychol 1987; 21:133–146 [A]

207. McLean PD, Hakstian AR: Clinical depression: comparative efficacy of outpatient treatments. J Consult Clin Psychol 1979; 47:818–836 [A]

208. Usaf SO, Kavanagh DJ: Mechanisms of improvement in treatment for depression: test of self-efficacy and performance model. J Cognitive Psychotherapy 1990; 4:51–70 [A]

209. Nezu AM, Perri MG: Social problem-solving therapy for unipolar depression: an initial dismantling investigation. J Consult Clin Psychol 1989; 57:408–413 [B]

210. Gallagher DE, Thompson LW: Treatment of major depressive disorder in older adult outpatients with brief psychotherapies. Psychotherapy: Theory, Research, and Practice 1982; 19:482–490 [A]

211. Gallagher-Thompson D, Hanley-Peterson P, Thompson LW: Maintenance of gains versus relapse following brief psychotherapy for depression. J Consult Clin Psychol 1990; 58:371–374 [A]

212. Beck TA, Rush AJ, Shaw BF, Emery G: Cognitive Therapy of Depression. New York, Guilford Press, 1979 [F]

213. Rush AJ, Hollon SD, Beck AT, Kovacs M: Depression: must pharmacotherapy fail for cognitive therapy to succeed? Cognitive Therapy and Research 1978; 2:199–206 [B]

214. Hollon SD, DeRubeis RJ, Seligman MEP: Cognitive therapy and the prevention of depression. Applied Preventive Psychol 1992; 1:89–95 [G]

215. Shea MT, Elkin I, Imber SD, Sotsky SM, Watkins JT, Collins JF, Pilkonis PA, Beckham E, Glass DR, Dolan RT, Parloff MB: Course of depressive symptoms over follow-up. Findings from the National Institute of Mental Health Treatment of Depression Collaborative Research Program. Arch Gen Psychiatry 1992; 49:782–787 [A]

216. Ross M, Scott M: An evaluation of the effectiveness of individual and group cognitive therapy in the treatment of depressed patients in an inner city health centre. J Royal College of General Practitioners 1985; 35:239–242 [A]

217. O'Leary KD, Beach SR: Marital therapy: a viable treatment for depression and marital discord. Am J Psychiatry 1990; 147: 183–186 [A]

218. Beach SRH, Sandeen EE, O'Leary KD: Depression in Marriage. New York, Guilford Press, 1990 [G]

219. Yager J: Patients with mood disorders and marital/family problems, in Annual Review of Psychiatry, vol 11. Edited by Tasman A. Washington, DC, American Psychiatric Press, 1992 [G]

220. Coyne JC: Inpatient family intervention, in Affective Disorders and the Family: Assessment and Treatment. Edited by Clarkin JF, Haas GL, Glick ID. New York, Guilford Press, 1988 [F]

221. Coyne JC, Kessler RC, Tal M, Turnbull J, Wortman CB, Greden JF: Living with a depressed person. J Consult Clin Psychol 1987; 55:347–352 [F]

222. Jacobson NS, Dobson K, Fruzzetti AE, Schmaling KB, Salusky S: Marital therapy as a treatment for depression. J Consult Clin Psychol 1991; 59:547–557 [A]

223. Regier DA, Farmer ME, Rae DS, Locke BZ, Keith SJ, Judd LL, Goodwin FK: Comorbidity of mental disorders with alcohol and other drug abuse. Results from the Epidemiologic Catchment Area (ECA) Study. JAMA 1990; 264:2511–2518 [C]

224. Blacker D, Tsuang MT: Contested boundaries of bipolar disorder and the limits of categorical diagnosis in psychiatry. Am J Psychiatry 1992; 149:1473–1483 [F]

225. Akiskal HS, Hirschfeld MA, Yerevanian BI: The relationship of personality to affective disorders. Arch Gen Psychiatry 1983; 40:801–810 [F]

226. van Gent EM, Vida SL, Zwart FM: Group therapy in addition to lithium therapy in patients with bipolar disorders. Acta Psychiatr Belg 1988; 88:405–418 [B]

227. Wulsin L, Bachop M, Hoffman D: Group therapy in manic-depressive illness. Am J Psychother 1988; 42:263–271 [F]

228. Graves JS: Living with mania: a study of outpatient group psychotherapy for bipolar patients. Am J Psychother 1993; 47:113–126 [B]

229. Shakir SA, Volkmar FR, Bacon S, Pfefferbaum A: Group psychotherapy as an adjunct to lithium maintenance. Am J Psychiatry 1979; 136:455–456 [B]

230. Volkmar FR, Bacon S, Shakir SA, Pfefferbaum A: Group therapy in the management of manic-depressive illness. Am J Psychother 1981; 35:226–234 [B]

231. Davenport YB, Ebert MH, Adland ML, Goodwin FK: Couples group therapy as an adjunct to lithium maintenance of the manic patient. Am J Orthopsychiatry 1977; 47:495–502 [G]

232. Ablon SL, Davenport YB, Gershon ES, Adland ML: The married manic. Am J Orthopsychiatry 1975; 45:854–866 [G]

233. Zarin DA, Pass TM: Lithium and the single episode: when to begin long-term prophylaxis for bipolar disorder. Med Care 1987; 25(12 suppl):S76–S84 [E]

234. Wehr TA: Sleep loss: a preventable cause of mania and other excited states. J Clin Psychiatry 1989; 50(Dec suppl):8–16 [F]

235. Gelenberg AJ: Catatonic syndrome. Lancet 1976; 1:1339–1341 [G]

236. Black DW, Winokur G, Nasrallah MA: Suicide in subtypes of major affective disorder: a comparison with general population suicide mortality. Arch Gen Psychiatry 1987; 44:878–880 [C]

237. Fawcett J, Scheftner W, Clark D, Hedeker D, Gibbons R, Coryell W: Clinical predictors of suicide in patients with major affective disorders: a controlled prospective study. Am J Psychiatry 1987; 144:35–40 [C]

238. Müller-Oerlinghausen B, Ahrens B, Grof E, Grof P, Lenz G, Schou M, Simhandl C, Thau K, Volk J, Wolf R, Wolf T: The effect of long-term lithium treatment on the mortality of patients with manic-depressive and schizoaffective illness. Acta Psychiatr Scand 1992; 86:218–222 [C]

239. Fetner HH, Geller B: Lithium and tricyclic antidepressants. Psychiatr Clin North Am 1992; 15:223–224 [F]

240. Hassanyeh F, Davison K: Bipolar affective psychosis with onset before age 16 years: report of 10 cases. Br J Psychiatry 1980; 137:530–539 [G]

241. Horowitz HA: Lithium and the treatment of adolescent manic depressive illness. Diseases of the Nervous System 1977; 38:480–483 [G]

242. Hsu LK, Starzynski JM: Mania in adolescence. J Clin Psychiatry 1986; 47:596–599 [B]

243. Strober M, Morrell W, Burroughs J, Lampert C, Danforth H, Freeman R: A family study of bipolar I disorder in adolescence. Early onset of symptoms linked to increased familial loading and lithium resistance. J Affect Disord 1988; 15:255–268 [C]

244. Alessi N, Naylor MW, Ghaziuddin M, Zubieta JK: Update on lithium carbonate therapy in children and adolescents. J Am Acad Child Adolesc Psychiatry 1994; 33:291–304 [F]

245. Campbell M, Perry R, Green WH: Use of lithium in children and adolescents. Psychosomatics 1984; 25:95–106 [G]

246. Bertagnoli MW, Borchardt CM: A review of ECT for children and adolescents. J Am Acad Child Adolesc Psychiatry 1990; 29:302–307 [F]

247. Carlson GA: Bipolar disorder in children and adolescents, in Psychiatric Disorders in Children and Adolescents. Edited by Garfinkle BD, Carlson GA, Weller EB. Philadelphia, WB Saunders, 1990 [F]

248. Cohen LS, Friedman JM, Jefferson JW, Johnson EM, Weiner ML: A reevaluation of risk of in utero exposure to lithium. JAMA 1994; 271:146–150 [F]

249. Lier L, Kastrup M, Rafaelsen OJ: Psychiatric illness in relation to childbirth and pregnancy, II: diagnostic profiles, psychosocial and perinatal aspects. Nord Psykitr Tidsskr 1989; 43:535–542 [F]

250. Lindhout D, Meinardi H. Spina bifida and in-utero exposure to valproate (letter). Lancet 1984; 2:396 [G]

251. Rosa FW: Spina bifida in infants of women treated with carbamazepine during pregnancy. N Engl J Med 1991; 324:674–677 [D]

252. Centers for Disease Control: Valproate: a new cause of birth defects—report from Italy and follow-up from France. Morbidity and Mortality Weekly Report 1983; 32:438–439 [C]

253. Pastuszak A, Schick-Boschetto B, Zuber C, Feldkamp M, Pinelli M, Sihn S, Donnenfeld A, McCormack M, Leen-Mitchell M, Woodland C, Gardner A, Hom M, Koren G: Pregnancy outcome following first-trimester exposure to fluoxetine (Prozac). JAMA 1993; 269:2246–2248 [C]

254. Schou M, Amdisen A, Steenstrup OR: Lithium and pregnancy–II: hazards to women given lithium during pregnancy and delivery. Br Med J 1973; 2:137–138 [G]

255. Marcos LR, Cancro R: Psychopharmacotherapy of Hispanic depressed patients: clinical observations. Am J Psychiatry 1982; 36:505–512 [G]

256. Escobar JI, Tuason VB: Antidepressant agents: a cross-cultural study. Psychopharmacol Bull 1980; 16:49–52 [B]

257. Ambelas A: Life events and mania: a special relationship? Br J Psychiatry 1987; 150:235–240 [G]

258. Swann AC, Secunda SK, Stokes PE, Croughan J, Davis JM, Koslow SH, Maas JW: Stress, depression, and mania: relationship between perceived role of stressful events and clinical and biochemical characteristics. Acta Psychiatr Scand 1990; 81:389–397 [C]

PRACTICE GUIDELINE FOR THE
Treatment of Patients With Panic Disorder

WORK GROUP ON PANIC DISORDER

Jack Gorman, M.D., Co-Chair
Katherine Shear, M.D., Co-Chair

Deborah Cowley, M.D.
C. Deborah Cross, M.D.
John March, M.D.
Walton Roth, M.D.
Michael Shehi, M.D.

▶ NOTE TO THE READER

In this practice guideline, treatment recommendations are discussed in sections IV and V and are summarized in section I. Data regarding the safety and efficacy of available treatments are reviewed in section III.

This practice guideline was approved in December 1997 and was published in *The American Journal of Psychiatry* in May 1998.

CONTENTS

INTRODUCTION

This guideline summarizes data to inform the psychiatrist of the care of patients with panic disorder. It begins at the point where the psychiatrist has diagnosed an adult patient as suffering from this disorder according to the criteria in DSM-IV (1) and has evaluated the patient for the existence of coexisting mental disorders. It also assumes that the psychiatrist or other physician has evaluated the patient for general medical conditions or other factors that may be causing or exacerbating the panic or that may affect its treatment. The guideline also briefly addresses issues specific to the treatment of panic disorder in children and adolescents.

The purpose of this guideline is to assist the psychiatrist in caring for a patient with panic disorder. It should be noted that many patients have conditions that cannot be completely described by the DSM-IV diagnostic category. The psychiatrist caring for a patient with panic disorder should consider, but not be limited to, the treatments recommended in this practice guideline. Psychiatrists care for patients with panic disorders in many different settings and serve a variety of functions; the recommendations in this guideline are primarily intended for psychiatrists who provide, or coordinate, the overall care of the patient with panic disorder.

DEVELOPMENT PROCESS

This practice guideline was developed under the auspices of the Steering Committee on Practice Guidelines. The process is detailed in the Appendix to this volume. Key features of the process include the following:

- a comprehensive literature review (description follows) and development of evidence tables
- initial drafting by a work group that included psychiatrists with clinical and research expertise in panic disorder
- the production of multiple drafts with widespread review, in which 20 organizations and over 100 individuals submitted comments (see section VII)
- approval by the APA Assembly and Board of Trustees
- planned revisions at 3- to 5-year intervals

The following computerized searches of relevant literature were conducted.

The first literature search was conducted by using MEDLINE and Psychological Abstracts, for the period of 1980–1994. The key words for the search were "panic disorder," "agoraphobia," "drug treatment," "non-drug treatment," and "combined modality treatment." A total of 825 citations were found.

A second search was conducted in MEDLINE for the period of 1980–1994 and used the key words "panic disorder" and "tricyclics," "MAO inhibitors," "benzodiazepines," "SSRI's and anticonvulsants," "behavioral and/or cognitive," "all other psychotherapy/psychoanalysis," and "children without adults and combined child and adult." In Psychological Abstracts the key words "panic disorder" and "psychosocial treatment" were used.

A third search was completed in MEDLINE for the period 1992–1996 and used the following key words: "panic disorder," "agoraphobia," "antidepressive agents," "tricyclic," "MAO inhibitors," "benzodiazepine," "anti-anxiety agents," "anticonvulsants," "behavior therapy," "psychotherapy/psychoanalysis," "children," and "psychosocial treatment."

I. SUMMARY OF RECOMMENDATIONS

▶ A. CODING SYSTEM

Each recommendation is identified as falling into one of three categories of endorsement, indicated by a bracketed Roman numeral following the statement. The three categories represent varying levels of clinical confidence regarding the recommendation:

[I] Recommended with substantial clinical confidence.
[II] Recommended with moderate clinical confidence.
[III] May be recommended on the basis of individual circumstances.

▶ B. GENERAL CONSIDERATIONS

Panic disorder, with or without agoraphobia, is a common psychiatric illness that can have a chronic course and be associated with significant morbidity. The care of patients with panic disorder involves a comprehensive array of approaches that are designed to reduce the frequency and severity of panic episodes, reduce morbidity, and improve patient functioning [I]. Modalities for which there is considerable evidence of efficacy in the treatment of panic disorder include psychotherapy, specifically cognitive behavioral therapies, and pharmacotherapy [I]. Other psychotherapies, including psychodynamic, are widely employed in conjunction with medication and/or elements of cognitive behavioral therapies on the basis of a clinical consensus that they are effective for some patients [II]. Considerations for choosing specific treatments among the various options are presented.

1. Choice of treatment setting

For most patients with panic disorder, treatment can be conducted on an outpatient basis and rarely requires hospitalization [I]. Examples of patients who may require inpatient treatment include individuals with comorbid depression who are at risk of suicide attempts or patients with comorbid substance use disorders who require detoxification.

Sometimes the first contact between patient and psychiatrist occurs in the emergency room or hospital to which a patient has been admitted for an acute panic episode. The psychiatrist may be able to make the diagnosis of panic disorder and initiate treatment in this setting after general medical conditions have been ruled out.

2. Formulation of a treatment plan

A comprehensive general medical and psychiatric evaluation should precede treatment to determine whether potential general medical and substance-induced conditions may be causing the panic symptoms, complicate treatment, or require specific interventions, especially with a patient who has a new onset of symptoms [I]. In addition, the assessment of developmental factors, psychosocial stressors and conflicts, social supports, and general living situation will aid the treatment [I]. The psychiatrist's evaluation of the patient's condition and the intended treatment should guide the choice of laboratory and diagnostic studies [I].

3. Psychiatric management

Psychiatric management forms the foundation of psychiatric treatment for patients with panic disorder and should be instituted for all patients in combination with specific treatments, such as medications and psychotherapy. The following are important components of psychiatric management for patients with panic disorder [I]: establishing and maintaining a therapeutic alliance; educating and reassuring the patient concerning panic disorder; evaluating particular symptoms and monitoring them over time; evaluating types and severity of functional impairment; identifying and addressing comorbid conditions; working with other health professionals; educating family members and enlisting their help when appropriate; enhancing treatment compliance; and working with the patient to address early signs of relapse. Many patients with panic disorder require a reliable treatment relationship because they relapse or have partial responses and benefit from extended periods of treatment, or because they intensely fear abandonment. For these reasons, it is helpful to be able to assure the patient of the continued availability of his or her psychiatrist.

4. Choice of treatment modalities to be used in conjunction with psychiatric management

Psychotherapy, specifically panic-focused cognitive behavioral therapy (CBT), and medications have both been shown to be effective treatments for panic disorder [I]. There is no convincing evidence that one modality is superior for all patients or for particular subpopulations of patients. The choice between psychotherapy and pharmacotherapy depends on an individualized assessment of the efficacy, benefits, and risks of each modality and the patient's personal preferences (including costs) [I]. In every case, the patient should be fully informed by the psychiatrist about the availability and relative advantages and disadvantages of CBT, antipanic medications, and other forms of treatment.

a) Cognitive behavioral therapy and other psychotherapies

CBT encompasses a range of treatments, each consisting of several elements, including psychoeducation, continuous panic monitoring, development of anxiety management skills, cognitive restructuring, and in vivo exposure. In practice, the types of therapy encompassed by CBT are often quite diverse. It is unknown whether certain elements are more effective for all patients or for specific patients. The efficacy of CBT for the treatment of panic disorder is supported by extensive and high-quality data. Other psychotherapies may be considered in conjunction with psychiatric management [III], but supplementation with (or replacement by) either CBT or an antipanic medication should be strongly considered if there is no significant improvement within 6–8 weeks.

b) Pharmacotherapy

There are four classes of medications that have been shown to be effective: selective serotonin reuptake inhibitors (SSRIs), tricyclic antidepressants (TCAs), benzodiazepines, and monoamine oxidase inhibitors (MAOIs) [I]. Medications from all four classes have been found to have roughly comparable efficacy [II]. Choosing a medication from among these classes is generally guided by considerations of adverse effects and the physician's understanding of the patient's personal preferences (including costs) and other aspects of the clinical situation [I]. For many patients, SSRIs are likely to have the most favorable balance of efficacy and adverse effects. Although SSRIs carry a risk of sexual side effects, they lack the cardiovascular side effects, anticholinergic side effects, and toxicity associated with overdose that occur with TCAs and MAOIs. SSRIs also lack the potential for physiologic dependency associated with benzodiazepines. TCAs can be tolerated by most patients, although generally not as well as SSRIs. The risks of cardiovascular and anticholinergic side effects of TCAs should be considered, especially for the elderly or patients with general medical problems. Benzodiazepines may be used preferentially in situations in which very rapid control of symptoms is critical (e.g., the patient is about to quit school, lose a job, or require hospitalization). However, the risks of long-term benzodiazepine use, including physiologic dependence, should also be considered. Benzodiazepine use is generally contraindicated for patients with a history of substance use disorder. Although MAOIs are effective, they are generally reserved for patients who do not respond to other treatments because of the risk of hypertensive crises and necessary dietary restrictions. SSRIs are likely to be more expensive than TCAs or benzodiazepines because of the lack of generic preparations.

5. Other treatment considerations

a) Combined medication and psychotherapy

Studies comparing the efficacy of combined antipanic medication and CBT with the efficacy of either modality alone have produced conflicting results. Currently, it is not possible to identify which patients might benefit more from combination therapy. Combined antipanic medication and CBT may be especially useful for patients with severe agoraphobia and those who show an incomplete response [III].

b) Determining the length of treatment

With either CBT or antipanic medication, the acute phase of treatment lasts approximately 12 weeks [II]. After this time, many clinicians reduce the frequency of CBT and then gradually discontinue treatment when the patient is judged to be stable. It is not known whether a second round of CBT is effective for patients who relapse or whether "booster" CBT sessions may prevent relapse.

If a medication has been used, a trial of discontinuation may be attempted after 12–18 months of maintenance therapy if the patient has experienced significant or full improvement [III]. Many patients will partially or fully relapse when medication is discontinued and may benefit from prolonged periods of treatment [III]. Although data on the percentage of patients that remain well after medication discontinuation have been widely divergent, evidence suggests that it is between 30% and 45% (2). Patients who relapse are generally given medication again and/or offered CBT. Patients who remain panic free should be encouraged to contact their psychiatrists in the future at the first sign of the reemergence of panic attacks.

Patients who show no improvement within 6–8 weeks with a particular treatment should be reevaluated with regard to diagnosis, the need for a different treatment, or the need for a combined treatment approach [III]. Patients who do not respond as expected to medication or CBT or who have repeated relapses should be evaluated for possible addition of a psychodynamic or other psychotherapeutic intervention.

c) Use of benzodiazepines for early symptom control, in combination with another treatment modality

It may take several weeks of treatment before patients begin to experience noticeable benefits from either CBT or pharmacotherapy. For some patients with severe panic attacks or high levels of anticipatory anxiety, concomitant benzodiazepine use may be helpful [III]. It may be appropriate to minimize the dose and duration when benzodiazepines are used in this manner, because of potential risks (e.g., physiologic dependence).

d) Comorbidities and other clinical features influencing treatment

Comorbid psychiatric illness, concurrent general medical illnesses, and certain demographic or psychosocial features of patients with panic disorder may have important influences on treatment. Prevalent comorbid psychiatric factors that should be considered include suicidality, substance use, mood disorders, other anxiety disorders, personality disorders, and significant dysfunction in personal, social, or vocational areas. Specific psychosocial therapies (including psychodynamic psychotherapy) may be useful to address comorbid disorders or environmental or psychosocial stressors in patients with panic disorder and are frequently used in conjunction with CBT and/or antipanic medications. Important general medical conditions that may be seen with, or confused with, panic disorder include an array of cardiovascular, pulmonary, neurologic, endocrinologic, and gastrointestinal conditions. Special treatment considerations are necessary for pediatric and geriatric patients with panic disorder. Details concerning the influence of these factors on the treatment of patients with panic disorder are found in section V.

II. DISEASE DEFINITION, NATURAL HISTORY, AND EPIDEMIOLOGY

▶ A. DIAGNOSIS OF PANIC DISORDER

The essential features of panic disorder consist of a mixture of characteristic signs and symptoms that persist for at least 1 month. The symptoms include recurrent panic attacks and persistent concern about having another attack or worry about the implications and consequences of the attacks. Panic attacks are discrete periods of intense fear or discomfort, accompanied by at least four of the 13 somatic or cognitive symptoms defined by DSM-IV. An attack has an abrupt onset and reaches a peak usually within 10 minutes. It is often accompanied by a sense of imminent danger and an urge to escape.

Panic disorder must be distinguished from other conditions that can have panic symptoms as an associated feature. These conditions include other mental disorders (e.g., specific phobias, posttraumatic stress disorder, or separation anxiety disorder), the direct effects of substances, including over-the-counter medications (e.g., caffeine or stimulants), withdrawal from a substance (e.g., withdrawal from sedative-hypnotics), or certain general medical conditions (e.g., hyperthyroidism). For further discussion of these issues, see DSM-IV.

▶ B. SPECIFIC FEATURES OF PANIC DISORDER

1. Cross-sectional issues

There are a number of important clinical and psychosocial features to consider in a cross-sectional evaluation. First, because there is such variance in the types and duration of attacks that may occur with panic disorder, the psychiatrist should consider other possible diagnoses. The psychiatrist should assess the patient for the presence of life-threatening behaviors, the degree to which the panic disorder interferes with the patient's ability to conduct his or her daily routine or to care for self and others, and the presence of a substance use disorder or a depressive disorder.

2. Longitudinal issues

Because of the variable nature of panic disorder, it is necessary to consider a number of longitudinal issues when evaluating the patient. These include the fluctuations in this chronic condition, the development of complications, and the response to prior treatments.

C. NATURAL HISTORY AND COURSE

Several types of panic attacks may occur. The most common is the unexpected attack, defined as one not associated with a known situational trigger. Individuals may also experience situationally predisposed panic attacks (which are more likely to occur in certain situations but do not necessarily occur there) or situationally bound attacks (which occur almost immediately on exposure to a situational trigger). Other types of panic attacks include those that occur in particular emotional contexts, those involving limited symptoms, and nocturnal attacks.

Patients with panic disorder may also have agoraphobia, in which case they experience anxiety and avoidance of places or situations where escape or help may be unavailable if they have panic symptoms. Typical situations eliciting agoraphobia include traveling on buses, subways, or other public transportation and being on bridges, in tunnels, or far from home. Many patients who develop agoraphobia find that situational attacks become more common than unexpected attacks.

Panic attacks vary in their frequency and intensity. It is not uncommon for an individual to experience numerous moderate attacks for months at a time or to experience frequent attacks daily for a short period (e.g., a week), with months separating subsequent periods of attack.

Individuals with panic disorder commonly have anxiety about the recurrence of panic attacks or symptoms or about the implications or consequences. Panic disorder, especially with agoraphobia, may lead to the loss or disruption of interpersonal relationships, especially as individuals struggle with the impairment or loss of social role functioning and the issue of responsibility for symptoms.

Examples of the disrupting nature of panic disorder include the fear that an attack is the indicator of a life-threatening illness despite medical evaluation indicating otherwise or the fear that an attack is a sign of emotional weakness. Some individuals experience the attacks as so severe that they take such actions as quitting a job to avoid a possible attack. Others may become so anxious that they eventually avoid most activities outside their homes. Evidence from one naturalistic follow-up study of patients in a tertiary-care setting suggests that at 4–6 years posttreatment about 30% of individuals are well, 40%–50% are improved but symptomatic, and the remaining 20%–30% have symptoms that are the same or slightly worse (3, 4).

D. EPIDEMIOLOGY AND ASSOCIATED FEATURES

Epidemiologic data collected from a variety of countries have documented similarities in lifetime prevalence (1.6%–2.2%), age at first onset (20s), higher risk in females (about twofold), and symptom patterns of panic disorder (5). While the full-blown syndrome is usually not present until early adulthood, limited symptoms often occur much earlier. Several investigators have documented cases of panic disorder prepubertally (6).

One-third to one-half of individuals diagnosed with panic disorder in community samples also have agoraphobia, although a much higher rate of agoraphobia is encountered in clinical samples (5). Among individuals with panic disorder, the lifetime prevalence of major depression is 50%–60% (7). For individuals with both panic disorder and depression, the onset of depression precedes the onset of panic disorder in one-third of this population, while the onset of depression coincides with or follows the onset of panic disorder in the remaining two-thirds. Approximately one-third of patients with panic disorder are depressed when they present for treatment (7).

Epidemiologic studies have clearly documented the morbidity associated with panic disorder. In the Epidemiologic Catchment Area study, subjects with panic symptoms or disorders, as compared to other disorders, were the most frequent users of emergency medical services and were more likely to be hospitalized for physical problems (8). Patients with panic disorder, especially with comorbid depression, were at higher risk for suicide attempts (9), impaired social and marital functioning, use of psychoactive medication, and substance abuse (10).

Family studies using direct interviews of relatives and family history studies have shown that panic disorder is highly familial. Results from studies conducted in different countries (United States, Belgium, Germany, Australia) have shown that the median risk of panic disorder is eight times as high in the first-degree relatives of probands with panic disorder as in the relatives of control subjects (11). A recent family data analysis showed that forms with early onsets (at age 20 or before) were the most familial, carrying a more than 17 times greater risk (12). Results from twin studies have suggested a genetic contribution to the disorder (13, 14).

III. TREATMENT PRINCIPLES AND ALTERNATIVES

▶ A. PSYCHIATRIC MANAGEMENT

Psychiatric management consists of a comprehensive array of activities and interventions that should be instituted by psychiatrists for all patients with panic disorder, in combination with specific treatment modalities. Patients with panic disorder frequently fear that panic attacks represent catastrophic medical events. In addition, they may live in a nearly constant state of apprehension and may be severely limited by phobic avoidance. For such reasons, reassurance, education, and support are important components of psychiatric management, along with accurate diagnosis that takes into account all the elements of a patient's individual symptom pattern. The psychiatrist should help the patient cope with the effects that panic disorder sometimes has on family members and with the possibility that the disorder may be chronic, requiring long-term treatment.

The specific components of psychiatric management include performing a diagnostic evaluation; evaluating the particular symptoms; evaluating types and severity of functional impairment of the individual patient; establishing and maintaining a therapeutic alliance; monitoring the patient's psychiatric status; providing education to the patient and, when appropriate, to the family about panic disorder; working with non-psychiatric physicians the patient consults; enhancing treatment compliance; and working with the patient to address early signs of relapse.

1. Performing a diagnostic evaluation

Patients with panic symptoms should receive a thorough diagnostic evaluation both to determine whether a diagnosis of panic disorder is warranted and to reveal the presence of other psychiatric or general medical conditions. Evaluation of a patient with panic disorder frequently involves a number of physicians. The psychiatrist with responsibility for the care of the patient should oversee the evaluation. The general principles and components of a complete psychiatric evaluation have been outlined in the American Psychiatric Association's *Practice Guideline for Psychiatric Evaluation of Adults* (15; included in this volume). This should include a history of the present illness and current symptoms; past psychiatric history; general medical history and history of substance use disorders; personal history (e.g., psychological development, response to life transitions and major life events); social, occupational, and family history; review of the patient's medications; review of systems; mental status examination; physical examination; and diagnostic tests as indicated.

2. Evaluating particular symptoms

Although patients with panic disorder share common features of the illness, there are important interindividual differences. The frequency of panic attacks varies widely among patients, and the constellation of symptoms for each attack also differs. Some patients complain, for example, of attacks that primarily involve cardiovascular symptoms, such as palpitations, chest pain, and paresthesia, while others are more overwhelmed by cognitive symptoms, such as depersonalization and the fear of "losing one's mind." The amount of anticipatory anxiety and the degree of phobic avoidance also vary from patient to patient. Many patients with panic disorder are not highly avoidant; at the opposite extreme are patients who will not leave the house without a trusted companion. It is critical to be sensitive to these individual differences in the elements of panic disorder among patients for two reasons. First, it is important for the patient to feel that the psychiatrist understands accurately the patient's individual experience of panic. Second, treatment may be influenced by the particular constellation of symptoms and other problems of a given patient.

Therefore, it is important to carefully assess the frequency and nature of a patient's panic attacks. It is helpful for patients to monitor their panic attacks, using techniques such as keeping a daily diary, in order to gather data regarding the relationship of panic symptoms to internal stimuli (e.g., emotions) and external stimuli (e.g., substances, particular situations or settings). Such monitoring can be therapeutic.

3. Evaluating types and severity of functional impairment

The degree of functional impairment varies considerably among patients with panic disorder. It is increasingly recognized that resolution of panic attacks, even though they are the core symptom of panic disorder, may be insufficient to warrant the term "clinical remission." As already mentioned, some patients have such high levels of anticipatory anxiety that even when the panic attacks are gone they continue to live restricted lives because of fear. Varying levels of phobic avoidance also determine the degree of impairment experienced by patients with panic disorder. The avoidance of common situations and places, such as driving, restaurants, shopping malls, and elevators, is a cardinal symptom of panic disorder and obviously leads to considerable inability to function in both social and work roles. Sometimes a patient is more focused on the attacks themselves and relegates phobic avoidance to secondary importance. There are situations in which phobic avoidance becomes such a routine part of the patient's life that both the patient and the family are actually reluctant to see it remit. A patient who is homebound because of panic disorder, for example, may have assumed all of the household chores for the family for years. Remission of this kind of phobic avoidance leads to the desire to engage in activities outside of the home, thus leaving a gap. Without recognizing this, family members can tacitly undermine a potentially successful treatment to avoid disrupting their ingrained patterns. In dealing with phobic avoidance and the range of functional impairment seen in patients with panic disorder it is critical to determine exactly what the patient defines as a satisfactory outcome. The patient should be encouraged to define a desirable level of functioning for himself or herself. Treatment of panic disorder should include substantial effort to alleviate or minimize phobic avoidance. Even after the panic attacks have subsided, the patient may continue to have significant limitations in activities that need to be addressed in treatment.

4. Establishing and maintaining a therapeutic alliance

By the very nature of the illness, many patients with panic disorder are extremely anxious about all treatment interventions. Panic disorder is usually a chronic, long-term condition for which adherence to a treatment plan is important. Hence, a strong treatment alliance is crucial. It is often the case that the treatment of panic disorder involves asking the patient to do things that may be frightening and uncomfortable, such as confronting phobic situations. Here again, a strong treatment alliance is necessary to support the patient in doing these things. Patients with panic disorder are generally very sensitive to separations and need to know that the psychiatrist will be available to answer questions in case of emergencies. Careful attention to the patient's fears and wishes with regard to his or her treatment is essential in establishing and maintaining the therapeutic alliance. Management of the therapeutic alliance should include an awareness of transference and countertransference phenomena and requires sensitive management by the psychiatrist, even if not directly addressed.

5. Monitoring the patient's psychiatric status

As treatment progresses, the different elements of panic disorder often resolve at different points. Usually, panic attacks are controlled first, but subthreshold panic attacks may linger and require further treatment. The fear that attacks may occur in the future often continues even after the attacks themselves appear to have ceased. The psychiatrist should continue to monitor the status of all of the symptoms with which the patient originally presented and should monitor the success of the treatment plan on an ongoing basis.

Finally, many illnesses, including depression and substance use disorders, co-occur with panic disorder at higher rates than are seen in the general population. Depression can develop even during successful treatment of panic disorder. Failure to recognize an emergent depression can seriously compromise therapeutic outcome.

6. Providing education to the patient and, when appropriate, to the family

Many patients with panic disorder believe they are suffering from a disorder of an organ system other than the central nervous system. They may fervently believe they have heart or lung disease. On the other hand, the significant others of patients with panic disorder frequently insist that absolutely nothing is wrong with the patient, using as evidence the fact that extensive medical testing has yielded unremarkable results (16). Under these circumstances, the patient becomes demoralized and isolated while the family can become angry or rejecting. Educating both the family and the patient and emphasizing that panic disorder is a real illness requiring support and treatment can be critical in some situations. Regardless of the method of treatment selected, successful therapies of panic disorder usually begin by explaining to the patient that the attacks themselves are not life threatening; the family may be helped to understand that panic attacks are terrifying to the patient and that the disorder, unless treated, is debilitating.

7. Working with other physicians

Patients with panic disorder often have long-standing relationships with other physicians. Because the patient is often convinced that the panic attacks represent serious abnormalities of other organ systems, a variety of general medical physicians may be involved. Psychiatric management usually requires two approaches in such cases. First, the psychiatrist may be called on to educate nonpsychiatric physicians about the ability of panic attacks to masquerade as many other general medical conditions. Although a general medical evaluation is necessary to rule out important treatable general medical conditions, there is usually little to be gained from extensive medical testing. Attempting to diagnose and treat a variety of nonspecific medical complaints sometimes only delays initiation of treatment of the panic disorder itself. Second, nonpsychiatric physicians can become frustrated with patients with panic disorder. The psychiatrist may need to intervene to ensure that the patient with panic disorder continues to receive an appropriate level of medical care from the primary care physician and medical specialists.

8. Enhancing treatment compliance

The treatment of panic disorder involves confronting many things that the patient fears. Patients are often afraid of medically adverse events; hence, they fear taking medication and are very sensitive to all somatic sensations induced by them. Some psychotherapies require the patient to confront phobic situations and often to keep careful records of anxious thoughts. These can also cause an initial increase in anxiety for the patient. The anxiety produced by treatment may lead to noncompliance. Patients stop taking medication abruptly or fail to complete required assignments during behavioral therapy. Recognition of this possibility guides the physician to design an approach to treatment that encourages the patient to articulate his or her fears. The treatment must be conducted in a completely supportive environment so that missed sessions and lapses in taking medication or carrying out behavioral and cognitive tasks are understood as part of the illness or as manifestations of issues in the therapist-patient relationship.

Family members may play a helpful role in improving treatment compliance. If compliance is not improved with discussion of fears, reassurance, nonpunitive acceptance, educational measures, and similar measures, it may be an indication of more complex resistance that is out of the patient's awareness and may be an indication for a psychodynamic treatment approach.

9. Working with the patient to address early signs of relapse

Studies have shown that panic disorder can be a chronic illness. Sometimes, an exacerbation of symptoms can occur even while the patient is undergoing treatment. This can be disconcerting and needs to be dealt with in two ways: by reassuring the patient that fluctuations in symptom levels can occur during treatment before an acceptable level of remission is reached and by evaluating whether changes in the treatment plan are warranted. Although treatment works for most patients to reduce the burden of panic disorder, patients may continue to have lingering symptoms, including occasional panic attacks of minor severity and residual avoidance. Depression can occur at any time. Relapse following treatment cessation is also always possible. Patients need to be instructed that panic disorder sometimes recurs and that if it does it is important to initiate treatment quickly to avoid the onset of complications such as phobic avoidance (17). The patient should know that he or she is welcome to contact the psychiatrist and that rapid reinitiation of treatment almost always results in improvement.

B. INTERPRETING RESULTS FROM STUDIES OF TREATMENTS FOR PANIC DISORDER

1. Measurement of outcomes

In the following sections the available data on the efficacy of treatments for panic disorder are reviewed. Short-term efficacy has usually been evaluated in 6–12-week clinical trials by observing the change in symptom ratings over the course of treatment. These outcome measures all assess a variety of panic and phobia symptoms, generally derived from the DSM-IV definition of panic attacks. Both the patient and the clinician can be asked to rate the presence and severity of a patient's symptoms. Patients have been designated as "panic free" if they do not have a sufficient number of panic symptoms to meet the DSM-IV criteria for panic disorder. However, patients labeled as "panic free" may not necessarily be free of all panic symptoms (i.e., symptom free). Another outcome measure that has been employed to assess short-term treatment response is the proportion of patients achieving remission (usually defined as the absence of panic attacks within a specified period of time).

The long-term efficacy of treatments has been measured in terms of relapse rates among panic-free or symptom-free patients receiving treatment over the course of several years. A variety of definitions of relapse have been used, based on the emergence of a certain number of symptoms or based on the percentage of change in scores on symptom rating scales. In some studies, requests for or use of additional treatment have been considered indicative of relapse; while such outcome measures may reflect an intervention's effect on patient functioning, as well as symptoms, they may also be affected by other clinical and nonclinical factors.

2. Issues in study design and interpretation

When evaluating clinical trials of medications for panic disorder, it is important to take into consideration whether a placebo group was used, the type of placebo, and the response rate in the placebo group. Response rates as high as 75% have been observed among patients receiving placebo in clinical trials of patients with panic disorder (18). High placebo response rates could explain much of the observed treatment effect in uncontrolled trials or make significant treatment effects more difficult to detect in controlled trials. It is also important to consider the dose of medication(s) employed in pharmacologic trials.

When evaluating studies of psychosocial treatments, such as CBT, which consist of multiple elements, it may be difficult to know which elements are responsible for producing beneficial outcomes. It is also important to consider the nature of the elements that were used. For example, although the types of CBT used in recent trials have been rigorously defined and have been similar, they have not been identical (19–21).

Another factor to consider is the use of medications that are not prescribed as part of the treatment protocol. For example, patients in studies of CBT may be using prescription medications that are not controlled for. In addition, patients in medication studies may be taking additional doses of the tested medications or other antipanic medications (either explicitly, as doses taken as needed, or surreptitiously). Studies that monitor such occurrences have shown rates as high as 33% (22).

► C. SPECIFIC PSYCHOSOCIAL INTERVENTIONS

Psychosocial interventions, such as psychotherapy, have traditionally been the predominant psychiatric treatment for patients with panic disorder. However, unlike medication therapies, it has been more difficult to clearly define aspects of psychosocial therapies, such as the elements they consist of and the "doses." Only recently have some psychosocial treatments been more formally operationalized and evaluated.

At the present time, cognitive behavioral treatments for panic disorder have been the most well studied. Other forms of psychotherapy are widely used for patients with panic disorder but have undergone less empirical testing. These treatments may be very different from cognitive behavioral interventions. One important difference is that many forms of psychotherapy focus broadly on the patient's current life and history, rather than more narrowly on panic-related symptoms.

1. Cognitive behavioral therapy

a) Goals
CBT is a symptom-oriented approach to the treatment of panic disorder. The treatments employed in recent clinical trials contain the following key components:

- psychoeducation
- continuous panic monitoring
- breathing retraining
- cognitive restructuring focused on correction of catastrophic misinterpretation of bodily sensations
- exposure to fear cues

The types of therapy encompassed by CBT are likely to be more diverse, and such diverse approaches have not been studied.

(1) Psychoeducation
CBT always begins with one or more sessions for the purpose of psychoeducation. The aims of such sessions are to identify and name the patient's symptoms, provide a direct explanation of the basis for the symptoms, and outline a plan for the treatment. The initial education for patients is generally imparted in a didactic fashion. Exercises that actually evoke panic symptoms, such as hyperventilation, may be useful for illustrating the role of interoceptive (i.e., internal) cues in panic disorder.

(2) Continuous panic monitoring
Patients are also instructed to continuously monitor their panic attacks and record their anxious cognitions, using techniques such as keeping a daily diary. Patients are

informed that this will help in the assessment of the frequency and nature of their panic attacks and provide data regarding the relationship of panic symptoms to internal stimuli (e.g., emotions) and external stimuli (e.g., substances).

(3) Breathing retraining

Next, the therapist introduces an anxiety management technique, such as abdominal breathing, to control the physiologic reactivity. The patient is asked to practice this technique daily.

(4) Cognitive restructuring

These techniques are used to identify and counter fear of bodily sensations. Most commonly, such thinking involves overestimation of the probability of a negative consequence and catastrophic thinking about the meaning of such sensations. Patients are encouraged to consider the evidence and to think of alternative possible outcomes following the experience of the bodily cue. Part of this process involves identifying the likely origin of the feared sensations and/or any misinformation about the meaning of the sensations. The cognitive restructuring component of CBT is usually conducted by using a Socratic teaching method.

(5) Exposure to fear cues

The final and central component of the treatment involves actual exposure to fear cues. In order to conduct such exposure, the therapist frequently works with the patient to identify a hierarchy of fear-evoking situations. The degree of anxiety elicited in each of these situations is graded on a 0–10 scale, and several situations that evoke anxiety at each level are documented. The patient is then asked to enter situations, usually at the low end of the hierarchy, on a regular (usually daily) basis until the fear has attenuated. The situation that arouses the next level of anxiety is then targeted. Employing more intense initial exposures and not proceeding in a graduated manner, referred to as "flooding," has also been used (23). Examples of exposures to panic cues are having patients run in place, spin in a desk chair, and breathe through a straw. The cues for panic attacks are generally interoceptive, while those for agoraphobia may be either interoceptive or environmental (24). Interoceptive exposures are usually conducted in the therapist's office and at home in naturalistic situations. Agoraphobic exposure is best carried out in the actual situation(s).

b) Efficacy

CBT efficacy studies have generally involved either cognitive behavioral treatment (as just described) or cognitive therapy. Studies of agoraphobia use behavioral exposure treatment (25, 26). A recent presentation of data from 26 subjects supports the efficacy of combining these approaches (27).

Twelve randomized controlled trials of CBT for panic disorder were identified and reviewed (19–21, 28–36). The length of treatment varied from 4 weeks to 16 weeks, and the number of subjects per cell varied from nine to 34. The degree of agoraphobia was none to mild in most of the studies. The control treatment was a wait list in five of these, a relaxation component alone in five, supportive psychotherapy in three, and a placebo medication in two. The results are shown in table 1. The results in the control conditions suggest that length of treatment and perhaps the specific interventions used may be important in determining efficacy. However, more data are necessary before firm conclusions can be drawn. Also of note, 38% of the patients in the eight studies for which medication data were given were taking some medications that were not specifically part of the study protocols (range, 0%–70%).

TABLE 1. Results of 12 Randomized Controlled Studies of Cognitive Behavioral Therapy for Patients With Panic Disorder

Treatment	Response rate (%)
Cognitive behavioral therapy (12–15 weeks)	
Intent to treat	66
Completers	78
Control treatments	
Wait list	26
Relaxation only	
Intent to treat	45
Completers	56
Placebo	
Intent to treat	34
Completers	33
Supportive psychotherapy completers	
16 weeks	78
8 weeks	25
4 weeks	8

Several studies have examined the use of one component of CBT, behavioral exposure, for specifically agoraphobia symptoms in patients with panic disorder (35, 37–41). These studies support the efficacy of behavioral treatment in reducing phobic symptoms for patients who are able and willing to complete a treatment program of a few months. Patients who were virtually homebound were included in some of these studies, indicating that there is no need to reserve this treatment for milder or less chronic cases.

Long-term follow-ups of panic disorder range from 6 months to 8 years (20, 29, 33, 36–38, 42, 43). The three studies that included at least 1 year of follow-up showed promising results, with an average of 88% of subjects remaining panic free. However, a closer look at the results in one study indicates that the percentage of patients who remained panic free throughout the 24-month period was only about 50%, and only 21% were panic free and had achieved "high end-state functioning" consistently throughout the follow-up period (43). "High end-state functioning" refers to a low severity of overall panic disorder symptoms, including anticipatory anxiety, limited-symptom episodes, and phobic symptoms in addition to panic attacks. These follow-up results are comparable to those found in medication treatment follow-up studies. One review of a series of studies also indicated that the improvement in agoraphobia and in disability after exposure therapy persists for 4 to 8 years (44).

c) Adverse effects

Cognitive behavioral exposure is a relatively benign type of intervention. However, exposure to feared situations does initially increase anxiety, and this could be considered an adverse effect. Sometimes the patient develops dependence on the therapist, which may need to be addressed. Another limitation of CBT is that it may not address other psychological problems that patients with panic disorder may have. While these problems may be less prominent than the panic disorder symptoms for many patients, some patients present with serious current and/or ongoing environmental stresses and/or other comorbid psychiatric disorders. For these patients, panic symptom relief may be less helpful, or even relatively unimportant, as a focus of treatment.

d) Implementation issues

(1) Patient acceptance

CBT requires considerable time and discipline on the part of the patient. Exercises must be practiced daily, and monitoring must be done continuously. In addition, patients must be willing to confront feared situations. Approximately 10%–30% of patients are unable or unwilling to complete these requirements (19, 29, 30, 33). The treatment is far less effective for these patients. Despite these limitations, however, data from several studies (39, 45, 46) indicate that more patients with panic disorder who seek treatment are willing to accept a nonmedication approach than medication.

(2) Group treatment

CBT for panic disorder is usually provided individually, in approximately 12 sessions, but there is evidence that group treatments may be equally effective (33, 47–51). Exposure treatments for patients with agoraphobia are often conducted in groups, and this approach has been used in many studies documenting efficacy. In addition, the inclusion of the spouse or significant other in agoraphobic treatment has been studied and found to enhance treatment efficacy (52). In this couples approach, the support person is included in psychoeducation sessions and is given a role as an assistant in exposure exercises.

(3) Withdrawal of anxiolytics

The discontinuation of benzodiazepines, such as alprazolam or clonazepam, for patients with panic disorder is often accompanied by withdrawal symptoms and relapse into panic disorder. Several studies have shown that using adjunctive CBT in this clinical situation results in successful discontinuation of the benzodiazepine for significantly more patients (53–55).

2. Psychodynamic psychotherapy

a) Goals

Psychodynamic psychotherapy is based on the concept that symptoms result from mental processes that may be outside of the patient's conscious awareness and that elucidating these processes can lead to remission of symptoms (56, 57). Moreover, in order to lessen vulnerability to panic, the psychodynamic therapist considers it necessary to identify and alter core conflicts (56). The goals of psychodynamic psychotherapy range considerably and may be more ambitious and require more time to achieve than those of a more symptom-focused treatment approach. There are some case reports of brief dynamic psychotherapies that took no longer than CBT to achieve reasonable treatment goals for patients with panic disorder (58–61). One recent study compared CBT to an emotion-focused brief psychotherapy and showed them to be equivalent (62). When combined with short-term symptomatic treatment, this approach may produce optimal long-term outcome for some patients.

b) Efficacy

There are no published reports of randomized controlled trials evaluating the efficacy of this approach for panic disorder. Studies documenting a role for both recent and early life events in the development of panic disorder, as well as a number of studies showing that patients with panic disorder remember the behavior and attitudes of their parents as more overprotective and less caring than do control subjects, provide indirect support for some aspects of the theory. One study documented the usefulness of psychodynamic psychotherapy as an adjunct to medication for outpatients with and without agoraphobia (63). In a second study (35), the control treatment of reflective listening produced results equivalent to those for CBT. In addition, a number of anecdotal case reports of successful psychodynamic treatment appear in the literature. Most of these are reports of isolated cases rather than systematic consecutive case series, and reliable, validated outcome measures were not used. Milrod et al. (56) have published a treatment manual for panic-focused psychodynamic psychotherapy, and a pilot test of outcome and of the ability of trained psychoanalysts to follow this manual is currently under way. An ongoing randomized controlled trial uses a manualized psychodynamically informed approach called "emotion-focused treatment." However, this treatment also contains cognitive, behavioral, and experiential components and differs substantially from the treatment described by Milrod et al.

c) Adverse effects

In general, psychodynamic psychotherapy has relatively few side effects. As with any psychotherapy, psychological dependency must be skillfully managed so as to facilitate treatment rather than prolong it unduly.

d) Implementation issues

In psychodynamic psychotherapy, the successful emotional and cognitive understanding of the various elements of psychic conflict (impulses, conscience and internal standards that are often excessively harsh, psychological defensive patterns, and realistic concerns) and reintegration of these elements in a more realistic and adaptive way may result in symptom resolution and fewer relapses. To achieve this insight and acceptance, the therapist places the symptoms in the context of the patient's life history and current realities and extensively uses the therapeutic relationship to focus on unconscious symptom determinants.

There are a variety of methods for conducting dynamic psychotherapy (64). Generally, the clinical approach of dynamic psychiatrists is less directive than that of behavioral therapists or psychopharmacologists. In a psychodynamic psychotherapy, it is important to consider the risks and benefits of substituting the therapist's executive functions for those of the patient. Transference considerations and the patient's freedom to associate into unexpected material must be taken into account. Some CBT techniques can be combined with psychodynamic techniques (56, 65). Clinically, as with other treatment approaches, patient factors are important determinants of the length and intensity of appropriate treatment and of specific interventions the psychiatrist may employ.

3. Combined treatments

Investigators have examined use of the combination of medication and CBT for patients with panic disorder and agoraphobia. Several short-term treatment studies have shown that the combination of the TCA imipramine with one component of CBT, behavioral exposure, may be superior to either treatment alone (66–72). Another study showed that the SSRI paroxetine plus cognitive therapy worked significantly better for patients with panic disorder than cognitive therapy plus placebo (73).

There has been one study of the combination of psychodynamic psychotherapy with medication (63). This study suggested that psychodynamic psychotherapy may improve the long-term outcome of medication-treated patients.

4. Group therapy

Reports in the literature of group therapy in the treatment of panic disorder have consisted primarily of cognitive behavioral approaches. Telch et al. (33) found a greater proportion of panic-free subjects among those who had been given group CBT than among delayed-treatment control subjects (85% versus 30%); the authors concluded that the improvements with group CBT were comparable to those in studies of individually administered CBT and pharmacologic treatment. Fifteen patients who had incomplete responses to pharmacotherapy were treated by Pollack et al. (74) with 12 weeks of group CBT and had subsequent improvements in the number of panic attacks and in scores on the Clinical Global Impression. CBT was also used concurrently with medication in a group setting for acute treatment of panic disorder (75).

Mindfulness meditation is an additional treatment proposed for panic disorder (76). This treatment is administered in a group format and includes an attention-focusing component and relaxation strategies. In one study, an 8-week trial of mindfulness meditation resulted in significant reductions in ratings of anxiety symptoms and panic attacks (77). However, it has not been compared to other, proven treatments. A 3-year follow-up showed continued beneficial effects. Other types of groups, such as medication support groups and consumer-run self-help groups, can also provide useful adjunctive experiences for patients with panic disorder.

5. Marital and family therapy

Some of the earliest theories of agoraphobia postulated an interpersonal basis for the symptoms, and some researchers have investigated the possibility that the results of behavioral treatment of agoraphobia can be enhanced by treatment of the couple or family system. While the issue has not been studied directly, patients with panic disorder without agoraphobia have symptoms that can disrupt day-to-day patterns of relationships and may place a family member in a caretaker or rescuer role. Increased dependency needs of patients with panic disorder may lead to frustration in family members, and relationships may be jeopardized. Empirical studies of the quality of marital relationships have provided mixed results; some investigators have reported that patients with agoraphobia and their spouses are not different from happily married couples (78, 79), while others show problems (80). Several studies have documented increased marital distress in some patients following successful treatment for agoraphobia (81, 82), although in general these investigators found treatment to improve marital satisfaction. In summary, there seems to be a subgroup of these patients who experience marital and/or other family distress and may benefit from a family intervention (83).

There is no published research on the use of marital or family therapy alone or with medication for the treatment of panic or agoraphobia, so no conclusions can be drawn about the potential efficacy of such an approach. Education of family members about the nature of the illness and inclusion of the spouse in the treatment may be helpful. There is a small literature exploring the benefits of including the spouse in treatment. Overall, it is clear that such a strategy is not detrimental, and results are mixed as to whether it helps. Two studies by the same research group (84, 85) show the superiority of treatment that includes the spouse as co-therapist over treatment without spouse involvement. One study (86) documented further improvement by addition of communication skills training.

6. Patient support groups

Patient support groups are very helpful for some patients suffering from panic disorder. Patients have the opportunity to learn that they are not unique in experiencing panic attacks and to share ways of coping with the illness. Support groups may also have a positive effect in encouraging patients to confront phobic situations. Finally, family members of patients with panic disorder may benefit from the educational aspects of patient support groups. In deciding to refer a patient to a support group, however, it is imperative that the psychiatrist obtain information about the nature of the group and the credentials of its leader(s). Support groups are not a substitute for effective treatment; rather, they are complementary.

▶ D. PHARMACOLOGIC INTERVENTIONS

Medications have been known to be useful in the treatment of panic disorder for over 30 years. Most studies have focused on their ability to stop or reduce the frequency of panic attacks, but many have also addressed the effect of medication on anticipatory anxiety, phobic avoidance, associated depression, and global function. Medications from several classes have been shown to be effective. As discussed in section III.B, when interpreting results from trials of pharmacologic interventions, it is important to consider whether a placebo group was used and the response rate in the placebo group.

1. Selective serotonin reuptake inhibitors

a) Goals

The primary goals of SSRI therapy of panic disorder are to reduce the intensity and frequency of panic attacks, to reduce anticipatory anxiety, and to treat associated depression. Often, successful therapy with SSRIs also leads to a reduction in phobic avoidance.

b) Efficacy

Four SSRIs are now available in the United States: fluoxetine, sertraline, paroxetine, and fluvoxamine. Clinical trials indicating that each of them is effective for panic disorder have now been completed.

Results of one multicenter double-blind, randomized trial that compared two doses of fluoxetine (10 mg/day and 20 mg/day) with placebo have been presented (87). Reductions in panic symptoms, measured by using several instruments, were significantly greater for patients treated with 20 mg/day of fluoxetine than those given placebo. Fluoxetine at 10 mg/day showed superiority over placebo for only a few assessments of panic symptoms. Two open studies of fluoxetine treatment for panic disorder have been published. Gorman et al. (88) found that of 16 patients whose fluoxetine dose began at 10 mg/day and was raised in 10 mg/day increments each week, only 44% eventually responded to fluoxetine (mean dose among responders was 27.1 mg/day); however, 90% of the nonresponders had been unable to tolerate the side effects. Schneier et al. (89), initiating fluoxetine treatment at 5 mg/day and using a more conservative titration schedule with 25 patients, found that 76% had moderate to marked improvements (median dose among responders was 20 mg/day).

Results from two multicenter randomized, double-blind, placebo-controlled trials of sertraline have been presented at recent public meetings but had not been published by 1996. Wolkow et al. (90) reported that patients treated with sertraline had a significantly greater reduction in panic attack frequency than those given placebo (79% versus 59% reduction). Similarly, Baumel et al. (91) found a significantly greater reduction in panic attack frequency for patients given sertraline than for those given placebo (77% versus 51% reduction).

Paroxetine, which has received approval from the U.S. Food and Drug Administration (FDA) for treatment of panic disorder, has been studied in several placebo-controlled trials. One double-blind trial compared paroxetine plus cognitive therapy to placebo plus cognitive therapy; significantly more patients in the paroxetine group (82% versus 50%) achieved a 50% reduction in panic attack frequency (73). Ballenger et al. (92) compared placebo to three doses of paroxetine; the percentages of patients given paroxetine at daily doses of 40 mg, 20 mg, and 10 mg and patients given placebo who were subsequently panic free were 86%, 65%, 67%, and 50%, respectively (only the difference between 40-mg paroxetine and placebo was statistically significant). In another double-blind trial (93), 367 patients were randomly assigned to paroxetine, clomipramine, or placebo. Paroxetine (at a mean final dose of 39 mg/day) was found to be superior to placebo and comparable to clomipramine (mean final dose of 92 mg/day).

Several controlled trials of fluvoxamine for panic disorder have also been published. In one (94), more patients who had been given fluvoxamine than placebo were panic free (61% versus 36%). Black et al. (32) compared fluvoxamine to a modified form of cognitive therapy and to placebo; there were more panic-free patients in the fluvoxamine group (81%) than in either the cognitive therapy (50%) or placebo (39%) group (only the difference between fluvoxamine and placebo was significant). In other studies fluvoxamine has proved to be better than maprotiline and an experimental serotonin-blocking medication, ritanserin (95, 96). Citalopram, an SSRI available in Europe, was studied in one double-blind trial in which 475 patients were randomly assigned to citalopram (10–15 mg/day, 20–30 mg/day, or 40–60 mg/day), clomipramine (60–90 mg/day), or placebo (97). Citalopram at 20–30 or 40–60 mg/day was significantly superior to placebo; citalopram at 20–30 mg/day was more effective than 40–60 mg/day and comparable to clomipramine.

Although the database for SSRI therapy of panic disorder is not yet as extensive as that for either imipramine or alprazolam, there are sufficient controlled trials available to state that these medications have demonstrated short-term efficacy in treating panic attacks. A meta-analysis (98) of 27 studies involving 2,348 patients in randomized, prospective, double-blind, placebo-controlled trials suggested that the effect size for improvement with SSRIs in panic disorder is significantly greater than for alprazolam or imipramine.

c) Side effects

SSRIs are safer than TCAs. They are not lethal in overdose and have few serious effects on cardiovascular function. Because they lack clinically significant anticholinergic effects, they can be prescribed to patients with prostatic hypertrophy or narrow-angle glaucoma. Because elimination of SSRIs involves hepatic metabolism, doses need to be adjusted for patients with liver disease and dysfunction.

The main side effects of SSRIs are headaches, irritability, nausea and other gastrointestinal complaints, insomnia, sexual dysfunctions, increased anxiety, drowsiness, and tremor. There are scattered reports in the literature of extrapyramidal side effects, but these have not been observed in large multicenter trials and may be idiosyncratic. There is no evidence that SSRIs increase suicidal or violent behavior.

There are a number of published case reports of a withdrawal syndrome caused by the abrupt discontinuation of SSRIs (99). Black et al. (32) abruptly withdrew fluvoxamine from patients with panic disorder after 8 months of treatment. A withdrawal syndrome characterized by dizziness, incoordination, headache, irritability, and nausea began within 24 hours, peaked at day 5 after withdrawal, and was generally resolved by day 14.

d) Implementation issues

(1) Dose

As is the case with tricyclics, some patients with panic disorder experience an initial feeling of increased anxiety, jitteriness, shakiness, and agitation when beginning treatment with an SSRI. For that reason, the initial dose should be lower than that usually prescribed to patients with depression. Louie et al. (100), for example, found that patients with both panic disorder and major depression were less tolerant of higher doses of fluoxetine than patients with major depression alone. The recommended starting doses for SSRIs are as follows: fluoxetine, 10 mg/day or less; sertraline, 25 mg/day; paroxetine, 10 mg/day; and fluvoxamine, 50 mg/day. In the few published studies, fluoxetine has been found to be effective at doses ranging between 5 and 80 mg/day. Recent case reports suggest that for some patients fluoxetine taken in doses as low as 1–2 mg/day may be effective (101). For paroxetine, in a clinical trial the lowest dose that was significantly superior to placebo was 40 mg/day, although some patients did respond to lower doses (92). For sertraline, a fixed-dose study suggests that doses of 50, 100, and 200 mg/day are equally effective for panic disorder (102). Fluvoxamine has been found effective in doses up to 300 mg/day. It is recommended that the initial low dose of the SSRI be maintained for several days and then increased to a more standard daily dose (e.g., 20 mg of fluoxetine or paroxetine, 50 mg of sertraline, 150 mg of fluvoxamine). Patients who fail to respond after several weeks may then do better with a further dose increase.

(2) Length of treatment

Studies of SSRI therapy for panic disorder have been conducted over 6 to 12 weeks and even longer periods. It is generally accepted that response does not occur for at least 4 weeks, and some patients will not realize full response for 8 to 12 weeks.

There are few data on the optimum length of treatment following response. Gergel et al. (103) selected patients who had responded to paroxetine in an acute-phase trial and randomly assigned them to placebo or 10, 20, or 40 mg/day of paroxetine for a 12-week maintenance period. After the maintenance phase, there was a significantly higher rate of relapse among the responders who had crossed over to placebo than those whose paroxetine treatment had been maintained (30% versus 5%).

LeCrubier et al. (93) evaluated the efficacy of paroxetine, clomipramine, and placebo for patients who completed a 12-week double-blind trial and then chose to continue receiving the randomly assigned treatment for an additional 36 weeks. Compared with the placebo-treated patients, the paroxetine patients experienced significantly greater reductions in panic symptoms, and a larger proportion remained free of panic attacks throughout the long-term study. There were no significant differences in efficacy between paroxetine and clomipramine.

If the medications are to be discontinued after prolonged use, it is recommended that the SSRI dose be tapered over several weeks. It is not clear whether this is necessary for fluoxetine, which has the longest half-life of any medication in the class.

2. Tricyclic antidepressants

a) Goals

The primary goals of TCA therapy of panic disorder are to reduce the intensity and frequency of panic attacks, to reduce anticipatory anxiety, and to treat associated depression. Successful tricyclic therapy also leads to a reduction in phobic avoidance.

b) Efficacy

The first controlled study documenting the efficacy of the tricyclic imipramine in blocking panic attacks was conducted by Klein and published in 1964 (104). In this study, imipramine was superior to placebo for antipanic effect and for change in the Clinical Global Impression (CGI). Since then, 15 controlled trials (16, 66, 105–117) have shown that imipramine is effective in reducing panic. After treatment with imipramine, 45%–70% of the patients were found to be panic free, compared to 15%–50% of those receiving placebo. In addition, patients with panic disorder who were treated with imipramine had less phobic avoidance and anticipatory anxiety than those receiving placebo. Typically, patients treated with imipramine realize a substantial reduction in panic after a minimum of 4 weeks of treatment; antipanic effect may not be fully experienced until 8 to 12 weeks of therapy. Anticipatory anxiety usually responds after the panic attacks have been reduced, and phobic avoidance is the last to be affected.

Given the equivalency of tricyclic agents in treating depression, there is little reason to expect tricyclics other than imipramine to work less well for panic disorder. However, very few controlled studies have evaluated other tricyclics for panic disorder. Lydiard et al. (18) found desipramine to be superior to placebo for a global measure of phobic avoidance and score on the Hamilton Rating Scale for Anxiety, but there was only a trend toward superiority ($p<0.09$) on the CGI. Although 85% of the desipramine-treated patients had reductions in panic attacks, this was not significantly different from the 76% for the placebo-treated patients. One double-blind comparative study showed the tricyclic maprotiline to be less effective than the SSRI fluvoxamine (118).

Two studies have shown that clomipramine is at least as effective as imipramine. There are anecdotal reports that clomipramine is actually somewhat more effective than imipramine; however, the evidence from the few studies that have directly compared the two is equivocal. In one double-blind, placebo-controlled study (106), clomipramine (mean dose, 109 mg/day) was superior to both imipramine (mean dose, 124 mg/day) and placebo in panic reduction and decrease in score on the Hamilton anxiety scale. In a nonblind, uncontrolled trial, Cassano et al. (119) did not find significant differences between clomipramine (mean dose, 128 mg/day) and imipramine (mean dose, 144 mg/day).

c) Side effects

The major adverse side effects common to all tricyclic medications and reported in studies of panic disorder treatment are 1) anticholinergic: dry mouth, constipation, difficulty urinating, increased heart rate, and blurry vision; 2) increased sweating; 3) sleep disturbance; 4) orthostatic hypotension and dizziness; 5) fatigue and weakness; 6) cognitive disturbance; 7) weight gain, especially for long-term users; and 8) sexual dysfunction (120). Higher doses are associated with a higher dropout rate in research studies. For example, Mavissakalian and Perel (110) reported that among subjects treated with an average of 35, 99, and 200 mg/day of imipramine, the dropout rates due to drug side effects were 6%, 15%, and 36%, respectively. TCAs should not be prescribed for patients with panic disorder who also have acute narrow-angle glaucoma or clinically significant prostatic hypertrophy. Patients with cardiac conduction abnormalities may experience a severe or fatal arrhythmia with tricyclics. Overdoses with TCAs can lead to significant cardiac toxicity and fatality; for this reason, TCAs may be suboptimal for suicidal patients. Elderly patients may be at increased risk of falls because of orthostatic hypotension caused by tricyclics.

d)   Implementation issues

(1) Dose

Clinicians have often noticed, and research studies have occasionally shown, that some patients with panic disorder are exquisitely sensitive to both the beneficial and adverse effects of tricyclics. Zitrin et al. (66) found that 20% of the patients in their study could not tolerate doses higher than 10 mg/day but still experienced panic blockade. Lydiard et al. (18) also reported an initial supersensitivity in some patients with panic disorder. Patients sometimes experience a stimulant-like response, including anxiety, agitation, or insomnia, when treatment with antidepressant medication of any class is initiated. For this reason, it is recommended that tricyclics be started for patients with panic disorder at doses substantially lower than those for patients with depression or other psychiatric conditions. One common strategy is to begin with only 10 mg/day of imipramine and gradually titrate the dose upward over the ensuing weeks.

Few studies have rigorously addressed the optimum dose of tricyclic medication for panic disorder. In most research studies, the mean final dose is approximately 150 mg/day and the maximum final dose is up to 300 mg/day. Mavissakalian and Perel (110) randomly assigned patients with panic disorder to low-dose (mean, 35 mg/day), medium-dose (mean, 99 mg/day), and high-dose (mean, 200 mg/day) imipramine. They found that both the medium and high doses were superior to placebo in reducing panic and not significantly different from each other; the low dose was no more effective than placebo. Given these findings, it is reasonable to titrate the imipramine dose of patients with panic disorder to approximately 100 mg/day and wait for at least 4 weeks to see whether there is a response. If tolerated, the dose can then be increased to as high as 300 mg/day if initial response is either absent or inadequate.

There is a suggestion in the literature that clomipramine may be effective in somewhat lower doses than imipramine. Clomipramine can generally be used effectively with doses less than 150 mg/day. Given the results of the studies by Modigh et al. (106) and Cassano et al. (119), it may be reasonable to administer clomipramine in a dose range of 25–150 mg/day.

(2) Length of treatment

Most controlled trials of tricyclics for the treatment of panic disorder were for a minimum of 8 weeks, and exactly when the patients began to respond has not always been reported. There is general clinical agreement that, similar to the situation with treatment of depression, it may take at least 4 weeks of tricyclic treatment for onset of antipanic effects; patients may not respond until 6 or even 8 weeks, and some additional response has been seen through 12 or more weeks. It is reasonable to wait for at least 6 weeks from initiation of tricyclic treatment, with at least 2 of those weeks at full dose, before deciding whether a tricyclic is effective for a patient with panic disorder. If there is some response at this point, the clinician and patient may wait longer to see how full the response will be by 8 to 12 weeks.

There are few long-term studies of tricyclic treatment for panic disorder in the literature. Cassano et al. (112) continued to treat patients with imipramine or placebo for 6 months after an acute-phase 8-week study and found that imipramine was still superior to placebo for panic reduction. Curtis et al. (113) also maintained patients on a regimen of placebo or imipramine for up to 8 months after acute 8-week treatment and found that the placebo-treated patients had more panic attacks and phobic avoidance and were more likely to drop out of treatment during the maintenance phase. In two small studies, Mavissakalian and Perel (121, 122) assessed the relapse rates of patients nonrandomly assigned to either a) discontinuation of imipramine following 6 months of full-dose imipramine plus 1 year of half-dose imipramine maintenance treatment or b) discontinuation following 6 months of acute imipramine treatment alone. They found significantly less relapse among the patients who had been in treatment for 18 months than among those who had been treated for 6 months. These studies suggest that maintenance treatment is beneficial for at least a year after a patient has achieved a response to a tricyclic. The exact relapse rate following discontinuation of imipramine or other tricyclic therapy is also not known (123, 124).

3. Benzodiazepines

a) Goals

The primary goals of benzodiazepine therapy of panic disorder are to reduce the intensity and frequency of panic attacks and to reduce anticipatory anxiety. Often, successful benzodiazepine therapy also leads to a reduction in phobic avoidance.

b) Efficacy

Alprazolam has been studied more extensively than any other benzodiazepine for the treatment of panic disorder and is approved by the FDA for the treatment of panic disorder. Eleven trials of alprazolam treatment of panic disorder were reviewed, including the Cross-National Collaborative Panic Study, which involved more than 1,000 patients randomly assigned to imipramine, alprazolam, or placebo (125). Nine of the trials were double blind, and seven were placebo controlled. Two meta-analyses of studies on alprazolam treatment for panic disorder were also reviewed.

In six of the seven double-blind, placebo-controlled trials, alprazolam was found to be superior to placebo in the treatment of panic attacks (113, 126–130), while the other one did not assess panic attacks as an outcome measure (131). The percentages of patients who were panic free (generally assessed over a 1-week period) at end point were 55%–75% for alprazolam (at doses of 5–6 mg/day) and 15%–50% for placebo. These percentages represent the "intention to treat" proportions (i.e., the panic-free proportion of the patients who were originally assigned to receive active treatment or placebo at the start of the trial); the differences between the completers were less striking or nonsignificant because of higher dropout rates for the nonresponders in the placebo groups. Alprazolam was superior to placebo in reducing phobic avoidance in five of the six studies in which it was assessed, disability in five of five studies, anticipatory anxiety in three of three studies, and Hamilton anxiety scale scores in six of seven studies. In most of the studies, patients with primary current major depression were excluded and the level of phobic avoidance was moderate.

Four of the 11 trials compared alprazolam to imipramine. Three of these were double blind. Alprazolam and imipramine were comparable in efficacy for panic attacks, phobias, Hamilton anxiety scores, disability, and CGI ratings. There were more dropouts in the imipramine group in three of the four studies.

These data support the efficacy of alprazolam (especially in the 5–6 mg/day range) in treating multiple dimensions of illness in patients with panic disorder who do not have primary current major depression.

Twelve studies regarding other benzodiazepines were also reviewed (126, 128, 132–141), and they support the short-term efficacy of other benzodiazepines for panic disorder. The agents studied include clonazepam (effective in the one double-blind, placebo-controlled trial), diazepam (effective in two of two trials, both double blind and one placebo controlled), and lorazepam (equivalent to alprazolam in three of three double-blind trials). One study showed superiority of imipramine over chlordiazepoxide.

These studies suggest that other benzodiazepines (at least diazepam, clonazepam, and lorazepam), when given in equivalent doses, may be as effective as alprazolam in the treatment of panic disorder.

There was one controlled trial of alprazolam as an adjunct to imipramine for the first 4 to 6 weeks of treatment (115). The subjects taking alprazolam showed a more rapid therapeutic response, but this was not associated with a lower percentage of treatment dropout. In addition, 10 of 17 patients taking alprazolam were unable to taper from 1.5 mg/day to discontinuation in 2 weeks after 4 to 6 weeks of treatment.

c) Side effects

The adverse effects of benzodiazepines in patients with panic disorder appear similar to those reported when benzodiazepines are used for other indications and include primarily sedation, fatigue, ataxia, slurred speech, memory impairment, and weakness. Some sedation or drowsiness occurred in 38%–75% of alprazolam-treated subjects and 11%–21% of those taking placebo. Memory problems were reported by up to 15% of patients taking alprazolam and 8.5% of patients taking placebo in the Cross-National Collaborative Panic Study. However, patients may not recognize their own cognitive impairment. It is prudent to be cautious about prescribing benzodiazepines to elderly patients or those with pretreatment cognitive impairment. The risk of falls for the elderly and the increased risk of motor vehicle accidents related to benzodiazepine use should also be considered. Among patients with histories of substance abuse or dependence, benzodiazepine use may aggravate symptoms and should be avoided. In general, however, benzodiazepines seem to be well tolerated in patients with panic disorder with very few serious side effects.

Major concerns about benzodiazepine tolerance and withdrawal have been raised. According to the report of the APA Task Force on Benzodiazepine Dependence, Toxicity, and Abuse, "There are no data to suggest that long-term therapeutic use of benzodiazepines by patients commonly leads to dose escalation or to recreational abuse" (142). However, benzodiazepines may still be underused because of an inappropriate fear of addiction. The studies of long-term alprazolam treatment for panic disorder show that the doses patients use at 32 weeks of treatment are similar to those used at 8 weeks, indicating that, as a group, patients with panic disorder do not escalate alprazolam doses or display tolerance to alprazolam's therapeutic effects, at least in the first 8 months of treatment. However, studies of dose escalation following longer periods of benzodiazepine use are generally lacking.

Six studies regarding discontinuation of alprazolam for patients with panic disorder were reviewed. These studies demonstrated that significant numbers of these patients (ranging from 33% to 100%) are unable to complete a taper of the medication after 6 weeks to 22 months of treatment. One study (143) showed that alprazolam causes significantly more withdrawal symptoms, recurrent panic attacks, and failure to complete the taper than imipramine, and another (144) suggested that patients with panic disorder have more difficulty during tapering of alprazolam than do those with generalized anxiety disorder, even when the patients in both groups are treated with similar doses. Difficulties during taper seem most severe during the last half of the taper period and the first week after the taper is completed. In many instances, it is difficult to determine the extent to which symptoms are due to withdrawal, rebound, or relapse.

The one study comparing diazepam to alprazolam for panic disorder indicated that both are no different from placebo during gradual tapering of the first half of the dose

(145). With abrupt discontinuation of the remaining dose, however, alprazolam caused significantly more anxiety, relapse, and rebound. In general, apart from this one study, the issue of discontinuation of benzodiazepines with short versus long half-lives or high versus low potency has not been adequately addressed in relation to panic disorder. The APA task force report on benzodiazepines (142) suggests that there are more difficulties with short-half-life, high-potency compounds. However, studies by Schweizer, Rickels, Weiss, and Zavodnick (129, 143) of benzodiazepine-treated patients showed no significant effect of half-life on the results of a gradual taper but greater withdrawal severity after abrupt discontinuation with compounds having shorter half-lives and with higher daily doses. These studies, although not involving patients with panic disorder specifically, suggest that half-life is less of a factor, or in fact may not be important, given a gradual taper schedule.

Thus, there is no evidence for significant dose escalation in patients with panic disorder (75). However, withdrawal symptoms and symptomatic rebound are commonly seen with discontinuation of alprazolam after as little as 6 to 8 weeks of treatment. These discontinuation effects appear more severe than those following taper of imipramine and may be more severe in patients with panic disorder than in those with generalized anxiety disorder. This would argue for tapering benzodiazepines very slowly for patients with panic disorder, probably over 2–4 months and at rates no higher than 10% of the dose per week (2, 146). Withdrawal symptoms can occur throughout the taper and may be especially severe toward the end of the taper. The decision of when to attempt a benzodiazepine taper may be influenced by factors such as the presence of psychosocial stressors or supports, the stability of comorbid conditions, and the availability of alternative treatment options.

d) Implementation issues

(1) Dose
The manufacturer's recommendation for alprazolam treatment of panic disorder notes that doses above 4 mg/day are usually necessary and that doses up to 10 mg/day are sometimes required. However, very few studies have empirically evaluated dose requirements. Two studies (22, 105) compared alprazolam doses of 6 mg/day and 2 mg/day. The study by Uhlenhuth et al. (105) showed a significant advantage for the higher dose in producing a panic-free state. The study by Lydiard et al. (22) showed very little difference between the higher and lower doses (absence of panic attacks at study end in 65% of patients taking higher dose, 50% taking lower dose, but only 15% taking placebo). However, the rates of surreptitious benzodiazepine use for the lower-dose (23%) and placebo (35%) patients were considerably greater than the rate for the patients taking the higher alprazolam dose (4%), perhaps suggesting that the patients did not find the lower dose or placebo clinically effective. Lydiard and colleagues found that adverse side effects were more pronounced at the higher dose than at the lower dose of alprazolam. Given these findings, it is necessary to be flexible in choosing the alprazolam dose for an individual patient. Most patients require three to four doses per day to avoid breakthrough or rebound symptoms, although some may achieve symptom control with two doses of alprazolam per day. The dose should be titrated up to 2–3 mg/day at first, but an increase to 5–6 mg/day will be necessary for some patients.

In one multicenter dose-ranging trial (147), patients with panic disorder were randomly assigned to placebo or one of five fixed doses (0.5, 1.0, 2.0, 3.0, or 4.0 mg/day) of clonazepam. During 6 weeks of treatment, the minimum effective dose was 1.0 mg/day, and daily doses of 1.0 mg/day and higher were equally effective in reducing the number of panic attacks. The investigators concluded that daily doses of 1.0 to 2.0 mg of clonazepam offered the best balance of therapeutic benefits and side effects. Because of its relatively long half-life, clonazepam can usually be administered once or twice a day.

The dosing of other benzodiazepines in the treatment of panic disorder is less well established. In controlled studies, lorazepam has been given at doses of about 7 mg/day, usually two or three times daily. Diazepam doses ranged from 5 to 40 mg/day in two published trials.

Results of several studies suggest a relationship between alprazolam blood levels and treatment response (148, 149). Monitoring blood levels of alprazolam may be useful for dose adjustment, although this is not routinely done.

(2) Length of treatment

Alprazolam had an earlier onset of action than imipramine in three controlled trials. Clinicians and patients often note some reduction in panic within the first week of treatment, although full blockade of panic attacks can take several weeks.

As with TCA treatment of panic disorder, there are very few data indicating the optimum length of maintenance therapy for responders to benzodiazepines. Two published trials have compared maintenance imipramine, alprazolam, and placebo treatment, and both suggest that imipramine may be superior. In the study by Cassano et al. (112), imipramine and alprazolam patients fared equally well in terms of panic reduction during a 6-month maintenance phase, but the imipramine-treated patients had less phobic avoidance. There were more alprazolam dropouts during the maintenance phase than during the 8-week acute treatment phase, while the number of imipramine dropouts did not differ between the two phases. Curtis et al. (113) found that from month 4 through the end of an 8-month maintenance phase patients taking imipramine had virtually no panic attacks, while alprazolam-treated patients continued to experience infrequent panic attacks. On all other measures, however, the two medications performed equally well. In a third investigation, by Lepola et al. (150), patients who had been treated with alprazolam (N=27) and imipramine (N=28) in a 9-week trial were then followed for 3 years in a naturalistic study. Significantly more alprazolam users than imipramine users were found to be still using their original medication after 3 years (74% versus 32%). The authors pointed out that it is difficult to know whether this difference is attributable to a better long-term response among the imipramine users than among the alprazolam users, a greater degree of intolerable side effects for the imipramine users, or greater difficulty in discontinuing treatment among the alprazolam users due to physiologic dependence.

4. Monoamine oxidase inhibitors

a) Goals

The primary goals of MAOI therapy of panic disorder are to reduce the intensity and frequency of panic attacks, to reduce anticipatory anxiety, and to treat associated depression. Often, successful therapy with MAOIs also leads to a reduction in phobic avoidance.

b) Efficacy

There have been virtually no studies involving the use of MAOIs since the introduction of the panic disorder diagnosis in DSM-III in 1980. It is therefore nearly impossible to cite controlled trials in which MAOIs that are approved for use in the United States and currently manufactured (i.e., phenelzine and tranylcypromine) have been used for the specific treatment of panic disorder with or without agoraphobia. Even the most modern and rigorous study (151) involved the use of phenelzine for the treatment of "phobic neurosis" (152). The commonly held belief that MAOIs are actually more potent antipanic agents than tricyclics has never been convincingly proven in the scientific literature and is only supported by clinical anecdote.

Two studies have looked at the effectiveness of a reversible inhibitor of monoamine oxidase A (RIMA) for panic disorder. No medication in the RIMA class is currently approved for use in the United States, but at least one, moclobemide, is widely used in Europe and Canada. These medications do not generally require adherence to the tyramine-free diet that is mandatory for patients treated with phenelzine or tranylcypromine. Both studies, one a double-blind comparison of brofaromine to clomipramine (153) and the other an open study of brofaromine (154), showed antipanic and antiphobic efficacy.

c) Side effects

Adverse side effects are clearly a major concern with MAOI therapy. The complexity of these medications suggests that they should be prescribed by physicians with experience in monitoring MAOI treatment.

The main risk of taking an MAOI is hypertensive crisis secondary to ingestion of tyramine. Hence, patients taking phenelzine or tranylcypromine must adhere to the special low-tyramine diet. Certain medications, including but not limited to sympathomimetic amines, decongestants, the over-the-counter medication dextromethorphan, and meperidine, must not be used with MAOIs. Another serious drug-drug interaction to be avoided is the "serotonergic syndrome" that can occur from the use of MAOIs with SSRIs (155). Even when the risk of hypertensive crisis is obviated by strict adherence to dietary and medication restrictions, MAOIs have substantial adverse effects. These include hypotension (sometimes leading to syncope), weight gain, hypomania, sexual dysfunction, paresthesia, sleep disturbance, myoclonic jerks, dry mouth, and edema.

d) Implementation issues

(1) Dose
Doses of phenelzine in controlled trials for panic-disorder-like illnesses have tended to be low, often no higher than 45 mg/day. Some authors have commented that higher doses may be more effective. Doses of phenelzine up to 90 mg/day and of tranylcypromine up to 70 mg/day are said by experienced clinicians to be necessary for some patients with panic disorder.

(2) Length of treatment
The onset of the antipanic effect of MAOIs generally follows the same time course as that for tricyclics. Patients rarely get significant benefit before several weeks have elapsed, and periods up to 12 weeks may be necessary before the full effectiveness of the medication can be judged.

No maintenance studies of MAOIs for panic disorder have been published. Hence, the optimal length of treatment, to provide the least chance of relapse, is not established.

5. Other antidepressants

a) Venlafaxine

One small controlled trial at a single site, drawn from a larger multicenter trial, showed that venlafaxine (mean dose, 150 mg/day) was effective for treating panic disorder (156). A published series of four cases of patients with panic disorder indicated that venlafaxine at relatively low doses (50–75 mg/day) may be effective and well tolerated (157).

b) Trazodone

One double-blind study (158) in which 74 patients with panic disorder were assigned to trazodone, imipramine, or alprazolam showed trazodone to be less effective than either imipramine or alprazolam. However, in a single-blind study (159) in which 11 patients with panic disorder were treated with trazodone, panic symptoms improved significantly from a baseline period of placebo treatment.

c) Bupropion

Bupropion has been found to be effective in the treatment of depression. Proposed mechanisms of action include dopaminergic and noradrenergic agonist effects. Although there have been several small clinical trials using bupropion for patients with panic disorder, there is general consensus that it is not effective in alleviating either the somatic or psychological symptoms of panic attacks. It may have a role as an adjunctive treatment for patients with panic disorder who suffer sexual dysfunction as a side effect of other antidepressant medications, but it nevertheless may be potentially "overenergizing" for this specific patient group (160).

d) Nefazodone

One retrospective analysis of a randomized, placebo-controlled trial evaluated the effectiveness of nefazodone and imipramine among patients with comorbid panic disorder and major depression (161). Patients treated with nefazodone experienced significantly greater reductions in panic symptoms than placebo-treated patients; imipramine treatment was not found to be significantly better than placebo. An open-label trial examined nefazodone treatment among patients with panic disorder and concurrent depression or depressive symptoms (162). Panic symptoms were judged to be much or very much improved in 71% of the patients treated with nefazodone.

6. Anticonvulsants

There are limited data concerning the use of anticonvulsant medication in the treatment of panic disorder. In case reports, carbamazepine has been reported to improve panic attacks in patients with EEG abnormalities (163). However, the only controlled trial of carbamazepine suggested that it is not superior to placebo in reducing panic attack frequency (164). One crossover study showed significantly greater improvement in panic symptoms during periods of treatment with valproate than during treatment with placebo (165). A few reports, mostly findings from small numbers of subjects in uncontrolled studies or anecdotal reports on a few subjects, also suggest that valproate is an effective treatment for panic disorder (166). In these studies, valproate was well tolerated, but the adverse side effects included gastrointestinal dysfunction, weight gain, dizziness, nausea, sedation, and alopecia. A single case report indicated that gabapentin was effective for a patient with panic disorder.

7. Other agents

a) Conventional antipsychotic medications

Conventional antipsychotic medications are rarely appropriate in the treatment of un-complicated panic disorder. There is no evidence that they are effective, and the risk of neurological side effects outweighs any potential benefit. There is interest, but no evidence, in the possibility that clozapine may be useful for extremely refractory cases of panic disorder. At present, however, this cannot be recommended.

b) β Blockers

The limited number of controlled trials that have been conducted with β-adrenergic blocking agents in panic disorder have provided mixed results. Noyes et al. (133) compared the efficacy of diazepam and propranolol for 21 patients with panic dis-order in a double-blind crossover study. Findings revealed that 18 of the 21 patients responded "moderately" to diazepam but only seven of the 21 responded to propra-nolol. As the sole agent, the β blocker did not appear to be effective in alleviating pho-bic symptoms or panic attacks, despite adequate peripheral blockade. Munjack et al. (167) compared the effectiveness of alprazolam, propranolol, and placebo for 55 pa-tients with panic disorder and agoraphobia. This study also showed superiority of al-prazolam over propranolol: 75% of the alprazolam patients met the criterion of zero panic attacks after 5 weeks, compared with 37% of the propranolol group and 43% of the placebo patients. Ravaris et al. (168) also compared propranolol with alprazolam, but the results demonstrated that alprazolam and propranolol provided similar effects in suppressing panic attacks and reducing avoidance behaviors; the only difference in this study was the more rapid onset of action of alprazolam. One open-label, case report study (169) indicated a possible additive effect of the combination of propra-nolol and alprazolam. No subsequent clinical trials have addressed the issue of com-bination therapy with these agents.

c) Calcium channel blockers

The cardiovascular symptoms associated with panic attacks include palpitations, fa-cial flushing, light-headedness, paresthesia, presyncopal disturbances, and tachycar-dia, which have been attributed to autonomic instability. Calcium channel blockers have been used increasingly to offset these physical manifestations in anxious pa-tients. Successful results have been achieved with regard to complaints of palpitations and hyperventilation. Calcium channel blockers have particular potential for patients with mitral valve prolapse, especially when echocardiographic data are correlated with physical manifestations of autonomic hyperactivity. Data from controlled clinical studies that delineate a specific efficacy of calcium channel blockers in panic disorder or other anxiety disorders are very limited. Klein and Uhde (170) conducted one dou-ble-blind crossover study of verapamil involving 11 patients with panic disorder. When treated with verapamil, the patients had statistically significant, although clin-ically modest, reductions in the number of panic attacks and severity of anxiety symp-toms. Use of these agents as anxiety treatments is mostly based on empirical assumptions related to cardiovascular effects or on case study reports. More investi-gation is needed to determine their role in panic amelioration, whether as a first-line treatment or as an adjunctive modality.

d) Inositol

Benjamin et al. (171) reported efficacy for inositol in a small, placebo-controlled trial involving 21 patients. The dose was 12 g/day, and the side effects were reported as minimal.

e) Clonidine

Few clinical trials with clonidine for the treatment of panic disorder and other anxiety disorders have been conducted. The controlled trials that have been done were limited to relatively small groups, and the results were equivocal with regard to efficacy. Uhde et al. (172) evaluated clonidine for patients with panic disorder and noted that it was more effective than placebo in reducing anxiety as measured by the Spielberger State-Trait Anxiety Inventory (173), Zung Anxiety Scale (174), and patient reports of frequency of anxiety symptoms. Hoehn-Saric et al. (175) studied the effect of clonidine on 23 patients with generalized anxiety disorder and panic disorder. They observed that clonidine was superior to placebo in relieving psychic and somatic symptoms, but of the 14 patients with panic disorder, three worsened with this agent. Hoehn-Saric et al. also noted that clonidine was not "as good as classical anxiety agents." There was a high frequency of side effects; 95% of the patients reported undesirable effects by week 12. Results from another study indicate that if there are therapeutic effects of clonidine for patients with panic disorder, they may be transient. Uhde et al. (172) gave intravenous clonidine or placebo to patients with panic disorder and healthy control subjects. After 1 hour, they found that clonidine was significantly more effective at reducing anxiety symptoms than placebo and that patients with panic disorder had a significantly greater reduction in anxiety symptoms than the control subjects. However, among 18 patients with panic disorder given oral clonidine for an average of 10 weeks, there was no difference in anxiety symptom scores assessed before and at the end of treatment.

f) Buspirone

Buspirone has been demonstrated to be effective in the long-term treatment of psychic and somatic symptoms of generalized anxiety disorder. Thus far, however, very limited information is available regarding the efficacy of buspirone for panic disorder. Sheehan et al. (176) reported that buspirone was not superior to placebo on any outcome measure in patients with panic disorder. This study was similar in outcome to a previous study (177), which also showed that buspirone did not seem to affect the symptoms of panic disorder.

IV. DEVELOPMENT OF A TREATMENT PLAN FOR THE INDIVIDUAL PATIENT

▶ A. CHOOSING A SITE OF TREATMENT

The treatment of panic disorder is generally conducted entirely on an outpatient basis, and the condition by itself rarely warrants hospitalization. Occasionally, the first contact between patient and psychiatrist occurs in the emergency room or the hospital when the patient has been admitted in the midst of an acute panic episode. The patient may even be admitted by emergency room staff to rule out myocardial infarction or other serious general medical events. In such cases, the psychiatrist may be able to make the diagnosis of panic disorder and initiate treatment once other general medical conditions have been ruled out. Because panic disorder is frequently comorbid with depression and appears to elevate the risk of suicide attempts by depressed patients, it may also be necessary to hospitalize the depressed patient with panic disorder when suicidal ideation is of clinical concern. The treatment of panic disorder along with the treatment of depression is then initiated on an inpatient basis. Similarly, patients with panic disorder frequently have comorbid substance use disorders, which can occasionally require inpatient detoxification. Once again, the treatment of panic can be initiated in the hospital before discharge to outpatient care. Rarely, hospitalization is required in very severe cases of panic disorder with agoraphobia when administration of outpatient treatment has been ineffective or is impractical. For example, a housebound patient may require more intensive and closely supervised CBT in the initial phase of therapy than that provided by outpatient care (178, 179).

B. FORMULATION OF A TREATMENT PLAN

Before treatment for panic disorder is initiated, a general medical and psychiatric evaluation should be conducted (15). Psychiatrists should consider potential general medical and substance-induced causes of panic symptoms, especially when caring for patients who have a new onset of symptoms. Diagnostic studies and laboratory tests should be guided by the psychiatrist's evaluation of the patient's condition and by the choice of treatment. Attention should be given to the patient's psychosocial stressors, social supports, and general living situation.

1. Psychiatric management

Once the diagnosis of panic disorder is made, the patient is informed of the diagnosis and educated about panic disorder, its clinical course, and its complications. Regardless of the ultimate treatment modality selected, it is important to reassure the patient that panic attacks reflect real physiologic events (e.g., the heart rate does increase, blood pressure usually goes up, and other physical changes occur) but that these changes are not dangerous acutely. To evaluate the frequency and nature of a patient's panic attacks, patients may be encouraged to monitor their symptoms by using techniques such as keeping a daily diary.

It is also extremely important when formulating the treatment plan to address the presence of any of the many conditions that are frequently comorbid with panic disorder. Continuing medical evaluation and management are a crucial part of the treatment plan. In some cases, treatment of these comorbid conditions may even take precedence over treatment of the panic attacks. For example, patients with serious substance abuse may need detoxification and substance abuse treatment before it is possible to institute treatment for panic disorder.

Regardless of the treatment modality, it is often helpful to involve family members and significant others when appropriate and possible. In many cases, panic disorder is not well understood by family members, who may accuse the patient of overreacting or even of malingering. In other cases, supportive and understanding family members may wish to participate in treatment by, for example, helping with exposure exercises. Educating family members and enlisting their help and support can be very helpful.

Family and supportive therapy may also be employed along with other psychosocial and pharmacologic treatments for panic disorder. This provides the necessary environment for improvement and helps resolve interpersonal issues that may have arisen as a direct result of panic attacks and avoidance behaviors.

Because patients with panic disorder often fear separations and being alone, many experience great comfort from having easy access to the treating psychiatrist. It is often important for a psychiatrist who treats patients with panic disorder to be very available to patients in the early phase of treatment, before the panic resolves. In general, these patients are very reassured by knowing their physicians are available. If the patient becomes overly dependent on the psychiatrist, the dependency should be addressed directly and nonjudgmentally in the treatment, rather than through physician unavailability. The psychiatrist should attend to the treatment of personality disorders in patients with panic disorder. Sometimes the symptoms of comorbid personality disorders are so prominent that they interfere with symptom-based treatment of panic disorder. In this case, psychodynamic psychotherapy may be indicated.

2. Choice of specific treatment modalities

As noted earlier, there are two methods that have been extensively studied and proven to be effective treatments for panic disorder: CBT and antipanic medication. Considerations that may help guide the choice between CBT and medication as the treatment modality include their comparable efficacies, differences in risks and benefits, differences in costs, the availability of clinicians trained in CBT, and patient preferences. The psychiatrist should remember that the best-studied treatments for panic disorder target specific symptoms, whereas the physician must treat the patient. This means that in some cases, less well-studied psychosocial treatment (e.g., psychodynamic psychotherapy, family therapy) may be the treatment of choice, for example, when symptoms of a personality disorder or extensive psychological conflicts are prominent in the clinical picture.

a) Considerations in choice of modality

(1) Efficacy

Direct comparisons of the efficacy of CBT and antipanic medications have been conducted, and some CBT researchers have found CBT to be superior (30, 39), while some pharmacotherapy studies have shown medication to be superior (32). Results from a large four-site study documented that the two treatments perform equally well (180). This is in line with the conclusions of the NIMH consensus development panel in 1991 that either of these treatments could be considered standard and that there was not sufficient evidence that either was superior to the other (181).

(2) Risks and benefits

The specific advantages and risks associated with CBT and pharmacotherapy may help guide the choice of which treatment to initiate. CBT lacks the adverse side effects of medications and the danger of developing physiological dependency on certain drugs. However, CBT requires patients to perform "homework" or confront feared situations, which approximately 10%–30% of patients have been found to be unwilling or unable to complete (19, 29, 30, 33). In addition, CBT may not be readily available to patients in some areas.

The advantages of pharmacotherapies include their ready availability, the need for less effort by the patient, and their more rapid onset (especially for benzodiazepines). Medications may be associated with a lower likelihood of psychological dependence on the therapist. Each class of antipanic medications (TCAs, MAOIs, SSRIs, and benzodiazepines) is associated with specific side effects, which must be considered (see discussion of choosing among the medication classes in section IV.B.2.b.2).

(3) Costs

Several factors influence the costs of treatment. In the case of CBT, these factors include the duration and frequency of treatment, the ability to maintain treatment gains, and any requirements for additional psychosocial or pharmacologic treatment. For antipanic medications, factors affecting cost include the choice and dose of antipanic agent, the availability of generic preparations, duration of treatment, the probability of relapse following discontinuation, requirements for additional pharmacotherapy or psychosocial treatment, and costs of treating medication-related side effects.

(4) Patient preferences

In most cases, the decision to use medication, CBT, another form of psychotherapy, or a combination of treatments is highly individualized. Informed patients may consider the evidence for a treatment's efficacy, particular advantages, risks and side effects, or costs.

b) Types of modalities

(1) CBT and other psychotherapies

Specific elements of CBT are reviewed in section III.C.1.a. Panic-focused CBT is generally administered in weekly sessions for approximately 12 weeks. The patient must be willing to fulfill "homework" assignments that include breathing exercises, recording anxious cognitions, and confronting phobic situations.

Clinicians have often reported that sessions with significant others help to relieve stress on families caused by panic attacks and phobias in the patient and thereby promote a supportive environment for the patient, which may facilitate compliance with CBT and other treatments. Cognitive behavioral approaches have been conducted in group formats with results similar to those for individual treatment.

There is evidence that many patients with panic disorder have complicating comorbid axis I and/or axis II conditions. Psychodynamic psychotherapy may be useful in reducing symptoms or maladaptive behaviors in these associated conditions. Such a treatment may also be a helpful adjunct for patients with panic disorder treated with medication who continue to experience difficulty with psychosocial stressors.

Using other psychosocial treatments in conjunction with psychiatric management may be helpful in addressing certain comorbid disorders or environmental or psychosocial stressors. However, there have been no controlled studies to support the efficacy of psychosocial treatments other than CBT, when used alone, for the treatment of panic disorder. Therefore, supplementation with or replacement by either CBT or antipanic medications should be strongly considered if no significant improvement in the panic symptoms occurs within 6–8 weeks.

(2) Medications

When pharmacotherapy has been selected, the choice of which class of medication to use may be informed by consideration of the relative efficacies of the various medication classes, differences in risks and benefits, differences in costs, and patient preferences, including the wish to conceive a child or continue with a pregnancy or nursing experience.

Because medications from all four classes—SSRIs, TCAs, benzodiazepines, and MAOIs—are roughly comparable in efficacy, the decision about which medication to choose for panic disorder mainly involves considerations of adverse side effects and cost. SSRIs are likely to be the best choice of pharmacotherapy for many patients with panic disorder because they lack significant cardiovascular and anticholinergic side effects and have no liability for physical dependency and subsequent withdrawal reactions.

The SSRIs carry a risk of sexual side effects and are also more expensive than tricyclics and benzodiazepines because generic preparations are not yet available. If cost is a consideration, it is important to note that tricyclics (particularly imipramine and clomipramine, for which most research has been conducted) and high-potency benzodiazepines (including alprazolam and clonazepam) are effective for panic disorder and that most patients can tolerate them. With tricyclics, consideration must be given to the possibility of cardiovascular and anticholinergic side effects. These are particularly troublesome for older patients and for patients with other medical problems. With benzodiazepines, consideration must be given to the fact that all of them will produce physical dependency in most patients. This may make it difficult for the patient to discontinue treatment. Also, benzodiazepines are generally contraindicated for patients with current or past substance use disorders.

Because many patients with panic disorder are hypersensitive to antidepressant medications at treatment initiation, it is recommended that doses approximately half of those given to depressed patients at the beginning of treatment be used for patients with panic disorder initially. The dose is then increased to a full therapeutic dose over subsequent days and as tolerated by the patient. TCAs, SSRIs, and MAOIs generally take 4 to 6 weeks to become effective for panic disorder. For this reason, high-potency benzodiazepines may be useful in situations where very rapid control of symptoms is critical. Because of their side effects and the need for dietary restrictions, MAOIs are generally reserved for patients who do not respond to other treatments.

(3) Combined medication and psychosocial treatment

The data regarding the efficacy of the combination of medications and CBT versus that of either modality alone are conflicting (66). Currently, it is not possible to identify which patients will benefit more from such combination therapy. Combining medication and CBT can be especially useful for patients with severe agoraphobia and for those who show an incomplete response to either treatment alone. In one study, combining psychodynamic psychotherapy with medication improved the long-term outcome of medication-treated patients (63). Psychodynamic psychotherapy is commonly used in conjunction with medication on the basis of a clinical consensus that it is effective for some patients.

3. Determining length of treatment

The acute phase of treatment with either CBT or medication generally lasts about 12 weeks. At the end of a successful acute phase, the patient should have markedly fewer and less intense panic attacks than before treatment. Ideally, panic attacks should be eliminated entirely. In addition, the patient should worry less about panic attacks and should experience minimal or no phobic avoidance. This is roughly the time required to realize the full benefit of either treatment.

After the acute phase of treatment with CBT, the frequency of visits is generally decreased, and they are eventually discontinued within several months. Some, but not all, studies indicate that long-term remission is possible, lasting several years after the completion of successful CBT. The efficacy of a second round of CBT for patients who relapse or "booster" CBT sessions for preventing relapse has not been studied.

There are very few systematic studies that indicate the optimal length of antipanic medication therapy. There is evidence that response to antipanic medication continues while the patient continues to take medication. Studies vary in the rate of relapse following medication discontinuation, but most show that relapse is common. It is generally believed, although not yet documented with research findings, that re-institution of medication aborts relapse. The general recommendation has been to maintain medication treatment for at least 1 year after response and then to attempt discontinuation, with close follow-up of the patient from this point. Relapsing patients should then begin taking medication again. There is preliminary evidence that longer periods of initial treatment with medication may decrease the risk of relapse when the medication is stopped. It is not known whether continuing treatment with medication indefinitely for patients who relapse after discontinuation is beneficial.

Patients are likely to show some improvement with either medication or CBT within 6–8 weeks (although full response may take longer). Patients who show no improvement within 6–8 weeks with a particular treatment should be reevaluated with regard to diagnosis, the need for a different treatment, or the need for combined treatment. Patients who do not respond as expected to medication or CBT, or who have repeated relapses, should be evaluated for possible addition of a psychodynamic or other psychosocial intervention.

4. Use of benzodiazepines for early symptom control, in combination with a different treatment modality

Nonbenzodiazepine antipanic medication and CBT often take weeks before beneficial effects are realized, and some patients express an urgent need for a diminution of high levels of anticipatory anxiety and for some reduction in the severity of panic attacks. This can usually be accomplished by administering a benzodiazepine.

However, the potential benefits of benzodiazepines during the initial stages of treatment with another modality should be balanced against the potential risks. First, the patient may attribute all of the response he or she obtains in the course of treatment for panic disorder to the initial administration of the benzodiazepine. Even when antipanic medication or CBT has probably started to work, the patient may still believe that the benzodiazepine is the effective agent. The patient may then have difficulty discontinuing the benzodiazepine. Second, cognitive behavioral therapists and other clinicians are concerned that benzodiazepines may relieve anxiety to such an extent that the patient loses motivation to follow all of the steps of CBT. Finally, even after relatively brief periods of benzodiazepine treatment—often only a few weeks—some patients experience withdrawal reactions upon discontinuation. Such patients may believe that they are experiencing a relapse into panic disorder and have great difficulty stopping use of the benzodiazepine.

For these reasons, when benzodiazepines are used during the initial stages of treatment with another modality, patients should be reassured that more definitive treatment will be likely to work in a few weeks. Avoiding unnecessarily high doses of benzodiazepines and asking the patient to take these medications only when needed may help avoid the development of steady-state benzodiazepine levels and the risk of dependency.

V. CLINICAL FEATURES INFLUENCING TREATMENT

The following sections review data pertinent to the treatment of individuals with panic disorder who have specific clinical features that may alter the general treatment considerations that are discussed in section IV. These sections are necessarily brief and are not intended to stand alone as a set of treatment recommendations. The recommendations reviewed in section IV, including the use of psychiatric management, generally apply unless otherwise indicated.

A. PSYCHIATRIC FACTORS

1. Suicidality

Both older follow-up studies of anxiety disorders and more recent investigations of panic disorder have demonstrated a higher than average rate of suicide attempts in patients with a lifetime history of these disorders (9, 182, 183). In a large epidemiological study of over 18,000 adults, Weissman et al. (9) found that 20% of individuals with a history of panic disorder and 12% of those with a history of panic attacks had attempted suicide. A high risk of suicidal ideation and attempts in patients with panic disorder has been confirmed in several studies (184–186) but not in others examining uncomplicated panic disorder or controlling for comorbid conditions (187, 188). In addition, Fawcett et al. (189), in a study of 954 patients with major depression, found that the presence of comorbid panic attacks was one determinant of suicide in the first year of follow-up.

It remains unclear whether uncomplicated panic disorder, especially panic without agoraphobia, is associated with a high risk of suicide attempts (186–188, 190) and whether suicide attempts by individuals with panic disorder are actually related to or caused by panic symptoms, as opposed to being a result of comorbid conditions. Comorbid psychiatric disorders clearly increase the risk of suicide in patients with panic disorder. In particular, comorbid lifetime major depression, alcohol or substance abuse or dependence, personality disorders, and brief depressive symptoms increase the risk of suicide attempts, as do younger age, earlier onset of illness, greater severity of illness, and a past history of suicide attempts or psychiatric hospitalization (9, 183–185, 191, 192).

The high rate of suicide attempts by patients with panic disorder is of considerable clinical significance, even if most or all of the increased risk is attributable to lifetime comorbidity. The vast majority of patients with panic disorder have current or past comorbid axis I or axis II disorders. Thus, uncomplicated panic disorder is relatively uncommon. Furthermore, comorbid conditions may go undetected in busy clinical settings. Thus, it is important to be aware that patients presenting with panic disorder are at high risk for lifetime suicidal ideation and attempts. All patients presenting with panic attacks should be asked about suicidal ideation and past suicide attempts and about conditions likely to increase risk and to require specific treatment, such as depression and substance abuse. When significant depression and/or suicidal ideation exist, appropriate antidepressant therapy should be initiated and a decision made about whether the patient can be safely treated as an outpatient. When substance abuse is present, this must become a primary focus of clinical attention, and every effort to treat the substance abuse must be made.

2. Comorbid substance use disorder

In clinical and epidemiological studies, patients with panic disorder with or without agoraphobia have higher than average rates of cocaine, alcohol, and sedative abuse and dependence (193–196). Cocaine, other stimulants, and marijuana have been reported to precipitate panic attacks in adolescents and adults (197–199). Some individuals may self-medicate panic and anxiety symptoms by using alcohol and sedatives. However, heavy alcohol use, acute alcohol withdrawal, and more prolonged subacute withdrawal may cause or exacerbate panic (193, 200). Individuals who are ataxic and tremulous may not venture out because of their embarrassment, insecurity, or disability. These actions may mimic panic disorder or agoraphobia. Patients with both panic disorder and substance abuse or dependence have a poorer prognosis than those with either disorder alone (193, 200).

Since a significant proportion of patients presenting with panic attacks or agoraphobia have a history of substance abuse or dependence, which may cause or aggravate their symptoms, clinicians should be careful to screen for substance use disorders in this population. Flashbacks induced by current or past use of inhalants or hallucinogens can cause panic-disorder-type symptoms. Treatment of the substance use disorder is essential. It is unclear whether specific antipanic treatment is necessary for patients with primary substance abuse. Several panic attacks during the early weeks of abstinence, decreasing in frequency, often warrant no treatment other than support and reassurance until the attacks abate (201, 202). However, if the panic attacks continue and increase over several weeks, the diagnosis of panic disorder is warranted. If a patient is not relieved of ongoing panic attacks, it is likely that he or she will resume substance abuse (203–207). In treating panic symptoms in dually diagnosed patients, benzodiazepines should be avoided whenever possible, in favor of psychotherapy and/or antidepressants. A history of abuse of other substances, both licit and illicit, is associated with a higher prevalence of benzodiazepine abuse, a greater euphoric response to benzodiazepines, and a higher rate of unauthorized use of alprazolam during treatment for panic disorder (208, 209). The potential benefits of other medications for panic should be weighed against possible interactions with alcohol and other medications, resulting in, for instance, lowering of the seizure threshold (for tricyclics) or hyper- or hypotensive reactions (for MAOIs).

The use of a number of legal substances, such as nicotine, caffeine, and sympathomimetics (e.g., nasal decongestants), may also worsen panic attacks and interfere with treatment response (210–212).

3. Comorbid mood disorder

Panic disorder often coexists with bipolar disorder or unipolar depression. Bowen et al. (213) reported that of 108 patients with panic disorder, 11% had comorbid unipolar depression and 23% had comorbid bipolar disorder. Savino et al. (214) found that of 140 patients with panic, 23% had comorbid unipolar depression and 11% had comorbid bipolar disorder.

Many studies indicate that patients with panic disorder and comorbid mood disorders exhibit greater impairment, more hospitalizations, a higher rate of suicide attempts, and generally more psychopathology than patients with pure panic disorder (213). In addition, patients with panic disorder and comorbid affective disorders generally respond less well to traditional treatments for panic disorder.

A significant proportion of patients with panic disorder complain of overstimulation when treated with antidepressants (both tricyclics and SSRIs), and the attrition rate due to side effects or nonresponse is high. Such medications, therefore, are most efficaciously introduced at low doses and slowly increased. If both panic disorder and depression are present, it is important that a patient's treatment regimen include specific antipanic treatments.

4. Other anxiety disorders

Panic attacks are part of the hallmark cluster of symptoms in panic disorder, but they do occur in other illnesses. Patients with posttraumatic stress disorder (PTSD), obsessive-compulsive disorder (OCD), generalized anxiety disorder, and specific and social phobias also sometimes report occasional panic attacks. Identification of triggers for panic attacks is important, since a patient can be misdiagnosed with panic disorder and considered treatment resistant if this is not done.

Other comorbid anxiety disorders complicate the picture as well. PTSD, as just mentioned, may present with a series of panic attacks (215, 216), and PTSD patients may meet specific criteria for panic disorder concomitantly. In addition, patients with PTSD often present with PTSD, panic disorder, and a third or fourth disorder (217–223). More specific treatments may be required to offset other profound symptoms in PTSD. OCD is yet another anxiety disorder that may present concomitantly with panic disorder (224) and is frequently a diagnostic oversight, in part because of the reticence of patients to talk about their experiences. Because phobias and avoidant behavior are common in panic disorder, phobic disorders and panic disorder also frequently occur as comorbid conditions. They have similar responses to MAOIs, SSRIs, and perhaps other antidepressants. Specific phobias are more responsive to specific cognitive behavioral treatments than is the phobic avoidance associated with panic disorder. In summary, panic attacks may be experienced in several anxiety disorders, either as a response to specific triggers or as part of a complicated pattern of comorbid conditions that would require very specific, tailored multimodal therapy for optimal recovery. Although the pharmacotherapeutic considerations may be similar in these conditions, specificity of treatment may make the difference between full response, partial response, and perceived refractoriness.

5. Comorbid personality disorders

About 40% to 50% of patients with the diagnosis of panic disorder additionally meet the criteria for one or more axis II disorders (225–227).

The personality disorders most frequently observed in panic disorder patients are three from the anxious cluster: avoidant, obsessive-compulsive, and dependent (228–230). In addition, patients with panic disorder often show traits from other personality disorders, such as affective instability (from borderline personality disorder) and hypersensitivity to people (from paranoid personality disorder) (225).

Some studies suggest that patients with panic disorder and comorbid personality disorders may improve less or be subject to greater relapse following medication treatment (225, 228–231) or exposure therapy (42, 232–234). However, in one study (235), patients with panic disorder and comorbid personality disorders benefited as much from CBT as did patients with panic disorder without comorbid personality disorders, and in another study (236), there were no differences in treatment effect between patients with and without comorbid personality disorders after statistical adjustment for agoraphobic avoidance and frequency of panic attacks.

The therapist may need to spend more time with patients who have personality disorders in order to strengthen the therapeutic relationship and to develop a hierarchy of specific treatment goals. Psychodynamically informed management and/or formal psychodynamic treatment may be helpful for patients with panic disorder and personality disorders who have not responded to panic-focused treatments alone.

▶ B. CONCURRENT GENERAL MEDICAL CONDITIONS

Panic attacks are associated with prominent physical symptoms and may be misinterpreted as general medical conditions by patients and/or physicians. Some general medical conditions (and/or effects of medications prescribed to treat them) may manifest themselves as panic symptoms, and general medical illness may be associated with comorbid panic disorder. A complete assessment for patients with panic disorder includes a general medical evaluation as delineated in the *Practice Guideline for Psychiatric Evaluation of Adults* (15; included in this volume). Such careful assessment, when results are negative, is reassuring for patients who fear serious physical illness. In the case of a patient who is diagnosed with a general medical condition, a decision must be made regarding the relationship between that condition and the panic disorder. If the medical condition or treatment is considered to be involved in the etiology of the panic symptoms, the treatment of panic disorder should be delayed until the general medical condition is treated and/or the medication discontinued. However, there may be a general medical condition that is not directly causing the panic disorder. Studies show that panic and other anxiety disorders are more prevalent in medically ill patients than in the population at large. Conditions that have been specifically associated with panic disorder, but not etiologically, include irritable bowel syndrome, migraine, and pulmonary disease (237–239). Acute onset of a wide range of medical conditions may also be associated with the development of an anxiety disorder. When a coexisting general medical condition is present, it is important to treat the panic disorder, since panic symptoms may exacerbate the associated general medical condition. Data from some studies suggest that panic disorder and phobic anxiety may increase the risk of mortality in patients with cardiovascular disease (182, 240). In general, treatment of panic disorder in patients with irritable bowel syndrome, pulmonary disease, or migraine is not different from treatment of uncomplicated panic disorder. In fact, studies have documented improvement in respiratory symptoms and amelioration of irritable bowel symptoms upon treatment with SSRIs, even when full-blown panic disorder is not present. If renal or liver damage is present or if there is general debilitation from general medical illness, the medication dose should be adjusted appropriately.

C. DEMOGRAPHIC VARIABLES

1. Child and adolescent population

The following section contains a brief overview of the available data regarding the treatment of children and adolescents with panic disorder. Unless stated otherwise, the general considerations discussed in section IV of this guideline apply to children; this is especially true of the importance of psychiatric management. Information and recommendations regarding the etiology, diagnosis, and assessment of panic disorder are beyond the scope of this section. The reader is referred to the American Academy of Child and Adolescent Psychiatry's *Practice Parameters for the Assessment and Treatment of Children and Adolescents With Anxiety Disorders* (241) for a more detailed discussion. Finally, the treatments reviewed are those for which the results of formal clinical trials have been published. Given the paucity of such data in the child and adolescent literature, many treatment plans will necessarily include components that are not well studied. For example, child and adolescent psychiatrists frequently find that a treatment plan requires attention to developmental issues (from psychological and physiological perspectives) and the involvement of multiple systems (e.g., schools, family, and community).

Panic disorder occurs in children and, more commonly, adolescents; panic disorder often is preceded by or co-occurs with separation anxiety disorder. This section reviews the literature on the treatment of pediatric panic disorder.

The literature on panic disorder in youth is considerably less robust than that for adults (242), and much controversy attends the relationship between separation anxiety disorder and panic disorder (243–245). Experts generally agree that treatment of panic disorder in children is similar to treatment of panic disorder in adults: cognitive behavioral psychotherapy and, where necessary, pharmacotherapy. Because family involvement in symptoms is common, family-based treatment strategies are often necessary. The literature regarding the psychodynamic treatment of children and adolescents tends to be focused on broader categories of anxiety disorders.

In one study of adolescents (246), panic disorder was reported to have a prevalence of 0.6% (girls, 0.7%; boys, 0.4%). Fewer than half of the young persons with panic disorder in this study had received treatment for panic disorder symptoms. The incidence of so-called limited-symptom panic attacks in young adolescents is somewhat greater and shows a steep increase with the onset of puberty (247). Panic disorder also occurs before puberty, although the true prevalence is unknown. Whether prepubertal or postpubertal, the presentation of panic disorder in young persons appears to be quite similar to that in adults, with the caveat that younger children show more separation anxiety symptoms (6).

Panic disorder is commonly accompanied by a variety of specific phobias, including fear of the dark, monsters, kidnappers, bugs, small animals, heights, and open or closed-in spaces. Nighttime fears, resistance to going to bed, difficulty falling asleep alone or sleeping through the night alone, and nightmares involving separation themes are not uncommon. These specific phobic symptoms may be common triggers for panic or separation anxiety and therefore are responsible for many of the avoidance and ritualized anxiety-reducing behaviors seen in patients with both separation anxiety disorder and panic disorder (242). Children with panic disorder also show high rates of comorbidity with other anxiety disorders and with depression (248). In younger children, separation anxiety disorder precedes depression in approximately two-thirds of the cases and may form the nidus for recurrent affective illness and panic disorder if left untreated (249).

The terms "school phobia" and "school refusal" are sometimes treated as reflecting panic disorder, even though not all children with school refusal show panic disorder and not all children with panic disorder manifest school refusal (250, 251). Moreover, while many school-refusing children do show significant separation anxiety, others are "phobic" school refusers, i.e., they are phobic of something within the school context and not fearful of leaving home or family (252, 253). Children also may refuse to go to school because of depressive disorders, conduct disorder, family problems, learning disabilities, or unrecognized mild retardation.

There is limited empirical research supporting the efficacy of any type of treatment of panic disorder in the pediatric population (242). Unfortunately, the pediatric literature primarily comprises uncontrolled studies, which are reviewed here.

Only a few published studies have addressed the treatment of panic disorder in children with cognitive behavioral techniques, and of these, there are no studies of contrasting groups. Only one study used a single-case design. Ollendick (254) applied standard treatments for panic disorder in adults (36, 255) to four adolescents with DSM-III-R panic disorder using a multiple-baseline-across-subjects design. In all cases, the panic attacks were eliminated, agoraphobia was reduced, and the ability to handle future "panicogenic" situations was enhanced.

Medication management strategies that are effective for adults with panic disorder have received anecdotal support for use with children and adolescents, but no treatment has shown conclusive support. Scattered case reports (256, 257) and case series (258, 259) suggest that standard TCAs, SSRIs, and the high-potency benzodiazepines alprazolam and clonazepam may be useful in treating pediatric panic disorder.

2. Geriatric population

Although anxiety symptoms and disorders are among the most common psychiatric ailments experienced by older adults, epidemiologic studies suggest that the prevalence of panic disorder in later life may be lower than that for midlife (260). A vigorous search for alternative and comorbid diagnoses, especially general medical conditions and effects of general medical pharmacologic agents, should be undertaken for elderly patients presenting with new panic symptoms. There have been few prospective clinical trials of anxiety disorder treatments for the elderly to document systematically the efficacy of standard medications and/or psychosocial treatments for this age group. If medication is used, the required dose may be lower than that for younger patients. The medication dose should be very low to begin, and medication increases should be slower and more limited than with younger adults. (Additional information will be provided in the forthcoming practice guideline on geriatric psychiatry.)

3. Gender

Panic disorder is more common in women for reasons that are not yet fully understood. In the Epidemiologic Catchment Area Study, the lifetime prevalence of panic disorder was twice as high in women as in men (261). The treatment of pregnant and nursing women raises certain specific concerns regarding the use of antipanic medications. A careful evaluation of the risks associated with frequently used medications has recently been reviewed by Altshuler et al. (262).

4. Cultural issues

Relatively little research has been done on anxiety disorders in African Americans. The National Institute of Mental Health Epidemiologic Catchment Area Study (263) and the National Comorbidity Survey (264) provide somewhat conflicting data on the prevalence of anxiety disorders. The Epidemiologic Catchment Area Study indicated that African Americans have a higher lifetime prevalence of agoraphobia but not panic disorder, while the National Comorbidity Survey found no racial differences in the prevalence of any anxiety disorder (264–266). Although the prevalences may be similar, racial differences in help seeking and symptom presentation may result in underrecognition and misdiagnosis. In one study (267), researchers identified panic disorder in 25% of a group of minority psychiatric outpatients of whom none had received this diagnosis from their clinicians. There is some evidence of a different clinical presentation of panic disorder in African Americans; specifically, there are associations with isolated sleep paralysis (268) and hypertension (269, 270). Studies show that African American patients in primary care report more severe somatic symptoms and have a higher prevalence of panic disorder than whites (271) and that African Americans are more likely to seek help in medical than in mental health facilities (272, 273).

VI. RESEARCH DIRECTIONS

A substantial amount of research has been devoted to the description of the phenomenology and treatment of panic disorder in recent years. Because of this, treatment of panic disorder is generally quite successful. These guidelines reveal, however, a number of areas in which further research would be most desirable.

Although the diagnosis of panic disorder is fairly straightforward, it is increasingly clear that a large proportion of patients with panic disorder also suffer from other anxiety disorders, depression, substance use disorders, and personality disorders. We have relatively little information on the optimal ways of treating these combinations of conditions or the extent to which comorbidity affects prognosis and whether the observed high rates of comorbidity are due to chance or fundamental overlaps in psychopathology. Hence, a thorough understanding of the relationship between panic disorder and other psychiatric disorders is needed.

In addition, while the start of a successful treatment for a patient with panic disorder may include reassurance that panic attacks are not medically catastrophic events, there are emerging data indicating that patients with phobic anxiety may have higher long-term rates of cardiovascular morbidity and mortality. It is not yet clear whether this association applies to individuals with a true diagnosis of panic disorder and, if it does, whether treatment diminishes the risk. Clearly, research about the long-term health risks that may be associated with panic disorder is needed.

We have very little scientifically accumulated information about panic disorder in childhood. It has been argued that separation anxiety in childhood is a precursor for panic disorder, but this has not been systematically substantiated. The epidemiology of panic disorder in childhood has not been well studied, nor has the optimal therapeutic approach been established.

These guidelines review a number of effective interventions for panic disorder, including pharmacotherapy and psychotherapy. Treatments are highly successful when measured in terms of the rate of panic attack blockade. On the other hand, studies continue to show that blocking panic attacks is only part of the solution to panic disorder and that many patients continue to suffer from associated features of the illness, including anticipatory anxiety and phobic avoidance. Very few long-term studies have been conducted to inform clinicians about how long treatment should last before there can be a reasonable certainty that response can be sustained. It is not known, for example, whether there is a length of medication exposure after which the patient with panic disorder will have a low chance for relapse. Similarly, it is not clear whether "booster" sessions of CBT are useful.

Even in selecting the first treatment for a new patient with panic disorder, there is uncertainty. Rigorous studies have shown that both medications and CBT are better than control treatments for panic disorder and approximately equal to each other. We do not yet know whether some individuals respond better to either CBT or medications and, if so, how to identify them. Further, it is not yet known whether combinations of medication and CBT are more effective than either treatment alone. Within the pharmacotherapy options, many medications have been shown to be effective, but few studies have elucidated whether there are advantages of one class over another, how benzodiazepines should properly be used if combined with antidepressants, or the best options for patients with refractory cases. CBT generally involves a "package" of several techniques, but it is not certain whether all of them are necessary or even beneficial.

Psychodynamic therapies and psychoanalysis are widely used for patients with panic disorder. Research is clearly needed to document the rates of response of patients with panic disorder to psychodynamically based treatments. This kind of research is clearly possible and deserves attention. Furthermore, whether psychodynamic treatments combined with medication or CBT offer any advantage over any of these treatments alone needs to be explored.

Finally, the treatment of any medical illness has a greater likelihood of success if it addresses fundamental pathological processes. Preclinical science is rapidly providing important insights into the biology of fear, and these findings must be translated into the clinical arena. This promises to open the way to highly specific antipanic therapies that will be improvements even over the very successful treatments we already have.

VII. INDIVIDUALS AND ORGANIZATIONS THAT SUBMITTED COMMENTS

David A. Adler, M.D.
Dick Baldwin, M.D.
James Ballenger, M.D.
Richard Balon, M.D.
Patricia L. Baltazar, Ph.D.
David H. Barlow, M.D., Ph.D.
Monica A. Basco, Ph.D.
William Bebchuk, M.D.
J. Gayle Beck, Ph.D.
Bernard D. Beitman, M.D.
Carl C. Bell, M.D.
Dinesh Bhugra, M.D.
Charles H. Blackinton, M.D.
Jack Blaine, M.D.
Barton J. Blinder, M.D., Ph.D.
David Brook, M.D.
Oliver G. Cameron, M.D., Ph.D.
Carlyle Chan, M.D.
Norman A. Clemens, M.D.
Christopher C. Colenda, M.D., M.P.H.
Michelle G. Craske, Ph.D.
Dorynne Czechowicz, M.D.
Jonathan Davidson, M.D.
Dave M. Davis, M.D.
Ted Dinan, M.D., Ph.D.
Kim A. Eagle, M.D.
James M. Ellison, M.D., M.P.H.
Frederick Engstrom, M.D.
Ann Maxwell Eward, Ph.D.
Harvey H. Falit, M.D.
Edward D. Frohlich, M.D.
Glen Gabbard, M.D.
David T. George, M.D.
William Goldman, M.D.
Sheila Hafter Gray, M.D.
Michael K. Greenberg, M.D.
William M. Greenberg, M.D.
George T. Grossberg, M.D.

Daniel W. Hicks, M.D.
Mac Horton, M.D.
Richard Justman, M.D.
Nalani V. Juthani, M.D.
Gary Kaplan, M.D.
Robert A. Kimmich, M.D.
Donald F. Klein, M.D.
Lawrence Kline, M.D.
Ronald R. Koegler, M.D.
Barry J. Landau, M.D.
Susan Lazar, M.D.
Henrietta Leonard, M.D.
Robert Liberman, M.D.
Francis G. Lu, M.D.
Henry Mallard, M.D.
Barton J. Mann, M.D.
V. Manohar, M.D.
John C. Markowitz, M.D.
Isaac Marks, M.D.
Ronald L. Martin, M.D.
Matis Mavissakalian, M.D.
Joseph Mawhinney, M.D.
Michael Mayo-Smith, M.D.
Christopher J. McLaughlin, M.D.
Barbara Milrod, M.D.
Jerome Motto, M.D.
Marvin Nierenberg, M.D.
Philip T. Ninan, M.D.
Russell Noyes, M.D.
David Osser, M.D.
Mark H. Pollack, M.D.
C. Alec Pollard, Ph.D.
Charles W. Portney, M.D.
Elizabeth Rahdert, Ph.D.
Penny Randall, M.D.
Michelle Riba, M.D.
Vaughn Rickert, Psy.D.
Barbara Rosenfeld, M.D.

Peter Roy-Byrne, M.D.
Pedro Ruiz, M.D.
Carlotta Schuster, M.D.
John J. Schwab, M.D.
Warren Seides, M.D.
Susan Simmons-Alling, M.S., R.N., C.S.
William Sledge, M.D.
Herbert Smokler, M.D.
David Spiegel, M.D.
Roger F. Suchyta, M.D.
Eva Szigethy, M.D., Ph.D.
Gerald Tarlow, Ph.D.
William R. Tatomer, M.D.
David M. Tobolowsky, M.D.

Mauricio Tohen, M.D., Dr.P.H.
Samuel M. Turner, Ph.D.
Robert M. Ward, M.D.
Naimah Weinberg, M.D.
Myrna Weissman, Ph.D.
Joseph Westermeyer, M.D.,
    M.P.H., Ph.D.
R. Reid Wilson, Ph.D.
Thomas Wise, M.D.
Earl Witenberg, M.D.
Sherwyn Woods, M.D., Ph.D.
Jesse H. Wright, M.D.
Roberto Zarate, M.D.
Howard Zonana, M.D.

American Academy of Addiction Psychiatry
American Academy of Child and Adolescent Psychiatry
American Academy of Neurology
American Academy of Pediatrics
American Association of Suicidology
American College of Cardiology
American Geriatric Society
American Nurses Association
American Psychoanalytic Association
American Psychosomatic Society
American Society of Addiction Medicine
American Society of Clinical Pathologists
Association for Academic Psychiatry
Association for the Advancement of Behavior Therapy
Association of Gay and Lesbian Psychiatrists
Baltimore/Washington Society for Psychoanalysis
Group for the Advancement of Psychiatry
National Institute on Drug Abuse
Royal College of Psychiatrists
Society for Adolescent Medicine

VIII. REFERENCES

The following coding system is used to indicate the nature of the supporting evidence in the summary recommendations and references:

[A]   *Randomized clinical trial.* A study of an intervention in which subjects are prospectively followed over time; there are treatment and control groups; subjects are randomly assigned to the two groups; both the subjects and the investigators are blind to the assignments.

[B]   *Clinical trial.* A prospective study in which an intervention is made and the results of that intervention are tracked longitudinally; study does not meet standards for a randomized clinical trial.

[C]   *Cohort or longitudinal study.* A study in which subjects are prospectively followed over time without any specific intervention.

[D]   *Case-control study.* A study in which a group of patients is identified in the present and information about them is pursued retrospectively or backward in time.

[E]   *Review with secondary data analysis.* A structured analytic review of existing data, e.g., a meta-analysis or a decision analysis.

[F]   *Review.* A qualitative review and discussion of previously published literature without a quantitative synthesis of the data.

[G]   *Other.* Textbooks, expert opinion, case reports, and other reports not included above.

1. American Psychiatric Association: Diagnostic and Statistical Manual of Mental Disorders, 4th ed (DSM-IV). Washington, DC, APA, 1994 [G]

2. Ballenger JC, Pecknold J, Rickels K, Sellers EM: Medication discontinuation in panic disorders. J Clin Psychiatry 1993; 54(Oct suppl):15–21, discussion 22–24 [F]

3. Katschnig H, Amering M, Stolk JM, Ballenger JC: Predictors of quality of life in a long-term follow-up study of panic disorder patients after a clinical drug trial. Psychopharmacol Bull 1996; 32:149–155 [C]

4. Roy-Byrne PP, Cowley DS: Course and outcome in panic disorder: a review of recent follow-up studies. Anxiety 1995; 1:150–160 [F]

5. Weissman MM, Bland RC, Canino GJ, Faravelli C, Greenwald S, Hwu HG, Joyce PR, Karam EG, Lee CK, Lellouch J, Lepine JP, Newman SC, Oakley-Browne MA, Rubio-Stipec M, Wells JE, Wickramaratne PJ, Wittchen HA, Yeh EK: The cross-national epidemiology of panic disorder. Arch Gen Psychiatry 1997; 54:305–309 [E]

6. Moreau D, Weissman MM: Panic disorder in children and adolescents: a review. Am J Psychiatry 1992; 149:1306–1314 [F]

7. Lesser IM, Rubin RT, Rifkin RP, Swinson RP, Ballenger JC, Burrows GD, DuPont RL, Noyes R, Pecknold JC: Secondary depression in panic disorder and agoraphobia, II: dimensions of depression symptomatology and their response to treatment. J Affect Disord 1989; 16:49–58 [B]

8. Klerman G, Weissman MM, Ouellette R, Johnson J, Greenwald S: Panic attacks in the community: social morbidity and health care utilization. JAMA 1991; 265:742–746 [E]

9. Weissman MM, Klerman GL, Markowitz JS, Ouellette R: Suicidal ideation and attempts in panic disorder and attacks. N Engl J Med 1989; 321:1209–1214 [C]

10. Markowitz JS, Weissman MM, Ouellette R, Lish JD, Klerman GL: Quality of life in panic disorder. Arch Gen Psychiatry 1989; 46:984–992 [B]

11. Knowles JA, Weissman MM: Panic disorder and agoraphobia, in American Psychiatric Press Review of Psychiatry, vol 14. Edited by Oldham JM, Riba MB. Washington, DC, American Psychiatric Press, 1995, pp 383–404 [G]

12. Goldstein RB, Wickramarante PJ, Horwath E, Weissman MM: Familial aggregation and phenomenology of "early"-onset (at or before age 20 years) panic disorder. Arch Gen Psychiatry 1997; 54:271–278 [C]

13. Kendler KS, Neale MC, Kessler RC, Heath AC, Eaves LJ: A test of the equal-environment assumption in twin studies of psychiatric illness. Behav Genet 1993; 23:21–27 [D]

14. Kendler KS, Neale MC, Kessler RC, Heath AC, Eaves LJ: Panic disorder in women: a population-based twin study. Psychol Med 1993; 23:387–406 [D]

15. American Psychiatric Association: Practice Guideline for Psychiatric Evaluation of Adults. Am J Psychiatry 1995; 152(Nov suppl):63–80 [G]

16. Cross-National Collaborative Panic Study SPI: Drug treatment of panic disorder: comparative efficacy of alprazolam, imipramine, and placebo. Br J Psychiatry 1992; 160:191–202, discussion 202–205; correction 1993; 161:724 [A]

17. Barlow DH, Craske MG: Mastery of Your Anxiety and Panic II. Albany, NY, Graywind Publications, 1994 [G]

18. Lydiard RB, Morton WA, Emmanuel NP, Zealberg JJ, Laraia MT, Stuart GW, O'Neil PM, Ballenger JC: Preliminary report: placebo-controlled, double-blind study of the clinical and metabolic effects of desipramine in panic disorder. Psychopharmacol Bull 1993; 29:183–188 [A]

19. Barlow DH, Craske MG, Cerney JA, Klosko JS: Behavioral treatment of panic disorder. Behavior Therapy 1989; 20:261–282 [A]

20. Clark DM, Salkovskis PM, Hackmann A, Middleton H, Anastasiades P, Gelder M: A comparison of cognitive therapy, applied relaxation and imipramine in the treatment of panic disorder. Br J Psychiatry 1994; 164:759–769 [A]

21. Beck AT, Sokol L, Clark DA, Berchick R, Wright F: A crossover study of focused cognitive therapy for panic disorder. Am J Psychiatry 1992; 149:778–783 [A]

22. Lydiard RB, Lesser IM, Ballenger JC, Rubin RT, Laraia M, DuPont R: A fixed-dose study of alprazolam 2 mg, alprazolam 6 mg, and placebo in panic disorder. J Clin Psychopharmacol 1992; 12:96–103 [A]

23. Fiegenbaum W: Long-term efficacy of ungraded versus graded massed exposure in agoraphobics, in Panic and Phobias 2: Treatments and Variables Affecting Course and Outcome. Edited by Hand I, Wittchen H-U. Berlin, Springer-Verlag, 1988, pp 83–88 [G]

24. Barlow DH: Anxiety and Its Disorders: The Nature and Treatment of Anxiety and Panic. New York, Guilford Press, 1988 [G]

25. Chambless DL, Gillis MM: Cognitive therapy of anxiety disorders. J Consult Clin Psychol 1993; 61:248–260 [E]

26. Clum GA, Suris R: A meta-analysis of treatments for panic disorder. J Consult Clin Psychol 1993; 61:317–326 [E]

27. Hofmann SG, Lehman CL, Barlow DH: How specific are specific phobias? J Behav Ther Exp Psychiatry 1997; 28:233–240 [C]

28. Margraf J, Gobel M, Schneider S: Cognitive-Behavioral Treatments for Panic Disorder, vol 5. Amsterdam, Swets and Zeitlinger, 1990 [G]

29. Craske MG, Brown TA, Barlow DH: Behavioral treatment of panic disorder: a two-year follow-up. Behavior Therapy 1991; 22:289–304 [D]

30. Klosko JS, Barlow DH, Tassinari R, Cerny JA: A comparison of alprazolam and behavior therapy in treatment of panic disorder. J Consult Clin Psychol 1990; 58:77–84 [A]

31. Clark DB, Agras WS: The assessment and treatment of performance anxiety in musicians. Am J Psychiatry 1991; 148:598–605 [A]

32. Black DW, Wesner R, Bowers W, Gabel J: A comparison of fluvoxamine, cognitive therapy and placebo in the treatment of panic disorder. Arch Gen Psychiatry 1993; 50:44–50 [A]

33. Telch MJ, Lucas JA, Schmidt NB, Hanna HH, Jaimez LT, Lucas RA: Group cognitive-behavioral treatment of panic disorder. Behav Res Ther 1993; 31:279–287 [A]

34. Craske MG, Rodriguez BI: Behavioral treatment of panic disorders and agoraphobia. Prog Behav Modif 1994; 29:1–26 [A]

35. Shear MK, Pilkonis PA, Cloitre M, Leon AC: Cognitive behavioral treatment compared with nonprescriptive treatment of panic disorder. Arch Gen Psychiatry 1994; 51:395–401 [A]

36. Ost LG, Westling BE: Applied relaxation vs cognitive behavior therapy in the treatment of panic disorder. Behav Res Ther 1995; 33:145–158 [A]

37. Ost LG, Westling BE, Hellstrom K: Applied relaxation exposure in vivo and cognitive methods in the treatment of panic disorder with agoraphobia. Behav Res Ther 1993; 31:383–394 [A]

38. van den Hout M, Arntz A, Hoekstra R: Exposure reduced agoraphobia but not panic and cognitive therapy reduced pain but not agoraphobia. Behav Res Ther 1994; 32:447–451 [A]

39. Marks IM, Swinson RP, Basoglu M: Alprazolam and exposure alone and combined in panic disorder with agoraphobia. Br J Psychiatry 1993; 162:776–787 [B]

40. Swinson RP, Soulios C, Cox BJ, Kuch K: Brief treatment of emergency room patients with panic attacks. Am J Psychiatry 1992; 149:944–946 [A]

41. Swinson RP, Fergus KD, Cox BJ, Wickwire K: Efficacy of telephone-administered behavioral therapy for panic disorder. Behav Res Ther 1995; 33:465–469 [B]

42. Fava GA, Zielezny M, Savron G, Grandi S: Long-term effects of behavioural treatment for panic disorder with agoraphobia. Br J Psychiatry 1995; 166:87–92 [B]

43. Brown TA, Barlow DH: Long term outcome of cognitive behavioral treatment of panic disorder. J Consult Clin Psychol 1995; 63:754–765 [B]

44. O'Sullivan G, Marks IM: Long-term outcome of phobic and obsessive compulsive disorders after exposure: a review chapter, in The Treatment of Anxiety: Handbook of Anxiety, vol 4. Edited by Noyes R, Roth M, Burrows G. Amsterdam, Elsevier, 1990, pp 82–108 [G]

45. Barlow DH: Cognitive-behavioral therapy for panic disorder: current status. J Clin Psychiatry 1997; 58(suppl 2):32–36 [F]

46. Shear MK, Barlow D, Gorman J, Woods S: Multicenter treatment study of panic disorder. Presented at the 36th annual meeting of the American College of Neuropsychopharmacology, Kamuela, Hawaii, Dec 8–12, 1997 [A]

47. Neron S, Lacroix D, Chaput Y: Group vs individual cognitive behaviour therapy in panic disorder: an open clinical trial with a six month follow-up. Can J Behavioral Sci 1995; 27:379–392 [C]

48. Cerny JA, Barlow DH, Craske MG, Himadi WG: Couples treatment of agoraphobia: a two-year follow-up. Behavior Therapy 1987; 18:401–415 [C]

49. Craske MG, Rowe M, Lewin M, Noriega-Dimitri R: Interoceptive exposure versus breathing retraining within cognitive-behavioural therapy for panic disorder with agoraphobia. Br J Clin Psychol 1997; 36(part 1):85–99 [A]

50. Hoffart A, Thornes K, Hedley LM: DSM-III-R axis I and II disorders in agoraphobic inpatients before and after psychosocial treatment. Psychiatry Res 1995; 56:1–9 [C]

51. Lidren D, Watkins P, Gould R, Clum G, Asterino M, Tulloch H: A comparison of bibliotherapy and group therapy in the treatment of panic disorder. J Consult Clin Psychol 1994; 62:865–869 [B]

52. Carter MM, Turovsky J, Barlow DH: Interpersonal relationships in panic disorder with agoraphobia: a review of empirical evidence. Clin Psychol: Science and Practice 1994; 1:25–34 [F]

53. Spiegel DA, Bruce TJ, Gregg SF, Nuzzarello A: Does cognitive behavior therapy assist slow-taper alprazolam discontinuation in panic disorder? Am J Psychiatry 1994; 151: 876–881 [A]

54. Otto MW, Pollack MH, Sachs GS, Reiter SR, Meltzer-Brody S, Rosenbaum JF: Discontinuation of benzodiazepine treatment: efficacy of cognitive-behavioral therapy for patients with panic disorder. Am J Psychiatry 1993; 150:1485–1490 [A]

55. Spiegel DA, Bruce TJ: Benzodiazepines and exposure-based cognitive behavior therapies for panic disorder: conclusion from combined treatment trials. Am J Psychiatry 1997; 154:773–781 [F]

56. Milrod B, Busch F, Cooper A, Shapiro T: Manual of Panic-Focused Psychodynamic Psychotherapy. Washington, DC, American Psychiatric Press, 1997 [G]

57. Kohut H: Thoughts on narcissism and narcissistic rage. Psychoanal Study Child 1972; 27:360–400 [G]

58. Bash M: Doing Brief Psychotherapy. New York, Basic Books, 1995 [G]

59. Gray JA: The neuropsychiatry of anxiety. Br J Psychol 1978; 69:417–434 [G]

60. Sifneos PE: The current status of individual short-term dynamic psychotherapy and its future: an overview. Am J Psychother 1984; 38:472–483 [G]

61. Sifneos PE: Short-term dynamic psychotherapy for patients with physical symptomatology. Psychother Psychosom 1984; 42:48–51 [F]

62. Shear MK: Psychotherapeutic issues in long-term treatment of anxiety disorder patients. Psychiatr Clin North Am 1995; 18:885–894 [F]

63. Wiborg IM, Dahl AA: Does brief dynamic psychotherapy reduce the relapse rate of panic disorder? Arch Gen Psychiatry 1996; 53:689–694 [A]

64. Beitman BD, Goldfried MR, Norcross JC: The movement toward integrating the psychotherapies: an overview. Am J Psychiatry 1989; 146:138–147 [G]

65. Shear MK, Weiner K: Psychotherapy for panic disorder. J Clin Psychiatry 1997; 58(suppl 2):38–43 [G]

66. Zitrin CM, Klein DF, Woerner MG: Treatment of agoraphobia with group exposure in vivo and imipramine. Arch Gen Psychiatry 1980; 37:63–72 [A]

67. Zitrin CM, Klein DF, Woerner MG, Ross DC: Treatment of phobias, I: comparison of imipramine hydrochloride and placebo. Arch Gen Psychiatry 1983; 40:125–138 [A]

68. Marks IM, Gray S, Cohen D, Hill R, Mawson D, Ramm E, Stern RS: Imipramine and brief therapist-aided exposure in agoraphobics having self-exposure homework. Arch Gen Psychiatry 1983; 40:153–162 [A]

69. Mavissakalian M, Michelson L, Dealy RS: Pharmacological treatment of agoraphobia: imipramine vs imipramine with programmed practice. Br J Psychiatry 1983; 143:348–355 [A]

70. Telch MJ, Agras WS, Taylor CB, Roth WT, Gallen CC: Combined pharmacological and behavioral treatment for agoraphobia. Behav Res Ther 1985; 23:325–335 [A]

71. Mavissakalian M, Michelson L: Relative and combined effectiveness of therapist-assisted in vivo exposure and imipramine. J Clin Psychiatry 1986; 47:117–122 [B]

72. Mavissakalian M, Michelson L: Two-year follow-up of exposure and imipramine treatment of agoraphobia. Am J Psychiatry 1986; 143:1106–1112 [B]

73. Oehrberg S, Christiansen PE, Behnke K: Paroxetine in the treatment of panic disorder: a randomized double-blind placebo-controlled study. Br J Psychiatry 1995; 167:374–379 [A]

74. Pollack MH, Otto MW, Kaspi SP, Hammerness PG, Rosenbaum JF: Cognitive behavior therapy for treatment-refractory panic disorder. J Clin Psychiatry 1994; 55:200–205 [B]

75. Nagy LM, Krystal JH, Woods SW: Clinical and medication outcome after short-term alprazolam and behavioral group treatment of panic disorder: 2.5 year naturalistic follow-up. Arch Gen Psychiatry 1989; 46:993–999 [B, C]

76. Kabat-Zinn J, Massion AO, Kristeller J, Peterson LG, Fletcher KE, Pbert L, Lenderking WR, Santorelli SF: Effectiveness of a meditation-based stress reduction program in the treatment of anxiety disorders. Am J Psychiatry 1992; 149:936–943 [B]

77. Miller JJ, Fletcher K, Kabat-Zinn J: Three-year follow-up and clinical implications of a mindfulness meditation-based stress reduction intervention in the treatment of anxiety disorders. Gen Hosp Psychiatry 1995; 17:192–200 [D]

78. Buglass D, Clarke J, Henderson AS, Kreitman N: A study of agoraphobic housewives. Psychol Med 1977; 7:73–86 [D]

79. Arrindell WA, Emmelkamp PM: Marital adjustment, intimacy and needs in female agoraphobics and their partners: a controlled study. Br J Psychiatry 1986; 149:592–602; correction 1987; 150:273 [D]

80. Lange A, van Dyck R: The function of agoraphobia in the marital relationship. Acta Psychiatr Scand 1992; 85:89–93 [E]

81. Hafner RJ: Predicting the effects on husbands of behaviour therapy for wives' agoraphobia. Behav Res Ther 1984; 22: 217–226 [C]

82. Milton F, Hafner J: The outcome of behavior therapy for agoraphobia in relation to marital adjustment. Arch Gen Psychiatry 1979; 36:807–811 [B]

83. Jacobson NS, Holtzworth-Monroe A, Schmaling KB: Marital therapy and spouse involvement in the treatment of depression, agoraphobia, and alcoholism. J Consult Clin Psychol 1989; 57:5–10 [F]

84. Himadi WG, Cerny JA, Barlow DH, Cohen S, O'Brien GT: The relationship of marital adjustment to agoraphobia treatment outcome. Behav Res Ther 1986; 24:107–115 [C]

85. Barlow DH, O'Brien GT, Last CG: Couples treatment of agoraphobia. Behavior Therapy 1984; 15:41–58 [C]

86. Arnow BA, Taylor CB, Agras WS: Enhancing agoraphobia treatment outcome by changing couple communication patterns. Behavior Therapy 1985; 16:452–467 [C]

87. Lydiard RB, Pollack MH, Judge R, Michelson D, Tamura R: Fluoxetine in panic disorder: a placebo-controlled study. Presented at the 10th Congress of the European College of Neuropsychopharmacology, Vienna, Sept 13–17, 1997 [A]

88. Gorman JM, Liebowitz MR, Fyer AJ, Goetz D, Campeas RB, Fyer MR, Davies SO, Klein DF: An open trial of fluoxetine in the treatment of panic disorder. J Clin Psychopharmacol 1987; 7:319–332 [B]

89. Schneier FR, Liebowitz MR, Davies SO, Fairbanks J, Hollander E, Campeas R, Klein DF: Fluoxetine in panic disorder. J Clin Psychopharmacol 1990; 10:119–121 [B]

90. Wolkow R, Apter J, Clayton A, Coryell W, Cunningham L, McEntee W, O'Hair D, Pollack M, Rausch J, Stewart R, Weisler R: Double-blind flexible dose study of sertraline and placebo in patients with panic disorder. Presented at the XX Congress of the Collegium Internationale Neuro-Psychopharmacologicum, Melbourne, Australia, June 23–27, 1996 [A]

91. Baumel B, Bielski R, Carman J, Hegel M, Houck C, Linden R, Nakra B, Ota K, Pohl R, Wolkow R: Double-blind comparison of sertraline and placebo in patients with panic disorder. Ibid [A]

92. Ballenger JC, Wheadon DE, Steiner M, Bushnell W, Gergel IP: Double-blind, fixed-dose, placebo-controlled study of paroxetine in the treatment of panic disorder. Am J Psychiatry 1998; 155:36–42 [A]

93. LeCrubier Y, Bakker A, Dunbar G, Judge R: A comparison of paroxetine, clomipramine and placebo in the treatment of panic disorder. Acta Psychiatr Scand 1997; 95:145–152 [A]

94. Hoehn-Saric R, McLeod DR, Hipsley PA: Effect of fluvoxamine on panic disorder. J Clin Psychopharmacol 1993; 13: 321–326 [B]

95. de Beurs E, van Balkom AJ, Lange A, Koele P, van Dyck R: Treatment of panic disorder with agoraphobia: comparison of fluvoxamine, placebo, and psychological panic management combined with exposure and of exposure in vivo alone. Am J Psychiatry 1995; 152:683–691 [B]

96. Westenberg HG, den Boer JA: Selective monoamine uptake inhibitors and a serotonin antagonist in the treatment of panic disorder. Psychopharmacol Bull 1989; 25:119–123 [B]

97. Wade AG, Lepola U, Koponen HJ, Pedersen V, Pedersen T: The effect of citalopram in panic disorder. Br J Psychiatry 1997; 170:549–553 [A]

98. Boyer W: Serotonin uptake inhibitors are superior to imipramine and alprazolam in alleviating panic attacks: a meta-analysis. Int Clin Psychopharmacol 1995; 10:45–49 [E]

99. Lejoyeux M, Ades J: Antidepressant discontinuation: a review of the literature. J Clin Psychiatry 1997; 58(July suppl): 11–16 [G]

100. Louie AK, Lewis TB, Lannon RA: Use of low-dose fluoxetine in major depression and panic disorder. J Clin Psychiatry 1993; 54:435–438 [C]

101. Emmanuel NP, Crosby C, Ware MR, Lydiard RB: The efficacy of once-a-week fluoxetine dosing in the treatment of panic disorder, in 1996 Annual Meeting New Research Program and Abstracts. Washington, DC, American Psychiatric Association, 1996, p 252 [G]

102. DuBoff E, England D, Ferguson JM, Londborg PD, Rosenthal MH, Smith W, Weise C, Wolkow RM: Sertraline in the treatment of panic disorder. Presented at the 8th Congress of the European College of Neuropsychopharmacology, Venice, Sept 30 to Oct 4, 1995 [A]

103. Gergel I, Burnham D, Kumar R: Treatment of panic disorder with paroxetine. Presented at the 6th World Congress of Biological Psychiatry, Nice, France, June 22–27, 1997 [A]

104. Klein D: Delineation of two drug-responses for anxiety syndromes. Psychopharmacologia 1964; 5:397–408 [A]

105. Uhlenhuth EH, Matuzas W, Glass RM, Easton C: Response of panic disorder to fixed doses of alprazolam or imipramine. J Affect Disord 1989; 17:261–270 [A]

106. Modigh K, Westberg P, Eriksson E: Superiority of clomipramine over imipramine in the treatment of panic disorder: a placebo-controlled trial. J Clin Psychopharmacol 1992; 12:251–261 [A]

107. Andersch S, Rosenberg NK, Kullingsjo H, Ottoson JQ, Hanson L, Lorentzen K, Mellergard M, Rasmussen S, Rosenberg R: Efficacy and safety of alprazolam, imipramine, and placebo in treating panic disorder: a Scandinavian multicenter study. Acta Psychiatr Scand Suppl 1991; 365:18–27 [A]

108. Mavissakalian M, Perel J: Imipramine in the treatment of agoraphobia: dose-response relationships. Am J Psychiatry 1985; 142:1032–1036 [A]

109. Mavissakalian MR, Perel JM: Imipramine dose-response relationship in panic disorder with agoraphobia. Arch Gen Psychiatry 1989; 46:127–131 [A]

110. Mavissakalian MR, Perel JM: Imipramine treatment of panic disorder with agoraphobia: dose ranging and plasma level-response relationships. Am J Psychiatry 1995; 152:673–682 [A]

111. Maier W, Roth SM, Argyle N, Buller R, Lavori P, Brandon S, Benkert O: Avoidance behaviour: a predictor of the efficacy of pharmacotherapy in panic disorder? Eur Arch Psychiatry Clin Neurosci 1991; 241:151–158 [A]

112. Cassano GB, Toni C, Musetti L: Treatment of panic disorder, in Synaptic Transmission. Edited by Biggio G, Concas A, Costa E. New York, Raven Press, 1992, pp 449–461 [A]

113. Curtis GC, Massana J, Udina C, Ayuso JL, Cassano GB, Perugi G: Maintenance drug therapy of panic disorder. J Psychiatr Res 1993; 27(suppl 1):127–142 [A]

114. Keller MB, Lavori PW, Goldenberg IM, Baker LA, Pollack MH, Sachs GS, Rosenbaum JF, Deltito JA, Leon A, Shear K, Klerman GL: Influence of depression on the treatment of panic disorder with imipramine, alprazolam, imipramine. J Affect Disord 1993; 28:27–38 [A]

115. Woods S, Nagy LM, Koleszar AS, Krystal JH, Heninger GR, Charney DS: Controlled trial of alprazolam supplementation during imipramine treatment of panic disorder. J Clin Psychopharmacol 1991; 12:32–38 [A]

116. Mellergard M, Lorentzen K, Bech P, Ottoson JQ, Rosenberg R: A trend analysis of changes during treatment of panic disorder with alprazolam and imipramine. Acta Psychiatr Scand Suppl 1991; 365:28–32 [A]

117. Pollack MH, Otto MW, Sachs GS, Leon A, Shear MK, Deltito JA, Keller MB, Rosenbaum JF: Anxiety psychopathology predictive of outcome in patients with panic disorder and depression treated with imipramine, alprazolam, and placebo. J Affect Disord 1994; 30:273–281 [A]

118. Den Boer JA, Westenberg HG: Effect of a serotonin and noradrenaline uptake inhibitor in panic disorder: a double-blind comparative study with fluvoxamine and maprotiline. Int Clin Psychopharmacol 1988; 3:59–74 [B]

119. Cassano GB, Petracca A, Perugi G, Nisita C, Musetti L, Mengali F, McNair DM: Clomipramine for panic disorder, I: the first 10 weeks of a long-term comparison with imipramine. J Affect Disord 1988; 14:123–127 [B]

120. Monteiro WO, Noshirvani HF, Marks IM: Anorgasmia from clomipramine in obsessive-compulsive disorder: a controlled trial. Br J Psychiatry 1987; 151:107–112 [B]

121. Mavissakalian M, Perel JM: Clinical experiments in maintenance and discontinuation of imipramine therapy in panic disorder with agoraphobia. Arch Gen Psychiatry 1992; 49:318–323 [B]

122. Mavissakalian M, Perel JM: Protective effects of imipramine maintenance treatment in panic disorder with agoraphobia. Am J Psychiatry 1992; 149:1053–1057 [B]

123. Sheehan DV: Tricyclic antidepressants in the treatment of panic and anxiety disorders. Psychosomatics 1986; 27:10–16 [F]

124. Fyer AJ, Liebowitz MR, Gorman JM, Campeas R, Levin A, Davies SO, Goetz D, Klein DF: Discontinuation of alprazolam treatment in panic patients. Am J Psychiatry 1987; 144:303–308 [B]

125. Klerman GL: Overview of the Cross-National Collaborative Panic Study. Arch Gen Psychiatry 1988; 45:407–412 [F]

126. Dunner DL, Ishiki D, Avery DH, Wilson LG, Hyde TS: Effect of alprazolam and diazepam in anxiety and panic attacks in panic disorder: a controlled study. J Clin Psychiatry 1986; 47:458–460 [B]

127. Ballenger JC, Burrows GD, DuPont RL Jr, Lesser IM, Noyes R Jr, Pecknold JC, Rifkin A, Swinson RP: Alprazolam in panic disorder and agoraphobia: results from a multicenter trial, I: efficacy in short-term treatment. Arch Gen Psychiatry 1988; 45:413–422 [A]

128. Tesar GE, Rosenbaum JF, Pollack MH, Otto MW, Sachs GS, Herman JB, Cohen LS, Spier SA: Double-blind, placebo-controlled comparison of clonazepam and alprazolam for panic disorder. J Clin Psychiatry 1991; 52:69–76 [A]

129. Schweizer E, Rickels K, Weiss S, Zavodnick S: Maintenance drug treatment of panic disorder, I: results of a prospective, placebo-controlled comparison of alprazolam and imipramine. Arch Gen Psychiatry 1993; 50:51–60 [A]

130. Dager SR, Roy-Byrne P, Hendrickson H, Cowley DS, Avery DH, Hall KC, Dunner DL: Long-term outcome of panic states during double-blind treatment and after withdrawal of alprazolam and placebo. Ann Clin Psychiatry 1992; 4:251–258 [A]

131. Chouinard G, Annable L, Fontaine R, Solyom L: Alprazolam in the treatment of generalized anxiety and panic disorders: a double-blind placebo-controlled study. Psychopharmacology (Berl) 1982; 77:229–233 [B]

132. McNair DM, Kahn RJ: Imipramine compared with a benzodiazepine for agoraphobia, in Anxiety: New Research and Changing Concepts. Edited by Klein DF, Rabkin J. New York, Raven Press, 1981, pp 69–80 [B]

133. Noyes RJ, Anderson DJ, Clancy J, Crowe RR, Slymen DJ, Ghoneim MM, Hinrichs JV: Diazepam and propranolol in panic disorder and agoraphobia. Arch Gen Psychiatry 1984; 41:287–292 [A]

134. Schweizer E, Rickels K: Failure of buspirone to manage benzodiazepine withdrawal. Am J Psychiatry 1986; 143:1590–1592 [B]

135. Schweizer E, Case WG, Rickels K: Benzodiazepine dependence and withdrawal in elderly patients. Am J Psychiatry 1989; 146:529–531 [B]

136. Schweizer E, Clary C, Dever AI, Mandos LA: The use of low-dose intranasal midazolam to treat panic disorder: a pilot study. J Clin Psychiatry 1992; 53:19–22 [B]

137. Charney DS, Woods SW: Benzodiazepine treatment of panic disorder: a comparison of alprazolam and lorazepam. J Clin Psychiatry 1989; 50:418–423 [B]

138. Pyke RE, Greenberg HS: Double-blind comparison of alprazolam and adinazolam for panic and phobia disorders. J Clin Psychopharmacol 1989; 9:15–21 [B]

139. Savoldi F, Somenzini G, Ecari U: Etizolam versus placebo in the treatment of panic disorder with agoraphobia: a double-blind study. Curr Med Res Opin 1990; 12:185–190 [A]

140. Beaudry P, Fontaine R, Chouinard G: Bromazepam, another high-potency benzodiazepine for panic attacks (letter). Am J Psychiatry 1984; 141:464–465 [G]

141. Noyes R, Borrows GD, Reich JH, Judd FK, Garvey M, Morman TR, Cook BL, Marriot P: Diazepam versus alprazolam for the treatment of panic disorder. J Clin Psychiatry 1996; 57:349–355 [A]

142. Benzodiazepine Dependence, Toxicity, and Abuse: A Task Force Report of the American Psychiatric Association. Washington, DC, APA, 1990 [G]

143. Rickels K, Schweizer E, Weiss S, Zavodnick S: Maintenance drug treatment for panic disorder, II: short- and long-term outcome after drug taper. Arch Gen Psychiatry 1993; 50:61–68 [B]

144. Klein E, Colin V, Stolk J, Lenox RH: Alprazolam withdrawal in patients with panic disorder and generalized anxiety disorder: vulnerability and effect of carbamazapine. Am J Psychiatry 1994; 151:1760–1766 [A]

145. Noyes R Jr, Garvey MJ, Cook B, Suelzer M: Controlled discontinuation of benzodiazepine treatment for patients with panic disorder. Am J Psychiatry 1991; 148:517–523 [B]

146. Pecknold JC, Swinson RP: Taper withdrawal studies with alprazolam inpatients with panic disorder and agoraphobia. Psychopharmacol Bull 1986; 22:173–176 [A]

147. Rosenbaum JF, Moroz G, Bowden CL: Clonazepam in the treatment of panic disorder with or without agoraphobia: a dose-response study of efficacy, safety, and discontinuance. J Clin Psychopharmacol 1997; 17:390–400 [A]

148. Lesser IM, Lydiard RB, Antal E, Rubin RT, Ballenger JC, DuPont R: Alprazolam plasma concentrations and treatment response in panic disorder and agoraphobia. Am J Psychiatry 1992; 149:1556–1562 [A]

149. Greenblatt DJ, Harmatiz JS, Shader RI: Plasma alprazolam concentrations: relation to efficacy and side effects in the treatment of panic disorder. Arch Gen Psychiatry 1993; 50: 715–722 [B]

150. Lepola UM, Rimon RH, Riekkinen PJ: Three-year follow-up of patients with panic disorder after short-term treatment with alprazolam and imipramine. Int Clin Psychopharmacol 1993; 8:115–118 [B]

151. Sheehan DV, Claycomb JB, Kouretas N: Monoamine oxidase inhibitors: prescription and patient management. Int J Psychiatry Med 1980–1981; 10:99–121 [G]

152. American Psychiatric Association: Diagnostic and Statistical Manual of Mental Disorders, 2nd ed (DSM-II). Washington, DC, APA, 1968 [G]

153. Bakish D, Saxena BM, Bowen R, D'Souza J: Reversible monoamine oxidase-A inhibitors in panic disorder. Clin Neuropsychopharmacol 1993; 16(suppl 2):S77–S82 [A]

154. Garcia-Borreguero D, Lauer CJ, Ozdaglar A, Wiedemann K, Holsboer F, Krieg JC: Brofaromine in panic disorder: a pilot study with a new reversible inhibitor of monoamine oxidase-A. Pharmacopsychiatry 1992; 25:261–264 [B]

155. van Harten J: Clinical pharmacokinetics of selective serotonin reuptake inhibitors. Clin Pharmacokinet 1993; 24:203–220 [F]

156. Pollack MH, Worthington JJ, Otto MW, Maki KM, Smoller JW, Manfro GG, Rudolph R, Rosenbaum JF: Venlafaxine for panic disorder: results from a double-blind, placebo-controlled study. Psychopharmacol Bull 1996; 32:667–670 [A]

157. Geracioti JD: Venlafaxine treatment of panic disorder: a case series. J Clin Psychiatry 1995; 56:408–410 [G]

158. Charney DS, Woods SW, Goodman WK, Rifkin B, Kinch M, Aiken B, Quadrino LM, Heninger GR: Drug treatment of panic disorder: the comparative efficacy of imipramine, alprazolam, and trazodone. J Clin Psychiatry 1986; 47:580–586 [B]

159. Mavissakalian M, Perel J, Bowler K, Dealy R: Trazodone in the treatment of panic disorder and agoraphobia with panic attacks. Am J Psychiatry 1987; 144:785–787 [B]

160. Sheehan DV, Davidson J, Manschreck T, Van Wyck Fleet J: Lack of efficacy of a new antidepressant (bupropion) in the treatment of panic disorder with phobias. J Clin Psychopharmacol 1983; 3:28–31 [G]

161. Zajecka JM: The effect of nefazodone on comorbid anxiety symptoms associated with depression: experience in family practice and psychiatric outpatient settings. J Clin Psychiatry 1996; 57(2 suppl):10–14 [A]

162. DeMartinis NA, Schweizer E, Rickels K: An open-label trial of nefazodone in high comorbidity panic disorder. J Clin Psychiatry 1996; 57:245–248 [B]

163. Keck PE Jr, McElroy SL, Friedman LM: Valproate and carbamazepine in the treatment of panic and posttraumatic stress disorders, withdrawal states, and behavioral dyscontrol syndromes. J Clin Psychopharmacol 1992; 12(1 suppl):36S–41S [F]

164. Uhde TW, Stein MB, Post RM: Lack of efficacy of carbamazepine in the treatment of panic disorder. Am J Psychiatry 1988; 145:1104–1109 [B]

165. Lum M, Fontaine R, Elie R, Ontiveros A: Divalproex sodium's antipanic effect in panic disorder: a placebo-controlled study. Biol Psychiatry 1990; 27(9A):164A [A, B]

166. Woodman CL, Noyes R: Panic disorder: treatment with valproate. J Clin Psychiatry 1994; 55:134–136 [B]

167. Munjack DJ, Crocker B, Cabe D, Brown R, Usigli R, Zulueta A, McManus M, McDowell D, Palmer R, Leonard M: Alprazolam, propranolol, and placebo in the treatment of panic disorder and agoraphobia with panic attacks. J Clin Psychopharmacol 1989; 9:22–27 [A]

168. Ravaris CL, Friedman MJ, Hauri PJ, McHugo GJ: A controlled study of alprazolam and propranolol in panic-disordered and agoraphobic outpatients. J Clin Psychopharmacol 1991; 11:344–350 [A]

169. Shehi M, Patterson WM: Treatment of panic attacks with alprazolam and propranolol. Am J Psychiatry 1984; 141:900–901 [B]

170. Klein E, Uhde TW: Controlled study of verapamil for treatment of panic disorder. Am J Psychiatry 1988; 145:431–434 [A]

171. Benjamin J, Levine J, Fux M, Aviv A, Levy D, Belmaker RH: Double-blind, placebo-controlled, crossover trial of inositol treatment for panic disorder. Am J Psychiatry 1995; 152:1084–1086 [A]

172. Uhde TW, Stein MB, Vittone BJ, Siever LJ, Boulenger JP, Klein E, Mellman TA: Behavioral and physiologic effects of short-term and long-term administration of clonidine in panic disorder. Arch Gen Psychiatry 1989; 46:170–177 [A, B]

173. Spielberger CD: State-Trait Anxiety Inventory. Palo Alto, Calif, Consulting Psychologists Press, 1985 [G]

174. Zung WWK: A rating instrument for anxiety disorders. Psychosomatics 1971; 12:371–379 [G]

175. Hoehn-Saric R, Merchant AF, Keyser ML, Smith VK: Effects of clonidine on anxiety disorders. Arch Gen Psychiatry 1981; 38:1278–1282 [B]

176. Sheehan DV, Raj AB, Harnett-Sheehan K, Soto S, Knapp E: The relative efficacy of high-dose buspirone and alprazolam in the treatment of panic disorder: a double-blind placebo-controlled study. Acta Psychiatr Scand 1993; 88:1–11 [A]

177. Sheehan DV, Raj A, Sheehan KH, Soto S: Is buspirone effective for panic disorder? J Clin Psychopharmacol 1990; 10:3–11 [A]

178. Pollard CA: Inpatient treatment of complicated agoraphobia and panic disorder. Hosp Community Psychiatry 1987; 38:951–958 [B]

179. Pollard HJ, Pollard CA: Follow-up study of an inpatient program for complicated agoraphobia and panic disorder. Anxiety Disorders Practice J 1993; 1:37–40 [C]

180. Cottraux J, Note ID, Cungi C, Legeron P, Heim F, Chneiweiss L, Bernard G, Bouvard M: A controlled study of cognitive behaviour therapy with buspirone or placebo in panic disorder with agoraphobia. Br J Psychiatry 1995; 167:635–641 [A]

181. Wolfe BE, Maser JD (eds): Treatment of Panic Disorder: A Consensus Development Conference. Washington, DC, American Psychiatric Press, 1994 [G]

182. Coryell W, Noyes R, Clancy J: Excess mortality in panic disorder. Arch Gen Psychiatry 1982; 39:701–703 [D]

183. Noyes R: Suicide and panic disorder: a review. J Affect Disord 1991; 22:1–11 [F]

184. Warshaw MG, Massion AO, Peterson LG, Pratt LA, Keller MB: Suicidal behavior in inpatients with panic disorder: retrospective and prospective data. J Affect Disord 1995; 34:235–247 [C, D]

185. Lepine JP, Chignon M, Teherani M: Suicide attempts in patients with panic disorder. Arch Gen Psychiatry 1993; 50:144–149 [D]

186. Johnson J, Weissman MM, Klerman GL: Panic disorder comorbidity and suicide attempts. Arch Gen Psychiatry 1990; 47:805–808 [D]

187. Beck AT, Steer RA, Snaderson WC, Skeie TM: Panic disorder and suicidal ideation and behavior: discrepant findings in psychiatric outpatients. Am J Psychiatry 1991; 148:1195–1199 [D]

188. Hornig CD, McNally RJ: Panic disorder and suicide attempt: a reanalysis of data from the Epidemiologic Catchment Area study. Br J Psychiatry 1995; 167:76–79 [D]

189. Fawcett J, Scheftner WA, Fogg L, Clark DC, Young MA, Hedeker D, Gibbons R: Time-related predictors of suicide in major affective disorder. Am J Psychiatry 1990; 147:1189–1194 [C]

190. Mannuzza S: Panic disorder and suicide attempts. J Anxiety Disord 1992; 6:261–274 [D]

191. Cox BJ, Direnfeld DM, Swinson RP, Norton GR: Suicidal ideation and suicide attempts in panic disorder and social phobia. Am J Psychiatry 1994; 151:882–887 [D]

192. Friedman S, Jones JC, Chernen L, Barlow DH: Suicidal ideation and suicide attempts among patients with panic disorder: a survey of two outpatient clinics. Am J Psychiatry 1992; 149:680–685 [D]

193. Kushner MG, Sher KJ, Beitman BD: The relation between alcohol problems and the anxiety disorders. Am J Psychiatry 1990; 147:685–695 [F]

194. Anthony JC, Tien AY, Petronis KR: Epidemiological evidence on cocaine use and panic attacks. Am J Epidemiol 1989; 129:543–549 [C]

195. Mirin SM, Weiss RD, Griffin ML, Michael JL: Psychopathology in drug users and their families. Compr Psychiatry 1991; 32:36–51 [E]

196. Nunes E, Quitkin B, Berman C: Panic disorder and depression in female alcoholics. J Clin Psychiatry 1988; 49:441–443 [F]

197. Aronson TA, Craig TJ: Cocaine precipitation of panic disorder. Am J Psychiatry 1986; 143:643–645 [D]

198. Pallanti S, Mazzi D: MDMA (Ecstasy) precipitation of panic disorder. Biol Psychiatry 1992; 32:91–95 [G]

199. Moran C: Depersonalization and agoraphobia associated with marijuana use. Br J Med Psychol 1986; 59:187–196 [B]

200. Cowley DS: Alcohol abuse, substance abuse, and panic disorder. Am J Med 1992; 92(suppl 1A):41S–48S [F]

201. Brown SA, Irwin M, Schuckit MA: Changes in anxiety among abstinent male alcoholics. J Stud Alcohol 1991; 52:55–61 [B]

202. Thevos AK, Johnston AL, Latham PK, Randall CL, Adinoff B, Malcolm R: Symptoms of anxiety in inpatient alcoholics with and without DSM-III-R anxiety diagnoses. Alcohol Clin Exp Res 1991; 15:102–105 [B]

203. George DT, Nutt DJ, Dwyer BA, Linnoila M: Alcoholism and panic disorder: is the comorbidity more than coincidence? Acta Psychiatr Scand 1990; 81:97–107 [F]

204. Cox BJ, Norton GR, Swinson RP, Endler NS: Substance abuse and panic-related anxiety: a critical review. Behav Res Ther 1990; 28:385–393 [E]

205. Anthenelli RM, Schuckit MA: Affective and anxiety disorders and alcohol and drug dependence: diagnosis and treatment. J Addict Dis 1993; 12:73–87 [F]

206. Tucker P, Westermeyer J: Substance abuse in patients with comorbid anxiety disorder. Am J Addictions 1995; 4:226–233 [C]

207. Westermeyer J, Tucker P: Comorbid anxiety disorder and substance disorder. Am J Addictions 1995; 4:97–106 [C]

208. Ciraulo DA, Sands BF, Shader RI: Critical review of liability for benzodiazepine abuse among alcoholics. Am J Psychiatry 1988; 145:1501–1506 [F]

209. Shelton RC, Harvey DS, Stewart PM, Loosen PT: Alprazolam in panic disorder: a retrospective analysis. Prog Neuropsychopharmacol Biol Psychiatry 1993; 17:423–434 [E]

210. Lucas PB, Pickar D, Kelsoe J, Rapaport M, Pato C, Hommer D: Effects of the acute administration of caffeine in patients with schizophrenia. Biol Psychiatry 1990; 28:35–40 [B]

211. Leibenluft E, Fiero PL, Bartko JJ, Moul DE, Rosenthal NE: Depressive symptoms and the self-reported use of alcohol, caffeine, and carbohydrates in normal volunteers and four groups of psychiatric outpatients. Am J Psychiatry 1993; 150:294–301 [E]

212. Boulenger J-P, Uhde TW, Wolff EA, Post RM: Increased sensitivity to caffeine in patients with panic disorder. Arch Gen Psychiatry 1984; 41:1067–1071 [D]

213. Bowen R, South M, Hawkes J: Mood swings in patients with panic disorder. Can J Psychiatry 1994; 39:91–94 [G]

214. Savino M, Perugi G, Simonini E, Soriani A, Cassano GB, Akiskal HS: Affective comorbidity in panic disorder: is there a bipolar connection? J Affect Disord 1993; 28:155–163 [D, G]

215. Marks IM: Fears, Phobias, and Rituals. New York, Oxford University Press, 1987 [G]

216. Marks IM: Agoraphobia, panic disorder and related conditions in the DSM-IIIR and ICD-10. J Psychopharmacol 1987; 1:6–12 [G]

217. Herve C, Gaillard M, Roujas F, Huguenard P: Alcoholism in polytrauma. J Trauma 1986; 26:1123–1126 [E]

218. Boudewyns PA, Woods MG, Hyer L, Albrecht JW: Chronic combat-related PTSD and concurrent substance abuse: implications for treatment of this frequent "dual diagnosis." J Trauma Stress 1991; 4:549–560 [D]

219. Davidson J, Kudler H, Smith R: Treatment of posttraumatic stress disorder with amitriptyline and placebo. Arch Gen Psychiatry 1990; 47:259–266 [A]

220. Davidson JR, Kudler HS, Saunders WB, Smith RD: Symptom and comorbidity patterns in World War II and Vietnam veterans with posttraumatic stress disorder. Compr Psychiatry 1990; 31:162–170 [D]

221. Pitman RK, Altman B, Greenwald E: Psychiatric complications during flooding therapy for posttraumatic stress disorder. J Clin Psychiatry 1991; 52:17–20 [G]

222. Dansky BS, Roitzsch JC, Brady KT, Saladin ME: Posttraumatic stress disorder and substance abuse: use of research in a clinical setting. J Trauma Stress 1997; 10:141–148 [C]

223. Cottler LB, Compton WM III, Mager D, Spitznagel EL, Janca A: Posttraumatic stress disorder among substance users from the general population. Am J Psychiatry 1992; 149:664–670 [E]

224. Greist JH, Jefferson JW: Panic Disorder and Agoraphobia: A Guide, 2nd revised ed. Middleton, Wis, Dean Foundation for Health, Research, and Education, 1993 [G]

225. Mavissakalian M: The relationship between panic disorder/agoraphobia and personality disorders. Psychiatr Clin North Am 1990; 13:661–684 [F]

226. Brooks RB, Baltazar PL, McDowell DE, Munjack DJ, Bruns JR: Personality disorders co-occurring with panic disorder with agoraphobia. J Personality Disorders 1991; 5:328–336 [D]

227. Pollack MH, Otto MW, Rosenbaum JF, Sachs GS: Personality disorders in patients with panic disorder: association with childhood anxiety disorders, early trauma, comorbidity, and chronicity. Compr Psychiatry 1992; 33:78–83 [C]

228. Reich JH: DSM-III personality disorders and the outcome of treated panic disorder. Am J Psychiatry 1988; 145:1149–1152 [B]

229. Reich J, Troughton E: Frequency of DSM-III personality disorders in patients with panic disorder: comparison with psychiatric and normal control subjects. Psychiatry Res 1988; 26:89–100 [A]

230. Reich JH, Vasile RG: Effect of personality disorders on the treatment outcome of axis I conditions: an update. J Nerv Ment Dis 1993; 181:475–484 [F]

231. Green M, Curtis GC: Personality disorders and panic patients: response to termination of antipanic medication. J Personal Disord 1988; 2:303–314 [B]

232. Chambless DL, Renneberg B, Goldstein A, Gracely EJ: MCMI-diagnosed personality disorders among agoraphobic outpatients: prevalence and relationship of severity and treatment outcome. J Anxiety Disord 1992; 6:195–211 [D]

233. Marchand A, Goyer LR, Mainguy N: L'impact de la presence de troubles de la personnalité, sur la réponse au traitement behavioral-cognitif du trouble panique avec agoraphobie. Science et Comportement 1992; 22:149–161 [B]

234. Black DW, Wesner RB, Gabel J, Bowers W, Monahan P: Predictors of short-term treatment response in 66 patients with panic disorder. J Affect Disord 1994; 30:233–241 [A]

235. Dreessen L, Arntz A, Luttels C, Sallaerts S: Personality disorders do not influence the results of cognitive behavioral therapies for anxiety disorders. Compr Psychiatry 1994; 35:265–274 [B]

236. Keijsers GPJ, Hoogduin CAL, Schapp CPDR: Prognostic factors in the behavioral treatment of panic disorder with and without agoraphobia. Behavior Therapy 1994; 25:689–708 [B]

237. Karajgi B, Rifkin A, Doddi S, Kolli R: The prevalence of anxiety disorders in patients with chronic obstructive pulmonary disease. Am J Psychiatry 1990; 147:200–201 [D]

238. Kaplan DS, Masand PS, Gupta S: The relationship of irritable bowel syndrome (IBS) and panic disorder. Ann Clin Psychiatry 1996; 8:81–88 [D]

239. Lydiard RB, Greenwald S, Weissman MM, Johnson J, Drossman DA, Ballenger JC: Panic disorder and gastrointestinal symptoms: findings from the NIMH Epidemiologic Catchment Area project. Am J Psychiatry 1994; 151:64–70 [E]

240. Kawachi I, Colditz GA, Ascherio A, Rimm E, Giovannucci E, Stampfer MJ, Willett WC: Prospective study of phobic anxiety and risk of coronary heart disease in men. Circulation 1994; 89:1992–1997 [C]

241. American Academy of Child and Adolescent Psychiatry: Practice Parameters for the Assessment and Treatment of Children and Adolescents With Anxiety Disorders. J Am Acad Child Adolesc Psychiatry 1997; 36(10 suppl):69S–84S [G]

242. Black B: Separation anxiety disorder and panic disorder, in Anxiety Disorders in Children and Adolescents. Edited by March J. New York, Guilford Press, 1995, pp 212–234 [G]

243. Black B, Robbins D: Panic disorder in children and adolescents. J Am Acad Child Adolesc Psychiatry 1990; 29:36–44 [F]

244. Kearney CA, Silverman WK: The panic disorder controversy continues. J Am Acad Child Adolesc Psychiatry 1991; 30:852–853 [G]

245. Kearney CA, Silverman WK: Let's not push the "panic" button: a critical analysis of panic and panic disorder in adolescents. Clin Psychol Rev 1992; 12:293–305 [E]

246. Whitaker A, Johnson J, Shaffer D, Rapoport JL, Kalikow K, Walsh BT, Davies M, Braiman S, Dolinsky A: Uncommon troubles in young people: prevalence estimates of selected psychiatric disorders in a nonreferred adolescent population. Arch Gen Psychiatry 1990; 47:487–496 [D]

247. Hayward C, Killen JD, Hammer LD, Lift IF, Wilson DM, Simmonds B, Taylor CB: Pubertal stage and panic attack history in sixth- and seventh-grade girls. Am J Psychiatry 1992; 149:1239–1243 [D]

248. Curry J, Murphy L: Comorbidity of anxiety disorders, in Anxiety Disorders in Children and Adolescents. Edited by March J. New York, Guilford Press, 1995, pp 301–317 [G]

249. Kovacs M, Feinberg TL, Crouse-Novak MA, Paulauskas SL, Finkelstein R: Depressive disorders in childhood, I: a longitudinal prospective study of characteristics and recovery. Arch Gen Psychiatry 1984; 41:229–237 [B]

250. Bernstein GA: Comorbidity and severity of anxiety and depressive disorders in a clinic sample. J Am Acad Child Adolesc Psychiatry 1991; 30:43–50 [C]

251. Last CG, Francis G, Hersen M, Kazdin AE, Strauss CC: Separation anxiety and school phobia: a comparison using DSM-III criteria. Am J Psychiatry 1987; 144:653–657 [D]

252. Last CG, Strauss CC: School refusal in anxiety-disordered children and adolescents. J Am Acad Child Adolesc Psychiatry 1990; 29:31–35 [D]

253. Gittelman-Klein R, Klein DF: School phobia: diagnostic considerations in the light of imipramine effects. J Nerv Ment Dis 1973; 156:199–215 [B]

254. Ollendick TH: Cognitive behavioral treatment of panic disorder and agoraphobia in adolescents: a multiple baseline design analysis. Behavior Therapy 1995; 26:517–531 [E]

255. Barlow DH: Effectiveness of behavior treatment for panic disorder with and without agoraphobia, in Treatment of Panic Disorder: A Consensus Development Conference. Edited by Wolfe BE, Maser JD. Washington, DC, American Psychiatric Press, 1994, pp 105–120 [G]

256. Ballenger JC, Carek DJ, Steele JJ, Cornish-McTighe D: Three cases of panic disorder with agoraphobia in children. Am J Psychiatry 1989; 146:922–924 [G]

257. Biederman J: Clonazepam in the treatment of prepubertal children with panic-like symptoms. J Clin Psychiatry 1987; 48(Oct suppl):38–42 [B]

258. Birmaher B, Waterman GS, Ryan N, Cully M: Fluoxetine for childhood anxiety disorders. J Am Acad Child Adolesc Psychiatry 1994; 33:993–999 [B]

259. Kutcher SP, MacKenzie S: Successful clonazepam treatment of adolescents with panic disorder. J Clin Psychopharmacol 1988; 8:299–301 [G]

260. Blazer D, George LK, Hughes D: The epidemiology of anxiety disorders: an age comparison, in Anxiety and the Elderly: Treatment and Research. Edited by Salzman C, Lebowitz BD. New York, Springer, 1991, pp 17–30 [G]

261. Eaton WW, Dryman A, Weissman MM: Panic and phobia, in Psychiatric Disorders in America. Edited by Robins LN, Regier DA. New York, Free Press, 1991, pp 155–179 [G]

262. Altshuler LL, Cohen L, Szuba MP, Burt VK, Gitlin M, Mintz J: Pharmacologic management of psychiatric illness during pregnancy: dilemmas and guidelines. Am J Psychiatry 1996; 153:592–606 [F]

263. Regier DA, Myers JK, Kramer M, Robins LN, Blazer DG, Hough RL, Eaton WW, Locke BZ: The NIMH Epidemiologic Catchment Area program: historical context, major objectives, and study population characteristics. Arch Gen Psychiatry 1984; 41:934–941 [G]

264. Kessler RC, McGonagle KA, Zhao S, Nelson CB, Hughes M, Eshleman S, Wittchen HU, Kendler KS: Lifetime and 12 month prevalence of DSM-III-R psychiatric disorders in the United States: results from the National Comorbidity Survey. Arch Gen Psychiatry 1994; 51:8–19 [C]

265. Blazer D, George LK, Landerman R, Pennybacker M, Melville ML, Woodbury M, Manton KG, Jordan K, Locke B: Psychiatric disorders: a rural/urban comparison. Arch Gen Psychiatry 1985; 42:651–656; correction 1986; 43:1142 [G]

266. Horwath E, Johnson J, Hornig CD: Epidemiology of panic disorder in African-Americans. Am J Psychiatry 1993; 150:465–469 [D]

267. Paradis CM, Friedman S, Lazar RM, Grubea J, Kesselman M: Use of a structured interview to diagnose anxiety disorders in a minority population. Hosp Community Psychiatry 1992; 43:61–64 [G]

268. Bell CC, Shakoor B, Thompson B, Dew D, Hughley E, Mays R, Shorter-Gooden K: Prevalence of isolated sleep paralysis in black subjects. J Natl Med Assoc 1984; 76:501–508 [D]

269. Neal AM, Smucker WD: The presence of panic disorder among African American hypertensives: a pilot study. J Black Psychol 1994; 20:29–35 [D]

270. Bell CC, Hildreth CJ, Jenkins EJ, Carter C: The relationship of isolated sleep paralysis and panic disorder to hypertension. J Natl Med Assoc 1988; 80:289–294 [D]

271. Brown C, Schulberg HC, Madonia MJ: Clinical presentations of major depression by African Americans and whites in primary medical care practice. J Affect Disord 1996; 41:181–191 [A]

272. Neighbors HW: Seeking help for personal problems: black Americans' use of health and mental health services. Community Ment Health J 1985; 21:156–166 [D]

273. Cooper-Patrick L, Crum RM, Ford DE: Characteristics of patients with major depression who received care in general medical and specialty mental health settings. Med Care 1994; 32:15–24 [E]

PRACTICE GUIDELINE FOR THE
Treatment of Patients With Eating Disorders
Second Edition

WORK GROUP ON EATING DISORDERS

Joel Yager, M.D., Chair

Arnold Andersen, M.D.
Michael Devlin, M.D.
Helen Egger, M.D.
David Herzog, M.D.
James Mitchell, M.D.
Pauline Powers, M.D.
Alayne Yates, M.D.
Kathryn Zerbe, M.D.

▶ NOTE TO THE READER

In this practice guideline, treatment recommendations are discussed in sections II and V and are summarized in section I. Data regarding the safety and efficacy of available treatments are reviewed in section IV.

This practice guideline was first published in February 1993. This updated revision was approved in July 1999 and was published in *The American Journal of Psychiatry* in January 2000.

CONTENTS

I. EXECUTIVE SUMMARY

▶ ## A. CODING SYSTEM

Each recommendation is identified as falling into one of three categories of endorsement, indicated by a bracketed Roman numeral following the statement. The three categories represent varying levels of clinical confidence regarding the recommendations:

[I] Recommended with substantial clinical confidence.
[II] Recommended with moderate clinical confidence.
[III] May be recommended on the basis of individual circumstances.

▶ ## B. GENERAL CONSIDERATIONS

Patients with eating disorders display a broad range of symptoms that frequently occur along a continuum between those of anorexia nervosa and bulimia nervosa. The care of patients with eating disorders involves a comprehensive array of approaches. These guidelines contain the clinical factors that need to be considered when treating a patient with anorexia nervosa or bulimia nervosa.

1. Choosing a site of treatment

Evaluation of the patient with an eating disorder prior to initiating treatment is essential for determining the appropriate setting of treatment. The most important physical parameters that affect this decision are weight and cardiac and metabolic status [I]. Patients should be psychiatrically hospitalized before they become medically unstable (i.e., display abnormal vital signs) [I]. The decision to hospitalize should be based on psychiatric, behavioral, and general medical factors [I]. These include rapid or persistent decline in oral intake and decline in weight despite outpatient or partial hospitalization interventions, the presence of additional stressors that interfere with the patient's ability to eat (e.g., intercurrent viral illnesses), prior knowledge of weight at which instability is likely to occur, or comorbid psychiatric problems that merit hospitalization.

Most patients with uncomplicated bulimia nervosa do not require hospitalization. However, the indications for hospitalization for these patients can include severe disabling symptoms that have not responded to outpatient treatment, serious concurrent general medical problems (e.g., metabolic abnormalities, hematemesis, vital sign changes, and the appearance of uncontrolled vomiting), suicidality, psychiatric disturbances that warrant hospitalization independent of the eating disorders diagnosis, or severe concurrent alcohol or drug abuse.

Factors influencing the decision to hospitalize on a psychiatric versus a general medical or adolescent/pediatric unit include the patient's general medical status, the skills and abilities of local psychiatric and general medical staffs, and the availability of suitable intensive outpatient, partial and day hospitalization, and aftercare programs to care for the patient's general medical and psychiatric problems.

2. Psychiatric management

Psychiatric management forms the foundation of treatment for patients with eating disorders and should be instituted for all patients in combination with other specific treatment modalities. Important components of psychiatric management for patients with eating disorders are as follows: establish and maintain a therapeutic alliance; coordinate care and collaborate with other clinicians; assess and monitor eating disorder symptoms and behaviors; assess and monitor the patient's general medical condition; assess and monitor the patient's psychiatric status and safety; and provide family assessment and treatment [I].

3. Choice of specific treatments for anorexia nervosa

Goals in the treatment of anorexia nervosa include restoring healthy weight (i.e., weight at which menses and ovulation in females, normal sexual drive and hormone levels in males, and normal physical and sexual growth and development in children and adolescents are restored); treating physical complications; enhancing patients' motivations to cooperate in the restoration of healthy eating patterns and to participate in treatment; providing education regarding healthy nutrition and eating patterns; correcting core maladaptive thoughts, attitudes, and feelings related to the eating disorder; treating associated psychiatric conditions, including defects in mood regulation, self-esteem, and behavior; enlisting family support and providing family counseling and therapy where appropriate; and preventing relapse.

a. Nutritional rehabilitation/counseling

A program of nutritional rehabilitation should be established for all patients who are significantly underweight [I]. Healthy target weights and expected rates of controlled weight gain (e.g., 2–3 lb/week for most inpatient and 0.5–1 lb/week for most outpatient programs) should be established. Intake levels should usually start at 30–40 kcal/kg per day (approximately 1000–1600 kcal/day) and should be advanced progressively. This may be increased to as high as 70–100 kcal/kg per day during the weight gain phase. Intake levels should be 40–60 kcal/kg per day during weight maintenance and for ongoing growth and development in children and adolescents. Patients who have higher caloric intake requirements may be discarding food, be vomiting, be exercising frequently, have increased nonexercise motor activity (e.g., fidgeting), or have truly higher metabolic rates. Vitamin and mineral supplements may also be beneficial for patients (e.g., phosphorus supplementation may be particularly useful to prevent serum hypophosphatemia).

It is essential to monitor patients medically during refeeding [I]. Monitoring should include assessment of vital signs as well as food and fluid intake and output; electrolytes (including phosphorus); and the presence of edema, rapid weight gain (associated primarily with fluid overload), congestive heart failure, and gastrointestinal symptoms, particularly constipation and bloating. Cardiac monitoring may be useful, especially at night, for children and adolescents who are severely malnourished (weight <70% of the standard body weight). Physical activity should be adapted to the food intake and energy expenditure of the patient.

Nutritional rehabilitation programs should also attempt to help patients deal with their concerns about weight gain and body image changes, educating them about the risks of their eating disorder and providing ongoing support to patients and their families [I].

b. Psychosocial interventions

The establishment and maintenance of a psychotherapeutically informed relationship is beneficial [II]. Once weight gain has started, formal psychotherapy may be very helpful. There is no clear evidence that any specific form of psychotherapy is superior for all patients. Psychosocial interventions need to be informed by understanding psychodynamic conflicts, cognitive development, psychological defenses, and complexity of family relationships as well as the presence of other psychiatric disorders. Psychotherapy alone is generally not sufficient to treat severely malnourished patients with anorexia nervosa. Ongoing treatment with individual psychotherapeutic interventions is usually required for at least a year and may take 5–6 years because of the enduring nature of many of the psychopathologic features of anorexia nervosa and the need for support during recovery.

Both the symptoms of eating disorders and problems in familial relationships that may be contributing to the maintenance of disorders may be alleviated by family and couples psychotherapy [II]. Group psychotherapy is sometimes added as an adjunctive treatment for anorexia nervosa; however, care must be taken to avoid patients competing to be the thinnest or sickest member or becoming excessively demoralized through observing the difficult, chronic course of other patients in the group.

c.   Medications

Treatment of anorexia nervosa should not rely on psychotropic medications as the sole or primary treatment [I]. An assessment of the need for antidepressant medications is usually best made following weight gain, when the psychological effects of malnutrition are resolving. These medications should be considered for the prevention of relapse among weight-restored patients or to treat associated features of anorexia nervosa, such as depression or obsessive-compulsive problems [II].

4.   Choice of specific treatments for bulimia nervosa

a.   Nutritional rehabilitation/counseling

Nutritional counseling as an adjunct to other treatment modalities may be useful for reducing behaviors related to the eating disorder, minimizing food restriction, increasing the variety of foods eaten, and encouraging healthy but not excessive exercise patterns [I].

b.   Psychosocial interventions

A comprehensive evaluation of individual patients, their cognitive and psychological development, psychodynamic issues, cognitive style, comorbid psychopathology, patient preferences, and family situation is needed to inform the choice of psychosocial interventions [I]. Cognitive behavioral psychotherapy is the psychosocial treatment for which the most evidence for efficacy currently exists, but controlled trials have also shown interpersonal psychotherapy to be very useful. Behavioral techniques (e.g., planned meals, self-monitoring) may also be helpful. Clinical reports have indicated that psychodynamic and psychoanalytic approaches in individual or group format may be useful once bingeing and purging are improving. Patients with concurrent anorexia nervosa or severe personality disorders may benefit from extended psychotherapy.

Whenever possible, family therapy should be considered, especially for adolescents still living with parents or older patients with ongoing conflicted interactions with parents or other family members [II].

c.   Medications

For most patients, antidepressant medications are effective as one component of an initial treatment [I]. Selective serotonin reuptake inhibitors (SSRIs) are currently considered to be the safest antidepressants and may be especially helpful for patients with significant symptoms of depression, anxiety, obsessions, or certain impulse disorder symptoms or for those patients who have had a suboptimal response to previous attempts at appropriate psychosocial therapy. Other antidepressant medications from a variety of classes can reduce the symptoms of binge eating and purging and may help prevent relapse among patients in remission.

While tricyclic and monoamine oxidase inhibitor (MAOI) antidepressants can be used to treat bulimia nervosa, tricyclics should be used with caution for patients who may be at high risk for suicide attempts, and MAOIs should be avoided for patients with chaotic binge eating and purging.

Emerging evidence has shown that a combination of psychotherapeutic interventions and medication results in higher remission rates and therefore should be considered when initiating treatment for patients with bulimia nervosa [II].

II. DEVELOPING A TREATMENT PLAN FOR THE INDIVIDUAL PATIENT

The following are recommendations for developing a treatment plan for individual patients with eating disorders. A number of factors should be considered when developing the treatment plan. Table 1 provides guidance for these clinical dimensions (1).

A. CHOOSING A SITE OF TREATMENT

The services available for the treatment of eating disorders can range from intensive inpatient settings (in which subspecialty general medical consultation is readily available), through partial hospital and residential programs, to varying levels of outpatient care (from which the patient can receive general medical treatment, nutritional counseling, and/or individual, group, and family psychotherapy). Pretreatment evaluation of the patient is essential for determining the appropriate setting of treatment (2). Weight and cardiac and metabolic status are the most important physical parameters for determining choice of setting. Generally, patients who weigh less than approximately 85% of their individually estimated healthy weights have considerable difficulty gaining weight in the absence of a highly structured program. Those weighing less than about 75% of their individually estimated healthy weights are likely to require a 24-hour hospital program. Once weight loss is severe enough to cause the indications for immediate medical hospitalization, treatment may be less effective, refeeding may entail greater risks, and prognosis may be more problematic than when intervention is provided earlier. Knowledge about gray matter deficits that result from malnutrition and persist following refeeding also point to the need for earlier rather than later effective interventions. Therefore, hospitalization should occur before the onset of medical instability as manifested by abnormal vital signs. The decision to hospitalize should be based on psychiatric and behavioral grounds, including rapid or persistent decline in oral intake; decline in weight despite maximally intensive outpatient or partial hospitalization interventions; the presence of additional stressors—such as intercurrent viral illnesses—that may additionally interfere with the patient's ability to eat; prior knowledge of weight at which instability is likely to occur; and comorbid psychiatric problems that merit hospitalization.

Indications for immediate medical hospitalization include marked orthostatic hypotension with an increase in pulse of >20 bpm or a drop in blood pressure of >20 mm Hg/minute standing, bradycardia below 40 bpm, tachycardia over 110 bpm, or inability to sustain body core temperature (e.g., temperatures below 97.0°F). Most severely underweight patients, those with physiological instability, and many children and adolescents whose weight loss, while rapid, has not been as severe as in adult patients nonetheless require inpatient medical management and comprehensive treatment for support of weight gain. Guidelines for treatment settings are provided in table 1.

Although most patients with uncomplicated bulimia nervosa do not require hospitalization, indications for hospitalization can include severe disabling symptoms that have not responded to adequate trials of competent outpatient treatment, serious concurrent general medical problems (e.g., metabolic abnormalities, hematemesis, vital sign changes, or the appearance of uncontrolled vomiting), suicidality, psychiatric disturbances that would warrant the patient's hospitalization independent of the eating disorders diagnosis, or severe concurrent alcohol or drug abuse.

Legal interventions, including involuntary hospitalization and legal guardianship, may be necessary to ensure the safety of treatment-reluctant patients whose general medical conditions are life-threatening (3). Decisions to hospitalize on a psychiatric versus general medical or adolescent/pediatric unit depend on the patient's general medical status, the skills and abilities of local psychiatric and general medical staffs, and the availability of suitable programs to care for the patient's general medical and psychiatric problems (4). Some evidence suggests that patients treated in eating disorders inpatient specialty units have better outcomes than patients treated in general inpatient settings that lack expertise and experience in treating patients with eating disorders (5).

Partial hospitalization and day hospital programs are being increasingly used in attempts to decrease the length of some inpatient hospitalizations; for milder cases, these programs are being increasingly used in place of hospitalization. However, such programs may not be appropriate for patients with lower initial weights (e.g., those who are ≤75% of average weight for height). In clinical practice, failure of outpatient treatment is one of the most frequent indications for more intensive treatment, either day/partial hospital or inpatient. In deciding whether to treat in a partial hospitalization program, the patient's level of motivation to participate in treatment and ability to work in a group setting should be considered (6, 7).

Patients with high motivation to comply with treatment, cooperative families, brief symptom duration, and who are less than 20% below healthy body weight may benefit from treatment in outpatient settings, but only if they are carefully monitored and if they and their families understand that a more restrictive setting may be necessary if persistent progress is not evident in a few weeks (8–10). Careful monitoring includes at least weekly (and often two to three times a week) postvoiding gowned weighings, which may also include measurement of urine specific gravity together with orthostatic vital signs and temperatures. While patients treated in the outpatient setting can remain with their families and continue to attend school or work, these advantages must be balanced against the risks of failure to progress in recovery.

▶ B. PSYCHIATRIC MANAGEMENT

Psychiatric management includes a broad range of tasks that are performed by the psychiatrist or that the psychiatrist should ensure are provided to the patient with an eating disorder. These should be instituted for all patients with eating disorders in combination with other specific treatment modalities.

TABLE 1. Level of Care Criteria for Patients With Eating Disorders[a]

	Level of Care[b]				
Characteristic	Level 1: Outpatient	Level 2: Intensive Outpatient	Level 3: Partial Hospitalization (Full-Day Outpatient Care)	Level 4: Residential Treatment Center	Level 5: Inpatient Hospitalization
Medical complications	Medically stable to the extent that more extensive medical monitoring, as defined in levels 4 and 5, is not required			Medically stable to the extent that intravenous fluids, nasogastric tube feedings, or multiple daily laboratory tests are not needed	For adults: heart rate <40 bpm; blood pressure <90/60 mm Hg; glucose <60 mg/dl; potassium <3 meq/liter; electrolyte imbalance; temperature <97.0 °F; dehydration; or hepatic, renal, or cardiovascular organ compromise requiring acute treatment. For children and adolescents: heart rate in the 40s; orthostatic blood pressure changes (>20-bpm increase in heart rate or >10–20-mm Hg drop); blood pressure below 80/50 mm Hg; hypokalemia or hypophosphatemia
Suicidality	No intent or plan			Possible plan but no intent	Intent and plan
Weight as % of healthy body weight (for children, determining factor is rate of weight loss)[c]	>85%	>80%	>75%	<85%	<75% (for children and adolescents: acute weight decline with food refusal even if not <75% below healthy body weight)
Motivation to recover, including cooperativeness, insight, and ability to control obsessive thoughts	Fair to good	Fair	Partial; preoccupied with ego-syntonic thoughts more than 3 hours a day; cooperative	Poor to fair; preoccupied with ego-syntonic thoughts 4–6 hours a day; cooperative with highly structured treatment	Very poor to poor; preoccupied with ego-syntonic thoughts; uncooperative with treatment or cooperative only in highly structured environment
Comorbid disorders (substance abuse, depression, anxiety)	Presence of comorbid condition may influence choice of level of care				Any existing psychiatric disorder that would require hospitalization

TABLE 1. Level of Care Criteria for Patients With Eating Disorders[a] (continued)

Characteristic	Level 1: Outpatient	Level 2: Intensive Outpatient	Level 3: Partial Hospitalization (Full-Day Outpatient Care)	Level 4: Residential Treatment Center	Level 5: Inpatient Hospitalization
			Level of Care[b]		
Structure needed for eating/gaining weight	Self-sufficient		Needs some structure to gain weight	Needs supervision at all meals or will restrict eating	Needs supervision during and after all meals or nasogastric/special feeding
Impairment and ability to care for self; ability to control exercise		Able to exercise for fitness, but able to control compulsive exercising	Structure required to prevent patient from compulsive exercising	Complete role impairment, cannot eat and gain weight by self; structure required to prevent patient from compulsive exercising	
Purging behavior (laxatives and diuretics)			Can greatly reduce purging in non-structured settings; no significant medical complications such as ECG abnormalities or others suggesting the need for hospitalization	Can ask for and use support or use skills if desires to purge	Needs supervision during and after all meals and in bathrooms
Environmental stress		Others able to provide adequate emotional and practical support and structure	Others able to provide at least limited support and structure	Severe family conflict, problems, or absence so as unable to provide structured treatment in home, or lives alone without adequate support system	
Treatment availability/living situation		Lives near treatment setting		Too distant to live at home	

[a]Adapted from La Via et al. (1).

[b]One or more items in a category should qualify the patient for a higher level of care. These are not absolutes, but guidelines requiring the judgment of physicians.

[c]Although this table lists percentages of healthy body weight in relation to suggested levels of care, these are only approximations and do not correspond to percentages based on standardized tables. For any given individual, differences in body build, body composition and other physiological variables may result in considerable differences as to what constitutes a healthy body weight in relation to "norms." For some, a healthy body weight may be 110% of "standard," whereas for others it may be 98%. Each individual's physiological differences must be assessed and appreciated.

1. Establish and maintain a therapeutic alliance

At the very outset, clinicians should attempt to build trust, establish mutual respect, and develop a therapeutic relationship with the patient that will serve as the basis for ongoing exploration and treatment of the problems associated with the eating disorder. Eating disorders are frequently long-term illnesses that can manifest themselves in different ways at different points during their course; treating them often requires the psychiatrist to adapt and modify therapeutic strategies over time. During the course of treatment, patients with eating disorders may resist looking beyond immediate eating disorder symptoms to comorbid psychopathology and underlying psychodynamics. Psychiatrists should be mindful of the fact that the interventions they prescribe for individuals with anorexia nervosa create extreme anxieties in the patients. Encouraging them to gain weight asks for them to do the very thing of which they are most frightened. Recognizing and acknowledging to patients one's awareness of these effects can assist in building the therapeutic alliance and decrease the patients' perceptions that the psychiatrist just wants to make them fat and does not understand or empathize with their underlying emotions. Addressing these resistances may be important in allowing treatment to proceed through impasses as well as helping to ameliorate factors that serve to aggravate and maintain eating disorders (11).

Patients with eating disorders also present treating physicians with extraordinary challenges in understanding and working with countertransference reactions. Because these illnesses are often difficult to ameliorate with short-term interventions, they often evoke the feeling in treating clinicians that they have not done enough to change or alleviate the patient's plight. A frequent range of countertransference feelings include beleaguerment, demoralization, and excessive needs to change the patient with a chronic eating disorder. Some authorities have observed that the gender of the therapist plays a role in the particular kind of countertransference reactions that come into play (12–14). Concerns about choice of gender of the therapist may be tied to patient concerns about boundary violations and should be attended to in selecting health care providers (15, 16). In addition to gender differences, cultural differences between patients and therapists and between patients and other aspects of the care system may also influence the course and conduct of treatment and require mindful attention. Most authorities believe ongoing processing of one's countertransference reactions, sometimes with the help of a supervisor or consultant, can be useful in helping the therapist persevere and reconcile intense, troublesome countertransference reactions. Regardless of the theoretical base the clinician uses, countertransference reactions have been described by a wide variety of therapists who used differing clinical approaches (13, 14, 17–22).

Patients who have been sexually abused or who have otherwise been the victims of boundary violations are prone to stir a profound need to rescue the patient, which can occasionally result in a loosening of the therapeutic structure, loss of therapeutic boundary keeping, and a sexualized countertransference reaction. In some cases, these countertransference responses have led to overt sexual acting out and unethical treatment on the part of the therapist, which may not only compromise treatment but also severely harm the patient (23). Clear boundaries are critical in the treatment of all patients with eating disorders, not only those who have been sexually abused but also those who may have experienced other types of boundary intrusions regarding their bodies, eating behaviors, and other aspects of the self by family members and others.

2. Coordinate care and collaborate with other clinicians

An important task for the psychiatrist is to coordinate and, depending on expertise, oversee the care of patients with eating disorders. A variety of professionals may collaborate in the care and provide such services as nutritional counseling, working with the family, and establishing various individual and group psychotherapeutic, cognitive behavior, or behavior programs. Other physician specialists and dentists should be consulted when necessary for management of general medical (e.g., cardiac dysfunction) and dental complications. Particularly in treatment settings where the staff does not have training or experience dealing with patients with eating disorders, the provision of education and supervision by the psychiatrist can be crucial to the success of treatment (24).

3. Assess and monitor eating disorder symptoms and behaviors

The psychiatrist should make a careful assessment of the patient's eating disorder symptoms and behaviors (25). Obtaining a detailed report of a single day or using a calendar as a prompt may help elicit specific information, particularly regarding perceived intake. Having a meal together or observing a meal may provide useful information, permitting the clinician to observe difficulties patients may have in eating particular foods, anxieties that erupt in the course of a meal, and rituals concerning food (such as cutting, separating, or mashing) that they may feel compelled to perform. The patient's understanding of how the illness developed and the effects of any interpersonal problems on the onset of the eating disorder should be explored. Family history should be obtained regarding eating disorders and other psychiatric disorders, obesity, family interactions in relation to the patient's disorder, and attitudes toward eating, exercise, and appearance. It is essential not to articulate theory in order to blame or permit family members to blame one another or themselves. Rather, the point is to identify stressors whose amelioration may facilitate recovery. In the assessment of young patients, it may be helpful to involve parents, school personnel, and health professionals who routinely work with children. The complete assessment usually requires at least several hours, and often patients and their families may not initially reveal pertinent information about sensitive issues, even when directly questioned. Some important information may be uncovered only after a trusting relationship has been established and the patient is better able to accurately identify inner emotional states.

Formal measures are also available for the assessment of eating disorders, including self-report questionnaires and semistructured interviews. Representative examples are listed in table 2.

4. Assess and monitor the patient's general medical condition

A full physical examination should be performed by a physician familiar with common findings in patients with eating disorders, with particular attention to vital signs; physical and sexual growth and development (including height and weight); the cardiovascular system; and evidence of dehydration, acrocyanosis, lanugo, salivary gland enlargement, and scarring on the dorsum of the hands (Russell's sign). A dental examination should also be performed. It is generally useful to assess growth, sexual development, and general physical development in younger patients. The use of a pediatric growth chart may permit identification of patients who have failed to gain weight and who have growth retardation (26).

The need for laboratory analyses should be determined on an individual basis depending on the patient's condition or when necessary for making treatment decisions. Some laboratory assessments indicated for patients with eating disorders and for specific clinical features appear in table 3.

TABLE 2. Representative Instruments for Assessment of Eating Disorders

Instrument	Form of Administration	Comments	Reference(s)
Diagnostic Survey for Eating Disorders (DSED)	Can be used as self-report or semistructured interview	Twelve sections cover demographics, weight history and body image, dieting, binge eating, purging, exercise, related behaviors, sexual functioning, menstruation, medical and psychiatric history, life adjustment, and family history	Johnson C: Diagnostic Survey for Eating Disorders (DSED), in The Etiology and Treatment of Bulimia Nervosa. Edited by Johnson C, Connors M. New York, Basic Books, 1987
Eating Attitudes Test	Self-report	Brief (26-item), standardized, self-report screening test of symptoms and concerns characteristic of eating disorders; completion time: 5–10 minutes	Garner DM, Olmsted MP, Bohr Y, Garfinkel PE: The Eating Attitudes Test: psychometric features and clinical correlates. Psychol Med 1982; 12:871–878 Garner DM: Psychoeducational principles in the treatment of eating disorders, in Handbook for Treatment of Eating Disorders. Edited by Garner DM, Garfinkel PE. New York, Guilford Press, 1997, pp 145–177
Eating Disorders Examination (EDE)	Semistructured interview	Measures the presence and severity of eating disorder features and provides operational DSM-IV diagnoses	Fairburn CG, Cooper Z: The Eating Disorders Examination—12th ed, in Binge Eating: Nature, Assessment and Treatment. Edited by Fairburn CG, Wilson GT. New York, Guilford Press, 1993
EDE-Q4	Self-report	Self-report version of the EDE, designed for situations in which an interview cannot be used; validated against the EDE	Fairburn CG, Beglin SJ: The assessment of eating disorders: interview or self-report questionnaire? Int J Eat Disord 1994; 16:363–370

TABLE 2. Representative Instruments for Assessment of Eating Disorders *(continued)*

Instrument	Form of Administration	Comments	Reference(s)
Eating Disorders Inventory	Self-report	Standardized measure of psychological traits and symptom clusters presumed to have relevance to understanding and treatment of eating disorders; 11 subscales presented in 6-point, forced choice format; three scales assess attitudes and behaviors concerning eating, weight, and shape; eight more scales assess more general psychological traits; completion time: 20 minutes	Garner DM, Olmstead MJ, Polivy J: Development and validation of a multidimensional eating disorder inventory for anorexia nervosa and bulimia. Int J Eat Disord 1983; 2:15–34 Garner DM: The Eating Disorders Inventory—2 Professional Manual. Odessa, Fla, Psychological Assessment Resources, 1991 Garner DM: The Eating Disorders Inventory—2 (EDI-2), in Outcomes Assessments in Clinical Practice. Edited by Sederer LI, Dickey B. Baltimore, Williams & Wilkins, 1996, pp 92–96
Eating Disorders Questionnaire	Self-report	Questions address eating disorders symptoms, associated symptoms, time course, treatment	Mitchell JE, Hatsukami D, Eckert E, Pyle RL: The Eating Disorders Questionnaire. Psychopharmacol Bull 1985; 21:1025–1043
Questionnaire of Eating and Weight Patterns	Self-report	Measures the nature and quantity of binge eating to assess binge-eating disorder	Yanovski SZ: Binge eating disorder: current knowledge and future directions. Obesity Res 1993; 1:306–320 Nangle DW, Ghonson WG, Carr-Nangle RD, Engler LB: Binge eating disorder and the proposed DSM-IV criteria: psychometric analysis of the Questionnaire of Eating and Weight Patterns. Int J Eat Disord 1993; 16:147–157
Yale-Brown-Cornell Eating Disorder Scale	Clinical conducted interview	Includes a 65-item symptom checklist plus 19 questions, covering 18 general categories of rituals and preoccupations; requires 15 minutes or less to complete	Mazure CM, Halmi KA, Sunday SR, Romano SJ, Einhorn AN: Yale-Brown-Cornell Eating Disorder Scale: development, use, reliability and validity. J Psychiatr Res 1994; 28:425–445 Sunday SR, Halmi KA, Einhorn AN: The Yale-Brown-Cornell Eating Disorder Scale: a new scale to assess eating disorders symptomatology. Int J Eat Disord 1995; 18:237–245

TABLE 3. Laboratory Assessments for Patients With Eating Disorders

Assessment	Patient Indication
Basic analyses	Consider for all patients with eating disorders
Blood chemistry studies	
Serum electrolyte level	
Blood urea nitrogen (BUN) level	
Creatinine level	
Thyroid function test	
Complete blood count (CBC)	
Urinalysis	
Additional analyses	Consider for malnourished and severely symptomatic patients
Blood chemistry studies	
Calcium level	
Magnesium level	
Phosphorus level	
Liver function tests	
Electrocardiogram	
Osteopenia and osteoporosis assessments	Consider for patients underweight more than 6 months
Dual-energy X-ray absorptiometry (DEXA)	
Estradiol level	
Testosterone level in males	
Nonroutine assessments	Consider only for specific unusual indications
Serum amylase level	Possible indicator of persistent or recurrent vomiting
Luteinizing hormone (LH) and follicle-stimulating hormone (FSH) levels	For persistent amenorrhea at normal weight
Brain magnetic resonance imaging (MRI) and computerized tomography (CT)	For ventricular enlargement correlated with degree of malnutrition
Stool	For blood

5. Assess and monitor the patient's psychiatric status and safety

Attention should be paid to comorbid psychiatric disturbances, especially affective and anxiety disorders, suicidality, substance abuse, obsessive and compulsive symptoms, and personality disturbances. Shoplifting, stealing food, and self-mutilatory behaviors should be noted. A developmental history should attend to temperament, psychological, sexual and physical abuse, and sexual history. Psychological testing, particularly after nutritional rehabilitation, may clarify personality and neuropsychological disturbances. In addition to assessing behavioral and formal psychopathological aspects of the case, it is always useful to investigate psychodynamic and interpersonal conflicts that may be relevant to understanding and treating the patient's eating disorder.

6. Provide family assessment and treatment

Eating disorders impose substantial burdens on the families of patients. Parents often avoid recognizing that the child or adolescent is ill and may have difficulties in accepting the seriousness of the illness. Parents then often struggle with the belief that they have themselves caused the illness and need help overcoming their guilt so that they can face their children's needs. The feelings of guilt are exacerbated by the rejection of their parenting that is implicit in the child's refusal of nurturance in the form of food. Parents also have difficulties in accepting the need for treatment or requiring that their child accept treatment, since the child's protest that treatment is noxious only increases the parent's guilt. Parents typically become angry at their child's secretive purging, exercising, and other efforts to avoid food or burn off calories and may come to view the children as "manipulative" rather than desperate. Parents may increasingly avoid their responsibilities of providing meals within specific contexts that bind family relationships. They are often riddled with anxieties that their child will die and, depending on the family and gravity of the case, may go on to develop anger, exhaustion, and despair. The patient's and family's preoccupations, social concerns, and rituals may begin to orient and focus around the illness, particularly family interactions involving meals. Decisions concerning food may impact family get-togethers, social visits, vacations, and even vocational choices.

Assessment of the family is important whenever possible, particularly for patients living at home or those who are enmeshed with their families. Family assessment may be extremely useful for some patients in order to understand interactions that may contribute to ongoing illness or that may potentially facilitate recovery. Comprehensive treatment of the patient should include an assessment of the burden of the illness on the family, with support and education given to the family as part of the overall treatment.

C. CHOICE OF SPECIFIC TREATMENTS FOR ANOREXIA NERVOSA

The aims of treatment are to 1) restore patients to healthy weight (at which menses and normal ovulation in females, normal sexual drive and hormone levels in males, and normal physical and sexual growth and development in children and adolescents are restored); 2) treat physical complications; 3) enhance patients' motivations to cooperate in the restoration of healthy eating patterns and to participate in treatment; 4) provide education regarding healthy nutrition and eating patterns; 5) correct core dysfunctional thoughts, attitudes, and feelings related to the eating disorder; 6) treat associated psychiatric conditions, including defects in mood regulation, self-esteem, and behavior; 7) enlist family support and provide family counseling and therapy where appropriate; and 8) prevent relapse.

1. Nutritional rehabilitation

For patients who are markedly underweight, a program of nutritional rehabilitation should be established. Hospital-based programs should be considered, particularly for the most nutritionally compromised patients (e.g., those whose weight is less than 75% of the recommended weight for their height or for children and adolescents whose weight loss may not be as severe but who are losing weight at a rapid rate). Nutritional rehabilitation programs should establish healthy target weights and have expected rates of controlled weight gain (e.g., 2–3 lb/week for inpatient units and 0.5–1 lb/week for outpatient programs). Intake levels should usually start at 30–40 kcal/kg per day (approximately 1000–1600 kcal/day) and should be advanced progressively. During the weight gain phase, intake may be increased to as high as 70–100 kcal/kg per day for some patients. During weight maintenance and for ongoing growth and development in children and adolescents, intake levels should be 40–60 kcal/kg per day. Patients who require higher caloric intakes may be discarding food, vomiting, or exercising frequently or have more nonexercise motor activity such as fidgeting; others may have a truly elevated metabolic rate. In addition to calories, patients benefit from vitamin and mineral supplements (and in particular may require phosphorus before serum hypophosphatemia occurs). Medical monitoring during refeeding is essential and should include assessment of vital signs as well as food and fluid intake and output; monitoring of electrolytes (including phosphorus); and observation for edema, rapid weight gain associated primarily with fluid overload, congestive heart failure, and gastrointestinal symptoms, particularly constipation and bloating. For children and adolescents who are severely malnourished (weight <70% standard body weight) cardiac monitoring, especially at night, may be desirable. Physical activity should be adapted to the food intake and energy expenditure of the patient.

Other treatment options for nutritional rehabilitation include temporary supplementation or replacement of regular food with liquid food supplements. On occasion, nasogastric feedings may be required. In life-threatening or very unusual circumstances, parenteral feedings for brief periods may be considered; however, infection is always a risk with parenteral feedings in emaciated and potentially immunocompromised patients with anorexia nervosa. These forceful interventions should be considered only when patients are unwilling to cooperate with oral feedings; when the patient's health, physical safety, and recovery are being threatened; and after appropriate legal and ethical considerations have been taken into account.

Additional goals of nutritional rehabilitation programs include education, ongoing support, and helping patients deal with their concerns about weight gain and body image changes.

2. Psychosocial interventions

It is essential that psychosocial interventions incorporate an understanding of psychodynamic conflicts, cognitive development, psychological defenses, and the complexity of family relationships as well as the presence of other psychiatric disorders. Although research studies regarding psychotherapy treat different interventions as distinctly separate treatments, in practice there is frequent overlap. Most nutritional rehabilitation programs employ a milieu incorporating emotional nurturance and one of a variety of behavioral interventions (which involve a combination of reinforcers that link exercise, bed rest, and privileges to target weights, desired behaviors, and informational feedback). Other forms of individual psychotherapy are also used in the treatment of anorexia nervosa, initiated as the patient is gaining weight. However, there has been little formal study of the optimal role for either individual or group psychotherapy in treating anorexia nervosa. Because of the enduring nature of many of the psychopathologic features of anorexia nervosa and the need for support during recovery, ongoing treatment with individual psychotherapeutic interventions is frequently required for at least a year and may take 5–6 years (27).

Family therapy and couples psychotherapy are frequently useful for both symptom alleviation and alleviation of problems in familial relationships that may be contributing to the maintenance of the disorders. Some practitioners use group psychotherapy as an adjunctive treatment for anorexia nervosa, but caution must be taken that patients do not compete to be the thinnest or sickest patient or become excessively demoralized through bearing witness to the difficult, ongoing struggles of other patients in the group.

Programs that focus exclusively on the need for abstinence (e.g., 12-step programs) without attending to nutritional considerations or cognitive and behavioral deficits are not recommended as the sole initial treatment approach for anorexia nervosa; interventions based on addiction models blended with features of other psychotherapeutic approaches can be considered. Support groups led by professionals or advocacy organizations may be beneficial as adjuncts to other psychosocial treatment modalities.

3. Medications

Psychotropic medications should not be used as the sole or primary treatment for anorexia nervosa. In addition, medication therapy should not be used routinely during the weight restoration period. The role for antidepressants is usually best assessed following weight gain, when the psychological effects of malnutrition are resolving. However, these medications should be considered to prevent relapse among weight-restored patients or to treat associated features of anorexia nervosa, such as depression or obsessive-compulsive problems.

D. CHOICE OF SPECIFIC TREATMENTS FOR BULIMIA NERVOSA

1. Nutritional rehabilitation/counseling

A primary focus for nutritional rehabilitation concerns monitoring the patient's patterns of binge eating and purging. Most patients with bulimia nervosa are of normal weight, so nutritional restoration will not be a central focus of treatment. However, even among patients of normal weight, nutritional counseling as an adjunct to other treatment modalities may be useful for reducing behaviors related to the eating disorder, minimizing food restriction, increasing the variety of foods eaten, and encouraging healthy but not excessive exercise patterns.

2. Psychosocial interventions

Psychosocial interventions should be chosen on the basis of a comprehensive evaluation of the individual patient, considering cognitive and psychological development, psychodynamic issues, cognitive style, comorbid psychopathology, patient preferences, and family situation. With respect to short-term interventions for treating acute episodes of bulimia nervosa, cognitive behavioral psychotherapy is the psychosocial treatment for which the most evidence for efficacy currently exists. However, controlled trials have also shown interpersonal psychotherapy to be very useful for this disorder. Behavioral techniques, such as planned meals and self-monitoring, may also be helpful for initial symptom management and interrupting the binge-purge behaviors. There are clinical reports indicating that psychodynamic and psychoanalytic approaches in individual or group format are useful once bingeing and purging are improving. These approaches address developmental issues, identity formation, body image concerns, sexual and aggressive difficulties, affect regulation, gender role expectations, interpersonal conflicts, family dysfunction, coping styles, and problem solving. Some patients, such as those with concurrent anorexia nervosa or concurrent severe personality disorders, may benefit from extended psychotherapy.

Family therapy should be considered whenever possible, especially for adolescents still living with parents or older patients with ongoing conflicted interactions with parents. Patients with marital discord may benefit from couples therapy. Support groups and 12-step programs such as Overeaters Anonymous may be helpful as adjuncts to initial treatment of bulimia nervosa and for subsequent relapse prevention but are not recommended as the sole initial treatment approach for bulimia nervosa.

3. Medications

Antidepressants are effective as one component of an initial treatment program for most patients. Although antidepressant medications from a variety of classes can reduce symptoms of binge eating and purging and may help prevent relapse among patients in remission, SSRIs are safest. They may be especially helpful for patients with substantial symptoms of depression, anxiety, obsessions, or certain impulse disorder symptoms, or for patients who have failed or had a suboptimal response to previous attempts at appropriate psychosocial therapy. Dose levels of tricyclic and MAOI antidepressants for treating bulimia nervosa are similar to those used to treat depression; practitioners should try to avoid prescribing tricyclics to patients who may be suicidal and MAOIs to patients with chaotic binge eating and purging.

4. Combinations of psychosocial interventions and medications

In some research, the combination of antidepressant therapy and cognitive behavioral therapy results in the highest remission rates. Therefore, clinicians should consider a combination of psychotherapeutic interventions and medication when initiating treatment.

III. DISEASE DEFINITION, EPIDEMIOLOGY, AND NATURAL HISTORY

▶ A. CLINICAL FEATURES

The DSM-IV criteria for establishing the diagnosis of anorexia nervosa or bulimia nervosa appear in table 4 and table 5, respectively.

Although DSM-IV criteria allow clinicians to diagnose patients with a specific eating disorder, the symptoms frequently occur along a continuum between those of anorexia nervosa and those of bulimia nervosa. Weight preoccupation and excessive self-evaluation of weight and shape are primary symptoms in both anorexia nervosa and bulimia nervosa, and many patients demonstrate a mixture of both anorexic and bulimic behaviors. For example, up to 50% of patients with anorexia nervosa develop bulimic symptoms, and some patients who are initially bulimic develop anorexic symptoms (28). Atypical patients—who deny fear of weight gain, appraise their bodies as malnourished, and deny distorted perceptions of their bodies—are not uncommon among Asian patients (29). In one U.S. series (30), these atypical features were seen in about one-fifth of the patients admitted to a specialty eating disorder program.

Anorexia nervosa appears in two subtypes: restricting and binge-eating/purging; classification into subtypes is based on the presence of bulimic symptoms. Patients with anorexia nervosa can alternate between bulimic and restricting subtypes at different periods of their illness (31–36). Among the binge-eating/purging subtype of patients with anorexia nervosa, further distinctions can be made between those who both binge and purge and those who purge but do not objectively binge. Patients with bulimia nervosa can be subclassified into the purging subtype and the nonpurging subtype. Many patients, particularly in younger age groups, have combinations of eating disorder symptoms that cannot be strictly categorized as either anorexia nervosa or bulimia nervosa and are technically diagnosed as "eating disorder not otherwise specified" (37).

Patients with anorexia nervosa and bulimia nervosa often experience other associated psychiatric symptoms and behaviors. Individuals with anorexia nervosa often demonstrate social isolation. Depressive, anxious, and obsessional symptoms,

TABLE 4. DSM-IV Criteria for Anorexia Nervosa

Criterion	Description
A	Refusal to maintain body weight at or above a minimally normal weight for age and height (e.g., weight loss leading to maintenance of body weight less than 85% of that expected or failure to make expected weight gain during period of growth, leading to body weight less than 85% of that expected).
B	Intense fear of gaining weight or becoming fat, even though underweight.
C	Disturbance in the way in which one's body weight or shape is experienced, undue influence of body weight or shape on self-evaluation, or denial of the seriousness of the current low body weight.
D	In postmenarcheal females, amenorrhea, i.e., the absence of at least three consecutive menstrual cycles. (A woman is considered to have amenorrhea if her periods occur only following hormone, e.g., estrogen, administration.)
Specify type	
Restricting type	During the current episode of anorexia nervosa, the person has not regularly engaged in binge-eating or purging behavior (i.e., self-induced vomiting or the misuse of laxatives, diuretics, or enemas).
Binge-eating/ purging type	During the current episode of anorexia nervosa, the person has regularly engaged in a binge-eating or purging behavior (i.e., self-induced vomiting or the misuse of laxatives, diuretics, or enemas).

TABLE 5. DSM-IV Criteria for Bulimia Nervosa

Criterion	Description
A	Recurrent episodes of binge eating. An episode of binge eating is characterized by both of the following: (1) Eating, in a discrete period of time (e.g., within any 2-hour period), an amount of food that is definitely larger than most people would eat during a similar period of time and under similar circumstances. (2) A sense of lack of control over eating during the episode (e.g., a feeling that one cannot stop eating or control what or how much one is eating).
B	Recurrent inappropriate compensatory behavior in order to prevent weight gain, such as self-induced vomiting; misuse of laxatives, diuretics, enemas, or other medications; fasting; or excessive exercise.
C	The binge eating and inappropriate compensatory behaviors both occur, on average, at least twice a week for 3 months.
D	Self-evaluation is unduly influenced by body shape and weight.
E	The disturbance does not occur exclusively during episodes of anorexia nervosa.
Specify type	
Purging type	During the current episode of bulimia nervosa, the person has regularly engaged in self-induced vomiting or the misuse of laxatives, diuretics, or enemas.
Nonpurging type	During the current episode of bulimia nervosa, the person has used other inappropriate compensatory behaviors, such as fasting or excessive exercise, but has not regularly engaged in self-induced vomiting or the misuse of laxatives, diuretics, or enemas.

perfectionistic traits, and rigid cognitive styles as well as sexual disinterest are often present among restricting anorexic patients (38). Early in the course of illness, patients with anorexia nervosa often have limited recognition of their disorder and experience their symptoms as ego-syntonic; this is sometimes accompanied by corresponding limited recognition by the family. Depressive, anxious, and impulsive symptoms as well as sexual conflicts and disturbances with intimacy are often associated with bulimia nervosa. Although patients with bulimia nervosa are likely to recognize their disorder, shame frequently prevents them from seeking treatment at an early stage (39–42). Patients with anorexia nervosa of the binge-eating/purging subtype are sometimes suicidal and self-harming. In one subgroup of patients with bulimia nervosa (the "multi-impulsive" bulimic patients), significant degrees of impulsivity (manifested as stealing, self-harm behaviors, suicidality, substance abuse, and sexual promiscuity) have been observed (43).

Some of the clinical features associated with eating disorders may result from malnutrition or semistarvation (44, 45). Studies of volunteers who have submitted to semistarvation and semistarved prisoners of war report the development of food preoccupation, food hoarding, abnormal taste preferences, binge eating, and other disturbances of appetite regulation as well as symptoms of depression, obsessionality, apathy, irritability, and other personality changes. In patients with anorexia nervosa, some of these starvation-related state phenomena, such as abnormal taste preference, may completely reverse with refeeding, although it may take considerable time after weight restoration for them to abate completely (46). However, some of these symptoms may reflect both preexisting and enduring traits, such as obsessive-compulsiveness, which are then further exacerbated by semistarvation and, therefore, may only be partially reversed with nutritional rehabilitation (47). Complete psychological assessments may not be possible until some degree of weight normalization is achieved (48). Although patients with bulimia nervosa may appear to be physically within the standards of healthy weight, they may also show psychological and biological correlates of semistarvation—such as depression, irritability, and obsessionality—and may be below a biologically determined set-point even at a weight considered to be "normal" according to population norms (49, 50).

Common physical complications of anorexia nervosa are listed in table 6. Amenorrhea of even a few months may be associated with osteopenia, which may progress to potentially irreversible osteoporosis and a correspondingly higher rate of pathological fractures (51–53). Pains in the extremities may signal stress fractures that may not be evident from examination of plain X-rays but whose presence may be signaled by abnormal bone scan results. Patients with anorexia nervosa who develop hypoestrogenemic amenorrhea in their teenage years that persists into young adulthood are at greatest risk for osteoporosis, since they not only lose bone mass but also fail to form bone at a critical phase of development. As a result, prepubertal and early pubertal patients are also at risk of permanent growth stunting (54). The areas most vulnerable to osteoporosis are the lumbar spine and hip.

Acute complications of anorexia nervosa include dehydration, electrolyte disturbances (with purging), cardiac compromise with various arrhythmias (including conduction defects and ventricular arrhythmias), gastrointestinal motility disturbances, renal problems, infertility, premature births, other perinatal complications, hypothermia, and other evidence of hypometabolism (55). Death from anorexia nervosa is often proximally due to cardiac arrest secondary to arrhythmias.

Common physical complications of bulimic behaviors are listed in table 7. The most serious physical complications occur in patients with chronic and severe pat-

TABLE 6. Physical Complications of Anorexia Nervosa

Organ System	Symptoms	Signs	Laboratory Test Results
Whole body	Weakness, lassitude	Malnutrition	Low weight/body mass index, low body fat percentage per anthropometrics or underwater weighing
Central nervous system	Apathy, poor concentration	Cognitive impairment; depressed, irritable mood	CT scan: ventricular enlargement; MRI: decreased gray and white matter
Cardiovascular and peripheral vascular	Palpitations, weakness, dizziness, shortness of breath, chest pain, coldness of extremities	Irregular, weak, slow pulse; marked orthostatic blood pressure changes; peripheral vasoconstriction with acrocyanosis	ECG: bradycardia, arrhythmias; Q-Tc prolongation (dangerous sign)
Skeletal	Bone pain with exercise	Point tenderness; short stature/arrested skeletal growth	X-rays or bone scan for pathological stress fractures; bone densitometry for bone mineral density assessment for osteopenia or osteoporosis
Muscular	Weakness, muscle aches	Muscle wasting	Muscle enzyme abnormalities in severe malnutrition
Reproductive	Arrested psychosexual maturation or interest; loss of libido	Loss of menses or primary amenorrhea; arrested sexual development or regression of secondary sex characteristics; fertility problems; higher rates of pregnancy and neonatal complications	Hypoestrogenemia; prepubertal patterns of LH, FSH secretion; lack of follicular development/dominant follicle on pelvic ultrasound
Endocrine, metabolic	Fatigue; cold intolerance; diuresis; vomiting	Low body temperature (hypothermia)	Elevated serum cortisol; increase in rT3 ("reverse" T3); dehydration; electrolyte abnormalities; hypophosphatemia (especially on refeeding); hypoglycemia (rare)
Hematologic	Fatigue; cold intolerance	Rare bruising/clotting abnormalities	Anemia; neutropenia with relative lymphocytosis; thrombocytopenia; low erythrocyte sedimentation rate; rarely clotting factor abnormalities
Gastrointestinal	Vomiting; abdominal pain; bloating; obstipation; constipation	Abdominal distension with meals; abnormal bowel sounds	Delayed gastric emptying; occasionally abnormal liver function test results
Genitourinary	Pitting edema		Elevated BUN; low glomerular filtration rate; greater formation of renal calculi; hypovolemic nephropathy
Integument	Change in hair	Lanugo	

TABLE 7. Physical Complications of Bulimia Nervosa

Organ System	Symptoms	Signs	Laboratory Test Results
Metabolic	Weakness; irritability	Poor skin turgor	Dehydration (urine specific gravity; osmolality); serum electrolytes: hypokalemic, hypochloremic alkalosis in those who vomit; hypomagnesemia and hypophosphatemia in laxative abusers
Gastrointestinal	Abdominal pain and discomfort in vomiters; occasionally automatic vomiting; obstipation; constipation; bowel irregularities and bloating in laxative abusers	Occasionally blood-streaked vomitus; vomiters may occasionally have gastritis, esophagitis, gastroesophageal erosions, esophageal dysmotility patterns (including gastroesophageal reflux, and, very rarely, Mallory-Weiss [esophageal or gastric tears]; may have increased rates of pancreatitis; chronic laxative abusers may show colonic dysmotility or melanosis coli	
Reproductive	Fertility problems	Spotty/scanty menstrual periods	May be hypoestrogenemic
Oropharyngeal	Dental decay; pain in pharynx; swollen cheeks and neck (painless)	Dental caries with erosion of dental enamel, particularly lingular surface of incisors; erythema of pharynx; enlarged salivary glands	X-rays confirm erosion of dental enamel; elevated serum amylase associated with benign parotid hyperplasia
Integument		Scarring on dorsum of hand (Russell's sign)	
Cardiomuscular (in ipecac abusers)	Weakness; palpitations	Cardiac abnormalities; muscle weakness	Cardiomyopathy and peripheral myopathy

terns of binge eating and purging and are most concerning in very-low-weight patients (56).

Laboratory abnormalities in anorexia nervosa may include neutropenia with relative lymphocytosis, abnormal liver function, hypoglycemia, hypercortisolemia, hypercholesterolemia, hypercarotenemia, low serum zinc levels, electrolyte disturbances, and widespread disturbances in endocrine function. Thyroid abnormalities may include low T_3 and T_4 levels, which are reversible with weight restoration and generally should not be treated with replacement therapy (57–60). Normal serum phosphorus values may be misleading, since they do not reflect total body phosphorus depletion (which is usually reflected in serum phosphorus only after refeeding has begun). In very severe cases of malnutrition, elevated serum levels of muscle enzymes associated with catabolism may be seen in more than one-half of the patients with anorexia nervosa (61).

MRI abnormalities reflect changes in the brain. White matter and cerebrospinal fluid volumes appear to return to the normal range following weight restoration. However, gray matter volume deficits, which correlate with the patient's lowest recorded body mass indices, may persist even after weight restoration (62–66). Some patients show persistent deficits in their neuropsychological testing results, which has been shown to be associated with poorer outcomes (67).

It is important to consider that laboratory findings in anorexia nervosa may be normal in spite of profound malnutrition. For example, patients may have low total body potassium levels even when serum electrolytes are normal and thus may be prone to unpredictable cardiac arrhythmias (68).

Laboratory abnormalities in bulimia nervosa may include electrolyte imbalances such as hypokalemia, hypochloremic alkalosis, mild elevations of serum amylase, and hypomagnesemia and hypophosphatemia, especially in laxative abusers (57, 69).

▶ B. NATURAL HISTORY AND COURSE

1. Anorexia nervosa

The percentage of individuals with anorexia nervosa who *fully* recover is modest. Although some patients improve symptomatically over time, a substantial proportion continue to have disturbances with body image, disordered eating, and other psychiatric difficulties (70). A review of a large number of carefully done follow-up studies conducted with hospitalized or tertiary referral populations at least 4 years after onset of illness show that the outcomes of about 44% of the patients could be rated as good (weight restored to within 15% of recommended weight for height; regular menstruation established), about 24% were poor (weight never reached within 15% of recommended weight for height; menstruation absent or at best sporadic), and about 28% of the outcomes fell between those of the good and poor groups; approximately 5% of the patients had died (early mortality). Overall, about two-thirds of patients continue to have enduring morbid food and weight preoccupation, and up to 40% have bulimic symptoms. Even among those who have good outcomes as defined by restoration of weight and menses, many have other persistent psychiatric symptoms, including dysthymia, social phobia, obsessive-compulsive symptoms, and substance abuse (71). In a carefully done 10–15-year follow-up study of adolescent patients hospitalized for anorexia nervosa—76% of whom met criteria for full recovery—time to recovery was quite protracted, ranging from 57 to 79 months depending on the definition of recovery (27, 30). Anorexic patients with atypical features, such as denying either a fear of gaining weight or a distorted perception of their bodies, had a somewhat better course (30). Mortality, which primarily resulted from cardiac arrest or suicide, has been found to increase with length of follow-up, reaching up to 20% among patients followed for more than 20 years (72). A 1995 meta-analysis suggests a 5.6% mortality rate per decade (73). However, in the aforementioned 10–15-year follow-up study of adolescents, in which patients received intensive treatment, no deaths were reported (27). Some studies estimate that death rates of young women with anorexia nervosa are up to 12 times those of age-matched women in the community and up to twice those of women with any other psychiatric disorders. However, these studies have involved clinical populations, and it is not clear what the corresponding community rates would be (73). Nevertheless, recent data suggest that of all psychiatric disorders, the greatest excess of patient mortality due to natural and unnatural causes is associated with eating disorders and substance abuse (74).

Poorer prognosis has been associated with initial lower minimum weight, the presence of vomiting, failure to respond to previous treatment, disturbed family relationships before illness onset, and marital status (being married) (75, 76). Patients with anorexia nervosa who purge are at much greater risk for developing serious general medical complications (77). In general, adolescents have better outcomes than adults, and younger adolescents have better outcomes than older adolescents (78–80). However, many of these prognostic indicators have not been consistently replicated and may be sturdier predictors of short-term but not long-term outcomes.

2. Bulimia nervosa

Very little is known about the long-term prognosis of patients with untreated bulimia nervosa. Over a 1- to 2-year period, a community sample reported modest degrees of spontaneous improvement, with roughly 25%–30% reductions in binge eating, purging, and laxative abuse (81, 82). The overall short-term success rate for patients receiving psychosocial treatment or medication has been reported to be 50%–70% (70). Relapse rates between 30% and 50% have been reported for successfully treated patients after 6 months to 6 years of follow-up, and some data suggest that slow improvement continues as the period of follow-up extends to 10–15 years (83–86). In a large study of the long-term course of bulimia nervosa patients 6 years after successful treatment in an intensive program (87), outcomes of 60% of the patients were rated as good, 29% were of intermediate success, and 10% were poor, with 1% deceased.

Patients who function well and have milder symptoms at the start of treatment, and who are therefore more likely to be treated as outpatients, often have a better prognosis than those who function poorly and whose disordered eating symptoms are of sufficient severity to merit hospitalization (88). Some studies suggest that higher frequency of pretreatment vomiting is associated with poor outcomes (89, 90). The importance of working on patients' motivation as a preliminary measure before starting other treatments has gained recent attention and has been found to impact the rapidity of response to care (5).

▶ C. EPIDEMIOLOGY

Estimates of the incidence or prevalence of eating disorders vary depending on the sampling and assessment methods. The reported lifetime prevalence of anorexia nervosa among women has ranged from 0.5% for narrowly defined to 3.7% for more broadly defined anorexia nervosa (91, 92). With regard to bulimia nervosa, estimates of the lifetime prevalence among women have ranged from 1.1% to 4.2% (93, 94).

Some studies suggest that the prevalence of bulimia nervosa in the United States may have decreased slightly in recent years (95). Eating disorders are more commonly seen among female subjects, with estimates of the male-female prevalence ratio ranging from 1:6 to 1:10 (although 19%–30% of the younger patient populations with anorexia nervosa are male) (96–98). The prevalence of anorexia nervosa and bulimia nervosa in children and younger adolescents is unknown.

In many other countries, there appears to be an overall increase in eating disorders, even in cultures in which the disorder is rare (99). Japan appears to be the only non-Western country that has had a substantial and continuing increase in eating disorders, with figures that are comparable to or above those found in the United States (100, 101). In addition, eating disorder concerns and symptoms appear to be increasing among Chinese women exposed to culture clashes and modernization in cities such as Hong Kong (102, 103). The prevalence of eating disorders appears to be increasing rapidly in other non-English-speaking countries such as Spain, Argentina, and Fiji (104–107).

In the United States, eating disorders appear to be about as common in young Hispanic women as in Caucasians, more common among Native Americans, and less common among blacks and Asians (108). However, several studies in the Southeastern United States (109, 110) have shown that many eating disorder behaviors are even more common among African American women than others. Black women are more likely to develop bulimia nervosa than anorexia nervosa and are more likely to purge with laxatives than by vomiting (111).

It has recently been suggested that in some patients, excessive exercise may precipitate the eating disorder (112, 113). Female athletes in certain sports such as distance running and gymnastics are especially vulnerable. Male bodybuilders are also at risk although the symptom picture often differs, since the bodybuilder may emphasize a wish to "get bigger" and may also abuse anabolic steroids.

First-degree female relatives of patients with anorexia nervosa have higher rates of anorexia nervosa (114) and bulimia nervosa (92, 115). Identical twin siblings of patients with anorexia nervosa or bulimia nervosa also have higher rates of these disorders, with monozygotic twins having higher concordance than dizygotic twins. The evidence regarding rates of bulimia nervosa in other first-degree female relatives remains unclear; some studies report a higher rate among first-degree female relatives while others do not (94). Families of patients with bulimia nervosa have been found to have higher rates of substance abuse (particularly alcoholism) (116, 117), but transmission of substance abuse in these families may be independent of transmission of bulimia nervosa (6). In addition, families of patients with bulimia nervosa have higher rates of affective disorders (116, 118) and obesity (119).

In the psychodynamic literature, patients with anorexia nervosa have been described as having difficulties with separation and autonomy (often manifested as enmeshed relationships with parents), affect regulation (including the direct expression of anger and aggression), and negotiating psychosexual development. These deficits may make women who are predisposed to anorexia nervosa more vulnerable to cultural pressures for achieving a stereotypic body image (17–19, 120, 121).

Patients with bulimia nervosa have been described as having difficulties with impulse regulation resulting from a dearth of parental (usually maternal) involvement. Bulimia nervosa has also been described as a dissociated self-state, as resulting from deficits in self-regulation, and as representing resentful, angry attacks on one's own body out of masochistic/sadistic needs (40, 41).

High rates of comorbid psychiatric illness are found in patients seeking treatment at tertiary psychiatric treatment centers. Comorbid major depression or dysthymia has been reported in 50%–75% of patients with anorexia nervosa (71) and bulimia nervosa (71, 122, 123). Estimates of the prevalence of bipolar disorder among patients with anorexia nervosa or bulimia nervosa are usually around 4%–6% but have been reported to be as high as 13% (124). The lifetime prevalence of obsessive-compulsive disorder (OCD) among anorexia nervosa cases has been as high as 25% (71, 125, 126), and obsessive-compulsive symptoms have been found in a large majority of weight-restored patients with anorexia nervosa treated in tertiary care centers (47). OCD is also common among patients with bulimia nervosa (122). Comorbid anxiety disorders, particularly social phobia, are common among patients with anorexia nervosa and patients with bulimia nervosa (71, 122, 123). Substance abuse has been found in as many as 30%–37% of patients with bulimia nervosa; among patients with anorexia nervosa, estimates of those with substance abuse have ranged from 12% to 18%, with this problem occurring primarily among those with the binge/purge subtype (71, 123).

Comorbid personality disorders are frequently found among patients with eating disorders, with estimates ranging from 42% to 75%. Associations between bulimia nervosa and cluster B and C disorders (particularly borderline personality disorder and avoidant personality disorder) and between anorexia nervosa and cluster C disorders (particularly avoidant personality disorder and obsessive-compulsive personality disorder) have been reported (127). Eating disorder patients with personality disorders are more likely than those without personality disorders to also have concurrent mood or substance abuse disorders (122). Comorbid personality disorders are significantly more common among patients with the binge/purge subtype of anorexia nervosa than the restricting subtype or normal weight patients with bulimia nervosa (128).

Sexual abuse has been reported in 20%–50% of patients with bulimia nervosa (129) and those with anorexia nervosa (130, 131), although sexual abuse may be more common in patients with bulimia nervosa than in those with the restricting subtype of anorexia nervosa (132–134). Childhood sexual abuse histories are reported more often in women with eating disorders than in women from the general population. Women who have eating disorders in the context of sexual abuse appear to have higher rates of comorbid psychiatric conditions than other women with eating disorders (134, 135).

IV. TREATMENT PRINCIPLES AND ALTERNATIVES

In the following sections, the available data on the efficacy of treatments for eating disorders are reviewed. Most studies have consisted of 6–12-week trials designed to evaluate the short-term efficacy of treatments. Unfortunately, there is a scarce amount of data on the long-term effects of treatment for patients with eating disorders, who often have a chronic course and variable long-term prognosis. Many studies also inadequately characterize the phase of illness when patients were first treated, e.g., early or late, which may have an impact on outcomes. In addition, most studies have examined the efficacy of treatments only on eating disorder symptoms; few have examined the effectiveness of treatments on associated features and comorbid conditions such as the persistent mood, anxiety, and personality disorders that are common among "real world" populations.

A variety of outcome measures are employed in trials for patients with eating disorders. Outcome measures in studies of patients with anorexia nervosa primarily are the amount of weight gained within specified time intervals or the proportion of patients achieving a specified percentage of ideal body weight, as well as the return of menses in those with secondary amenorrhea. Measures of the severity or frequency of eating disorder behaviors have also been reported. In studies of bulimia nervosa, outcome measures include reductions in the frequency or severity of eating disorder behaviors and the proportion of patients achieving elimination of or a specific reduction in eating disorder behaviors.

When interpreting the results of studies, particularly for psychosocial interventions that may consist of multiple elements, it may be difficult to identify the element(s) responsible for treatment effects. It is also important to keep in mind when comparing the effects of psychosocial treatments between studies that there may be important variations in the nature of the treatments delivered to patients.

▶ A. TREATMENT OF ANOREXIA NERVOSA

Anorexia nervosa is a complex, serious, and often chronic condition that may require a variety of treatment modalities at different stages of illness and recovery. Specific treatments include nutritional rehabilitation, psychosocial interventions, and medications; all may be used to correct malnutrition, culturally mediated distortions, and psychological, behavioral, and social deficits.

1. Nutritional rehabilitation

a. Goals

The goals of nutritional rehabilitation for seriously underweight patients are to restore weight, normalize eating patterns, achieve normal perceptions of hunger and satiety, and correct biological and psychological sequelae of malnutrition (136). In general, a healthy goal weight is the weight at which normal menstruation and ovulation are restored. For women who had healthy menses and ovulation in the past, one can estimate that healthy weight will be restored at approximately the same weight at which full physical and psychological vigor were present. Assuming that the patient was not obese to start with, restored healthy weight is unlikely to ever be much lower than that. Since some patients continue to menstruate even at low weight (91), and some others never regain menses, a minimum goal weight is often estimated as 90% of ideal weight for height according to standard tables. At that weight, 86% of patients resume menstruating (although not necessarily ovulating) within 6 months (137). Some studies have relied on pelvic sonography to demonstrate the return of a dominant follicle, which indicates that ovulation has returned (138). Others use anthropomorphic measures to estimate the percentage of body fat (approximately 20%–25%) usually needed for normal fertility (139). In premenarchal girls, a healthy goal weight is the weight at which normal physical and sexual development resumes. It is important to use pediatric growth charts to estimate what height and weight the patient might be expected to achieve.

b. Efficacy

Measures of nutritional status include several different standards of ideal body weight, which can be quite variable (140, 141). Some studies calculate the body mass index, a measure that has become standard in studies of obesity and increasingly in eating disorders research as well. This index is calculated with the formula (weight [in kg]/height [in meters]^2). Individuals with body mass indexes <18.5 are considered to be underweight, and body mass indexes ≤17.5, in the presence of the other diagnostic criteria, indicate anorexia nervosa. Body mass indexes are increasingly used in research studies, particularly to compare groups according to percentiles of the body mass index, which take into account height, sex, and age in their calculations (142). However, most clinicians still use standard tables to determine healthy body weights in relation to heights. In children and adolescents, growth curves should be followed and are most useful when longitudinal data are available, since extrapolations from cross-sectional data at one point in time can be misleading. Therefore, for most clinical work, it is reasonable to simply weigh the patient and gauge how far she is from her individually estimated healthy body weight (143).

The efficacy with which weight restoration can be achieved varies with treatment setting. For most severely underweight patients, e.g., patients whose weight is 25%–30% below healthy body weight at the start of treatment, little weight gain will be achieved with outpatient treatment. However, most inpatient weight restoration programs can achieve a weight gain of 2–3 lb/week without compromising the patient's safety. Weight at discharge in relation to the healthy target weight may vary depending on the patient's ability to feed herself, the patient's motivation and ability to participate in aftercare programs, and the adequacy of aftercare, including partial hospitalization. The closer the patient is to ideal body weight before discharge, the less the risk of relapse. Most outpatient programs find weight gain goals of 0.5–1 lb/week to be realistic, although gains of up to 2 lb/week have been reported in a partial hospital program in which patients are scheduled for 12 hours a day, 7 days a week (144). The latter is solely a step-down program, in which patients had been treated previously as inpatients. The clinicians running the program do not believe that it would work as effectively as a "step-up" program for never-hospitalized patients.

Considerable evidence suggests that with nutritional rehabilitation, other eating disorder symptoms diminish as weight is restored, although not necessarily to the point of disappearing. Clinical experience suggests that with weight restoration, food choices increase, food hoarding decreases, and obsessions about food decrease in frequency and intensity. However, it is by no means certain that abnormal eating habits will improve simply as a function of weight gain (76). There is general agreement that distorted attitudes about weight and shape are least likely to change and that excessive exercise may be one of the last of the behaviors associated with the eating disorder to abate.

Regular structured diets may also enable some patients with anorexia nervosa with associated binge-eating and purging behaviors to improve. For some patients, however, giving up severe dietary restrictions and restraints appears to increase binge-eating behavior, which is often accompanied by compensatory purging.

As weight is regained, changes in associated mood and anxiety symptoms can be expected. Initially, the apathy and lethargy associated with malnourishment may abate. As patients start to recover and feel their bodies getting larger, especially as they approach frightening magical numbers on the scale, they may experience a resurgence of anxious and depressive symptoms, irritability, and sometimes suicidal thoughts. These mood symptoms, non-food-related obsessional thoughts, and compulsive behaviors, while often not eradicated, usually decrease with sustained weight gain.

c. Side effects and toxicity

Although weight gain results in improvement in most of the physiological complications of semistarvation, including improvement in electrolytes, heart and kidney function, and attention and concentration, many adverse physiological and psychological symptoms may appear during weight restoration. Initial refeeding may be associated with mild transient fluid retention. However, patients who abruptly stop taking laxatives or diuretics may experience marked rebound fluid retention for several weeks, presumably from salt and water retention due to the elevated aldosterone levels associated with chronic dehydration. Refeeding edema and bloating are frequent occurrences. In rare instances, congestive heart failure may also develop (145).

Patients may experience abdominal pain and bloating with meals from the delayed gastric emptying that accompanies malnutrition. Excessively rapid refeeding and nasogastric or parenteral feeding may be particularly dangerous due to the potential of inducing severe fluid retention, cardiac arrhythmias, cardiac failure, delirium, or seizures, especially in those with the lowest weights (146, 147). Hypophosphatemia, which can be life threatening, can emerge during refeeding when reserves are depleted (148). Constipation can occur, which can progress to obstipation and acute bowel obstruction. As weight gain progresses, many patients also develop acne and breast tenderness. Many patients become unhappy and demoralized about resulting changes in body shape. Management strategies for dealing with these side effects include careful refeeding (to result in not more than 2–3 lb/week of weight gain aside from simple rehydration); frequent physical examinations; monitoring of serum electrolytes (including sodium, potassium, chloride, bicarbonate, calcium, phosphorus, and magnesium) in patients developing refeeding edema; and forewarning patients about refeeding edema. When nasogastric feeding is necessary, continuous feeding (i.e., over 24 hours) may be less likely than three to four bolus feedings a day to result in metabolic abnormalities or subjective discomfort and may be better tolerated by patients.

d. Implementation

Healthy target weights and expected rates of controlled weight gain should be established (e.g., 2–3 lb/week on inpatient units). Refeeding programs should be implemented in nurturing emotional contexts. Staff should convey to patients their intentions to take care of them and not let them die even when the illness prevents the patients from taking care of themselves. Staff should clearly communicate that they are not seeking to engage in control battles and are not trying to punish patients with aversive techniques. Some positive and negative reinforcements should be built into the program (e.g., required bed rest, exercise restrictions, or restrictions of off-unit privileges; these restrictions are reduced or terminated as target weights and other goals are achieved). Intake levels should usually start at 30–40 kcal/kg per day (approximately 1000–1600 kcal/day). Intake may have to be increased to as high as 70–100 kcal/kg per day for some patients during the weight gain phase. Intake levels during weight maintenance and as needed in children and adolescents for further growth and maturation should be set at 40–60 kcal/kg per day. Kaye and colleagues (149) found that weight-restored patients with anorexia nervosa often require 200–400 calories more than gender-, age-, weight-, and height-matched control subjects to maintain weight. Some of this difference may be due to higher rates of fidgeting and other non-exercise-related energy expenditure in these patients (150). Some patients who require higher caloric intakes are exercising frequently, vomiting, or discarding food, while others may have truly higher metabolic rates or other forms of energy expenditure, e.g., fidgeting. Dietitians can help patients choose their own meals and provide a structured food plan that ensures nutritional adequacy and makes certain that none of the major food groups are avoided.

Some patients are extremely unable to recognize their illness, accept the need for treatment, or tolerate the guilt that would accompany eating, even when performed to sustain their lives. On these rare occasions staff has to take over the responsibilities for providing life-preserving care. Nasogastric feedings are preferable to intravenous feedings and may be experienced positively by some patients—particularly younger patients—who may feel relieved to know that they are being cared for and who, while they cannot bring themselves to eat, are willing to allow physicians to feed them. Total parenteral feeding is required only very rarely and in life-threatening situations. Forced nasogastric or parenteral feeding can be accompanied by substantial dangers (e.g., severe fluid retention and cardiac failure from rapid refeeding), so these interventions should not be used routinely. In situations where involuntary forced feeding is considered, careful thought should be given to clinical circumstances, family opinion, and relevant legal and ethical dimensions of the patient's treatment.

General medical monitoring during refeeding should include assessment of vital signs, food and fluid intake, and output, if indicated, as well as observation for edema, rapid weight gain (associated primarily with fluid overload), congestive heart failure, and gastrointestinal symptoms. Minerals and electrolytes should also be closely monitored since hypophosphatemia and clinically significant electrolyte imbalances can be life-threatening. Serum potassium levels should be regularly monitored in patients who are persistent vomiters. Hypokalemia should be treated with oral potassium supplementation and rehydration. Serum phosphorus levels may drop precipitously during refeeding from the utilization of phosphorus during anabolism in the face of total body depletion. In such cases phosphorus supplementation will be necessary (146). Patients suspected of artificially increasing their weight should be weighed in the morning after voiding, wearing only a gown; their fluid intake also should be carefully monitored. Assessment of urine specimens obtained at the time of weigh-in for specific gravity may help ascertain the extent to which the measured weight reflects excessive water intake.

Physical activity should be adapted to the food intake and energy expenditure of the patient, taking into account bone mineral density and cardiac function. For the severely underweight, patient exercise should be restricted and always carefully supervised and monitored. Once a safe weight is achieved, the focus of an exercise program should be on physical fitness as opposed to expending calories. The focus on fitness should be balanced with restoring patients' positive relationships with their bodies—helping them to take back control and get pleasure from physical activities rather than being self-critically, even masochistically, enslaved to them. Staff should help patients deal with their concerns about weight gain and body image changes, since these are particularly difficult adjustments for patients to make.

Research that addresses the optimal length of hospitalization is sparse. Two studies have reported that hospitalized patients who are discharged at lower than their target weight subsequently relapse and are rehospitalized at higher rates than those who achieve their target weight. Often, these low-weight discharges were associated with brief lengths of stay. The closer the patient is to ideal weight at the time of discharge from the hospital, the lower the risk of relapse (151, 152). There is no available evidence to show that brief stays for anorexia nervosa are associated with good long-term outcomes.

2. Psychosocial treatments

a. Goals

The goals of psychosocial treatments are to help patients 1) understand and cooperate with their nutritional and physical rehabilitation, 2) understand and change the behaviors and dysfunctional attitudes related to their eating disorder, 3) improve their interpersonal and social functioning, and 4) address comorbid psychopathology and psychological conflicts that reinforce or maintain eating disorder behaviors. Achieving these goals often requires an initial enhancement of patients' motivation to change along with ongoing efforts to sustain this motivation.

b. Efficacy

Few systematic trials of psychosocial therapies have been completed, and a few others are under way. Most evidence for the efficacy of psychosocial therapies comes from case reports or case series (48). Additional evidence comes from the considerable clinical experience that suggests a well-conducted regimen of psychotherapy plays an important role in both ameliorating the symptoms of anorexia nervosa and preventing relapse.

Structured inpatient and partial hospitalization programs

Most inpatient programs employ one of a variety of behaviorally formulated interventions. These behavioral programs commonly provide a combination of nonpunitive reinforcers (e.g., empathic praise, exercise-related limits and rewards, bed rest and privileges linked to achieving weight goals and desired behaviors). Behavioral programs have been shown to produce good short-term therapeutic effects (153). One meta-analysis that compared behavioral psychotherapy programs to treatment with medications alone found that behavior therapy resulted in more consistent weight gain among patients with anorexia nervosa as well as shorter hospital stays (153). Some studies (154, 155) have shown that "lenient" behavioral programs, which utilize initial bed rest and the threat of returning the patient to bed if weight gain does not continue, may be as effective and perhaps in some situations more efficient than "strict" programs, in which meal-by-meal caloric intake or daily weight is tied precisely to a schedule of privileges (e.g., time out of bed, time off the unit, permission to exercise or receive visitors). The use of various modalities considered coercive by patients with anorexia nervosa, for whom control is of such importance, is an issue to be carefully considered. The setting of limits is developmentally appropriate in the management of adolescents and may help shape the patient's behavior in a healthy direction. It is essential for caregivers to be clear about their own intentions and empathic regarding the patients' impressions of being coerced. Caregivers should be seen as using techniques that are not meant as coercive measures but rather are components of a general medical treatment required for the patient's health and survival.

Individual psychotherapy

During the acute phase of treatment, the efficacy of specific psychotherapeutic interventions for facilitating weight gain remains uncertain. Clinical consensus suggests that during acute refeeding and while weight gain is occurring, it is virtually always beneficial to provide patients with individual psychotherapeutic management that is psychodynamically sensitive and informed and that provides empathic understanding, explanations, praise for positive efforts, coaching, support, encouragement, and other positive behavioral reinforcement. During the acute phase of treatment, as well as later on, seeing patients' families is also helpful. For patients who initially lack motivation, psychotherapeutic encounters that employ techniques based on motivational enhancement may help patients increase their awareness and desire for recovery.

On the other hand, attempts to conduct formal psychotherapy with starving patients—who are often negativistic, obsessional, or mildly cognitively impaired—may often be ineffective. Clinical consensus suggests that psychotherapy alone is generally not sufficient to treat severely malnourished patients with anorexia nervosa. While the value of establishing and maintaining a psychotherapeutically informed relationship is clearly beneficial, and psychotherapeutic sessions to enhance motivation and to further weight gain are likely to be helpful, the value of formal psychotherapy during the acute refeeding stage is uncertain (156). As yet, no controlled studies have reported whether cognitive behavior psychotherapy or other specific psychotherapeutic interventions are effective for nutritional recovery. Some practitioners have used various modalities of group psychotherapy programs adjunctively in the treatment of anorexia nervosa (157–159). However, practitioners have also found that group psychotherapy programs conducted during the acute phase among malnourished patients with anorexia nervosa may be ineffective and can sometimes have negative therapeutic effects (e.g., patients may compete for who can be thinnest or exchange countertherapeutic techniques on simulating weight gain or hiding food) (160).

However, once malnutrition has been corrected and weight gain has started, considerable agreement exists that psychotherapy can be very helpful for patients with anorexia nervosa. Although there has been little formal study of its effectiveness, psychotherapy is generally thought to be helpful for patients to understand 1) what they have been through; 2) developmental, family, and cultural antecedents of their illness; 3) how their illness may have been a maladaptive attempt to cope and emotionally self-regulate; 4) how to avoid or minimize risks of relapse; and 5) how to better deal with salient developmental and other important life issues in the future. At present there is no absolute weight or percentage of body fat that indicates when a patient is actually ready to begin formal psychotherapy. However, clinical experience shows that patients often display improved mood, enhanced cognitive functioning, and clear thought processes even before there is substantial weight gain. Many clinicians favor cognitive behavior psychotherapy for maintaining healthy eating behaviors and cognitive or interpersonal psychotherapy for inducing cognitive restructuring and promoting more effective coping (161, 162). Many clinicians also employ psychodynamically oriented individual or group psychotherapy after acute weight restoration to address underlying personality disorders that may contribute to the illness and to foster psychological insight and maturation (18, 19, 42, 121, 163). Thus, verbal or experiential psychotherapeutic interventions can begin as soon as the patient is no longer in a medically compromised state.

In a minority of patients whose refractory anorexia nervosa continues despite notable trials of nutritional rehabilitation, medications, and hospitalizations, more extensive psychotherapeutic measures may be undertaken in further efforts to engage and help motivate them, or, failing that, as compassionate care. This "difficult to treat" subgroup may represent an as yet poorly understood group of patients with malignant, chronic anorexia nervosa. Efforts made to understand and to engage the unique plight of such a patient may sometimes result in engagement in the therapeutic alliance such that the nutritional protocol may begin (18, 19, 120, 164). For patients who have difficulty talking about their problems, clinicians have also tried a variety of nonverbal therapeutic methods, such as creative arts and movement therapy programs, and have reported them to be useful (165). At various stages of recovery, occupational therapy programs may also enhance deficits in self-concept and self-efficacy (166, 167).

Family psychotherapy

Family therapy and couples psychotherapy are frequently useful for both symptom reduction and dealing with family relational problems that may contribute to maintaining the disorder. In one controlled study of patients with anorexia nervosa with onset at or before age 18 and a duration of fewer than 3 years, those treated with family therapy showed greater improvement 1 year after discharge from the hospital than those treated with individual psychotherapy. The 5-year follow-up study showed, quite remarkably, a continuing effect of family therapy (168, 169). The study also points out that family therapy may have more impact for adolescents with eating disorders than for adults. One limitation of this study was that patients were not assigned to receive both family and individual treatment, a combination frequently used in practice.

Particular help should be offered to patients with eating disorders who are themselves mothers. Attention should be paid to their mothering skills and to their offspring to minimize the risk of transmission of eating disorders (170–172).

Psychosocial interventions based on addiction models

Some clinicians consider that eating disorders may be usefully treated through addiction models, but no data from short- or long-term outcome studies that used these methods have been reported. Some concerns about addiction-oriented programs for eating disorders result from zealous and narrow application of the 12-step philosophy. Clinicians have reported encountering patients who, while attempting to resolve anorexia nervosa by means of 12-step programs alone, could have been greatly helped by adding conventional treatment approaches to the 12-step model, such as medications, nutritional counseling, and psychodynamic or cognitive behavior approaches. By limiting their attempts to recover to 12 steps alone, such patients not only deprive themselves of the potential benefits of conventional treatments but also may expose themselves to misinformation about nutrition and eating disorders offered by well-intentioned nonprofessionals encountered in these groups.

It is important for programs that employ these models to be equipped to care for patients with the substantial psychiatric and general medical problems that are often associated with eating disorders. Some programs attempt to blend features of addiction models, such as the 12 steps, with medical model programs that employ cognitive behavior approaches (173). However, no systematic data exist regarding the effectiveness of these approaches for any patients with anorexia nervosa.

Support groups

Support groups led by professionals or by advocacy organizations are available and provide patients and their families with mutual support, advice, and education about eating disorders. These groups may be of adjunctive benefit in combination with other treatment modalities. Patients and their families are increasingly using on-line web sites, news groups, and chat rooms as resources. While a substantial amount of worthwhile information and support are available in this fashion, lack of professional supervision may sometimes lead to misinformation and unhealthy dynamics among users. Clinicians should inquire about the use of electronic support and other alternative and complementary approaches and be prepared to discuss information and ideas that patients and their families have gathered from these sources.

c. Implementation

Although a variety of different management models are used for patients with anorexia nervosa, there are no data available on their efficacies. When competent to do so, the psychiatrist should manage both the general medical and psychiatric needs of the patient. Some programs routinely arrange for interdisciplinary team management (sometimes called split management) models of treatment, wherein a psychiatrist writes orders, handles administrative and general medical requirements, and prescribes behavioral techniques intended to change the disturbed eating and weight patterns. Other clinicians then provide the psychotherapeutic intervention (in the form of cognitive behavior psychotherapy, psychodynamic psychotherapy, or family therapy) with the patient alone or in a group. For this management model to work effectively, all personnel must work closely together, maintaining open communication and mutual respect to avoid reinforcing some patients' tendencies to play staff off each other, i.e., to split the staff.

An alternative interdisciplinary management approach has general medical care providers (e.g., specialists in internal medicine, pediatrics, adolescent medicine, and nutrition) manage general medical issues, such as nutrition, weight gain, exercise, and eating patterns, while the psychiatrist addresses the psychiatric issues. In adolescence, the biopsychosocial nature of anorexia nervosa and bulimia nervosa especially indicates the need for interdisciplinary treatment. Each aspect of care must be developmentally tailored to the treatment of adolescents (174).

3. Medications

a. Goals
Medications are used most frequently after weight has been restored to maintain weight and normal eating behaviors as well as treat psychiatric symptoms associated with anorexia nervosa.

b. Efficacy

Antidepressants
Studies of antidepressants for restoration of weight are limited, and these medications are not routinely used in the acute phase of treatment for severely malnourished patients. One recent controlled study (175) showed no advantage for adding fluoxetine to nutritional and psychosocial interventions in the treatment of hospitalized, malnourished patients with anorexia nervosa with respect to either the amount or the speed of weight recovery. Results from an uncontrolled trial (176) suggest that fluoxetine may help some treatment-resistant patients with weight restoration, but many patients will not be helped.

Antidepressants may be considered after weight gain when the psychological effects of malnutrition are resolving, since these medications have been shown to be helpful with weight maintenance (149). In one controlled trial, weight-restored patients with anorexia nervosa who took fluoxetine (average 40 mg/day) after hospital discharge had less weight loss, depression, and fewer rehospitalizations for anorexia nervosa during the subsequent year than those who received placebo. Few other controlled studies of antidepressant treatment of anorexia nervosa have been published. In an open outpatient study (177), those treated with psychotherapy plus citalopram did worse (losing several kilograms) than underweight anorexia nervosa patients treated with psychotherapy alone (whose weights dropped about 0.2 kg during the period of observation), which suggests that this SSRI medication was counterproductive for this population. In one study (178), lower-weight patients with the restricting subtype of anorexia who were receiving intensive inpatient treatment seemed to benefit, albeit to a small degree, from a combination of amitriptyline and cyproheptadine. In another study (179), no significant beneficial effect was observed from adding clomipramine to the usual treatment (although doses of only 50 mg/day were used).

SSRIs are commonly considered for patients with anorexia nervosa whose depressive, obsessive, or compulsive symptoms persist in spite of or in the absence of weight gain.

Other medications

Few controlled studies have been published on the use of other psychotropic medications for the treatment of anorexia nervosa. In one study (180), lithium carbonate resulted in no substantial benefit. Another study suggested no significant benefit for pimozide (181).

Other psychotropic medications are most often used to treat psychiatric symptoms that may be associated with anorexia nervosa. Examples include low doses of neuroleptics for marked obsessionality, anxiety, and psychotic-like thinking and antianxiety agents used selectively before meals to reduce anticipatory anxiety concerning eating (58, 182). Although there are no controlled studies to support effectiveness, eating disorders clinicians are increasingly using low doses of newer novel antipsychotic medications together with SSRIs or other new antidepressants in treating highly obsessional and compulsive patients with anorexia nervosa.

Other somatic treatments, ranging from vitamin and hormone treatments to electroconvulsive therapy, have been tried in uncontrolled studies. None has been shown to have specific value in the treatment of anorexia nervosa symptoms (183). Although estrogen replacement is sometimes used in anorexia nervosa patients with chronic amenorrhea to reduce calcium loss and thereby reduce the risks of osteoporosis (52), existing evidence in support of hormone replacement therapy for the treatment or prevention of osteopenia in women with anorexia nervosa is marginal at best. Estrogen replacement has not been evaluated in children or adolescents. Seeman and colleagues (184) reported that the lumbar bone mineral density of women with anorexia nervosa who were taking oral contraceptives was significantly higher than that of patients not supplemented with estrogen, although the bone mineral density in both groups remained below normal for age. In preliminary studies (185, 186), hormone replacement therapy did not effectively improve bone mass density. The only controlled trial to date that looked at the effects of estrogen administration on women with anorexia nervosa showed that estrogen-treated patients had no significant change in bone mass density compared to control subjects. However, a subgroup of the estrogen-treated patients whose initial body weight was less than 70% of their ideal weight had a 4.0% increase in mean bone density, whereas subjects of comparable body weight not treated with estrogen had a further 20.1% decrease in bone density. This finding suggests that hormone replacement therapy may help a subset of low-weight women with anorexia nervosa (54). At the same time, artificially inducing menses carries the risk of supporting or reinforcing a patient's denial that she does not need to gain weight. On the other hand, weight rehabilitation has been shown to be an effective means of increasing bone mineral density (51, 187). To summarize, estrogen alone does not generally appear to reverse osteoporosis or osteopenia, and unless there is weight gain, it does not prevent further bone loss. Before offering estrogen, many clinicians stress that efforts should first be made to increase weight and achieve resumption of normal menses (188).

Furthermore, at the present time there is no evidence that any of the new treatments for postmenopausal osteoporosis, such as biphosphonates, are effective for treating osteoporosis in patients with anorexia nervosa (189). However, studies concerning these medications, bone growth factors, and other investigative treatments are now under way. If fracture risk is substantial, patients should be cautioned to avoid high-impact exercises.

Pro-motility agents such as metoclopramide are commonly offered for the bloating and abdominal pains due to gastroparesis and premature satiety seen in the some patients.

c. Side effects and toxicity

Many clinicians report that malnourished depressed patients are more prone to side effects and less responsive to the beneficial effects of tricyclics, SSRIs, and other novel antidepressant medications than depressed patients of normal weight. For example, the use of tricyclics may be associated with greater risks of hypotension, increased cardiac conduction times, and arrhythmia, particularly in purging patients whose hydration may be inadequate and whose cardiac status may be nutritionally compromised. Although fluoxetine has been found to impair appetite and cause weight loss in normal weight and obese patients at higher doses, this effect has not been reported in anorexia nervosa patients treated with lower doses. Citalopram has been associated with additional weight loss in anorexia nervosa (177). Because of the reported higher seizure risk associated with bupropion in purging patients, this medication should not be used in such patients (190, 191).

Strategies to manage side effects include limiting the use of medications to patients with persistent depression, anxiety, or obsessive-compulsive symptoms; using low initial doses in underweight patients; and being very vigilant about side effects. Given other alternatives, tricyclic antidepressants should be avoided in underweight patients and in patients who are at risk for suicide. In patients for whom there is a concern regarding potential cardiovascular effects of medication, cardiovascular consultations to evaluate status and to advise on the use of medication may be helpful.

d. Implementation

Because anorexia nervosa symptoms and associated features such as depression may remit with weight gain, decisions concerning the use of medications should often be deferred until weight has been restored. Antidepressants can be considered for weight maintenance. The decision to use medications and which medications to choose will be determined by the remaining symptom picture (e.g., antidepressants are usually considered for those with persistent depression, anxiety, or obsessive-compulsive symptoms).

B. TREATMENT OF BULIMIA NERVOSA

Strategies for the treatment of bulimia nervosa include nutritional counseling and rehabilitation; psychosocial interventions (including cognitive behavior, interpersonal, behavioral, psychodynamic, and psychoanalytic approaches) in individual or group format; family interventions; and medications.

1. Nutritional rehabilitation

Reducing binge eating and purging are primary goals in treating bulimia nervosa. Because most patients described in the bulimia nervosa psychotherapy treatment literature have been of normal weight, weight restoration is usually not a focus of therapy as it is with patients with anorexia nervosa. Even if they are within statistically normal ranges, many patients with bulimia nervosa weigh less than their appropriate biologically determined set points (or set ranges) and may have to gain some weight to achieve physiological and emotional stability. These patients require the establishment of a pattern of regular, non-binge meals, with attention paid to increasing their caloric intake and expanding macronutrient selection. Although many patients with bulimia nervosa report irregular menses, improvement in menstrual function has not been systematically assessed in the available outcome studies.

Even among patients of normal weight, nutritional counseling can be used to accomplish a variety of goals, such as reducing behaviors related to the eating disorder, minimizing food restriction, correcting nutritional deficiencies, increasing the variety of foods eaten, and encouraging healthy but not excessive exercise patterns. There is some evidence that treatment programs that include dietary counseling and management as part of the program are more effective than those that do not (192).

2. Psychosocial treatments

a. Goals

The goals of psychosocial interventions vary and can include the following: reduction in, or elimination of, binge-eating and purging behaviors; improvement in attitudes related to the eating disorder; minimization of food restriction; increasing the variety of foods eaten; encouragement of healthy but not excessive exercise patterns; treatment of comorbid conditions and clinical features associated with eating disorders; and addressing themes that may underlie eating disorder behaviors such as developmental issues, identity formation, body image concerns, self-esteem in areas outside of those related to weight and shape, sexual and aggressive difficulties, affect regulation, gender role expectations, family dysfunction, coping styles, and problem solving.

b. Efficacy

Individual psychotherapy
Cognitive behavioral psychotherapy, specifically directed at the eating disorder symptoms and underlying cognitions in patients with bulimia nervosa, is the psychosocial intervention that has been most intensively studied and for which there is the most evidence of efficacy (43, 192–209). Significant decrements in binge eating, vomiting, and laxative abuse have been documented among some patients receiving cognitive behavior therapy; however, the percentage of patients who achieve full abstinence from binge/purge behavior is variable and often includes only a minority of patients (43, 193, 195–199, 201, 202, 204, 206). Among studies with control arms, cognitive behavior therapy has been shown to be superior to waiting list (43, 195, 198, 202), minimal intervention (206), or nondirective control (201) conditions. In most of the published cognitive behavior therapy trials, significant improvements in either self-reported (198, 210) or clinician-rated (200) mood have been reported.

In practice, many other types of individual psychotherapy are employed in the treatment of bulimia nervosa, such as interpersonal, psychodynamically oriented, or psychoanalytic approaches. Clinical experience also suggests that these approaches can help in the treatment of the comorbid mood, anxiety, personality, interpersonal, and trauma- or abuse-related disorders that frequently accompany bulimia nervosa (211). Evidence for the efficacy of these treatments for bulimia nervosa comes mainly from case reports and case series. Some modes of therapy, including the interpersonal and psychodynamic approaches, have also been studied in randomized trials as comparison treatments for cognitive behavior therapy or in separate trials (196, 199, 212). In general, these and other studies have shown interpersonal psychotherapy to be helpful. The specific forms of focused psychodynamic psychotherapy that have been studied in direct comparison to cognitive behavior therapy have generally not been as effective as cognitive behavior therapy in short-term trials (213, 214).

Behavioral therapy, which consists of procedures of exposure (e.g., to binge eating food) plus response prevention (e.g., inhibiting vomiting after eating), has also been considered as treatment for bulimia nervosa. However, the evidence regarding the efficacy of this approach is conflicting, as studies have reported enhanced (215), not significantly altered (216), and reduced (193) responses to cognitive behavior therapy when behavioral therapy was used as an adjunct. On the basis of results from a large clinical trial, and given its logistical complexity, exposure treatment does not appear to have additive benefits over a solid core of cognitive behavior therapy (115).

Very few studies have directly compared the effectiveness of various types of individual psychotherapy for treatment of bulimia nervosa. One study by Fairburn and colleagues that compared cognitive behavior therapy, interpersonal psychotherapy, and behavior therapy showed that all three treatments were effective in reducing binge-eating symptoms by the end of treatment, but cognitive behavior therapy was most effective in improving disturbed attitudes toward shape and weight and restrictive dieting (196, 197, 213, 214, 217, 218). However, at long-term follow-up (mean=5.8 years), the study found equal efficacy for interpersonal psychotherapy and cognitive behavior therapy on eating variables, attitudes about shape and weight, and restrictive dieting (218), which suggests that interpersonal psychotherapy patients had "caught up" in terms of benefits over time. An ongoing multicenter study (39) has basically replicated these findings.

Group psychotherapy
Group psychotherapy approaches have also been used to treat bulimia nervosa. A meta-analysis of 40 group treatment studies suggested moderate efficacy, with those studies that reported 1-year follow-up data reporting that improvement was typically maintained (205). There is some evidence that group treatment programs that include dietary counseling and management as part of the program are more effective than those that do not (192), and that frequent visits early in treatment (e.g., sessions several times a week initially) result in improved outcome (196, 197, 204). Many clinicians favor a combination of individual and group psychotherapy. Psychodynamic and cognitive behavior approaches may be combined. Group therapy may help patients to more effectively deal with the shame surrounding their disease as well as provide additional peer-based feedback and support.

Family and marital therapy
Family therapy has been reported to be helpful in the treatment of bulimia nervosa in a large case series, but more systematic studies are not available (207). Family therapy should be considered whenever possible, especially for adolescents who still live with their parents, older patients with ongoing conflicted interactions with parents, or patients with marital discord. For women with eating disorders who are mothers, parenting help and interventions aimed at assessing and, if necessary, aiding their children should be included (170–172).

Support groups/12-step programs
Considerable controversy exists regarding the role of 12-step programs as the sole intervention in the treatment of eating disorders, primarily because these programs do not address nutritional considerations or the complex psychological/behavioral deficits of patients with eating disorders. Twelve-step programs or other approaches that exclusively focus on the need for abstinence without attending to nutritional consid-

erations or behavioral deficits are not recommended as the sole initial treatment approach for bulimia nervosa.

Some patients have found Overeaters Anonymous and similar groups to be helpful as adjuncts to initial treatments or for preventing subsequent relapses (203, 219), but no data from short- or long-term outcome studies of these programs have been reported. Because of the great variability of knowledge, attitudes, beliefs, and practices from chapter to chapter and from sponsor to sponsor regarding eating disorders and their general medical and psychotherapeutic treatment, and because of the great variability of patients' personality structures, clinical conditions, and susceptibility to potential countertherapeutic practices, clinicians should carefully monitor patients' experiences with these programs.

c.   Side effects and toxicity

Patients occasionally have difficulty with certain elements of psychotherapy. For example, among patients receiving cognitive behavior therapy, some are quite resistant to self-monitoring while others have difficulty mastering cognitive restructuring. Many patients are initially resistant to changing their eating behaviors, particularly when it comes to increasing their caloric intake or reducing exercise. However, complete lack of acceptance of the approach appears to be rare, although this has not been systematically studied.

Management strategies to deal with potential negative effects of psychotherapeutic interventions include 1) careful pretreatment evaluation, during which time the therapist must assess and enhance the patient's level of motivation for change and identify appropriate candidates for a given approach and format (e.g., individual versus group); 2) being alert to a patient's reactions to and attitudes about the proposed treatment and listening to and discussing the patient's concerns in a supportive fashion; 3) ongoing monitoring of the quality of the therapeutic relationship; and 4) identification of patients for whom another treatment should be coadministered or given before psychotherapy begins (e.g., chemical dependency treatment for those actively abusing alcohol or other drugs, antidepressant treatment for patients whose depression makes them unable to become actively involved, more intensive psychotherapy for those with severe personality disorders, and group therapy for those not previously participating). Alternative strategies may be necessary to move the therapeutic process forward and to prevent abrupt termination of therapy.

d.   Implementation

A review of the literature shows that the way in which psychotherapy has been implemented varies, in some cases considerably. For cognitive behavior therapy, several controlled trials used fairly short-term, time-limited interventions, such as 20 individual psychotherapy sessions over 16 weeks, with two scheduled visits per week for the first 4 weeks (193, 196, 197, 213, 214, 217, 218, 220–222). Some investigators have examined whether more than one visit per week is needed, particularly early in treatment. In one study of group cognitive behavior psychotherapy (204), additional visits early in treatment or twice weekly visits throughout treatment were both superior regimens to one psychotherapy session per week.

A growing literature has suggested that cognitive behavior therapy can be administered successfully through self-help or guided self-help manuals, at times in association with pharmacotherapy (223–227). While such techniques are not yet sufficiently developed to recommend their acceptance as a primary treatment strategy, developments in this area may prove of great importance in providing treatment to patients who otherwise might not have access to adequate care. Clinicians unfamiliar with the cognitive behavior therapy approach may benefit from acquainting themselves with these treatment manuals and obtaining specialized training in cognitive behavior therapy to further help their bulimia nervosa patients by using such manuals in treatment (213, 228–233).

This section has presented the results of cognitive behavior therapy and other short-term treatments, since these treatments have been the subject of the preponderance of studies. However, the field is in great need of well-conducted studies that examine other treatment approaches, particularly psychodynamically informed therapies. In addition, most available studies report relatively short-term results. Better studies are needed of the long-term effectiveness of these as well as other psychotherapeutic approaches, particularly for the complex presentations with multiple comorbid conditions that are usually seen in psychiatric practice.

3. Medications

a. Goals
Medications, primarily antidepressants, are used to reduce the frequency of disturbed eating behaviors such as binge eating and vomiting. In addition, pharmacotherapy is employed to alleviate symptoms that may accompany disordered eating behaviors, such as depression, anxiety, obsessions, or certain impulse disorder symptoms.

b. Antidepressants

Efficacy
The observation that some patients with bulimia nervosa were clinically depressed led to the first uses of antidepressants in the acute phase of treatment (234). However, later randomized trials demonstrated that nondepressed patients also responded to these medications and that baseline presence of depression was not a predictor of medication response (235–237). Although wide variability exists across studies, reductions in binge eating and vomiting rates in the range of 50%–75% have been achieved with active medication (191, 238–252). The available studies also suggest that antidepressants improve associated comorbid disorders and complaints such as mood and anxiety symptoms. Some studies show improved interpersonal functioning with medication as well. Specific antidepressant agents that have demonstrated efficacy among patients with bulimia nervosa in double-blind, placebo-controlled studies include tricyclic compounds such as imipramine (234, 253), desipramine (235, 254–256), and amitriptyline (for mood but not eating variables) (236); the SSRI fluoxetine (242–244); several MAOIs, including phenelzine (237), isocarboxazid (257), and brofaromine (for vomiting but not binge eating) (258); and several other antidepressants, including mianserin (252), bupropion (191), and trazodone (250). (Bupropion, however, was associated with seizures in purging bulimic patients, so its use is not recommended.) One study (251) suggests that patients with atypical depression and bulimia nervosa may preferentially respond to phenelzine in comparison with imipramine. However, since MAOIs are potentially dangerous in patients with chaotic eating and purging, great caution should be exercised in their use for bulimia nervosa. To date, the only medication approved by the Food and Drug Administration for bulimia nervosa is fluoxetine.

Two trials have examined the utility of antidepressant maintenance therapy. One trial with fluvoxamine (240) demonstrated an attenuated relapse rate versus placebo in patients with bulimia nervosa who were on a maintenance regimen of the medication after leaving an inpatient treatment program; however, in the continuation arm of a clinical trial with desipramine (256), 29% of the patients entering that phase experienced a relapse within 4 months. Trials using fluoxetine for relapse prevention are currently under way.

Side effects and toxicity

Side effects vary widely across studies depending on the type of antidepressant medication used. For the tricyclic antidepressants, common side effects include sedation, constipation, dry mouth, and, with amitriptyline, weight gain (234–236, 253–255). The toxicity of tricyclic antidepressants in overdose, up to and including death, also dictates caution in patients who are at risk for suicide. In the first multicenter fluoxetine trial (242), the most common side effects at 60 mg/day were insomnia (30%), nausea (28%), and asthenia (23%). In the second multicenter study (244), the most common side effects were insomnia (35%), nausea (30%), and asthenia (21%). Sexual side effects are also common in patients receiving SSRIs. Studies using various other medications have reported substantial dropout rates, although attrition rates across clinical trials have varied dramatically, and the degree to which medication side effects are the cause of high dropout rates has not been defined. Other common contributors to dropping out of clinical trials may involve subtle interpersonal and psychodynamic factors in the physician-patient relationships, which if left unaddressed will also contribute to treatment resistance. The quality of collaboration between patient and clinician is key to success in medication trials (259).

For patients with bulimia nervosa who require mood stabilizers, lithium carbonate is problematic, since lithium levels may shift markedly with rapid volume changes. Both lithium carbonate and valproic acid frequently lead to undesirable weight gains. Selection of a mood stabilizer that avoids these problems may result in better compliance and effectiveness.

No clear risk factors for the development of side effects among patients with bulimia nervosa have been identified. As in most clinical situations, careful preparation of the patient regarding possible side effects and their symptomatic management if they develop should be employed (e.g., stool softeners for constipation).

Implementation

Often, several different antidepressant medications may have to be tried sequentially to achieve the optimum effect. Doses of tricyclic and MAOI antidepressants for treating patients with bulimia nervosa parallel those used to treat patients with depression, although fluoxetine at doses higher than those used for depression may be more effective for bulimic symptoms (e.g., 60–80 mg/day). The first multicenter fluoxetine study (242) demonstrated that 60 mg was clearly superior to 20 mg on most variables, and in the second study (244) all subjects receiving active medication started with 60 mg. The medication was surprisingly well tolerated at this dose, and many clinicians initiate treatment for bulimia nervosa with fluoxetine at the higher dose, titrating downward if necessary due to side effects.

In cases where symptoms do not respond to medication, it is important to assess whether the patient has taken the medication shortly before vomiting. Serum levels of medication may be obtained to determine whether presumably effective levels have actually been achieved. One study (235) suggested that desipramine serum levels similar to those targeted in depression studies are most therapeutic in patients with bulimia nervosa, but in general serum level/response data have not been presented.

There are few reports on the use of antidepressant medications in the maintenance phase. Available data suggest high rates of relapse while taking medication and possibly higher rates when medications are withdrawn (256). In the absence of more systematic data, most clinicians recommend continuing antidepressant therapy for a minimum of 6 months and probably for a year in most patients with bulimia nervosa.

c. Other medications

A number of other medications have been used experimentally for bulimia nervosa without evidence of efficacy, including fenfluramine (239) and lithium carbonate (245). Fenfluramine has now been taken off the market because of associations between its use (mainly in combination with phentermine) and cardiac valvular abnormalities. Lithium continues to be used occasionally as an adjunct for the treatment of comorbid conditions. The opiate antagonist naltrexone has been studied in three randomized trials at doses used for narcotic addiction and for relapse prevention in alcohol abuse (50–120 mg/day). The results consistently show that the medication is not superior to placebo in the reduction of bulimic symptoms (238, 246, 249). In a small, double-blind crossover study involving higher doses (e.g., 200–300 mg/day), naltrexone did appear to have some efficacy. Further studies using these dose ranges are needed. However, there have been mixed reports concerning the risk of hepatotoxicity with the use of high doses (247, 248, 260).

4. Combinations of psychosocial and medication treatment

Six studies have examined the relative efficacy of psychotherapy, medication, or both in the treatment of bulimia nervosa. In the first study (261), intensive group cognitive psychotherapy (45 hours of therapy over 10 weeks) was superior to imipramine alone in reducing symptoms of binge eating and purging and symptoms of depression. Imipramine plus intensive group cognitive behavior therapy did not improve the outcome on eating variables but did improve depression and anxiety variables. In the second study (262), patients in group cognitive behavior therapy improved more than those receiving desipramine alone. Some advantage was also seen for combination therapy on some variables, such as dietary restraint. The third study (263), which compared fluoxetine treatment, cognitive behavior therapy, and combination therapy, favored cognitive behavior therapy alone and suggested little benefit for combination therapy. Results of this study are difficult to interpret because of a high attrition rate (50% by the 1-month follow-up). In the fourth study (264), cognitive behavior therapy was superior to supportive psychotherapy; active medication (consisting of desipramine, followed by fluoxetine if abstinence from binge eating and purging was not achieved) was superior to placebo in reducing eating disorder behaviors. The combination of cognitive behavior therapy and active medication resulted in the highest abstinence rates. The use of sequential medication in this study addressed a limitation of earlier studies in that typically when one antidepressant fails, a clinician tries other agents, which often result in better antidepressant efficacy than seen with the first medication alone. In the fifth study (241), no advantage was found for the use of fluoxetine over placebo in an inpatient setting, although both groups improved significantly. In the sixth study (265), combination treatment with desipramine and cognitive behavior therapy was terminated prematurely because of a high dropout rate.

In conclusion, the studies suggest that target symptoms such as binge eating and purging and attitudes related to the eating disorder generally respond better to cognitive behavior therapy than pharmacotherapy (261–263), with at least two studies

(262, 264) showing that the combination of cognitive behavior therapy and medication is superior to either alone. Two of the studies suggest a greater improvement in mood and anxiety variables when antidepressant therapy is added to cognitive behavior therapy (261, 264). Of note, many experienced clinicians do not find cognitive behavior therapy to be as useful as described by researchers. This may be due to several factors, including clinician inexperience or discomfort with the methods or differences between patients seen in the community and those who have participated as research subjects in these studies.

V. CLINICAL AND ENVIRONMENTAL FEATURES INFLUENCING TREATMENT

A. OTHER IMPORTANT CLINICAL FEATURES OF EATING DISORDERS

1. Eating disorder not otherwise specified

Eating disorder not otherwise specified is a commonly used diagnosis, given to nearly 50% of patients with eating disorders who present to tertiary care eating disorders programs. Eating disorder not otherwise specified appears to be particularly common among adolescents. This heterogeneous group of patients largely consists of subsyndromal cases of anorexia nervosa or bulimia nervosa (e.g., those who fail to meet one criterion, such as not having 3 months of amenorrhea or having fewer binge eating episodes per week than required for strictly defined diagnosis). One variant of eating disorder not otherwise specified consists of abusers of weight reduction medications who are trying to lose excessive amounts of weight for cosmetic reasons. In general, the nature and intensity of treatment depends on the symptom profile and severity of impairment, not the DSM-IV diagnosis.

One diagnosis within the eating disorder not otherwise specified category is binge-eating disorder. Although it is not an approved DSM-IV diagnosis at this time, there are research criteria listed in DSM-IV, which consist of disturbances in one or more of the following spheres: behavioral (e.g., binge eating), somatic (e.g., obesity is common although not required), and psychological (e.g., body image dissatisfaction, low self-esteem, depression) (8). Although binge-eating disorder appears to be relatively rare in community cohorts (2% prevalence), it is common among patients seeking treatment for obesity at hospital-affiliated weight programs (30% prevalence) (266). About one-third of these patients are male. Binge-eating disorder occurs much more frequently in adults than in adolescents. Strategies for the treatment of binge-eating disorder include nutritional counseling and dietary management; individual or group behavioral, cognitive behavior, interpersonal, or psychodynamic psychotherapy; and medications.

a. Nutritional rehabilitation and counseling; effect of diet programs on weight

Very-low-calorie diets in patients with binge-eating disorder have been associated with substantial initial weight losses, with over one-third of these patients maintaining their weight loss 1 year after treatment (267–270). Very-low-calorie diets employed together with group behavioral weight control have been effective in reducing binge eating during the period of fasting but may be less effective during or following re-feeding (267, 268, 270). However, since such dieting may disinhibit eating and lead to compensatory overeating and binge eating (271), and since chronic calorie restriction can also increase symptoms of depression, anxiety, and irritability (46), new alternative therapies that use a nondiet approach by focusing on self-acceptance, improving body image, better nutrition and health, and increased physical movement and not on weight loss have been developed (272–274). Studies that compared traditional behavioral weight loss programs with nondieting programs have found similar rates of maintained weight loss, with the nondiet programs also producing significant reductions in symptoms related to binge eating, depression, anxiety, bulimia, drive for thinness, and body dissatisfaction (275, 276). Patients with histories of repeated weight loss attempts followed by weight gain (so-called "yo-yo" dieting) or patients with an early onset of binge eating might benefit from following programs that focus on decreasing binge eating rather than weight loss (277, 278).

b. Psychosocial treatments

Cognitive behavior therapy, behavior therapy, and interpersonal therapy have all been associated with binge frequency reduction rates of two-thirds or more and significant abstinence rates during active treatment. However, deterioration during the follow-up period has been observed with all three forms of psychotherapy. Behavior therapy, but not cognitive behavior therapy, has generally been associated with a significant initial weight loss that is then partially regained during the first year following treatment (279–287). This pattern of weight regain after initial weight loss is common in all general medical and psychological treatments for obesity, not only for obesity associated with binge-eating disorder. One 6-year study (288) that followed intensively treated patients with binge-eating disorder found that approximately 57% had good outcomes, 35% intermediate outcomes, and 6% had poor outcomes; 1% had died. Self-help programs using self-guided professionally designed manuals have been effective in reducing the symptoms of binge-eating disorder in the short run for some patients and may sometimes have long-term benefit (289). Addiction-based 12-step approaches, self-help organizations, or treatment programs based on the Alcoholics Anonymous model have been tried, but no systematic outcome studies of these programs are available.

c. Medications

It must be pointed out that medication treatment studies of binge-eating disorder have generally reported very high placebo response rates (around 70%) (238, 290). These high placebo response rates suggest that great caution is needed in evaluating claims of effective treatments, particularly in studies that use only a waiting list control condition.

Medications, primarily antidepressants, have been used in the treatment of binge-eating disorder and related syndromes. Tricyclic antidepressants and fluvoxamine have been associated with reductions of 63%–90% in binge frequency during 2–3 months of treatment (238, 291–293). Naltrexone has been associated with a decrease in binge frequency on the same order (73%), although this rate did not differ from the response to placebo (238). Patients tend to relapse after medication is discontinued (290, 293).

Although the appetite suppressant medications fenfluramine and dexfenfluramine have also been found to significantly reduce binge frequency (290), their use has been associated with serious adverse events, including a 23-fold increase in the risk of developing primary pulmonary hypertension when used for longer than 3 months (294). Very recent studies suggest that patients taking the combination of fenfluramine and phentermine may be at greater risk of heart valve deformation and pulmonary hypertension; as a result, fenfluramine has been withdrawn from the market (294–297). Studies in animals indicate that fenfluramine and dexfenfluramine may be associated with persistent serotonergic neurotoxicity (298, 299).

d. Combined psychosocial and medication treatment strategies

In most studies, the co-administration of medication with psychotherapy has been found to be associated with significantly more weight loss than with psychotherapy alone (280, 300).

2. Chronicity of eating disorders

Many patients who have a chronic course of anorexia nervosa, extending for a decade or more, are unable to maintain a healthy weight and suffer from chronic depression, obsessionality, and social withdrawal. Individualized treatment planning and careful case management are necessary for such chronic patients. Treatment may require consultation with other specialists, repeated hospitalizations, partial hospitalizations, residential care, individual or group therapy, other social therapies, trials of various medications as indicated, and, occasionally, ECT in patients who are seriously depressed. Communication among professionals is especially important throughout the outpatient care of such patients. With chronic patients, small progressive gains and fewer relapses may be the goals of psychological interventions. More frequent outpatient contact and other supports may sometimes help prevent further hospitalizations. Expectations for weight gain with hospitalization may be more modest for chronic patients. Achieving a safe weight compatible with life rather than a healthy weight may be all that is possible. Focusing on quality-of-life issues, rather than change in weight or normalization of eating, and providing compassionate care may be all one can realistically achieve (21, 301).

▶ B. OTHER PSYCHIATRIC FACTORS

1. Substance abuse/dependence

Substance abuse/dependence is common among women with eating disorders (6). Among individuals with bulimia nervosa, 22.9% have been observed to meet criteria for alcohol abuse (302). Substance abuse appears to be less common among restricting patients with anorexia nervosa than among those having the binge-eating/purge type (123, 303, 304). For example, one recent prospective, longitudinal study (305) found bulimic anorectic women to be seven times more likely to develop substance abuse problems than restricting anorectic patients. Patients with comorbid substance abuse and eating disorders appear to have more severe problems with impulsivity in general, including greater risks of shoplifting, suicide gestures, and laxative abuse (135, 304, 306). Available studies indicate that eating disorder patients with a history of prior but currently inactive substance abuse respond to standard therapies in the same manner as those without such a history (307–309) and do not appear to experience exacerbations of their substance abuse disorders after successful treatment (308). However, the presence of a currently active comorbid substance abuse problem does have implications for treatment. A study of 70 patients with comorbid eating disorders and substance abuse found that the associated axis III medical disorders reflected complications of both eating disorders and substance abuse disorders. Patients with comorbid eating and substance abuse disorders required longer inpatient stays and were less compliant with treatment following hospitalization than those with substance abuse disorders alone (310). Where treatment staff are competent to treat both disorders, concurrent treatment should be attempted.

2. Mood and anxiety disorders

A very high percentage of treatment-seeking patients with eating disorders report a lifetime history of unipolar depression (124, 311, 312). Nutritional insufficiency and weight loss often predispose patients to symptoms of depression (46). Depressed individuals with an eating disorder experience greater levels of anxiety, guilt, and obsessionality, but less social withdrawal and lack of interest, than depressed individuals without eating disorders (313). Several studies suggest that the presence of comorbid depression at initial presentation has minimal or no predictive value for treatment outcome (84). However, the experience of many clinicians suggests that severe depression can impair a patient's ability to become meaningfully involved in psychotherapy and may dictate the need for medication treatment for the mood symptoms from the beginning of treatment.

Lifetime prevalence rates for anxiety disorders also appear to be higher for patients with both anorexia nervosa and bulimia nervosa, but rates for specific anxiety disorders vary (122). In patients with anorexia nervosa, social phobia and OCD are the anxiety disorders most commonly described. For those with bulimia nervosa, comorbid presentations of social phobia, OCD, or simple phobia are most often described. Overanxious disorders of childhood are also common in both anorexia nervosa and bulimia nervosa and precede the onset of these eating disorders (314). Although there is no clear evidence that comorbid anxiety disorders impact significantly on eating disorder treatment outcome, such comorbid problems should be addressed in treatment planning.

3. Personality disorders

The reported prevalence of personality disorders has varied widely across eating disorders and across studies. Individuals with anorexia nervosa tend to have higher rates of cluster C personality disorders, while normal weight patients with bulimia nervosa are more likely to display features of cluster B disorders, particularly impulsive, affective, and narcissistic trait disturbances (128, 315–320). The presence of borderline personality disorder seems to be associated with a greater disturbance in eating attitudes, a history of more frequent hospitalizations, and the presence of other problems such as suicide gestures and self-mutilation (316, 320). The presence of borderline personality disorder is also associated with poorer treatment outcome and higher levels of psychopathology at follow up (321, 322). Although it has not yet been systematically studied, clinical consensus strongly suggests that the presence of a comorbid personality disorder, particularly borderline personality disorder, dictates the need for longer-term therapy that focuses on the underlying personality structure and dealing with interpersonal relationships in addition to the symptoms of the eating disorder.

4. Posttraumatic stress disorder (PTSD)

Available data on the extent of PTSD among patients with eating disorders are still limited. According to one national survey (323), the lifetime rate of PTSD was nearly 37% among women with bulimia nervosa, much higher than the rate of PTSD seen in community cohorts. There are higher rates of abuse history in patients with bulimia nervosa. Histories of trauma and PTSD are likely to be important in therapy and should be taken into consideration.

C. CONCURRENT GENERAL MEDICAL CONDITIONS

1. Type 1 diabetes mellitus

Eating disorder symptoms appear to be more common among females with diabetes mellitus than in the general population. Thus, a high index of suspicion for these disorders is warranted for those working with young female diabetic patients. The presentation of eating disorders in the context of diabetes mellitus may be substantially more complex than that seen with eating disorders alone, may require more interaction with general medical specialists, and may present as numerous general medical crises before the presence of the eating disorder is diagnosed and treated. There is good evidence that when bulimia nervosa or eating disorder not otherwise specified co-occur with diabetes mellitus, rates of diabetic complications are higher. Diabetics with eating disorders often underdose their insulin in order to lose weight. Out-of-control diabetics with bulimia nervosa may require a period of inpatient treatment for stabilization of both the diabetes mellitus and the disturbed eating (324, 325).

Parenthetically, poor compliance or underdosing with weight-inducing medications such as steroids, anticonvulsants, lithium, and other psychotropic medications necessary for the treatment of other conditions occurs often in patients with eating disorders and even in those with subclinical weight concerns.

2. Pregnancy

Eating disorders may begin de novo during pregnancy, but many patients get pregnant even while they are actively symptomatic with an eating disorder. The behaviors associated with eating disorders including inadequate nutritional intake, binge eating, purging by various means, and the use or abuse of some teratogenic medications (e.g., to varying degrees lithium, benzodiazepines, or divalproex) can all result in fetal or maternal complications (326). The care of a pregnant patient with an eating disorder is difficult and usually requires the collaboration of a psychiatrist and an obstetrician who specializes in high-risk pregnancies (327–330). Although some patients may be able to eat normally and decrease binge eating and purging during their pregnancy, it is best for the eating disorder to be treated before the pregnancy if possible. Among patients whose symptoms abate during pregnancy, there is some evidence that the eating disorder symptoms often recur after delivery (331). Although women with lifetime histories of anorexia nervosa may not have reduced fertility, they do appear to be at risk of a greater number of birth complications than comparison subjects and of giving birth to babies of lower birth weight (304). This is true both for women who are actively anorectic at the time of pregnancy as well as for women with a prior history of anorexia nervosa. Mothers with eating disorders may have more difficulties than others in feeding their babies and young children than other mothers and may need additional guidance, assistance, and monitoring of their mothering (170–172).

D. DEMOGRAPHIC VARIABLES

1. Male gender

Especially in bulimia subgroups, males with eating disorders who present to tertiary care centers may have more comorbid substance use disorders and more antisocial personality disorders than females. Like females, they are prone to osteoporosis (332). Although gender does not appear to influence the outcome of treatment, some aspects of treatment may need to be modified on the basis of gender. Open-blind studies suggest that normalizing testosterone in males during nutritional rehabilitation for anorexia nervosa may be helpful in increasing lean muscle mass, but definitive studies are not completed. Although studies in clinical samples have suggested that there might be a higher incidence of homosexuality among males with eating disorders (333, 334), this has not yet been confirmed epidemiologically. Nevertheless, since issues concerning sexual orientation are not uncommon among males with eating disorders seen in clinical settings, these issues should be considered in treatment (333). Where possible, therapy groups for males alone may address some of the specific needs of these patients and help them deal with the occasional stigmatization of males by females in treatment. Males with anorexia nervosa may require higher energy intakes (up to 4,000–4,500 kcal/day), since they normally have higher lean body mass and lower fat mass compared to females. And, since they are larger to begin with, males with anorexia nervosa often require much larger weight gains to get back to normal weight (335).

Of note, epidemiological prevalence studies of anorexia nervosa and bulimia nervosa indicate that in North America there are probably more males with bulimia nervosa than females with anorexia nervosa. Although eating disorders are much more prevalent in women, males with eating disorders are not rare and case series of males often report on hundreds of patients (333, 335). The stereotype that eating disorders are female illnesses may limit a full understanding of the scope and nature of problems faced by male patients with eating disorders.

2. Age

Although most eating disorders start while patients are in their teens and 20s, earlier and later onsets are encountered as well. In some patients with early onsets (i.e., between ages 7 and 12), obsessional behavior and depression are common. Children often present with physical symptoms such as nausea, abdominal pain, feeling full, or being unable to swallow; their weight loss can be rapid and dramatic. Children with early-onset anorexia nervosa may suffer from delayed growth (174, 336–340) and may be especially prone to osteopenia and osteoporosis (51, 52). In a few cases, exacerbations of anorexia nervosa and OCD-like symptoms have been associated with pediatric infection-triggered autoimmune neuropsychiatric disorders (341, 342). Bulimia nervosa under the age of 12 is rare.

Anorexia nervosa has been reported in elderly patients in their 70s and 80s, in whom the illness has generally been present for 40 or 50 years. In many cases the illness started after age 25 (so-called anorexia tardive). In some case reports, adverse life events such as deaths, marital crisis, or divorce have been found to trigger these older-onset syndromes. Fear of aging has also been described as a major precipitating factor in some patients (19, 343). Rates of comorbid depression have been reported to be higher among these patients in some studies but not in others (344).

3. Cultural factors

Specific pressures and values concerning weight and shape vary among different cultures. Strivings for beauty and acceptance according to the stereotypes they perceive in global-cast media are leading increasing numbers of women around the world to develop attitudes and eating behaviors associated with eating disorders (105, 345). Clinicians should engage these women in informed and sensitive discussions regarding their struggles and personal experiences about what it means to be feminine and what it means to be "perfect" in the modern world (346). Clinicians should be sensitive to and inquire as to how weight and shape concerns are experienced by patients, especially those who are minorities, from non-Western or other cultural backgrounds, or are transitioning and assimilating into Western societies.

4. Eating disorders in athletes

Eating disorders are more common among competitive athletes than the general age-matched population (347, 348). Female athletes are especially at risk in sports that emphasize a thin body or appearance, such as gymnastics, ballet, figure skating, and distance running. Males in sports such as bodybuilding and wrestling are also at greater risk. Certain antecedent factors such as cultural preoccupation with thinness, performance anxiety, and athlete self-appraisal may predispose a female athlete to body dissatisfaction, which often mediates the development of eating disorder symptoms (349). Parents and coaches of young athletes may support distorted shape and eating attitudes in the service of guiding the athlete to be more competitive.

Physicians working with adolescent and young adult athletes, particularly those athletes participating in the at-risk sports, must be alert to early symptoms of eating disorders. Simple screening questions about weight, possible dissatisfaction with appearance, amenorrhea, and nutritional intake on the day before evaluation may help identify an athlete who is developing an eating disorder. Early general medical and psychiatric intervention is key to prompt recovery.

Extreme exercise appears to be a risk factor for developing anorexia nervosa, especially when combined with dieting (112). A "female athlete triad" has been identified, consisting of disordered eating, amenorrhea, and osteoporosis (350). Similarly, an "overtraining syndrome" has been described: a state of exhaustion, depression, and irritability in which athletes continue to train but their performance diminishes (351). Both have been linked to the syndrome of "activity anorexia," which has been observed in animal models (352).

5. Eating disorders in high schools and colleges

Eating disorders are common among female high school and college students, and psychiatrists and other health and mental health professionals may be involved in their care in various ways. From a primary prevention perspective, health professionals may be called upon to provide information and education about eating disorders in classrooms, athletic programs, and assorted other extracurricular venues. The efficacy of such programs for the reduction of eating disorders is still uncertain (353, 354). Helping in early intervention, health professionals may serve as trainers, coordinators, and professional supports for peer counseling efforts conducted at school, in dormitories, and through other campus institutions. Through student health and student psychological services, they may serve as initial screeners and diagnosticians and help manage students with varying levels of severity of eating disorders (355).

On occasion psychiatrists may be called upon as clinicians and as agents of the school administration to offer guidance in the management of impaired students with serious eating disorders. In such situations the suggested guidelines for levels of care described in table 1 should be followed. Accordingly, to stay in school students must be treatable as outpatients. It is advisable that students be required to take a leave of absence if they are severely ill (355, 356). The student should be directed to inpatient hospital care if weight is 30% or more below an expected healthy weight, or if any of the other indications for hospitalization listed in table 1 are present.

For students with serious eating disorders who remain in school, the psychiatrist and other health providers should work with the school's administration toward developing policies and programs that make student attendance contingent upon participation in a suitable treatment program. For the severely ill student, the clinical team must include a general medical clinician who can gauge safety and monitor weight, vital signs, and laboratory indicators. For the student to be permitted to continue in school, these clinicians may require a minimum weight and other physical, behavioral, or laboratory target measures to ensure basic medical safety. An explicit policy should be developed specifying that clinicians have the final say regarding the student's participation in physically demanding activities such as organized athletics. Restrictions must be based on actual medical concerns. Procedures should be in compliance with the school's policies regarding management of students with psychiatric disabilities and the Americans with Disabilities Act (356).

VI. RESEARCH DIRECTIONS

Further studies of eating disorders are needed that address issues surrounding the epidemiology, causes, and course of illness. Areas of specific concern include:

1. Genetic and other biological, gender-related, psychological, familial, social, and cultural risk factors that contribute to the development of specific eating disorders, greater morbidity and higher mortality, treatment resistance, and risk of relapse.
2. Structure-function relationships associated with predisposing vulnerabilities, nutritional changes associated with the disorders, and changes in recovery examined through imaging studies.
3. The differential presentation of eating disorders across various developmental periods from early childhood through late adulthood.
4. Linkages between physiological and psychological processes of puberty and the onset of typical eating disorders.
5. The impact of various comorbid conditions (including mood, anxiety, substance abuse, obsessive-compulsive symptoms, personality disorders, PTSD, cognitive impairments, and other commonly encountered concurrent disorders) on course and treatment response.
6. The effect of exercise, including the role of extreme exercise, and food restriction in precipitating and maintaining eating disorders. Conversely, the possible protective effect of contemporary women's athletics on girls' eating and weight attitudes.
7. Further delineation and definition of eating disorder not otherwise specified and binge-eating disorder, with clarification of risk factors, morbidity, treatments, and prognosis.
8. Family studies on factors associated with onset and maintenance of eating disorders, as well as concerning the impact of eating disorders on other family members.
9. Culturally flexible diagnostic criteria to allow for the identification and treatment of the many "atypical" cases, which may represent a large number of eating disorders patients in non-Western societies.

Additional studies and assessments of new interventions are also needed, specifically with regard to

1. Primary prevention programs in schools and through the media.
2. Targeted prevention through screenings and risk-factor early intervention programs.
3. Improved guidelines for choice of treatment setting and selection of specific treatments on the basis of more refined clinical indicators and a better understanding of the stages of these disorders (including follow-up issues for short-term and long-term treatment studies).
4. Development and testing of newer biological agents affecting hunger, satiety, and energy expenditure as well as commonly associated psychiatric symptoms and conditions.
5. Development and testing of various individually administered and "bundled" individual and group psychotherapies including cognitive behavior, interpersonal, psychodynamic, psychoanalytic, and family therapies as well as nutritional therapies and other psychosocial therapies (creative arts, 12-step models, and professional or layperson-led support groups and self-help groups for patients and families).
6. Treatment outcome studies related to various systems or settings of care, including HMO versus fee for service; limitations of hospital or other intensive treatment resources due to managed care and other resource limitations; treatment in eating disorder specialty units versus general psychiatry treatment units; and impact of staff composition, professional background of providers, system or setting characteristics, and roles of primary care versus mental health providers in the treatment of eating disorders.
7. Further development and testing of professionally designed self-administered treatments by manuals and computer-based treatment programs.
8. Modifications of treatment required because of various comorbid conditions.
9. The impact of commonly used "alternative" and "complementary" therapies on the course of illness.
10. New methods for assessing and treating osteopenia, osteoporosis, and other long-term medical sequelae.
11. Further delineation of proper education and training for psychiatrists and other healthcare providers to deal with patients with eating disorders.

VII. INDIVIDUALS AND ORGANIZATIONS THAT SUBMITTED COMMENTS

Carl Bell, M.D.
Peter J. V. Beumont, M.D.
Cynthia Bulik, M.D.
Paula Clayton, M.D.
Scott Crow, M.D.
Dave M. Davis, M.D.
David R. DeMaso, M.D.
Judith Dogin, M.D.
Christopher G. Fairburn, Ph.D.
Aaron H. Fink, M.D.
Martin Fisher, M.D.
Sara Forman, M.D.
David M. Garner, M.D.
Neville H. Golden, M.D.
Joseph Hagan, M.D.
Allan S. Kaplan, M.D.
Debra K. Katzman, M.D.
Melanie A. Katzman, M.D.
Diane Keddy, M.S., R.D.
Thomas E. Kottke, M.D., M.S.P.H.

Richard Kreipe, M.D.
Elaine Lonegran, M.S.W., Ph.D.
Jerome A. Motto, M.D.
Diane Mickley, M.D.
Jean Bradley Rubel, Ph.D.
Marian Schienholtz, M.S.W.
Paul M. Schyve, M.D.
Reba Sloan, M.P.H., L.R.D.
Mae Sokol, M.D.
Joshua Sparrow, M.D.
Michael Strober, M.D.
Albert Stunkard, M.D.
Richard T. Suchinsky, M.D.
Jack Swanson, M.D.
Janet Treasure, M.D.
Joe Westermeyer, M.D.
Denise Wilfley, Ph.D.
Stephen Wonderlich, Ph.D.

American Academy of Pediatrics
American Association of Directors of Psychiatric Residency Training
American Association of Suicidology
American Dietetic Association (Sports, Cardiovascular and Wellness Nutritionists)
Anorexia Nervosa and Related Eating Disorders
American Group Psychotherapy Association
Black Psychiatrists of America
Center for Eating and Weight Disorders
Joint Commission on Accreditation of Health Care Organizations

VIII. REFERENCES

The following coding system is used to indicate the nature of the supporting evidence in the references:

[A] *Randomized clinical trial.* A study of an intervention in which subjects are prospectively followed over time; there are treatment and control groups; subjects are randomly assigned to the two groups; both the subjects and the investigators are blind to the assignments.

[B] *Clinical trial.* A prospective study in which an intervention is made and the results of that intervention are tracked longitudinally; study does not meet standards for a randomized clinical trial.

[C] *Cohort or longitudinal study.* A study in which subjects are prospectively followed over time without any specific intervention.

[D] *Case-control study.* A study in which a group of patients and a group of control subjects are identified in the present and information about them is pursued retrospectively or backward in time.

[E] *Review with secondary analysis.* A structured analytic review of existing data, e.g., a meta-analysis or a decision analysis.

[F] *Review.* A qualitative review and discussion of previously published literature without a quantitative synthesis of the data.

[G] *Other.* Textbooks, expert opinion, case reports, and other reports not included above.

1. LaVia M, Kaye WH, Andersen A, Bowers W, Brandt HA, Brewerton TD, Costin C, Hill L, Lilenfeld L, McGilley B, Powers PS, Pryor T, Yager J, Zucker ML: Anorexia nervosa: criteria for levels of care. Eating Disorders Research Society Annual Meeting, Boston, 1998 [G]

2. Crisp AH, Callender JS, Halek C, Hsu LK: Long-term mortality in anorexia nervosa: a 20-year follow-up of the St George's and Aberdeen cohorts. Br J Psychiatry 1992; 161:104–107 [C]

3. Appelbaum PS, Rumpf T: Civil commitment of the anorexic patient. Gen Hosp Psychiatry 1998; 20:225–230 [G]

4. Maxmen JS, Silberfarb PM, Ferrell RB: Anorexia nervosa: practical initial management in a general hospital. JAMA 1974; 229:801–803 [G]

5. Treasure J, Palmer RL: Providing specialized services for anorexia nervosa. Br J Psychiatry (in press) [D]

6. Kaye W, Kaplan AS, Zucker ML: Treating eating disorders in a managed care environment. Psychiatr Clin North Am 1996; 19:793–810 [F]

7. Kaplan AS, Olmsted MP: Partial hospitalization, in Handbook of Treatment for Eating Disorders, 2nd ed. Edited by Garner DM, Garfinkel PE. New York, Guilford Press, 1997, pp 354–360 [G]

8. American Psychiatric Association: Practice guideline for eating disorders. Am J Psychiatry 1993; 150:212–228 [I]

9. Andersen AE: Practical Comprehensive Treatment of Anorexia Nervosa and Bulimia. Baltimore, Md, Johns Hopkins University Press, 1985 [I]

10. Owen W, Halmi KA: Medical evaluation and management of anorexia nervosa, in Treatments of Psychiatric Disorders: A Task Force Report of the American Psychiatric Association, vol 1. Washington, DC, APA, 1989, pp 517–519 [I]

11. Kaplan AS, Garfinkel P: Difficulties in treating patients with eating disorders: a review of patient and clinician variables. Can J Psychiatry 1999 (in press) [G]

12. Wooley SC: Uses of countertransference in the treatment of eating disorders: a gender perspective, in Psychodynamic Treatment of Anorexia Nervosa and Bulimia. Edited by Johnson CL. New York, Guilford Press, 1991, pp 245–294 [G]

13. Zerbe KJ: Knowable secrets: transference and countertransference manifestations in eating disordered patients, in Treating Eating Disorders: Ethical, Legal, and Personal Issues. Edited by Vandereycken W, Beumont PJV. New York, New York University Press, 1998, pp 30–55 [G]

14. Zunino N, Agoos E, Davis WN: The impact of therapist gender on the treatment of bulimic women. Int J Eat Disord 1991; 10:253–263 [E]

15. Katzman MA, Waller G: Implications of therapist gender in the treatment of eating disorders: daring to ask the questions, in The Burden of the Therapist. Edited by Vandereycken W. London, Athelone Press, 1998, pp 56–79 [G]

16. Waller G, Katzman MA: Female or male therapists for women with eating disorders? a pilot study of expert opinions. Int J Eat Disord 1997; 22:111–114 [G]

17. Bloom C, Gitter A, Gutwill S: Eating Problems: A Feminist Psychoanalytic Treatment Model. New York, Basic Books, 1994 [G]

18. Zerbe KJ: The Body Betrayed: Women, Eating Disorders, and Treatment. Washington, DC, American Psychiatric Press, 1993 [G]

19. Zerbe KJ: Whose body is it anyway? understanding and treating psychosomatic aspects of eating disorders. Bull Menninger Clin 1993; 57:161–177 [F]

20. Werne J: Treating Eating Disorders. San Francisco, Jossey-Bass, 1996 [G]

21. Yager J: Patients with chronic, recalcitrant eating disorders, in Special Problems in Managing Eating Disorders. Edited by Yager J, Gwirtsman HE, Edelstein CK. Washington, DC, American Psychiatric Press, 1992, pp 205–231 [G]

22. Zerbe KJ: Integrating feminist and psychodynamic principles in the treatment of an eating disorder patient: implications for using countertransference responses. Bull Menninger Clin 1995; 59:160–176 [G]

23. Kaplan AS, Fallon P: Therapeutic boundaries in the treatment of patients with eating disorders. Fourth London International Conference on Eating Disorders, April 20–22, 1999, p 30 [G]

24. Andersen AE: Hospital Treatment of Anorexia Nervosa. Washington, DC, American Psychiatric Press, 1989 [I]

25. Kaplan AS: Medical and nutritional assessment, in Medical Issues and the Eating Disorders: The Interface. Edited by Kaplan AS, Garfinkel PE. New York, Brunner/Mazel, 1993, pp 1–16 [G]

26. Powers PS: Initial assessment and early treatment options for anorexia nervosa and bulimia nervosa. Psychiatr Clin North Am 1996; 19:639–655 [F]

27. Strober M, Freeman R, Morrell W: The long-term course of severe anorexia nervosa in adolescents: survival analysis of recovery, relapse, and outcome predictors over 10–15 years in a prospective study. Int J Eat Disord 1997; 22:339–360 [C]

28. Bulik C, Sullivan PF, Fear J, Pickering A: Predictors of the development of bulimia nervosa in women with anorexia nervosa. J Nerv Ment Dis 1997; 185:704–707 [G]

29. Lee S, Ho TP, Hsu LKG: Fat phobic and non-fat phobic anorexia nervosa—a comparative study of 70 Chinese patients in Hong Kong. Psychol Med 1993; 23:999–1004 [D]

30. Strober M, Freeman R, Morrell W: Atypical anorexia nervosa: separation from typical cases in course and outcome in a long-term prospective study. Int J Eat Disord 1999; 25:135–142 [C]

31. Beumont PJ, George GC, Smart DE: Dieters and vomiters and purgers in anorexia nervosa. Psychol Med 1976; 6:617–622 [C]

32. Casper RC, Eckert ED, Halmi KA, Goldberg SC, Davis JM: Bulimia: its incidence and clinical importance in patients with anorexia nervosa. Arch Gen Psychiatry 1980; 37:1030–1035 [C]

33. Garfinkel PE, Moldofsky H, Garner DM: The heterogeneity of anorexia nervosa: bulimia as a distinct group. Arch Gen Psychiatry 1980; 37:1036–1040 [C]

34. Kassett JA, Gwirtsman HE, Kaye WH, Brandt HA, Jimerson DC: Pattern of onset of bulimic symptoms in anorexia nervosa. Am J Psychiatry 1988; 145:1287–1288 [C]

35. Wilson CP, Hogan CC, Mintz IL: Fear of Being Fat: The Treatment Of Anorexia Nervosa and Bulimia, 2nd ed. Northvale, NJ, Jason Aronson, 1985 [F]

36. Wilson CP, Hogan CC, Mintz IL: Psychodynamic Technique in the Treatment of Eating Disorders. Northvale, NJ, Jason Aronson, 1992 [F]

37. Bunnell DW, Shenker IR, Nussbaum MP, Jacobson MS, Cooper P, Phil D: Subclinical versus formal eating disorders: differentiating psychological features. Int J Eat Disord 1990; 9:357–362 [D]

38. Zerbe KJ: The emerging sexual self of the patient with an eating disorder: implications for treatment. Eating Disorders: J Treatment and Prevention 1995; 3:197–215 [B]

39. Favazza AR, DeRosear L, Conterio K: Self-mutilation and eating disorders. Suicide Life Threat Behav 1989; 19:352–361 [G]

40. Johnson C, Connors ME: The Etiology and Treatment of Bulimia Nervosa. New York, Basic Books, 1987 [I]

41. Rizzuto A: Transference, language, and affect in the treatment of bulimarexia. Int J Psychoanal 1988; 69:369–387 [G]

42. Schwartz HJ: Bulimia: Psychoanalytic Treatment and Theory, 2nd ed. Madison, Conn, International Universities Press, 1990 [I]

43. Lacey H: Bulimia nervosa, binge-eating, and psychogenic vomiting: a controlled treatment study and long-term outcome. Br Med J 1983; 2:1609–1613 [A]

44. Casper RC, Davis JM: On the course of anorexia nervosa. Am J Psychiatry 1977; 134:974–978 [C]

45. Garfinkel PE, Kaplan AS: Starvation based perpetuating mechanisms in anorexia nervosa and bulimia. Int J Eat Disord 1985; 4:651–655 [E]

46. Keys A, Brozek J, Henschel A, Mickelsen O, Taylor HL: The Biology of Human Starvation. Minneapolis, University of Minnesota Press, 1950 [B]

47. Srinivasagam NM, Kaye WH, Plotnicov KH, Greeno C, Weltzin TE, Rao R: Persistent perfectionism, symmetry, and exactness after long-term recovery from anorexia nervosa. Am J Psychiatry 1995; 152:1630–1634 [C]

48. Garner DM, Garfinkel PE (eds): Handbook of Psychotherapy for Anorexia Nervosa and Bulimia. New York, Guilford Press, 1985 [G]

49. Fichter MM: Starvation-related endocrine changes, in Psychobiology and Treatment of Anorexia Nervosa and Bulimia Nervosa. Edited by Halmi KA. Washington, DC, American Psychopathological Association, 1992, pp 193–210 [G]

50. Fichter MM, Pirke KM, Pollinger J, Wolfram G, Brunner E: Disturbances in the hypothalamo-pituitary-adrenal and other neuroendocrine axes in bulimia. Biol Psychiatry 1990; 27:1021–1037 [D]

51. Bachrach LK, Guido D, Katzman DK, Litt IF, Marcus RN: Decreased bone density in adolescent girls with anorexia nervosa. Pediatrics 1990; 86:440–447 [C]

52. Bachrach LK, Katzman DK, Litt IF, Guido D, Marcus RN: Recovery from osteopenia in adolescent girls with anorexia nervosa. J Clin Endocrinol Metab 1991; 72:602–606 [B]

53. Rigotti NA, Neer RM, Skates SJ, Herzog DB, Nussbaum SR: The clinical course of osteoporosis in anorexia nervosa: a longitudinal study of cortical bone mass. JAMA 1991; 265:1133–1138 [B]

54. Klibanski A, Biller BM, Schoenfeld DA, Herzog DB, Saxe VC: The effects of estrogen administration on trabecular bone loss in young women with anorexia nervosa. J Clin Endocrinol Metab 1995; 80:898–904 [B]

55. Stewart DE, Robinson E, Goldbloom DS, Wright C: Infertility and eating disorders. Am J Obstet Gynecol 1990; 163:1196–1199 [C]

56. Beumont PJV, Kopec-Schrader EM, Lennerts W: Eating disorder patients at a NSW teaching hospital: a comparison with state-wide data. Aust NZ J Psychiatry 1995; 29:96–103 [G]

57. de Zwaan M, Mitchell JE: Medical complications of anorexia nervosa and bulimia nervosa, in Medical Issues and the Eating Disorders: The Interface. Edited by Kaplan AS, Garfinkel PE. New York, Brunner/Mazel, 1993, pp 60–100 [G]

58. Garfinkel PE, Garner DM: The Role of Drug Treatments for Eating Disorders. New York, Brunner/Mazel, 1987 [I]

59. Halmi KA: Anorexia nervosa and bulimia. Annu Rev Med 1987; 38:373–380 [F]

60. Herzog DB, Copeland PM: Eating disorders. N Engl J Med 1985; 313:295–303 [F]

61. Krieg JC, Pirke KM, Lauer C, Backmund H: Endocrine, metabolic, and cranial computed tomographic findings in anorexia nervosa. Biol Psychiatry 1988; 23:377–387 [G]

62. Golden NH, Ashtari M, Kohn MR, Patel M, Jacobson MS, Fletcher A, Shenker IR: Reversibility of cerebral ventricular enlargement in anorexia nervosa demonstrated by quantitative magnetic resonance imaging. J Pediatr 1996; 128:296–301 [B]

63. Katzman DK, Lambe EK, Mikulis DJ, Ridgley JN, Goldbloom DS, Zipursky RB: Cerebral gray matter and white matter volume deficits in adolescent girls with anorexia nervosa. J Pediatr 1996; 129:794–803 [D]

64. Kingston K, Szmukler G, Andrewes D, Tress B, Desmond P: Neuropsychological and structural brain changes in anorexia nervosa before and after refeeding. Psychol Med 1996; 26:15–28 [C]

65. Lambe EK, Katzman DK, Mikulis DJ, Kennedy S, Zipursky RB: Cerebral gray matter volume deficits after weight recovery from anorexia nervosa. Arch Gen Psychiatry 1997; 54:537–542 [C]

66. Swayze VW II, Andersen A, Arndt S, Rajarethinam R, Fleming F, Sato Y, Andreasen NC: Reversibility of brain tissue loss in anorexia nervosa assessed with a computerized Talairach 3-D proportional grid. Psychol Med 1996; 26:381–390 [C]

67. Hamsher K, Halmi KA, Benton AL: Prediction of outcome in anorexia nervosa from neuropsychological status. Psychiatry Res 1981; 4:79–88 [C]

68. Powers PS, Tyson IB, Stevens BA, Heal AV: Total body potassium and serum potassium among eating disorder patients. Int J Eat Disord 1995; 18:269–276 [G]

69. Mitchell JE, Pyle RL, Eckert ED, Hatsukami D, Lentz R: Electrolyte and other physiological abnormalities in patients with bulimia. Psychol Med 1983; 13:273–278 [G]

70. Herzog DB, Nussbaum KM, Marmor AK: Comorbidity and outcome in eating disorders. Psychiatr Clin North Am 1996; 19:843–859 [F]

71. Halmi KA, Eckert E, Marchi P, Sampugnaro V, Apple R, Cohen J: Comorbidity of psychiatric diagnoses in anorexia nervosa. Arch Gen Psychiatry 1991; 48:712–718 [C]

72. Theander S: Outcome and prognosis in anorexia nervosa and bulimia: some results of previous investigations compared with those of a Swedish long term study. J Psychiatr Res 1985; 19:493–508 [C]

73. Sullivan PF: Mortality in anorexia nervosa. Am J Psychiatry 1995; 152:1073–1074 [E]

74. Harris EC, Barraclough B: Excess mortality of mental disorder. Br J Psychiatry 1998; 173:11–53 [F]

75. Hsu LKG: Outcome and treatment effects, in Handbook of Eating Disorders. Edited by Beaumont PJV, Burrows BD, Casper RC. Amsterdam, Elsevier, 1987, pp 371–377 [I]

76. Hsu LKG: Eating Disorders. New York, Guilford Press, 1990 [I]

77. Russell G: Bulimia nervosa: an ominous variant of anorexia nervosa. Psychol Med 1979; 9:429–488 [E]

78. Kreipe RE, Churchill BH, Strauss J: Long-term outcome of adolescents with anorexia nervosa. Am J Dis Child 1989; 43:1322–1327 [C]

79. Nussbaum MP, Shenker IR, Baird D, Saravay S: Follow up investigation of patients with anorexia nervosa. J Pediatr 1985; 106:835–840 [C]

80. Steiner H, Mazer C, Litt IF: Compliance and outcome in anorexia nervosa. West J Med 1990; 153:133–139 [C]

81. Drewnowski A, Yee DK, Krahn DD: Dieting and Bulimia: A Continuum of Behaviors. Washington, DC, American Psychiatric Press, 1989 [G]

82. Yager J, Landsverk J, Edelstein CK: A 20-month follow-up study of 628 women with eating disorders, I: course and severity. Am J Psychiatry 1987; 144:1172–1177 [B]

83. Hsu LK, Sobkiewicz TA: Bulimia nervosa: a four to six year follow up. Psychol Med 1989; 19:1035–1038 [B]

84. Keel PK, Mitchell JE: Outcome in bulimia nervosa. Am J Psychiatry 1997; 154:313–321 [F]

85. Keel PK, Mitchell JE, Miller KB, Davis TL, Crow SJ: Long-term outcome of bulimia nervosa. Arch Gen Psychiatry 1998; 56:63–69 [E]

86. Luka LP, Agras WS, Schneider JA: Thirty month follow up of cognitive behavioral group therapy for bulimia (letter). Br J Psychiatry 1986; 148:614–615 [B]

87. Fichter MM, Quadflieg N: Six-year course of bulimia nervosa. Int J Eat Disord 1997; 22:361–384 [C]

88. Swift WJ, Ritholz M, Kalin NH, Kaslow N: A follow-up study of thirty hospitalized bulimics. Psychosom Med 1987; 49:45–55 [B]

89. Agras WS, Walsh T, Wilson G: A multisite comparison of cognitive behavior therapy (CBT) and interpersonal therapy (IPT) in the treatment of bulimia nervosa. Fourth London International Conference on Eating Disorders, April 20–22, 1999, p 61 [G]

90. Olmsted MP, Kaplan AS, Rockert W: Rate and prediction of relapse in bulimia nervosa. Am J Psychiatry 1994; 151:738–743 [C]

91. Garfinkel PE, Lin E, Goering P, Spegg C, Goldbloom D, Kennedy S, Kaplan AS, Woodside DB: Should amenorrhoea be necessary for the diagnosis of anorexia nervosa. Br J Psychiatry 1996; 168:500–506 [G]

92. Walters EE, Kendler KS: Anorexia nervosa and anorexic-like syndromes in a population-based female twin sample. Am J Psychiatry 1995; 152:64–71 [D]

93. Garfinkel PE, Lin E, Goering P, Spegg C, Goldbloom DS, Kennedy S, Kaplan AS, Woodside DB: Bulimia nervosa in a Canadian community sample: prevalence and comparison of subgroups. Am J Psychiatry 1995; 152:1052–1058 [C]

94. Kendler KS, MacLean C, Neale M, Kessler R, Heath A, Eaves L: The genetic epidemiology of bulimia nervosa. Am J Psychiatry 1991; 148:1627–1637 [H]

95. Heatherton TF, Nichols P, Mahamedi F, Keel P: Body weight, dieting, and eating disorder symptoms among college students, 1982 to 1992. Am J Psychiatry 1995; 152:1623–1629 [D]

96. Fosson A, Knibbs J, Bryant-Waugh R, Lask B: Early onset of anorexia nervosa. Arch Dis Childhood 1987; 62:114–118 [F]

97. Hawley RM: The outcome of anorexia nervosa in younger subjects. Br J Psychiatry 1985; 146:657–660 [C]

98. Higgs JF, Goodyer IN, Birch J: Anorexia nervosa and food avoidance emotional disorder. Arch Dis Childhood 1989; 64:346–351 [D]

99. Pate JE, Pumariega AJ, Hester C, Garner DM: Cross cultural patterns in eating disorders: a review. Am J Child Adolesc Psychiatry 1992; 31:802–809 [F]

100. Kiriike N, Nagata T, Tanaka M, Nishiwaki S, Takeuchi N, Kawakita Y: Prevalence of binge-eating and bulimia among adolescent women in Japan. Psychiatry Res 1988; 26:163–169 [D]

101. Nadaoka T, Oiji A, Takahashi S, Morioka Y, Kashiwakura M, Totsuka S: An epidemiological study of eating disorders in a northern area of Japan. Acta Psychiatr Scand 1996; 93:305–310 [D]

102. Davis C, Katzman MA: Chinese men and women in the USA and Hong Kong: body and self-esteem ratings as a prelude to dieting and exercise. Int J Eat Disord 1998; 23:99–102 [D]

103. Davis C, Katzman MA: Perfection as acculturation: psychological correlates of eating problems in Chinese male and female students living in the United States. Int J Eat Disord 1999; 25:65–70 [D]

104. Becker AE: Acculturation and Disordered Eating in Fiji. Washington, DC, American Psychiatric Press, 1999 [G]

105. Nasser M: Culture and Weight Consciousness. New York, Routledge, 1997 [G]

106. Toro J, Cervera M, Perez P: Body shape, publicity and anorexia nervosa. Social Psychiatry Psychiatr Epidemiol 1988; 23:132–136 [E]

107. Toro J, Nicolau R, Cervera M, Castro J, Blecua MJ, Zaragoza M, Toro A: A clinical and phenomenological study of 185 Spanish adolescents with anorexia nervosa. Eur Child Adolesc Psychiatry 1995; 4:165–174 [E]

108. Crago M, Shisslak CM, Estes LS: Eating disturbances among American minority groups: a review. Int J Eat Disord 1996; 19:239–248 [F]

109. Langer L, Warheit G, Zimmerman R: Epidemiological study of problem eating behaviors and related attitudes in the general population. Addict Behav 1992; 16:167–173 [D]

110. Warheit G, Langer L, Zimmerman R, Biafora F: Prevalence of bulimic behaviors and bulimia among a sample of the general population. Am J Epidemiol 1993; 137:569–576 [D]

111. Pumariega AJ, Gustavson CR, Gustavson JC: Eating attitudes in African-American women: the essence. Eating Disorders: J Treatment and Prevention 1994; 2:5–16 [D]

112. Davis C, Kennedy SH, Ravelski E, Dionne M: The role of physical activity in the development and maintenance of eating disorders. Psychol Med 1994; 24:957–967 [B]

113. Garner DM, Rosen LW, Barry D: Eating disorders among athletes: research and recommendations. Child Adolesc Psychiatr Clin North Am 1998; 7:839–857 [F]

114. Strober M, Lampert C, Morrell W, Burroughs J, Jacobs C: a controlled family study of anorexia nervosa: evidence of familial aggregation and lack of shared transmission with affective disorders. Int J Eat Disord 1990; 9:239–253 [B]

115. Bulik C, Sullivan P, Carter FA, McIntosh VV, Joyce PR: The role of exposure with response prevention in the cognitive behavioral therapy for bulimia nervosa. Psychol Med 1998; 28:611–623 [B]

116. Lilenfeld L, Kaye W, Greeno C, Merikangas KR, Plotnicov KH, Pollice C, Radhika R, Strober M, Bulik C, Nagy L: Psychiatric disorders in women with bulimia nervosa and their first-degree relatives: effects of comorbid substance dependence. Int J Eat Disord 1997; 22:253–264 [D]

117. Mitchell JE, Hatsukami D, Pyle R, Eckert E: Bulimia with and without a family history of drug use. Addict Behav 1988; 13:245–251 [C]

118. Hudson JI, Pope HG Jr, Yurgelun-Todd D, Jonas JM, Frankenburg FR: A controlled study of lifetime prevalence of affective and other psychiatric disorders in bulimic outpatients. Am J Psychiatry 1987; 144:1283–1287 [C]

119. Pyle RL, Mitchell JE, Eckert ED: Bulimia: a report of 34 cases. J Clin Psychiatry 1981; 42:60–64 [G]

120. Zerbe KJ: Feminist psychodynamic psychotherapy of eating disorders: theoretic integration informing clinical practice. Psychiatr Clin North Am 1996; 19:811–827 [F]

121. Zerbe KJ, March S, Coyne L: Comorbidity in an inpatient eating disorders population: clinical characteristics and treatment implications. Psychiatr Hospital 1993; 24:3–8 [D]

122. Braun DL, Sunday SR, Halmi KA: Psychiatric comorbidity in patients with eating disorders. Psychol Med 1994; 24:859–867 [C]

123. Herzog DB, Keller MB, Sacks NR, Yeh CJ, Lavori PW: Psychiatric comorbidity in treatment-seeking anorexics and bulimics. J Am Acad Child Adolesc Psychiatry 1992; 31:810–818 [D]

124. Hudson JI, Pope HG, Jonas JM, Yurgelun-Todd D: Phenomenologic relationship of eating disorders to major affective disorder. Psychiatry Res 1983; 9:345–354 [D]

125. Hecht H, Fichter MM, Postpeschil F: Obsessive-compulsive neuroses and anorexia nervosa. Int J Eat Disord 1983; 2:69–77 [D]

126. Kasvikis YG, Tsakiris F, Marks IM, Basogul M, Noshirvani HF: Past history of anorexia nervosa in women with obsessive compulsive disorder. Int J Eat Disord 1986; 5:1069–1076 [C]

127. Skodol AE, Oldham JM, Hyler SE, Kellman HD, Doidge N, Davies M: Comorbidity of DSM-III-R eating disorders and personality disorders. Int J Eat Disord 1993; 14:403–416 [D]

128. Herzog DB, Keller MB, Lavori PW, Kenny GM, Sacks NR: The prevalence of personality disorders in 210 women with eating disorders. J Clin Psychiatry 1992; 53:147–152 [G]

129. Bulik CM, Sullivan PF, Rorty M: Childhood sexual abuse in women with bulimia. J Clin Psychiatry 1989; 50:460–464 [C]

130. Schmidt U, Tiller J, Treasure J: Self-treatment of bulimia nervosa: a pilot study. Int J Eat Disord 1993; 13:273–277 [B]

131. Vize CM, Cooper PJ: Sexual abuse in patients with eating disorder patients with depression and normal controls: a comparative study. Br J Psychiatry 1995; 167:80–85 [D]

132. Pope HG Jr, Hudson JI: Is childhood sexual abuse a risk factor for bulimia nervosa? Am J Psychiatry 1992; 149:455–463 [E]

133. Rorty M, Yager J, Rossotto E: Childhood sexual physical and psychological abuse and their relationship to comorbid psychopathology in bulimia nervosa. Int J Eat Disord 1994; 16:317–334 [C]

134. Wonderlich SA, Brewerton TD, Jocic Z, Dansky BS, Abbott DW: Relationship of childhood sexual abuse and eating disorders. J Am Acad Child Adolesc Psychiatry 1997; 36:1107–1115 [F]

135. Wonderlich SA, Mitchell JE: Eating disorders and comorbidity: empirical, conceptual and clinical implications. Psychopharmacol Bull 1997; 33:381–390 [F]

136. Kaye WH, Gwirtsman H, Obarzanek E, George DT: Relative importance of calorie intake needed to gain weight and level of physical activity in anorexia nervosa. Am J Clin Nutr 1988; 47:989–994 [C]

137. Golden NH, Jacobson MS, Schebendach J, Solanto MV, Hertz SM, Shenker IR: Resumption of menses in anorexia nervosa. Arch Pediatr Adolesc Med 1997; 151:16–21 [C]

138. Treasure JL, Wheeler M, King EA, Gordon PA, Russell GF: Weight gain and reproductive function: ultrasonographic and endocrine features in anorexia nervosa. Clin Endocrinol 1988; 29:607–616 [C]

139. Frisch RE: Fatness and fertility. Sci Am 1988; 258:88–95 [F]

140. Metropolitan Life Insurance Company: 1983 Metropolitan height and weight tables. Stat Bull Metrop Life Found 1983; 64:3–9 [E]

141. Hamill PV, Johnston FE, Lemeshow S: Height and weight of youths 12–17 years, United States. Vital Health Stat 1 1973: 11:1–81 [C]

142. Hebebrand J, Himmelmann GW, Heseker H, Schafer H, Remschmidt H: Use of percentiles for the body mass index in anorexia nervosa: diagnostic, epidemiological and therapeutic considerations. Int J Eat Disord 1996; 19:359–369 [D]

143. Reiff DW, Reiff KKL: Set point, in Eating Disorders: Nutrition Therapy in the Recovery Process. Gaithersburg, Md, Aspen, 1992, pp 104–105 [G]

144. Guarda AS, Heinberg LJ: Effective weight-gain in step down partial hospitalization program for eating disorders. Annual Meeting of Academy for Eating Disorders, San Diego, 1999 [G]

145. Powers PS: Heart failure during treatment of anorexia nervosa. Am J Psychiatry 1982; 139:1167–1170 [G]

146. Kohn MR, Golden NH, Shenker IR: Cardiac arrest and delirium: presentations of the refeeding syndrome in severely malnourished adolescents with anorexia nervosa. J Adolesc Health 1998; 22:239–243 [G]

147. Scott M, Solomon, Kriby DF: The refeeding syndrome: a review. JPEN Parenter Enteral Nutr 1990; 14:90–97 [F]

148. Treasure J, Todd G, Szmukler G: The inpatient treatment of anorexia nervosa, in Handbook of Eating Disorders. Edited by Szmukler G, Dare C, Treasure J. Chichester, UK, John Wiley & Sons, 1995, pp 275–291 [G]

149. Kaye WH, Weltzin TE, Hsu LK, Bulik CM: An open trial of fluoxetine in patients with anorexia nervosa. J Clin Psychiatry 1991; 52:464–471 [G]

150. Levine JA, Eberhardt NL, Jensen MD: Role of nonexercise activity thermogenesis in resistance to fat gain in humans. Science 1999; 283:212–214 [B]

151. Baran SA, Weltzin TE, Kaye WH: Low discharge weight and outcome in anorexia nervosa. Am J Psychiatry 1995; 152:1070–1072 [C]

152. Halmi KA, Licinio-Paixao J: Outcome: hospital program for eating disorders, in 1989 Annual Meeting Syllabus and Proceedings Summary. Washington, DC, American Psychiatric Association, 1989, p 314 [G]

153. Agras WS: Eating Disorders: Management of Obesity, Bulimia and Anorexia Nervosa. Oxford, UK, Pergamon Press, 1987 [I]

154. Nusbaum JG, Drever E: Inpatient survey of nursing care measures for treatment of patients with anorexia nervosa. Issues Ment Health Nurs 1990; 11:175–184 [G]

155. Touyz SW, Beumont PJ, Glaun D, Phillips T, Cowie I: A comparison of lenient and strict operant conditioning programmes in refeeding patients with anorexia nervosa. Br J Psychiatry 1984; 144:517–520 [F]

156. Danziger Y, Carel CA, Tyano S, Mimouni M: Is psychotherapy mandatory during the actual refeeding period in the treatment of anorexia nervosa. J Adolesc Health Care 1989; 10:328–331 [B]

157. Duncan J, Kennedy SH: Inpatient group treatment, in Group Psychotherapy for Eating Disorders. Edited by Harper-Giuffre H, MacKenzie KR. Washington, DC, American Psychiatric Press, 1992, pp 149–160 [G]

158. Maxmen JS: Helping patients survive theories: the practice of an educative model. Int J Group Psychother 1984; 34:355–368 [G]

159. Yellowlees P: Group psychotherapy in anorexia nervosa. Int J Eat Disord 1988; 7:649–655 [G]

160. Maher MS: Group therapy for anorexia nervosa, in Current Treatment of Anorexia Nervosa and Bulimia. Edited by Powers PS, Fernandez RC. Basel, Switzerland, Karger, 1980, pp 265–276 [G]

161. Garner DM: Individual psychotherapy for anorexia nervosa. J Psychiatr Res 1985; 19:423–433 [F]

162. Hall A, Crisp AH: Brief psychotherapy in the treatment of anorexia nervosa: outcome at one year. Br J Psychiatry 1987; 151:185–191 [A]

163. Wilson CP, Mintz IL (eds): Psychosomatic Symptoms: Psychoanalytic Treatment of the Underlying Personality Disorder. Northvale, NJ, Jason Aronson, 1989 [F]

164. Dare C: The starving and the greedy. J Child Psychotherapy 1993; 19:3–22 [F]

165. Hornyak LM, Baker EK: Experiential Therapies for Eating Disorders. New York, Guilford Press, 1989 [G]

166. Breden AK: Occupational therapy and the treatment of eating disorders. Occupational Therapy in Health Care 1992; 8:49–68 [G]

167. Lim PY: Occupational therapy with eating disorders: a study on treatment approaches. Br J Occupational Therapy 1994; 57:309–314 [G]

168. Eisler I, Dare C, Russell G, Szmukler G, leGrange D, Dodge E: Family and individual therapy in anorexia nervosa: a 5-year follow-up. Arch Gen Psychiatry 1997; 54:1025–1030 [B]

169. Russell GF, Szmukler GI, Dare C, Eisler I: An evaluation of family therapy in anorexia nervosa and bulimia nervosa. Arch Gen Psychiatry 1987; 44:1047–1056 [A]

170. Agras WS, Hammer LD, McNicholas F: A prospective study of the influence of eating-disordered mothers on their children. Int J Eat Disord 1999; 25:253–262 [C]

171. Russell GF, Treasure J, Eisler I: Mothers with anorexia nervosa who underfeed their children: their recognition and management. Psychol Med 1998; 28:93–108 [D]

172. Stein A, Woolley H, Cooper SD, Fairburn CG: An observational study of mothers with eating disorders and their infants. J Child Psychol Psychiatry 1994; 35:733–748 [C]

173. Johnson CL, Taylor C: Working with difficult to treat eating disorders using an integration of twelve-step and traditional psychotherapies. Psychiatr Clin North Am 1996; 19:829–941 [F]

174. Fisher M, Golden NH, Katzman DK, Kreipe RE, Rees J, Schebendach J, Sigman G, Ammerman S, Hoberman HM: Eating disorders in adolescents: a background paper. J Adolesc Health 1995; 16:420–437 [F]

175. Attia E, Haiman C, Walsh BT, Flater SR: Does fluoxetine augment the inpatient treatment of anorexia nervosa? Am J Psychiatry 1998; 155:548–551 [A]

176. Gwirtsman HE, Guze BH, Yager J, Gainsley B: Fluoxetine treatment of anorexia nervosa: an open clinical trial. J Clin Psychiatry 1990; 51:378–382 [G]

177. Bergh C, Eriksson M, Lindberg G, Sodersten P: Selective serotonin reuptake inhibitors in anorexia. Lancet 1996; 348:1459–1460 [B]

178. Halmi KA, Eckert E, LaDu TJ, Cohen J: Anorexia nervosa: treatment efficacy of cyproheptadine and amitriptyline. Arch Gen Psychiatry 1986; 43:177–181 [A]

179. Lacey JH, Crisp AH: Hunger, food intake and weight: the impact of clomipramine on a refeeding anorexia nervosa population. Postgrad Med J 1980; 56(suppl 1):79–85 [A]

180. Gross HA, Ebert MH, Faden VB: A double-blind controlled study of lithium carbonate in primary anorexia nervosa. J Clin Psychopharmacol 1981; 1:376–381 [A]

181. Vandereycken W, Pierloot R: Pimozide combined with behavior therapy in the short-term treatment of anorexia nervosa: a double blind placebo-controlled cross-over study. Acta Psychiatr Scand 1982; 66:445–450 [A]

182. Wells LA, Logan KM: Pharmacologic treatment of eating disorders: a review of selected literature and recommendations. Psychosomatics 1987; 28:470–479 [F]

183. Garfinkel PE, Garner DM: Anorexia Nervosa: A Multidimensional Perspective. New York, Brunner/Mazel, 1982 [I]

184. Seeman E, Szmukler G, Formica C, Tsalamandris C, Mestrovic R: Osteoporosis in anorexia nervosa: the influence of peak bone density, bone loss, oral contraceptive use and exercise. J Bone Miner Res 1992; 7:1467–1474 [C]

185. Hegenroeder AC: Bone mineralization, hypothalamic amenorrhea, and sex steroid therapy in female adolescents and young adults. J Pediatr 1995; 126:683–689 [F]

186. Kreipe RE, Hicks DG, Rosier RN, Puzas JE: Preliminary findings on the effects of sex hormones on bone metabolism in anorexia nervosa. J Adolesc Health 1993; 14:319–324 [B]

187. Treasure JL, Russell GF, Fogelman I, Murby B: Reversible bone loss in anorexia nervosa. Br Med J (Clin Res Ed) 1987; 295:474–475 [D]

188. Emans SJ, Goldstein DP: Pediatric and Adolescent Gynecology, 3rd ed. Boston, Little, Brown, 1990 [G]

189. Grinspoon S, Baum H, Lee K, Anderson E, Herzog D, Klibanski A: Effects of short-term recombinant human insulin-like growth factor I administration on bone turnover in osteopenic women with anorexia nervosa. J Clin Endocrinol Metab 1996; 81:3864–3870 [B]

190. Physicians' Desk Reference, 46th ed. Montvale, NJ, Medical Economics, 1992 [G]

191. Horne RL, Ferguson JM, Pope HJ, Hudson JI, Lineberry CG, Ascher J, Cato A: Treatment of bulimia with bupropion: a multicenter controlled trial. J Clin Psychiatry 1988; 49:262–266 [A]

192. Laessle RG, Zoettle C, Pirke KM: Meta-analysis of treatment studies for bulimia. Int J Eat Disord 1987; 6:647–654 [E]

193. Agras WS, Schneider JA, Arnow B, Raeburn SD, Telch CF: Cognitive-behavioral and response prevention treatments for bulimia nervosa. J Consult Clin Psychol 1989; 57:215–221 [A]

194. Beck AT, Ward CH, Mendelson M, Mock J, Erbaugh J: An inventory for measuring depression. Arch Gen Psychiatry 1961; 4:561–571 [G]

195. Connors ME, Johnson CL, Stuckey MK: Treatment of bulimia with brief psychoeducational group therapy. Am J Psychiatry 1984; 141:1512–1516 [B]

196. Fairburn CG, Jones R, Peveler RC, Hope RA, O'Connor M: Psychotherapy and bulimia nervosa: longer-term effects of interpersonal psychotherapy, behavior therapy, and cognitive behavioral therapy. Arch Gen Psychiatry 1993; 50:419–428 [A]

197. Fairburn CG, Marcus MD, Wilson GT: Cognitive-behavioral therapy for binge eating and bulimia nervosa: a comprehensive treatment manual, in Binge Eating: Nature, Assessment, and Treatment. Edited by Fairburn CG, Wilson GT. New York, Guilford Press, 1993, pp 361–404 [G]

198. Freeman CP, Barry F, Dunkeld-Turnbull J, Henderson A: Controlled trial of psychotherapy for bulimia nervosa. Br Med J (Clin Res Ed) 1988; 296:521–525 [B]

199. Garner DM, Rockert W, Davis R, Garner MV, Olmsted MP, Eagle M: A comparison of cognitive-behavioral and supportive-expressive therapy for bulimia nervosa. Am J Psychiatry 1993; 150:37–46 [B]

200. Hamilton M: A rating scale for depression. J Neurol Neurosurg Psychiatry 1960; 23:56–62 [D]

201. Kirkley BG, Schneider JA, Agras WS, Bachman JA: Comparison of two group treatments for bulimia. J Consult Clin Psychol 1985; 53:43–48 [A]

202. Lee NF, Rush AJ: Cognitive-behavioral group therapy for bulimia. Int J Eat Disord 1986; 5:599–615 [A]

203. Malenbaum R, Herzog D, Eisenthal S, Wyshak G: Overeaters anonymous. Int J Eat Disord 1988; 7:139–144 [G]

204. Mitchell JE, Pyle RL, Pomeroy C, Zollman M, Crosby R, Sein H, Eckert ED, Zimmerman R: Cognitive-behavioral group psychotherapy of bulimia nervosa: importance of logistical variables. Int J Eat Disord 1993; 14:277–287 [B]

205. Oesterheld JR, McKenna MS, Gould NB: Group psychotherapy of bulimia: a critical review. Int J Group Psychother 1987; 37:163–184 [F]

206. Ordman AM, Kirschenbaum DS: Cognitive-behavioral therapy for bulimia: an initial outcome study. J Consult Clin Psychol 1985; 53:305–313 [B]

207. Schwartz RC, Barett MJ, Saba G: Family therapy for bulimia, in Handbook of Psychotherapy for Anorexia Nervosa and Bulimia. Edited by Garner DM, Garfinkel PE. New York, Guilford Press, 1985, pp 280–307 [G]

208. Vandereycken W: The addiction model in eating disorders: some critical remarks and a selected bibliography. Int J Eat Disord 1990; 9:95–102 [G]

209. Yager J, Landsverk J, Edelstein CK: Help seeking and satisfaction with care in 641 women with eating disorders I: patterns of utilization attributed change and perceived efficacy of treatment. J Nerv Ment Dis 1989; 177:632–637 [G]

210. Beck AT, Steer RA, Garbin MG: Psychometric properties of the BDI: twenty-five years of evaluation. Clin Psychol Rev 1988; 8:77–100 [G]

211. Root MPP: Persistent, disordered eating as a gender-specific, post-traumatic stress response to sexual assault. Psychotherapy 1991; 28:96–102 [G]

212. Laessle RG, Tuschl RJ, Kotthaus BC, Pirke JM: A comparison of the validity of three scales for the assessment of dietary restraint. J Abnorm Psychol 1989; 98:504–507 [E]

213. Fairburn CG: Cognitive behavioral treatment for bulimia, in Handbook of Psychotherapy for Anorexia Nervosa and Bulimia. Edited by Garner DM, Garfinkel PE. New York, Guilford Press, 1985, pp 160–192 [G]

214. Fairburn CG, Kirk J, O'Connor M, Cooper PJ: A comparison of two psychological treatments for bulimia nervosa. Behav Res Ther 1985; 24:629–643 [B]

215. Leitenberg H, Rosen J, Gross J, Nudelman S, Vara LS: Exposure plus response-prevention treatment of bulimia nervosa. J Consult Clin Psychol 1988; 56:535–541 [A]

216. Johnson C: Diagnostic survey for eating disorders in initial consultation for patients with bulimia and anorexia nervosa, in Handbook of Psychotherapy for Anorexia Nervosa and Bulimia. Edited by Garner DM, Garfinkel PE. New York, Guilford Press, 1985, pp 19–51 [G]

217. Fairburn CG: A cognitive behavioral approach to the treatment of bulimia. Psychol Med 1981; 11:707–711 [B]

218. Fairburn CG, Norman PA, Welch SL, O'Conner ME, Doll HA, Peveler RC: A prospective study of outcome in bulimia nervosa and the long-term effects of three psychological treatments. Arch Gen Psychiatry 1995; 52:304–312 [A]

219. Rorty M, Yager J: Why and how do women recover from bulimia nervosa? Int J Eat Disord 1993; 14:249–260 [D]

220. Fairburn CG, Jones R, Peveler RC: Three psychological treatments for bulimia nervosa. Arch Gen Psychiatry 1991; 48:453–469 [A]

221. Wilson GT, Eldredge KL, Smith D: Cognitive behavioral treatment with and without response prevention for bulimia. Behav Res Ther 1991; 29:575–583 [A]

222. Wilson GT, Rossiter E, Kleifield EI, Lindholm L: Cognitive-behavioral treatment of bulimia nervosa: a controlled evaluation. Behav Res Ther 1986; 24:277–288 [B]

223. Cooper PJ, Coker S, Fleming C: Self-help for bulimia nervosa: a preliminary report. Int J Eat Disord 1994; 16:401–404 [B]

224. Cooper PJ, Coker S, Fleming C: An evaluation of the efficacy of supervised cognitive behavioral self-help for bulimia nervosa. J Psychosom Res 1996; 40:281–287 [B]

225. Thiels C, Schmidt U, Treasure J, Garthe R, Troop N: Guided self-change for bulimia nervosa incorporating use of a self-care manual. Am J Psychiatry 1998; 155:947–953 [B]

226. Treasure J, Schmidt U, Troop N, Tiller J, Todd G, Keilen M, Dodge E: First step in managing bulimia nervosa: controlled trial of therapeutic manual. Br Med J 1994; 308:686–689 [B]

227. Treasure J, Schmidt U, Troop N, Tiller J, Todd G, Turnbull S: Sequential treatment for bulimia nervosa incorporating a self-care manual. Br J Psychiatry 1995; 167:1–5 [B]

228. Agras WS: Cognitive Behavior Therapy Treatment Manual for Bulimia Nervosa. Stanford, Calif, Stanford University School of Medicine, Department of Psychiatry and Behavioral Sciences, 1991 [F]

229. Agras WS, Apple R: Overcoming Eating Disorders—Therapist's Guide. San Antonio, Tex, Psychological Corp (Harcourt), 1998 [G]

230. Apple R, Agras WS: Overcoming Eating Disorders—Client Workbook. San Antonio, Tex, Psychological Corp (Harcourt), 1998 [G]

231. Boutacoff LI, Zollman M, Mitchell JE: Healthy Eating: A Meal Planning System—Group Treatment Manual. Minneapolis, University of Minnesota Hospital and Clinic, Department of Psychiatry, 1989 [G]

232. Mitchell JE, Eating Disorders Program Staff: Bulimia Nervosa: Individual Treatment Manual. Minneapolis, University of Minnesota Hospital and Clinic, Department of Psychiatry, 1989 [F]

233. Mitchell JE, Eating Disorders Program Staff: Bulimia Nervosa: Group Treatment Manual. Minneapolis, University of Minnesota Hospital and Clinic, Department of Psychiatry, 1991 [F]

234. Pope HG Jr, Hudson JI, Jonas JM, Yurgelun-Todd D: Bulimia treated with imipramine: a placebo-controlled, double-blind study. Am J Psychiatry 1983; 140:554–558 [A]

235. Hughes PL, Wells LA, Cunningham CJ, Ilstrup DM: Treating bulimia with desipramine: a double-blind placebo-controlled study. Arch Gen Psychiatry 1986; 43:182–186 [A]

236. Mitchell JE, Groat R: A placebo-controlled double-blind trial of amitriptyline in bulimia. J Clin Psychopharmacol 1984; 4:186–193 [A]

237. Walsh BT, Stewart JW, Roose SP, Gladis M, Glassman AH: Treatment of bulimia with phenelzine: a double-blind placebo controlled study. Arch Gen Psychiatry 1984; 41:1105–1109 [A]

238. Alger SA, Schwalberg MD, Bigaoutte JM, Michalek AV, Howard LJ: Effects of a tricyclic antidepressant and opiate antagonists on binge-eating behavior in normal weight bulimic and obese binge-eating subjects. J Clin Nutr 1991; 53:865–871 [A]

239. Fahy TA, Eisler I, Russell GFM: A placebo-controlled trial of d-fenfluramine in bulimia nervosa. Br J Psychiatry 1993; 162:597–603 [B]

240. Fichter MM, Kruger R, Rief W, Holland R, Dohne J: Fluvoxamine in prevention of relapse in bulimia nervosa: effects on eating-specific psychopathology. J Clin Psychopharmacol 1996; 16:9–18 [A]

241. Fichter MM, Leibl K, Rief W, Brunner E, Schmidt-Auberger S, Engel RR: Fluoxetine versus placebo: a double-blind study with bulimic inpatients undergoing intensive psychotherapy. Pharmacopsychiatry 1991; 24:1–7 [A]

242. Fluoxetine Bulimia Nervosa Collaborative Study Group: Fluoxetine in the treatment of bulimia nervosa. Arch Gen Psychiatry 1992; 49:139–147 [A]

243. Freeman CP, Morris JE, Cheshire KE, Davies F, Hamson M: A double-blind controlled trial of fluoxetine versus placebo for bulimia nervosa. Proceedings of the Third International Conference on Eating Disorders, New York, 1988 [A]

244. Goldstein DJ, Wilson MG, Thompson VL, Potvin JH, Rampey AH Jr (Fluoxetine Bulimia Nervosa Research Group): Long-term fluoxetine treatment of bulimia nervosa. Br J Psychiatry 1995; 166:660–666 [A]

245. Hsu LKG, Clement L, Santhouse R, Ju ESY: Treatment of bulimia nervosa with lithium carbonate: a controlled study. J Nerv Ment Dis 1991; 179:351–355 [A]

246. Igoin-Apfelbaum L, Apfelbaum M: Naltrexone and bulimic symptoms (letter). Lancet 1987; 2:1087–1088 [A]

247. Jonas JM, Gold MS: Naltrexone reverses bulimic symptoms (letter). Lancet 1986; 1:807 [G]

248. Jonas JM, Gold MS: Treatment of antidepressant-resistant bulimia with naltrexone. Int J Psychiatry Med 1986; 16:306–309 [B]

249. Mitchell JE, Christenson G, Jennings J, Huber M, Thomas B, Pomeroy C, Morley J: A placebo-controlled double-blind crossover study of naltrexone hydrochloride in outpatients with normal weight bulimia. J Clin Psychopharmacol 1989; 9:94–97 [A]

250. Pope HG Jr, Keck PE Jr, McElroy SL, Hudson JI: A placebo-controlled study of trazodone in bulimia nervosa. J Clin Psychopharmacol 1989; 9:254–259 [A]

251. Rothschild R, Quitkin HM, Quitkin FM, Stewart JW, Ocepek-Welikson K, McGrath PJ, Tricamo E: A double-blind placebo-controlled comparison of phenelzine and imipramine in the treatment of bulimia in atypical depressives. Int J Eat Disord 1994; 15:1–9 [A]

252. Sabine EJ, Yonace A, Farrington AJ, Barratt KH, Wakeling A: Bulimia nervosa: a placebo-controlled double-blind therapeutic trial of mianserin. Br J Clin Pharmacol 1983; 15:195S–202S [A]

253. Agras WS, Dorian B, Kirkley BG, Arnow B, Bachman J: Imipramine in the treatment of bulimia: a double-blind controlled study. Int J Eat Disord 1987; 6:29–38 [A]

254. Barlow J, Blouin J, Blouin A, Perez E: Treatment of bulimia with desipramine: a double blind crossover study. Can J Psychiatry 1988; 33:129–133 [A]

255. Blouin AG, Blouin JH, Perez EL, Bushnik T, Zuro C, Mulder E: Treatment of bulimia with fenfluramine and desipramine. J Clin Psychopharmacol 1988; 8:261–269 [A]

256. Walsh BT, Hadigan CM, Devlin MJ, Gladis M, Roose SP: Long-term outcome of antidepressant treatment for bulimia nervosa. Am J Psychiatry 1991; 148:1206–1212 [A]

257. Kennedy SH, Piran N, Warsh JJ, Prendergast P, Mainprize E, Whynot C, Garfinkel PE: A trial of isocarboxazid in the treatment of bulimia nervosa. J Clin Psychopharmacol 1988; 8:391–396; correction, 1989; 9:3 [A]

258. Kennedy SH, Goldbloom DS, Ralevski E, Davis C, D'Souza JD, Lofchy J: Is there a role for selective monoamine oxidase inhibitor therapy in bulimia nervosa? a placebo-controlled trial of brofaromine. J Clin Psychopharmacol 1993; 13:415–422 [A]

259. Raymond NC, Mitchell JE, Fallon P, Katzman MA: A collaborative approach to the use of medication, in Feminist Perspectives on Eating Disorders. Edited by Fallon P, Katzman MA, Wooley SC. New York, Guilford Press, 1994, pp 231–250 [G]

260. Marrazzi MA, Wroblewski JM, Kinzie J, Luby ED: High dose naltrexone in eating disorders—liver function data. Am J Addict 1997; 6:621–629 [B]

261. Mitchell JE, Pyle RL, Eckert ED, Hatsukami D, Zimmerman R, Pomeroy C: A comparison study of antidepressants and structured intensive group psychotherapy in the treatment of bulimia nervosa. Arch Gen Psychiatry 1990; 47:149–157 [A]

262. Agras WS, Rossiter EM, Arnow B, Schneider JA, Telch CF, Raeburn SD, Bruce B, Perl M, Koran LM: Pharmacologic and cognitive-behavioral treatment for bulimia nervosa: a controlled comparison. Am J Psychiatry 1992; 149:82–87 [A]

263. Goldbloom DS, Olmsted M, Davis R, Clewes J, Heinmaa M, Rockert W, Shaw B: A randomized controlled trial of fluoxetine and cognitive behavioral therapy for bulimia nervosa: short-term outcome. Behav Res Ther 1997; 35:803–811 [A]

264. Walsh BT, Wilson GT, Loeb KL, Devlin MJ, Pike KM, Roose SP, Fleiss J, Waternaux C: Medication and psychotherapy in the treatment of bulimia nervosa. Am J Psychiatry 1997; 154:523–531 [G]

265. Leitenberg H, Rosen JC, Wolf J, Vara LS, Detzer MJ, Srebnik D: Comparison of cognitive-behavior therapy and desipramine in the treatment of bulimia nervosa. Behav Res Ther 1994; 32:37–45 [A]

266. Spitzer RL, Devlin MJ, Walsh BT, Hasin D: Binge eating disorder: a multisite field trial of the diagnostic criteria. Int J Eat Disord 1992; 11:191–203 [D]

267. de Zwaan M, Mitchell JE, Mussell MP, Crosby RD: Does CBT improve outcomes in obese binge eaters participating in a very low-calorie diet treatment? Presented at the Eating Disorders Research Society annual meeting, Pittsburgh, PA, November 15–17, 1996 [B]

268. Telch CF, Agras WS: The effects of a very low calorie diet on binge eating. Behavior Therapy 1993; 24:177–193 [B]

269. Wadden TA, Foster GD, Letizia KA: Response of obese binge eaters to treatment by behavior therapy combined with very low calorie diet. J Consult Clin Psychol 1992; 60:808–811 [A]

270. Yanovski SZ, Gormally JF, Leser MS, Gwirtsman HE, Yanovski JA: Binge eating disorder affects outcome of comprehensive very-low-calorie diet treatment. Obesity Res 1994; 2:205–212 [B]

271. Polivy J, Herman CP: Dieting and binging: a casual analysis. Am Psychol 1985; 40:193–201 [F]

272. Carrier KM, Steinhardt MA, Bowman S: Rethinking traditional weight management programs: a 3-year follow-up evaluation of a new approach. J Psychol 1993; 128:517–535 [D]

273. Ciliska D: Beyond Dieting: Psychoeducational Interventions for Chronically Obese Women. New York, Brunner/Mazel, 1990 [G]

274. Kaplan AS, Ciliska D: The relationship between eating disorders and obesity: psychopathologic and treatment considerations. Psychiatr Annals 1999; 29:197–202 [B]

275. Goodrick GK, Poston WS II, Kimball KT, Reeves RS, Foreyt JP: Nondieting versus dieting treatment of overweight binge-eating women. J Consult Clin Psychol 1998; 66:363–368 [B]

276. Tanco S, Linden W, Earle T: Well-being and morbid obesity in women: a controlled therapy evaluation. Int J Eat Disord 1998; 23:325–339 [B]

277. Grilo CM: Treatment of obesity: an integrative model, in Body Image, Eating Disorders, and Obesity. Edited by Thompson JK. Washington, DC, American Psychological Association, 1996, pp 389–423 [G]

278. Marcus MD: Obese patients with binge-eating disorder, in The Management of Eating Disorders and Obesity. Edited by Goldstein DJ. Totowa, NJ, Humana Press, 1999, pp 125–138 [G]

279. Agras WS, Telch CF, Arnow B, Eldredge K, Detzer MJ, Henderson J, Marnell M: Does interpersonal therapy help patients with binge-eating disorder who fail to respond to cognitive-behavioral therapy? J Consult Clin Psychol 1995; 63:356–360 [B]

280. Agras WS, Telch CF, Arnow B, Eldredge K, Wilfley DE, Raeburn SD, Henderson S, Marnell M: Weight loss cognitive-behavioral and desipramine treatments in binge-eating disorder: an addictive design. Behavior Therapy 1994; 25:225–238 [A]

281. Carter FA, Bulik CM, Lawson RH, Sullivan PF, Wilson JS: Effect of mood and food cues on body image in women with bulimia and controls. Int J Eat Disord 1996; 20:65–76 [B]

282. Eldredge KL, Agras WS, Arnow B, Telch CF, Bell S, Castonguay L, Marnell M: The effects of extending cognitive-behavioral therapy for binge eating disorder among initial treatment nonresponders. Int J Eat Disord 1999; 21:347–352 [B]

283. Marcus MD, Wing RR: Cognitive treatment of binge eating, V: behavioral weight control in the treatment of binge eating disorder (letter). Ann Behav Med 1995; 17:S090 [A]

284. Peterson C, Mitchell JM, Engbloom S, Nugent S, Mussell MP, Miller JP: Group cognitive-behavioral treatment of binge eating disorder: a comparison of therapist-led versus self-help formats. Int J Eat Disord 1998; 24:125–136 [B]

285. Smith DE, Marcus MD, Kaye W: Cognitive-behavioral treatment of obese binge eaters. Int J Eat Disord 1992; 12:257–262 [B]

286. Telch CF, Agras WS, Rossiter EM, Wilfey D, Kenardy J: Group cognitive-behavioral treatment for the nonpurging bulimic: an initial evaluation. J Consult Clin Psychol 1990; 58:629–635 [B]

287. Wilfey DE, Agras WS, Telch CF, Rossiter EM, Schneider JA, Cole AG, Sifford LA, Raeburn SD: Group cognitive-behavioral therapy and group interpersonal psychotherapy for the nonpurging bulimic individual: a controlled comparison. J Consult Clin Psychol 1993; 61:296–305 [A]

288. Fichter MM, Quadflieg N, Gnutmann A: Binge-eating disorder: treatment outcome over a 6-year course. J Psychosom Res 1998; 44:385–405 [E]

289. Carter JC, Fairburn CG: Cognitive-behavioral self-help for binge eating disorder: a controlled effectiveness study. J Consult Clin Psychol 1998; 66:616–623 [B]

290. Stunkard A, Berkowitz R, Tanrikut C, Reiss E, Young L: d-Fenfluramine treatment of binge eating disorder. Am J Psychiatry 1996; 153:1455–1459 [A]

291. Gardiner HM, Freeman CP, Jesinger DK, Collins SA: Fluvoxamine: an open pilot study in moderately obese female patients suffering from atypical eating disorders and episodes of bingeing. Int J Obes Relat Metab Disord 1993; 17:301–305 [B]

292. Hudson JI, McElroy SL, Raymond NC, Crow S, Keck PE Jr, Carter WP, Mitchell JE, Strakowski SM, Pope HG Jr, Coleman BS, Jonas JM: Fluvoxamine in the treatment of binge-eating disorder: a multicenter placebo-controlled, double-blind trial. Am J Psychiatry 1998; 155:1756–1762 [A]

293. McCann UD, Agras WS: Successful treatment of nonpurging bulimia nervosa with desipramine: a double-blind, placebo-controlled study. Am J Psychiatry 1990; 147:1509–1513 [A]

294. Abenhaim L, Moride Y, Brenot F, Rich S, Benichou J, Kurz X, Higenbottam T, Oakley C, Wouters E, Aubier M, Simonneau G, Beguad B: Appetite-suppressant drugs and the risk of primary pulmonary hypertension. N Engl J Med 1996; 335:609–616 [D]

295. Connolly H, Crary J, McGoon M, Hensrud D, Edwards B, Edwards W, Schaff H: Valvular heart disease associated with fenfluramine-phentermine. N Engl J Med 1997; 337:581–588 [C]

296. Graham DJ, Green L: Further cases of valvular heart disease associated with fenfluramine-phentermine (letter). N Engl J Med 1997; 337:635 [G]

297. Mark EJ, Patalas ED, Chang HT, Evans RJ, Kessler SC: Fatal pulmonary hypertension associated with short-term use of fenfluramine and phentermine. N Engl J Med 1997; 337:602–606 [G]

298. McCann U, Hatzidimitriou G, Ridenour A, Fischer C, Yuan J, Katz J, Ricaurte G: Dexfenfluramine and serotonin neurotoxicity: further preclinical evidence that clinical caution is indicated. J Pharmacol Exp Ther 1994; 269:792–798 [G]

299. Ricaurte GA, Martello MB, Wilson MA, Molliver ME, Katz JL, Martello AL: Dexfenfluramine neurotoxicity in brains of non-human primates. Lancet 1991; 338:1487–1488 [G]

300. Marcus MD, Wing RR, Ewing L, Kern E, McDermott M, Gooding W: A double-blind, placebo-controlled trial of fluoxetine plus behavior modification in the treatment of obese binge-eaters and non-binge-eaters. Am J Psychiatry 1990; 147:876–881 [A]

301. Kerr A, Leszcz M, Kaplan AS: Continuing care groups for chronic anorexia nervosa, in Group Psychotherapy for Eating Disorders. Edited by Harper-Giuffre H, MacKenzie KR. Washington, DC, American Psychiatric Press, 1992, pp 261–272 [G]

302. Holderness C, Brooks-Gunn J, Warren M: Comorbidity of eating disorders and substance abuse: review of the literature. Int J Eat Disord 1994; 16:1–35 [F]

303. Bulik C, Sullivan P, Epstein L, McKee M, Kaye W, Dahl R, Weltzin T: Drug use in women with anorexia and bulimia nervosa. Int J Eat Disord 1992; 11:214–225 [D]

304. Bulik C, Sullivan P, Fear J, Pickering A, Dawn A, McCullin M: Fertility and reproduction in women with anorexia nervosa: a controlled study. J Clin Psychiatry 1999; 60:130–135 [B]

305. Strober M, Freeman R, Bower S, Rigali J: Binge-eating in anorexia nervosa predicts later onset of substance use disorder: a ten-year prospective, longitudinal follow-up of 95 adolescents. J Youth and Adolescence 1997; 25:519–532 [C]

306. Hatsukami D, Mitchell JE, Eckert E, Pyle R: Characteristics of patients with bulimia only, bulimia with affective disorder and bulimia with substance abuse problems. Addict Behav 1986; 11:399–406 [D]

307. Collings S, King M: Ten year follow-up of 50 patients with bulimia nervosa. Br J Psychiatry 1994; 165:80–87 [C]

308. Mitchell JE, Pyle RL, Eckert ED, Hatsukami D: The influence of prior alcohol and drug abuse problems on bulimia nervosa treatment outcome. Addict Behav 1990; 15:169–173 [D]

309. Strasser T, Pike K, Walsh B: The impact of prior substance abuse on treatment outcome for bulimia nervosa. Addict Behav 1992; 17:387–395 [C]

310. Westermeyer J, Specker S: Social resources and social function in comorbid eating and substance disorder: a matched-pairs study. Am J Addict (in press) [A]

311. Cooper PJ: Eating disorders and their relationship to mood and anxiety disorders, in Eating Disorders and Obesity: A Comprehensive Handbook. Edited by Brownell KD, Fairburn CG. New York, Guilford Press, 1995, pp 159–164 [G]

312. Edelstein CK, Yager J: Eating disorders and affective disorders, in Special Problems in Managing Eating Disorders. Edited by Yager J, Gwirtsman HE, Edelstein CK. Washington, DC, American Psychiatric Press, 1992, pp 15–50 [G]

313. Cooper PJ, Fairburn GG: The depressive symptoms of bulimia nervosa. Br J Psychiatry 1986; 148:268–274 [G]

314. Bulik C, Sullivan P, Fear J, Joyce PR: Eating disorders and antecedent anxiety disorders: a controlled study. Acta Psychiatr Scand 1997; 92:101–107 [B]

315. Bulik CM, Sullivan PF, Joyce PR, Carter FA: Temperament, character, personality disorder in bulimia nervosa. J Nerv Ment Dis 1995; 183:593–598 [B]

316. Johnson C, Tobin D, Enright A: Prevalence and clinical characteristics of borderline patients in an eating disordered population. J Clin Psychiatry 1989; 50:9–15 [D]

317. Vitousek K, Manke F: Personality variables and disorders in anorexia nervosa and bulimia nervosa. J Abnorm Psychol 1994; 103:137–147 [G]

318. Wonderlich SA: Personality and eating disorders, in Eating Disorders and Obesity: A Comprehensive Textbook. Edited by Brownell KD, Fairburn C. New York, Guilford Press, 1996, pp 171–176 [G]

319. Wonderlich SA, Mitchell JE: Eating disorders and personality disorders, in Special Problems in Managing Eating Disorders. Edited by Yager J, Gwirtsman HE, Edelstein CK. Washington, DC, American Psychiatric Press, 1992, pp 51–86 [G]

320. Wonderlich SA, Swift WJ: Borderline versus other personality disorders in the eating disorders: clinical description. Int J Eat Disord 1990; 9:629–638 [G]

321. Ames-Frankel J, Devlin MJ, Walsh BT, Strasser TJ, Sadik C, Oldham JM, Roose SP: Personality disorder diagnoses in patients with bulimia nervosa: clinical correlates and changes with treatment. J Clin Psychiatry 1992; 53:90–96 [C]

322. Johnson C, Tobin DL, Dennis A: Differences in treatment outcome between borderline and non-borderline bulimics at one-year follow-up. Int J Eat Disord 1990; 9:617–627 [B]

323. Dansky BS, Brewerton TD, Kilpatrick DG, O'Neil PM: The National Women's Study: relationship of victimization and posttraumatic stress disorder to bulimia nervosa. Int J Eat Disord 1997; 21:213–228 [D]

324. Rodin G, Daneman D, DeGroot J: The interaction of chronic medical illness and eating disorders, in Medical Issues and the Eating Disorders: The Interface. Edited by Kaplan AS, Garfinkel PE. New York, Brunner/Mazel, 1993, pp 179–181 [G]

325. Yager J, Young RT: Eating disorders and diabetes mellitus, in Special Problems in Managing Eating Disorders. Edited by Yager J, Gwirtsman HE, Edelstein CK. Washington, DC, American Psychiatric Press, 1992, pp 185–203 [G]

326. Powers PS: Management of patients with comorbid medical conditions, in Handbook of Treatment for Eating Disorders, 2nd ed. Edited by Garner DM, Garfinkel PE. New York, Guilford Press, 1997, pp 424–436 [G]

327. Brinch M, Isageer T, Tolstrup K: Anorexia nervosa and motherhood: reproduction pattern and mothering behavior of 50 women. Acta Psychiatr Scand 1988; 77:611–617 [C]

328. Rand CSW, Willis DC, Kuldau JM: Pregnancy after anorexia nervosa. Int J Eat Disord 1987; 6:671–674 [G]

329. Stewart DE, Raskin J, Garfinkel PE, MacDonald OL, Robinson GE: Anorexia nervosa, bulimia and pregnancy. Am J Obstet Gynecol 1987; 157:1194–1198 [C]

330. Treasure JL, Russell GF: Intrauterine growth and neonatal weight gain in babies of women with anorexia nervosa. Br Med J 1988; 296:1038–1039 [B]

331. Lacey H, Smith G: Bulimia nervosa: the impact of pregnancy on mother and baby. Br J Psychiatry 1987; 150:777–781 [D]

332. Powers PS, Spratt EG: Males and females with eating disorders. Eating Disorders: J Treatment and Prevention 1994; 2:197–214 [D]

333. Carlat DJ, Camargo CA Jr, Herzog DB: Eating disorders in males: a report on 135 patients. Am J Psychiatry 1997; 154:1127–1132 [G]

334. Fichter MM, Daser CC: Symptomatology, psychosexual development, and gender identity in 42 anorexic males. Psychol Med 1987; 17:409–418 [G]

335. Andersen AE: Males With Eating Disorders. New York, Brunner/Mazel, 1990 [G]

336. Golden NH, Kreitzer P, Jacobson MS, Chasalow FI, Schebendach J, Freedman SM, Shenker IR: Disturbances in growth hormone secretion and action in adolescents with anorexia nervosa. J Pediatr 1994; 125:655–660 [D]

337. Katzman DK, Zipursky RB: Adolescents with anorexia nervosa: the impact of the disorder on bones and brains. Ann NY Acad Sci 1997; 817:127–137 [F]

338. Katzman DK, Zipursky RB, Lambe EK, Mikulis DJ: A longitudinal magnetic resonance imaging study of brain changes in adolescents with anorexia nervosa. Arch Pediatr Adolesc Med 1997; 151:793–797 [C]

339. Nussbaum MP, Baird D, Sonnenblick M, Cowan K, Shenker IR: Short stature in anorexia nervosa patients. J Adolesc Health Care 1985; 6:453–455 [D]

340. Pfeiffer RJ, Lucas AR, Ilstrup DM: Effects of anorexia nervosa on linear growth. Clin Pediatr (Phila) 1986; 25:7–12 [G]

341. Henry MC, Perlmutter SJ, Swedo SE: Anorexia, OCD, and streptococcus. J Am Acad Child Adolesc Psychiatry 1999; 38:228–229 [G]

342. Sokol MS, Gray NS: Case study: an infection triggered, autoimmune subtype of anorexia nervosa. J Am Acad Child Adolesc Psychiatry 1997; 36:1128–1133 [G]

343. Gupta MA: Concerns about aging and a drive for thinness: a factor in the biopsychosocial model of eating disorders? Int J Eat Disord 1995; 18:351–357 [B]

344. Boast N, Coker E, Wakeling A: Anorexia nervosa of late onset. Br J Psychiatry 1992; 160:257–260 [G]

345. Davis C, Yager J: Transcultural aspects of eating disorders: a critical literature review. Cult Med Psychiatry 1992; 16:377–382 [G]

346. Katzman MA, Lee S: Beyond body image: the integration of feminist and transcultural theories in the understanding of self-starvation. Int J Eat Disord 1997; 22:385–394 [F]

347. Powers PS, Johnson C: Small victories: prevention of eating disorders among athletes. Eating Disorders: J Treatment and Prevention 1997; 4:364–377 [D]

348. Thompson RA, Sherman RT: Helping Athletes With Eating Disorders. Champaign, Ill, Human Kinetics, 1993 [G]

349. Williamson DA, Netemeyer RG, Jackman LP, Anderson DA, Funsch CL, Rabalais JY: Structural equation modeling for risk factors for the development of eating disorder symptoms in female athletes. Int J Eat Disord 1995; 17:387–393 [E]

350. Nattiv A, Agostini R, Drinkwater B, Yeager KK: The female athlete triad: the inter-relatedness of disordered eating, amenorrhea, and osteoporosis. Clin Sports Med 1994; 13:405–418 [G]

351. Yates A: Athletes, eating disorders and the overtraining syndrome, in Activity Anorexia: Theory, Research and Treatment. Edited by Epling W, Pierce W. Hillsdale, NJ, Lawrence Erlbaum Associates, 1996, pp 179–188 [G]

352. Epling W, Pierce W: Activity Anorexia: Theory, Research, Treatment. Hillsdale, NJ, Lawrence Erlbaum Associates, 1996 [G]

353. Mann T, Nolen-Hoesksema S, Huang K, Burgard D, Wright A, Hanson K: Are two interventions worse than none? joint primary and secondary prevention of eating disorders in college females. Health Psychol 1997; 16:215–225 [B]

354. Shisslak CM, Crago M, Estes LS, Gray N: Content and method of developmentally appropriate prevention programs, in The Developmental Psychopathology of Eating Disorders: Implications for Research, Prevention, and Treatment. Edited by Smolak L, Levine MP, Striegel-Moore RH. Mahwah, NJ, Lawrence Erlbaum Associates, 1996, pp 341–363 [E]

355. Glenn AA, Pollard JW, Denovcheck JA, Smith AF: Eating disorders on campus: a procedure for community intervention. J Counseling & Development 1986; 65:163–165 [G]

356. Coll KM: Mandatory psychiatric withdrawal from public colleges and universities: a review of potential legal violations and appropriate use. J College Student Psychotherapy 1991; 5:91–98 [E]

APPENDIX
Practice Guideline Development Process

I. BACKGROUND AND DEFINITION

In 1991, the American Psychiatric Association (APA), through its Assembly and Board of Trustees, embarked on the process of developing practice guidelines. Since its inception, the APA has generated, in many different formats, guidelines for psychiatric practice. *Practice guidelines* as defined by this project, however, are systematically developed documents appearing in a standardized format presenting patient care strategies to assist psychiatrists in clinical decision making. Importantly, although practice guidelines may be used for a variety of purposes, their primary purpose is to assist psychiatrists in their care of patients.

Both the American Medical Association (AMA) and the Institute of Medicine (IOM) have sought to define the key features necessary to ensure that practice guidelines are of high quality. The AMA's attributes apply to the development process, stating that practice parameters/guidelines should 1) be developed by or in conjunction with physician organizations, 2) explicitly describe the methodology and process used in their development, 3) assist practitioner and patient decisions about appropriate health care for specific clinical circumstances, 4) be based on current professional knowledge and reviewed and revised at regular intervals, and 5) be widely disseminated. The IOM's attributes are criteria for evaluating the finished product: validity, based on the strength of the evidence, expert judgment, and estimates of health and cost outcomes compared with alternative practices; reliability/reproducibility; clinical applicability and flexibility; clarity; attention to multidisciplinary concerns; timely updates; and documentation. Taken together, these prescriptives have essentially set national standards for guideline efforts.

II. TOPIC SELECTION

The APA Steering Committee on Practice Guidelines oversees the development of APA practice guidelines. The Steering Committee selects topics for practice guidelines according to the following criteria:

1. Degree of public importance (prevalence and seriousness)
2. Relevance to psychiatric practice
3. Availability of information and relevant data
4. Availability of work already done that would be useful in the development of a practice guideline
5. The area is one in which increased psychiatric attention and involvement would be helpful for the field

III. CONTRIBUTORS

APA practice guidelines are developed by a work group of psychiatrists in active clinical practice, including academicians or researchers who spend a significant percentage of their time in the clinical care of patients. Work group members are selected on the basis of their knowledge and experience in the topic area, their commitment to the integrity of the guideline development process as outlined by the AMA and IOM, and their representativeness of the diversity of American psychiatry.

Work group members are asked to decline participation if they feel there are possible conflicts of interest or biases that could impact their ability to maintain scientific objectivity. The following statement appears in every practice guideline to clarify this point:

> This practice guideline has been developed by psychiatrists who are in active clinical practice. In addition, some contributors are primarily involved in research or other academic endeavors. It is possible that through such activities some contributors have received income related to treatments discussed in this guideline. A number of mechanisms are in place to minimize the potential for producing biased recommendations due to conflicts of interest. The guideline has been extensively reviewed by members of the APA as well as by representatives from related fields. Contributors and reviewers have all been asked to base their recommendations on an objective evaluation of the available evidence. Any contributor or reviewer who has a potential conflict of interest that may bias (or appear to bias) his or her work has been asked to notify the APA Office of Quality Improvement and Psychiatric Services. This potential bias is then discussed with the work group chair and the chair of the Steering Committee on Practice Guidelines. Further action depends on the assessment of the potential bias.

The APA is listed as the "author" of practice guidelines, with individual contributions and reviewers acknowledged. Final editorial responsibility for practice guidelines rests with the Steering Committee and the Office of Quality Improvement and Psychiatric Services.

IV. EVIDENCE BASE

The evidence base for practice guidelines is derived from two sources—research studies and clinical consensus. Where gaps exist in the research data, evidence is derived from clinical consensus, obtained through extensive review of multiple drafts of each guideline (see section VI). Both research data and clinical consensus vary in their validity and reliability for different clinical situations; guidelines state explicitly the nature of the supporting evidence for specific recommendations so that readers can make their own judgments regarding the utility of the recommendations. The following coding system is used for this purpose:

[A] *Randomized clinical trial.* A study of an intervention in which subjects are prospectively followed over time; there are treatment and control groups; subjects are randomly assigned to the two groups; both the subjects and the investigators are "blind" to the assignments.

[B] *Clinical trial.* A prospective study in which an intervention is made and the results of that intervention are tracked longitudinally; study does not meet standards for a randomized clinical trial.

[C] *Cohort or longitudinal study.* A study in which subjects are prospectively followed over time without any specific intervention.

[D] *Case-control study.* A study in which a group of patients and a group of control subjects are identified in the present and information about them is pursued retrospectively or backward in time.

[E] *Review with secondary analysis.* A structured analytic review of existing data, e.g., a meta-analysis or a decision analysis.

[F] *Review.* A qualitative review and discussion of previously published literature without a quantitative synthesis of the data.

[G] *Other.* Textbooks, expert opinion, case reports, and other reports not included above.

The literature review process is explicitly described in the guideline, including statements concerning

1. Basic search strategy (e.g., key words, time period covered, research methodologies considered)
2. Sources for identifying studies (e.g., review articles, texts, abstracting and indexing services, Index Medicus, Sciences Citations Index, computer search services)
3. Criteria for selecting publications (e.g., number of relevant publications identified, whether all were reviewed, whether only prospective studies were selected)
4. Review methods (e.g., publications reviewed in their entirety, abstract review only)
5. Methods for cataloging reported outcomes (e.g., study design, sample characteristics, relevant findings)

The literature review will include other guidelines addressing the same topic, when available. Wherever possible, evidence tables are constructed to illustrate the data regarding risks and benefits for each treatment. In many cases, however, evidence tables are used only to assist in writing the text and do not appear in the guideline.

V. FORMAT

Each practice guideline is presented in a standardized format, with variations as appropriate (e.g., a guideline about psychiatric evaluation or a procedure may vary from that about a specific illness).

The outline for the second edition of *Practice Guideline for the Treatment of Patients With Major Depressive Disorder* and subsequent guidelines and revisions is as follows:

Part A. Treatment Recommendations
     I. Summary of Treatment Recommendations
     II. Formulation and Implementation of a Treatment Plan
     III. Specific Clinical Features Influencing the Treatment Plan
Part B. Background Information and Review of Available Evidence
     IV. Disease Definition, Epidemiology, Natural History and Course
     V. Review and Synthesis of Available Evidence

Part C. Future Research Needs
Individuals and Organizations That Submitted Comments
References

Section I provides an overview of the organization and scope of recommendations contained in subsequent sections, with each recommendation identified as falling into one of three categories of endorsement:

[I]   Recommended with substantial clinical confidence.
[II]   Recommended with moderate clinical confidence.
[III] May be recommended on the basis of individual circumstances.

Section II presents a synthesis of the information discussed in section V, directed at providing a framework for clinical decision making for the individual patient.

Section III addresses psychiatric, general medical, and demographic factors influencing treatment, including comorbidities. Relevant ethnic, cross-cultural, social, or extrinsic factors (e.g., cultural mores, family, support system, living situation, health care beliefs) that could potentially preclude or modify the practical application of guidelines and may play a role in health care decisions are emphasized.

Section IV presents the characteristics of the illness using current DSM criteria. Differential diagnosis, appropriate diagnostic procedures, aspects of the epidemiology and natural history with important treatment implications, and issues concerning special patient characteristics are outlined in this section.

Section V presents a review of the available data on all potential treatments, organized according to three broad categories: 1) psychiatric management, 2) psychosocial interventions, and 3) somatic interventions. For each treatment, this information is presented in a standard format:

a. Goals of treatment
b. Efficacy data
c. Side effects and safety
d. Implementation issues (e.g., patient selection, laboratory testing, dosing, frequency, duration)

Part C identifies directions for further research.

Immediately following the research directions is the list individuals and organizations that submitted substantive comments of guideline drafts.

Last, all references cited in the published guideline are listed.

VI. REVIEW, DISSEMINATION, AND UPDATES

Each practice guideline is extensively reviewed at multiple draft stages. Draft 1 is reviewed by the Steering Committee. Approximately 50 reviewers with expertise in the topic, representatives of approximately 100 related organizations, the APA Assembly, District Branches, Joint Reference Committee, Board of Trustees, Council on Quality Improvement, other components related to the subject area, and any APA member by request are given the opportunity to review and comment on each practice guideline prior to publication.

The development process may be summarized as follows:

Step 1: The Steering Committee on Practice Guidelines selects a small number of individuals to serve as the work group chair and members.

Step 2: The work group chair and Office of Quality Improvement and Psychiatric Services staff develop a preliminary outline, to be continuously revised and refined throughout subsequent steps in the development process.

Step 3: A literature search is conducted by APA and/or the work group. Relevant articles from the search are obtained, in abstract form or in entirety. The work group reviews these articles, codes them for study design, and constructs evidence tables for each treatment.

Step 4: Draft 1 is written based on evidence tables and outline.

Step 5: Draft 1 is circulated to the work group and Steering Committee for review and comment.

Step 6: Draft 2 is written based on comments received.

Step 7: Draft 2 is circulated to the work group, the Steering Committee, and approximately 50 reviewers with expertise in the subject area.

Step 8: Draft 3 is written based on comments received.

Step 9: Draft 3 is circulated to the work group, Steering Committee, 50 expert reviewers, the APA Board of Trustees, Assembly, Joint Reference Committee, Council on Quality Improvement, District Branches, individual members (open review available through District Branches), *The American Journal of Psychiatry,* and 100 representatives of related organizations.

Step 10: Draft 4 is written based on comments received.

Step 11: Draft 4 is submitted to the formal APA review and approval process (Council on Quality Improvement, Assembly, Board of Trustees).

After final approval by the Assembly and Board of Trustees, each practice guideline is widely disseminated. Practice guidelines are made available to all psychiatrists in a variety of ways, including publication in *The American Journal of Psychiatry.* Each practice guideline will be revised at 5- to 10-year intervals to reflect new knowledge in the field.

INDEX

Page numbers printed in **boldface** *type refer to tables or figures.*

Agoraphobia, and panic disorder, 573, 574, 580, 581, 584

Agranulocytosis, and clozapine, 332

AHCPR (Agency for Health Care Policy and Research), 87, 243, 244, 418

AIDS. *See also* HIV
delirium and, 41, 51, 54, 60
substance use disorders and, 156

AIDS-related dementia, and schizophrenia, 382

Akathisia, and antipsychotics, 322

Akinesia, and antipsychotics, 321

Alanine aminotransferase (ALT) levels, and tacrine, 100

Al-Anon, 188

Alateen, 188

Alcohol abuse and alcoholism. *See also* Substance use disorders and substance abuse
bipolar disorder and, 538
clinical factors influencing treatment of, 189–194
delirium and, **48**
dementia and, 85
elderly and, 180
ethnicity and, 378
major depressive disorder and, 442
medical problems and, 177
nicotine dependence and, 252, 258–259, 279–280
opioid-related disorders and, 208, 209
overview of treatment of, 182–183
panic disorder and, 603–604
pharmacologic treatments for, 184–185
psychosocial treatments for, 185–189
schizophrenia and, 373
settings for treatment of, 183–184
summary of recommendations on, 148–149

Alcohol and Alcohol Problems Science Database (National Institute on Alcohol Abuse and Alcoholism), 212, 213

Alcohol dementia, 193

Alcoholic hallucinosis, 193

Alcoholics Anonymous, 167, 168, 169, 188

Alcohol-induced peripheral myopathy, 192

Allergic effects, of antipsychotics, 326

Alliance for the Mentally Ill, 362

Alprazolam
panic disorder and, 590, 591–592, 593
schizophrenia and, 342

Alternative treatment settings, for schizophrenia, 306

Alzheimer's Association, 89, 92, 93, 122, 123

Alzheimer's disease. *See also* Dementia
definition of, 82–83
development process for practice guideline on, 74
diagnosis of, 83
factors modifying treatment decisions for, 118–123
introduction to, 73
prevalence of, 82
psychiatric management of, 86–94
psychotherapy and psychosocial treatments for, 94–96
research on, 123–124
sites for treatment of, 85–86
somatic treatment of, 96–115
summary of recommendations on, 75–80

Amantadine
Alzheimer's disease and related dementias and apathy, 79, 113
antipsychotics and, 321, **323**
cocaine-related disorders and, 195, 199
side effects of, 112

Amenorrhea, and eating disorders, 648

American Academy of Child and Adolescent Psychiatry, 303, 606

American Academy of Neurology, 87

American Journal of Psychiatry, 705

American Medical Association (AMA), 701

American Psychiatric Association. *See also* *Diagnostic and Statistical Manual of Mental Disorders,* Fourth Edition (DSM-IV)
confidentiality standards and, 22
development process for practice guidelines and, 701–705
Position Statement on Nicotine Dependence and, 243
practice guideline for geriatric psychiatry and, 97
Task Force on Benzodiazepine Dependence, Toxicity, and Abuse, 591, 592
Task Force on Electroconvulsive Therapy, 467

Americans with Disabilities Act, 678

Amitriptyline
eating disorders and, 662, 668, 669
side effects of, 112, 669

Asthma, and major depressive disorder, 450
Ataxia, and alcohol-related disorders, 193
Athletes, and eating disorders, 677
Attention deficit hyperactivity disorder, and bipolar disorder, 539
Atypical features
of eating disorders, 646, 651–652
of major depressive disorder, 441
Automobiles, driving and Alzheimer's disease and related dementias, 90–91, 115–116. *See also* Safety
Aversion therapy
nicotine dependence and, 260–261, 269
substance use disorders and, 166
Avoidance, and panic disorder, 575–576
Avoidant personality disorder, and major depressive disorder, 472
Azumolene, and neuroleptic malignant syndrome, 323

Barbiturates
alcohol-related disorders and, 191
antipsychotics and, 330
Basal ganglia strokes, and delirium, 57
Behavior. *See also* Aggression; Behavior therapy; Sexual behavior; Violence and violent behavior
delirium and, 48, 49
dementia and, 117
substance use disorders and, 153
Behavioral exposure treatment, for panic disorder, 580, 581
Behavioral family management, and bipolar disorder, 526
Behavior therapy. *See also* Behavior; Cognitive behavioral therapy; Multimodal behavior therapy
for alcohol-related disorders, 186–187
for Alzheimer's disease and related dementias, 76, 95
for bipolar disorder, 527
for cocaine-related disorders, 196
for eating disorders, 645, 659, 666, 672
for major depressive disorder, 471
for nicotine dependence, 247–248, 259–263, 276, 284
for opioid-related disorders, 204
for substance use disorders, 165–166
Benzodiazepines
alcohol abuse and, 149, 190, 191, 192, 194

Alzheimer's disease and related dementias and, 78, 79, 107–108, 115
bipolar disorder and, 520, 521, 537
clozapine and, 333
cocaine use disorders and, 150, 198
delirium and, 53–55, 58
electroconvulsive therapy and, 525
nicotine dependence and, 270
opioid-related disorders and, 208
panic disorder and, 571–572, 590–593, 601, 602, 604
schizophrenia and, 308, 341–343
side effects of, 54, 108, 342, 591–592
side effects of antipsychotics and, 322
substance use disorders and, 163, 164
Benztropine mesylate, and side effects of antipsychotics, **323**
Bereavement, and major depressive disorder, 445
Beta blockers
alcohol-related disorders and, 190, 191, 192
Alzheimer's disease and related dementias and, 78, 110
antipsychotics and, 330
nicotine dependence and, 270
panic disorder and, 596
side effects of antipsychotics and, 322
Bibliography on Smoking and Health (Centers for Disease Control and Prevention), 244
Binge eating disorder, 671
Binge-eating/purging subtype, of anorexia nervosa, 646, **647**
Bipolar disorder
clinical features influencing treatment of, 537–543
development process for practice guideline on, 501
diagnosis of, 503
eating disorders and, 654
electroconvulsive therapy and, 523–525
epidemiology of, 504–505
introduction to, 502
natural history and course of, 504
panic disorder and, 604
pharmacologic treatment of, 508–523, 544–545
psychiatric management of, 506–508, 544
psychosocial treatments for, 540–541

Cardiac disease. *See also* Cardiovascular
disease
major depressive disorder and, 450
schizophrenia and, 360, 381
Cardiopulmonary disorders, and delirium,
42
Cardiovascular disease. *See also* Cardiac
disease; Stroke
alcohol-related disorders and, 192
tobacco use and, 250, 281
Cardiovascular effects
of antipsychotics, 52–53
of electroconvulsive therapy, 467–468
of monoamine oxidase inhibitors, 463
pharmacotherapy for eating disorders
and, 664
of tricyclic antidepressants, 459
Caregivers
Alzheimer's disease and related
dementias and, 89, 91, 93, 116, 119,
122
delirium and, 48
eating disorders and, 659
Case formulation, and assessment of adults,
19–20
Case management, and schizophrenia,
349–350
Catatonia and catatonic symptoms
bipolar disorder and, 537–538
major depressive disorder and, 441
schizophrenia and, 308, 367
side effects of antipsychotics and, 321
Centers for Disease Control and Prevention,
244
Central nervous system. *See also* Neurologic
effects
alcohol-related disorders and disorders
of, 192–193
delirium and disorders of, **42**
Cerebrovascular disease, and dementia, 83
Chaperones, and physical examination by
psychiatrist, 19
Chelating agents, and Alzheimer's disease,
97, 103
Chemical aversion therapy, for substance
use disorders, 164
Child custody evaluations, 9
Children. *See also* Age; Parenting
benzodiazepines and, 54
bipolar disorder and, 504, 539, 540

cocaine-related disorders and
development of, 199
eating disorders and, 676
major depressive disorder and, 445–446
panic disorder and, 606–607
schizophrenia and, 303
secondhand smoke and illnesses in, 281
substance use disorders and, 178, 179
China, and eating disorders, 653
Chloral hydrate, and sleep disturbances, 79,
114, 115
Chlordiazepoxide
alcohol-related disorders and, 190
schizophrenia and, 342
Chlorpromazine
delirium and, 51, 60
schizophrenia and, 344, 365, 378
Cholinergic medications, and delirium, 55
Cholinesterase inhibitors, and Alzheimer's
disease, 98–100
Cigarette smoking. *See* Nicotine
dependence
Cimetidine, and antipsychotics, 330
Citalopram, and eating disorders, 664
Citric acid inhaler, and smoking cessation,
271
Clinical Assessment of Confusion—A
(CAC-A), 44
Clinical consultations, and adult psychiatric
evaluation, 8–9
Clinical Global Impression (CGI), 584, 590
*Clinical Practice Guideline on Smoking
Cessation* (AHCPR), 243, 244
Clinical remission, and panic disorder, 575
Clomipramine
eating disorders and, 662
panic disorder and, 588, 589
Clonazepam
Alzheimer's disease and related
dementias and, 108
bipolar disorder and, 521
panic disorder and, 590–591, 592–593
schizophrenia and, 342, 366
side effects of antipsychotics and, 322
Clonidine
alcohol-related disorders and, 190–191,
192
nicotine dependence and, 270, 272,
274–275, 276, 282
opioid use disorders and, 151, 203,
206–207

panic disorder and, 597
side effects of, 270
substance use disorders and, 163
Clozapine
Alzheimer's disease and related
dementias and, 78, 105, 107
bipolar disorder and, 521, 523
nicotine dependence and, 250–251
panic disorder and, 596
schizophrenia and, 307–308, 330–334,
344, 356, 366, 370, 372
side effects of, 105, 106, 308, 325, 332,
333
tardive dyskinesia and, 324, 325
Clubhouse model, of community treatment
for schizophrenia, 351
Cocaine Anonymous, 168, 197
Cocaine use disorders. *See also* Substance
use disorders and substance abuse
clinical features influencing treatment of,
197–199
opioid-related disorders and, 208, 209
overview of treatment for, 194
pharmacologic treatments for, 195–196
psychosocial treatments for, 196–197
summary of recommendations on,
149–150
treatment settings and, 194–195
Coding systems, for recommendations in
practice guidelines
Alzheimer's disease and related
dementias and, 75
bipolar disorder and, 543
delirium and, 37
eating disorders and, 631, 681
major depressive disorder and, 479–480
panic disorder and, 569
schizophrenia and, 305
substance use disorders and, 145
Cognition and cognitive impairments. *See
also* Memory and memory
impairments; Thoughts and thinking
alcohol-related disorders and, 192
Alzheimer's disease and related
dementias and, 76–77, 80, 83,
97–103, 110, 116
bipolar disorder and, 527–528
delirium and changes in, 39, 41, 50, 57
major depressive disorder and, 443
mental status examination and, 14–15
substance use disorders and, 153

Cognitive behavioral therapy. *See also*
Behavior therapy; Cognitive therapy
alcohol-related disorders and, 186
bipolar disorder and, 526
cocaine-related disorders and, 196
eating disorders and, 633, 645, 665,
667–668, 670, 672
major depressive disorder and, 470–471
opioid-related disorders and, 203–204
panic disorder and, 570, 579–582,
599–601
substance use disorders and, 165
Cognitive restructuring, and panic disorder,
580
Cognitive therapy. *See also* Cognitive
behavioral therapy
for Alzheimer's disease and related
dementias, 76, 95–96
for schizophrenia, 354
for substance use disorders, 165
Collateral sources
adult psychiatric evaluations and, 10, 17
clinical consultations and, 9
Colleges, and eating disorders, 677–678
Combined therapy. *See also*
Pharmacotherapy; Psychotherapy
bipolar disorder and, 583
eating disorders and, 634, 646, 670, 673
major depressive disorder and, 423, 427,
433, 437–438, 475
nicotine dependence and, 272, 276
panic disorder and, 571
Community mental health care, and
schizophrenia, 349–355
Community reinforcement therapy
cocaine-related disorders and, 196, 197
alcohol-related disorders and, 186–187
substance use disorders and, 165
Community resources, and Alzheimer's
disease, 92–93, 122. *See also* Social
service agencies
Comorbidity, of psychiatric disorders. *See
also* Complications; Medical conditions
alcohol-related disorders and, 191–193
Alzheimer's disease and related
dementias and, 110–113, 118–119
bipolar disorder and, 528, 538, 539
cocaine-related disorders and, 198–199
delirium and, 59–60
eating disorders and, 642, 653–654,
673–675

Dantrolene sodium, and neuroleptic malignant syndrome, 323

Day care. *See also* Day hospitalization
    Alzheimer's disease and, 119
    schizophrenia and, 357–358

Day hospitalization. *See also* Day care; Partial hospitalization
    for cocaine-related disorders, 197
    for eating disorders, 635
    for schizophrenia, 357

Daytime drowsiness, and antipsychotics, 320

Death, Alzheimer's disease and preparation for, 117. *See also* Mortality; Sudden death

Decision making
    Alzheimer's disease and, 94
    pharmacotherapy for schizophrenia and, 306, 362

Deinstitutionalization, and homelessness in schizophrenia patients, 377

Delirium
    associated features of, 40
    causes of, 42–43
    clinical features influencing treatment of, 59–61
    competency and consent issues and, 59
    definition and clinical features of, 39–40
    dementia and, 118
    development process for practice guideline on, 36
    differential diagnosis of, 40–41
    environmental and supportive interventions for, 49–50, 57
    epidemiology of, 41–42
    formal measures of, 43–45
    introduction to, 35
    psychiatric management of, 45–49, 57
    somatic interventions for, 51–57, 58–59
    summary of recommendations on, 37–38
    treatment plans for, 57–59

Delirium Rating Scale (DRS), 45, 51

Delirium Symptom Interview (DSI), 44–45

Delusions, and dementia, 81, 116

Dementia. *See also* Alzheimer's disease
    AIDS-related, 382
    alcohol-related disorders and, 193
    associated features of, 80–81
    definition of, 80
    delirium and, 40–41
    developmental process for practice guideline on, 74
    differential diagnosis of, 81–82
    factors modifying treatment decisions for, 118–123
    introduction to, 73
    major depressive disorder and, 450
    prevalence of, 82
    progressive, 82, 85, 90
    pseudodementia, 81, 110, 443
    psychiatric management of, 86–94
    psychotherapy and psychosocial treatments for, 94–96
    research on, 123–124
    sites of treatment for, 85–86
    somatic treatment of, 96–115
    specific types of, 82–85
    staging of, 82
    summary of recommendations on, 75–80
    vascular, 82, 83–84, 92

Dementia of the Alzheimer's type, 82–83

Demographic factors
    Alzheimer's disease and related dementias and, 122–123
    bipolar disorder and, 540–543
    eating disorders and, 675–678
    major depressive disorder and, 444–446, 448–450
    nicotine dependence and, 282–283
    panic disorder and, 606–608
    schizophrenia and, 377–381

Denial
    bipolar disorder and, 507
    substance use disorders and, 162

Denicotinized tobacco, 271

Dental complications, and eating disorders, 639

Dependency, and panic disorder, 584

Depot medications, and antipsychotics, 327–328, 364, 365

Depression. *See also* Major depressive disorder; Unipolar depression
    alcohol-related disorders and, 191–192
    Alzheimer's disease and dementia patients and, 78–79, 110–113, 117
    bipolar disorder and, 503, 534–535, 545–546
    eating disorders and, 653–654
    nicotine dependence and, 280
    panic disorder and, 574, 597, 603
    schizophrenia and, 374–375

Dermatologic side effects, of lithium, 512

Desferrioxamine, and Alzheimer's disease, 103

Desipramine
alcohol-related disorders and, 185
Alzheimer's disease and, 112, 113
cocaine-related disorders and, 195, 197, 198–199
eating disorders and, 668, 670
panic disorder and, 588
side effects of, 112

Detoxification. *See also* Withdrawal
alcohol abuse and, 148, 184, 194
bipolar disorder and substance abuse, 530
medical conditions and substance use disorders, 172
major depressive disorder and substance abuse, 442
opioid-related disorders and, 206–207
panic disorder and, 598

Developmental history
adult psychiatric evaluation and, 12
eating disorders and, 642

Dexfenfluramine, and eating disorders, 672, 673

Dextroamphetamine, and apathy in Alzheimer's patients, 113

Dextrose, and nicotine dependence, 271

Diabetes mellitus, and eating disorders, 675

Diagnosis. *See also* Adult psychiatric evaluation; Assessment; Differential diagnosis
of Alzheimer's disease, 83
of bipolar disorder, 503
clinical consultation and, 8
of delirium, 44–45
of eating disorders, 646–648, 651
emergency evaluation and provisional, 7
of major depressive disorder, 429–430, 452–454
of nicotine dependence, 248–251, 253–254
observations of patient behavior and, 18
of panic disorder, 572, 575
of substance use disorders, 153–154

Diagnostic and Statistical Manual of Mental Disorders, Fourth Edition (DSM-IV)
adult psychiatric evaluation and, 20
Alzheimer's disease and, 83, 104, 110
bipolar disorder and, 502, 504

delirium and, 35, 39
dementia and, 81, 84, 110
eating disorders and, 646, **647,** 671
major depressive disorder and, 419, **453**
nicotine dependence and, 243, 248, 250, **251,** 252, 254
opioid-related disorders and, 200
panic disorder and, 567, 572, 578
side effects of antipsychotics and, 321
substance dependence and, **249**
substance use disorders and, 143, 152–153
subtypes of schizophrenia and, 311

Diagnostic Survey for Eating Disorders (DSED), **640**

Diazepam
alcohol-related disorders and, 190
Alzheimer's disease and related dementias and, 107
panic disorder and, 590–591, 593, 596
schizophrenia and, 342

Diet
eating disorders and, 656, 671–672
monoamine oxidase inhibitors and tyramine-free, 102, 112, 434, 463, 594

Differential diagnosis. *See also* Diagnosis
adult psychiatric evaluation and, 19–20
bipolar disorder and, 503–504
delirium and, 40–41, 61
dementia and, 81–82
major depressive disorder and, 454

Diphenhydramine
opioid-related disorders and, 208
sleep disturbances and, 115

Disability evaluations, 9

Discharge
adult psychiatric evaluation and planning for, 9
emergency evaluation and, 8

Discontinuation, of treatment. *See also* Termination
for bipolar disorder, 510, 537, 547
for major depressive disorder, 428, 439–440, 476
for panic disorder, 571, 591–592

Disorganized subtype, of schizophrenia, 310–311

Disorientation, and delirium, 39, 50

Disulfiram, and alcohol-related disorders, 148, 163–164, 184–185

Electrocardiograms (ECGs)
   antipsychotic medications for delirium
      and, 38
   lithium and, 512
   schizophrenia and, 360
Electroconvulsive therapy (ECT)
   bipolar disorder and, 523–525, 531, 544
   delirium and, 56–57
   depression in Alzheimer's disease and
      dementia patients, 79, 113
   major depressive disorder and, 423, 433,
      436, 439, 467–468, 478
   schizophrenia and, 308, 344–345, 367,
      370
   side effects of, 344–345, 467–468, 524
Electroencephalograms (EEGs)
   anticonvulsants and, 343
   delirium and, 40, 45
   nicotine withdrawal and, 250
EMBASE, 36
Emergency management, of violence in
   schizophrenia patients, 376
Emergency psychiatric evaluation, of adults,
   7–8
Emergency room
   opioid-related disorders and, 205
   panic disorder and, 569, 597
Emetine, and chemical aversion treatment,
   164
Emotion-oriented treatments, for
   Alzheimer's disease and related
   dementias, 76, 95
Emotions, and delirium, 40, 50
Employment
   patient history and, 13
   schizophrenia and, 352–354
   substance use disorders and, 158
Enabling behavior, and substance use
   disorders, 181
Endocrine disorders
   alcohol-related disorders and, 192
   antipsychotics and, 325
Environmental interventions. *See also* Stress
   and stress management
   for bipolar disorder, 543
   for delirium, 38, 49–50, 57
Epidemiologic Catchment Area (ECA) study,
   182, 312, 454, 505, 574, 608
Epidemiology
   of bipolar disorder, 504–505
   of delirium, 41–42

   of eating disorders, 652–654
   of major depressive disorder, 454
   of nicotine dependence, 251–252,
      284–285
   of panic disorder, 573–574
   of schizophrenia, 312–313
   of substance use disorders, 154–155, 156
Epilepsy
   major depressive disorder and, 451
   valproate and, 516
Ergoloid mesylates, and Alzheimer's
   disease, 77, 97, 102–103
Estrogen replacement therapy
   Alzheimer's disease and, 97, 103
   anorexia nervosa and, 663
Ethnicity. *See also* Culture; Race
   adult psychiatric evaluation and, 21
   Alzheimer's disease and caregivers, 123
   bipolar disorder and, 542
   eating disorders and, 653
   major depressive disorder and, 445
   nicotine dependence and, 283
   schizophrenia and, 378
   substance use disorders and, 180
Evaluation. *See* Adult psychiatric evaluation
Evidence base, for practice guidelines,
   702–703
*Evidence Report on Treatment of
   Depression—Newer
   Pharmacotherapies,* 456
Excerpta Medica, 74
Exclusion criteria, and psychosocial
   interventions for schizophrenia, 348
Exercise. *See also* Recreational activity
   eating disorders and, 653, 658, 677
   nicotine dependence and, 263
Exploratory therapy, and schizophrenia, 346
Exposure therapy, for panic disorder, 580
Extrapyramidal side effects. *See also* Side
   effects
   of antipsychotics, 52, 53, 58, 320–323
   delirium in elderly and, 61
Extrapyramidal Symptom Rating Scale, 335

Factitious disorder, and dementia, 81
Fagerstrom Test for Nicotine Dependence,
   249, **250,** 254
Fairweather Lodge, and community care for
   schizophrenia, 350–351
Falls, and Alzheimer's disease, 89, 108, 121.
   See also Accidents; Hip fractures

major depressive disorder and, 431
substance use disorders and, 175
Homeopathic remedies, and nicotine
dependence, 271. *See also* Botanical
agents
Homosexuality, and eating disorders, 676
Hormone replacement therapy, and
anorexia nervosa, 663
Hospice care, and Alzheimer's disease, 117
Hospitalization. *See also* Day
hospitalization; Inpatient settings;
Involuntary hospitalization; Long-term
hospitalization; Partial hospitalization
alcohol abuse and, 148
bipolar disorder and, 530
delirium and, 41–42
eating disorders and, 631, 634–635,
636–637, 658
major depressive disorder and, 430, 431
opioid-related disorders and, 205
panic disorder and, 597–598
schizophrenia and, 306, 355–357, 361,
375, 376
substance use disorders and, 171–172
Human immunodeficiency virus. *See* HIV
Huntington's disease
delirium and, 57
dementia and, 85
Hypnosis, and nicotine dependence, 263
Hydroxyzine, and opioid-related disorders,
208
Hyperactive form, of delirium, 40
Hypertension
delirium and, **48**
major depressive disorder and, 451
monoamine oxidase inhibitors and crises
of, 463
Hyperthermia, and delirium, **48**
Hypoactive form, of delirium, 40
Hypoglycemia, and delirium, **48**
Hypokalemia, and anorexia nervosa, 658
Hypophosphatemia, and anorexia nervosa,
657
Hypotension, and antipsychotic
medications, 320
Hypothyroidism, and lithium, 512
Hypoxia, and delirium, **48**

Idiosyncratic side effects
of carbamazepine, 519
of lithium, 512–513

of valproate, 516–517
Imipramine
cocaine-related disorders and, 195
eating disorders and, 668
panic disorder and, 588, 589
side effects of, 112
Individual psychotherapy. *See also*
Psychotherapy
alcohol-related disorders and, 187
eating disorders and, 644, 659–660,
665–666
schizophrenia and, 346
substance use disorders and, 166
Indomethacin, and Alzheimer's disease, 103
Infectious diseases, and substance use
disorders, 177
Informed consent, and adult psychiatric
evaluation, 21
Initial interventions, for nicotine
dependence, 256–257
Inositol, and panic disorder, 596
Inpatient settings. *See also*
Hospitalization
adult psychiatric evaluation and, 9
Alzheimer's disease and related
dementias and, 85–86, 121–122
eating disorders and, 659
nicotine dependence and, 277
Insight-oriented therapy, for schizophrenia,
346
Insomnia. *See also* Sleep
bipolar disorder and, 537
nicotine patch and, 267
tricyclic antidepressants and, 461
Institute of Medicine (IOM), 701
Instrumental activities of daily living (IADL),
and functional assessment, 15
Integrated psychological therapy, 354
Intensive care units (ICUs), and delirium,
49–50
Intensive outpatient care, for eating
disorders, **636–637**
Interdisciplinary management, of eating
disorders, 662
Interepisode status, of major depressive
disorder, 455
Interictal delirium, 57
Interindividual differences, in panic
disorder, 575
Intermediate-potency antipsychotic agents,
and schizophrenia, 318

Interpersonal therapy
    bipolar disorder and, 526, 527
    cocaine-related disorders and, 196–197
    eating disorders and, 672
    major depressive disorder and, 471–472
    substance use disorders and, 167
Interviews
    adult psychiatric evaluation and, 15–16,
        16–17
    general psychiatric evaluation and, 7
Intoxication
    alcohol abuse and, 149, 189
    caffeine and, 259
    cocaine and, 150, 197–198
    opiates and, 151, 205–206
    substance use disorders and, 154, 159,
        161, 163
Intranasal use, of cocaine, 199
Involuntary hospitalization
    bipolar disorder and, 529
    eating disorders and, 635
    major depressive disorder and, 431
    schizophrenia and, 361
Isocarboxazide, and eating disorders, 668

Japan, and eating disorders, 653
Jaundice, antipsychotic-induced, 326
Job support, and schizophrenia, 352–353

Kidneys, and lithium, 512–513. *See also*
    Renal effects
Korsakoff's syndrome, 177, 193

LAAM, and opioid use disorders, 150, 151,
    164, 182, 201, 202–203
Labetalol, and cocaine-related disorders,
    198
Laboratory tests. *See also* Medical
    examination; Urine screening; White
    blood cell (WBC) count
    adult psychiatric evaluation and, 15
    Alzheimer's disease and related
        dementias and, 87
    delirium and, 45, **47**
    eating disorders and, 639, **642,** 651
    lithium and, 513–514
    schizophrenia and, 305, 360, 373
    substance use disorders and, 159
Language. *See* Culture; Speech

Legal issues. *See also* Informed consent;
        Involuntary hospitalization; Power of
        attorney
    adult psychiatric evaluation and, 21, 22
    Alzheimer's disease and, 93–94
    eating disorders and, 635
    substance use disorders and, 181–182
Length of treatment
    for nicotine dependence, 268
    for panic disorder, 571, 587, 589–90, 593,
        594, 601–602
    for substance use disorders, 147–148
Levothyroxine, and lithium, 512
Lewy body dementia, 61, 82, 84, 105
Light therapy
    bipolar disorder and, 523
    major depressive disorder and, 444,
        468–469
    premenstrual dysphoria and, 469
Lisuride, and neuroleptic malignant
    syndrome, 323
Lithium
    alcohol-related disorders and, 185, 192
    Alzheimer's disease and related
        dementias and, 78, 110
    bipolar disorder and, 509–514, 531–532,
        536, 538, 541
    carbamazepine and, 520
    cocaine-related disorders and, 198
    eating disorders and, 669, 670
    electroconvulsive therapy and, 525
    major depressive disorder and, 466
    schizophrenia and, 308, 340–341
    side effects of, 341, 540, 511–513, 669
    substance use disorders and, 164
Lithium withdrawal syndrome, and bipolar
    disorder, 510
Liver disease, and delirium, 60. *See also*
    Hepatic disease; Hepatic effects
Lobeline, and nicotine dependence, 265,
    268
Long-acting depot medications, for
    schizophrenia, 307, 327, 364, 365
Longitudinal features
    of bipolar disorder, 503–504
    of panic disorder, 573
    of substance use disorders, 154
Long-term care facilities
    adult psychiatric evaluation and, 10

Medical examination *(continued)*
Alzheimer's disease and related
dementias and, 86–87
carbamazepine and, 519
emergency psychiatric evaluation and, 8
nicotine dependence and, 255
panic disorder and, 598
Medical history. *See also* Medical conditions;
Physical status
adult psychiatric evaluation and, 11–12
carbamazepine and, 519
lithium and, 513, 514
substance use disorders and, 159
valproate and, 517
Medication-induced parkinsonism, and
antipsychotics, 321
Medication support groups. *See* Self-help
groups; Support groups
MEDLARS, 304, 418
MEDLINE, 23, 36, 56, 74, 212, 244, 304, 501,
568
Medroxyprogesterone, and Alzheimer's
disease and related dementias, 78, 110
Melancholia, and major depressive disorder,
454
Melatonin, and Alzheimer's disease, 97, 103
Memorial Delirium Assessment Scale
(MDAS), 45
Memory and memory impairments. *See also*
Cognition and cognitive impairments
benzodiazepines and, 591
delirium and, 39
dementia and, 80
electroconvulsive therapy and, 345, 467
Mentally Ill Chemical/Substance Abusers,
188
Mental retardation, and dementia, 81
Mental status examination. *See also*
Cognition and cognitive impairment;
Functional assessment and impairments
adult psychiatric evaluation and, 14–15
delirium and, **47**
Mepazine, and schizophrenia, 318
Metabolic disorders, and delirium, **42**
Methadone, and opioid use disorders, 150,
151, 163, 164, 182, 201–203, 204, 206,
210
Methylphenidate
Alzheimer's disease and, 113
nicotine dependence and, 271
Metoclopramide, and eating disorders, 664

Metoprolol, and dementia, 110
Mianserin, and eating disorders, 668
Mild impairment, and dementia, 82,
115–116
Military, and patient history, 13
Mindfulness meditation, and panic disorder,
584
Mini-Mental State examination, 51, 88, 98
Mirtazapine
major depressive disorder and, 458
side effects of, 462–463
Mixed episodes, and bipolar disorder,
535–536, 546
Moclobemide, and panic disorder, 594
Moderate impairment, and dementia, 82,
116–117
Molindone, and schizophrenia, 364
Monitoring
of Alzheimer's disease and related
dementias, 75, 87–88
of anorexia nervosa, 632
of bipolar disorder, 506, 514
of delirium, 46–47
of eating disorders, 635, 639, 642, 658
of major depressive disorder, 431
of nicotine dependence, 273–274, 278
of panic disorder, 576
of schizophrenia, 314, 349
of substance use disorders, 160–161
Monoamine oxidase inhibitors (MAOIs)
alcohol-related disorders and, 192
Alzheimer's disease and related
dementias and, 79, 102, 113
bipolar disorder and, 522
eating disorders and, 634, 646, 668, 669
major depressive disorder and, 423, **424,**
434, 436, 458, 466
opioid-related disorders and, 208
panic disorder and, 593–594
side effects of, 112, **447,** 463–464, 594,
669
washout times between trials of, **435**
Morbidity
bipolar disorder and, 504, 508
nicotine dependence and, 285
panic disorder and, 569
substance use disorders and, 156, 161
Morphine, and delirium, 56, 58
Mortality. *See also* Death; Sudden death
alcohol-related disorders and, 183–184,
189

bipolar disorder and, 504, 538
delirium and, 41–42
eating disorders and, 648, 652
nicotine dependence and, 250, 285
opioid-related disorders and, 200
schizophrenia and, 310
substance use disorders and, 156
Motivation. *See also* Motivational
enhancement therapy
eating disorders and level of care criteria,
636–637
nicotine dependence and tobacco use
cessation, 253, 254, 256, 273–275
Motivational enhancement therapy
nicotine dependence and, 256
substance use disorders and, 165
Motor disturbances, and dementia, 81. *See
also* Psychomotor activity
Multiaxial system, of diagnosis, 20
Multidisciplinary teams, and adult
psychiatric evaluation, 18
Multi-infarct dementia. *See* Vascular
dementia
Multimodal behavior therapy
nicotine dependence and, 260
substance use disorders and, 166
Multiple etiologies, of delirium, 43
Multiple-family groups, and schizophrenia,
347
Multiple substances. *See also* Polypharmacy
substance use disorders and, 176
withdrawal from, 161

Naloxone, and opioid use disorders, 151,
161, 205–206
Naltrexone
alcohol abuse and, 148, 184
eating disorders and, 670, 672
nicotine dependence and, 269
opioid use disorders and, 150, 163, 203,
207
side effects of, 203, 269
Narcissistic personality disorder, 444
Narcotic antagonists, 163
Narcotics Anonymous, 167, 168, 197, 205
National Alliance for the Mentally Ill, 529
National Cancer Institute, 257
National Comorbidity Survey, 608
National Depressive and Manic-Depressive
Association, 529
National Institute on Aging, 87

National Institute on Alcohol Abuse and
Alcoholism (NIAAA), 212, 213
National Institute of Mental Health, 87, 470,
471, 474
National Institute of Neurological and
Communication Disorders and Stroke,
87
National Institutes of Health, 87
NEECHAM Confusion Scale, 44
Nefazodone
major depressive disorder and, 458
panic disorder and, 595
side effects of, 112, 462
Negative symptoms, of schizophrenia,
310–311, 319, 321, 335, 372
Neonatal withdrawal syndrome, and
tricyclic antidepressants, 448
Neuroleptic malignant syndrome
antipsychotics and, 106, 323, 336
dementia and risk of, 78
ECT for delirium and, 56, 58–59
lithium and, 341
Neuroleptics
alcohol-related disorders and, 191
bipolar disorder and, 520–521
cocaine-related disorders and, 196
eating disorders and, 663
lithium and, 511
mania and, 509
substance use disorders and, 164
Neurological abnormalities, and delirium,
40
Neurologic effects. *See also* Central nervous
system
of antipsychotics, 320–325
of monoamine oxidase inhibitors, 464
of selective serotonin reuptake
inhibitors, 461
of tricyclic antidepressants, 460
Neurologic examination, and schizophrenia,
360
Nicotine Anonymous, 263
Nicotine dependence. *See also* Tobacco
assessment of, 253–255, 272–273
clinical features influencing treatment of,
279–284
development process for practice
guideline on, 244
diagnostic criteria for, 248–251
epidemiology of, 251–252
evidence ratings for, 245

Nicotine dependence *(continued)*
  introduction to, 243
  pharmacologic treatment of, **255,**
    274–275
  psychiatric management of, 255–259,
    273–275
  psychosocial therapies for, **255,** 259–263,
    274
  research on, 284–285
  somatic treatments for, 264–272
  summary of recommendations on,
    247–248
  target populations for, **243**
  treatment plan for, 272–279
Nicotine fading, 261–262
Nicotine gum, 247, 248, 264, 265, 266–267,
    268, 274, 276, 279
Nicotine inhalers, 265, 267
Nicotine lozenges, 265
Nicotine nasal spray, 248, 265, 266, 267,
    268, 276
Nicotine patch, 264–265, 266, 268, 274, 276,
    279
Nicotine replacement therapy, 247, 248,
    264–268, 272, 274, 278–279, 282, 283
Nonpurging subtype, of bulimia nervosa,
    647
Nonsteroidal anti-inflammatory agents
    (NSAIDs)
  Alzheimer's disease and, 97, 103
  lithium and, 511
Norepinephrine-serotonin modulators, and
    major depressive disorder, **424**
Nortriptyline
  Alzheimer's disease and related
    dementias and, 112, 113
  nicotine dependence and, 270
  side effects of, 112
NSAIDs. *See* Nonsteroidal anti-inflammatory
    agents
Nurses. *See* Staff
Nursing homes
  adult psychiatric evaluation and, 10
  Alzheimer's disease and related
    dementias and, 79–80, 94, 117, 120
  delirium and, 61
  schizophrenia and, 358
Nutritional rehabilitation and counseling,
    for eating disorders, 632, 633, 643–644,
    655, 664–665, 671–672

Nutritional supplements, and nicotine
    dependence, 271

Obesity, and eating disorders, 671
Observation, of patient behavior
  adult psychiatric evaluation and, 18–19
  delirium and, 49
Obsessive-compulsive disorder
  eating disorders and, 654, 674
  major depressive disorder and, 443
  panic disorder and, 604, 605
Obstructive uropathy, and major depressive
    disorder, 451
Occupation. *See* Employment; Vocational
    rehabilitation
Olanzapine
  Alzheimer's disease and, 105
  schizophrenia and, 307, 309, 336–338,
    363–364, 365
  side effects of, 105, 337
Oligomenorrhea, and antipsychotics, 325
Omnibus Budget Reconciliation Act of 1987,
    120
Open-ended questioning, and patient
    interview, 16
Ophthalmologic effects, of antipsychotics,
    326
Opiates, and delirium, 38, 56, 58. *See also*
    Opioid use disorders
Opioid antagonist treatment, 203
Opioid use disorders. *See also* Opiates;
    Substance use disorders and substance
    abuse
  clinical features influencing treatment of,
    151, 205–210
  overview of treatment of, 200–201
  pharmacologic treatment of, 150, 163,
    164, 182, 201–203
  psychosocial treatments for, 150–151,
    203–205
  treatment settings for, 150, 201
Oral contraceptives
  anorexia nervosa and, 663
  antidepressants and, 446, 448
  bipolar disorder and, 541
Osteoporosis, and eating disorders, 648, 663
Outcomes. *See also* Follow-up; Prognosis
  of bulimia nervosa, 652
  of panic disorder, 578
Outpatient settings
  adult psychiatric evaluation and, 10

Pharmacokinetics
  of carbamazepine, 518
  of lithium, 510–511
  of valproate, 515–516
Pharmacotherapy. *See also* Combined
    therapy; Discontinuation; Drug-drug
    interactions; Maintenance medication;
    Overdoses; Side effects; Somatic
    interventions; Toxins and toxicity;
    Withdrawal
  adult psychiatric evaluation during, 19
  alcohol-related disorders and, 148,
      184–185, 190
  bipolar disorder and, 508–523, 544–545
  cocaine use disorders and, 149, 195–196
  delirium and, **44**
  eating disorders and, 633–634, 645–646,
      662–664, 668–671, 672–673
  major depressive disorder and, 423–425,
      434–436, 439–440
  nicotine dependence and, 274–275,
      278–279
  opioid use disorders and, 150, 182,
      201–203
  panic disorder and, 570–571, 585–597,
      599
  schizophrenia and, 317–344
  substance abuse disorders and, 148,
      163–164, 184–185
  tobacco use cessation and blood levels
      of, **251**
Phenelzine
  Alzheimer's disease and, 113
  eating disorders and, 668
  panic disorder and, 594
  side effects of, 112
Phenothiazines
  schizophrenia and, **318**
  side effects of, 52
Phentermine, and eating disorders, 673
Phenylpropanolamine, and nicotine
    dependence, 271
Phenytoin, and alcohol-related disorders,
    191
Phobias. *See also* Phobic avoidance
  eating disorders and, 674
  panic disorder and, 605, 607
Phobic avoidance, and panic disorder, 576,
    605
Physical examination. *See* Medical
    examination

Physical status, and delirium, **47.** *See also*
    Medical conditions; Medical
    examination
Physicians, and panic disorder, 577
Physiological feedback, and nicotine
    dependence, 262
Physiologic dependence, and substance
    dependence, 153
Physostigmine
  anticholinergic effects of antipsychotics
      and, 320
  delirium and, 38, 55, 58
Pick's disease, and dementia, 84–85
Pindolol, and dementia, 110
Plasma levels, of antipsychotics, 307, 333,
    365, 366
Polydipsia
  lithium and, 512
  schizophrenia and, 311, 376–377
Polypharmacy. *See also* Multiple substances
  elderly patients and, 97, 381
  substance use disorders and, 176
Polyuria, and lithium, 512
Positive and Negative Symptoms Scale
    (PANSS), 334, 335
Positive symptoms, of schizophrenia,
    310–311, 312, 319, 335, 344
Postdelirium management, 49
Postictal delirium, 57
Postoperative patients, and delirium, 41
Postpartum period
  bipolar disorder and, 542
  major depressive disorder and, 449
Postpartum psychotic major depressive
    disorder, 449
Posttraumatic stress disorder
  eating disorders and, 674–675
  panic disorder and, 604, 605
Potassium levels
  anorexia nervosa and, 657
  lithium and, 512
Power of attorney, and Alzheimer's disease,
    94, 116
*Practice Guideline for Major Depressive
    Disorder in Adults,* 111, 523, 527, 534,
    535, 546
*Practice Guideline for Psychiatric
    Evaluation of Adults,* 87, 429, 575, 606
*Practice Guideline for Treatment of Patients
    With Bipolar Disorder,* 109, 341, 419,
    429

Psychodynamic psychotherapy *(continued)*
  panic disorder and, 582, 600
  substance use disorders and, 166
Psychoeducation. *See also* Education
  Alzheimer's disease and related
    dementias and, 76, 80, 91–92
  bipolar disorder and, 506–507, 526
  delirium and, 48–49, 50
  major depressive disorder and, 432, 445
  nicotine dependence and, 257, 263, 278
  panic disorder and, 576–577, 579, 584
  schizophrenia and, 314–315, 316, 346,
    347, 367
  substance use disorders and, 162
Psychological Abstracts, 568
Psychomotor activity, and delirium, 40.
    See also Motor disturbances
Psychosis
  Alzheimer's disease and related
    dementias and treatment of, 77–78,
    104–110, 117
  bipolar disorder and, 537–538
  major depressive disorder and, 441, 454
Psychosis-induced polydipsia, 311, 376–377
Psychosocial clubhouse, and schizophrenia,
    351
Psychosocial history
  adult psychiatric evaluation and, 12
  bipolar disorder and, 507–508, 530,
    540–543
  nicotine dependence and, 254, 282–283
  schizophrenia and, 377–381
Psychosocial treatments
  for alcohol-related disorders, 148–149,
    185–189
  for Alzheimer's disease and related
    dementias, 76, 94–96
  for bipolar disorder, 526, 540–541
  for cocaine use disorders, 149–150,
    196–197
  for eating disorders, 632–633, 644, 645,
    658–662, 665–668, 672
  for major depressive disorder, 469–475
  for nicotine dependence, **255,** 259–263,
    274, 278
  for opioid use disorders, 150–151,
    203–205
  for panic disorder, 579–585, 601
  for schizophrenia, 306, 309, 345–349,
    368–369
  for substance use disorders, 146, 164–169

Psychostimulants. *See also* Stimulants
  bipolar disorder and, 523
  side effects of, 112
Psychotherapy. *See also* Combined therapy;
    Family therapy; Group therapy;
    Individual psychotherapy;
    Interpersonal therapy; Psychodynamic
    psychotherapy; Supportive
    psychotherapy
  for Alzheimer's disease and related
    dementias, 76, 94–96
  for bipolar disorder, 525–529, 542
  for delirium, 49
  for eating disorders, 633, 644
  for major depressive disorder, 423, 426–
    427, 433, 436–437, 443, 448, 477–478
  for panic disorder, 570
  for schizophrenia, 367
Psychotic depression, and bipolar disorder,
    524, 535
PsycINFO, 36
PsycLIT, 23, 212–213, 244, 304
PTSD. *See* Posttraumatic stress disorder
Public health. *See also* Costs
  nicotine dependence and, 250
  substance use disorders and, 145, 151
Public policy, and tobacco use, 243
Puerperal psychosis, 449
Pulmonary disease, and tobacco use, 281
Purging behavior, and eating disorders,
    637, 646, **647**

QT interval, and antipsychotics, 53
Quality of life, and Alzheimer's disease, 93
Questionable impairments, and dementia,
    82
Questionnaire of Eating and Weight
    Patterns, **641**
Questionnaires, and patient interview, 17
Quetiapine
  Alzheimer's disease and, 105
  schizophrenia and, 307, 309, 336–337,
    339–340, 363–364, 365
  side effects of, 105, 339–340

Race. *See also* Ethnicity
  nicotine dependence and, 283
  panic disorder and, 608
  schizophrenia and, 378
  substance use disorders and, 156
Rapid cycling, and bipolar disorder, 504

Rapid smoking, as aversive therapy, 260–261

Rating scales. *See also* Measurement instruments

for severity of delirium symptoms, 45

patient interviews and, 17

Rational Recovery, 188

Reality orientation

Alzheimer's disease and, 95

schizophrenia and, 346

Reboxetine

major depressive disorder and, 458

side effects of, 463

Recognition and Initial Assessment of Alzheimer's Disease and Related Dementias (Agency for Health Care Policy and Research), 87

Recovery Incorporated, 354

Recreational activity, and Alzheimer's disease and related dementias, 76, 96. *See also* Exercise

Recurrence, of major depressive disorder, **428**, 455. *See also* Relapse

Reduction, in use of substances of abuse, 157–158

Referrals. *See also* Physicians

nicotine dependence and, 276

schizophrenia and, 316–317

Refractory anorexia nervosa, 660

Rehabilitation, and schizophrenia, 351–354

Rehospitalization rates, and schizophrenia, 317

Reinforcing effects, of abused substances, 163

Relapse. *See also* Recurrence

of alcohol-related disorders, 183, 188

cocaine-related disorders and prevention of, 196–197

of eating disorders, 652

of major depressive disorder, 432, 440

of nicotine dependence, 256, 259, 260, 262, 275–277

of panic disorder, 577–578, 589–590, 601–602

of schizophrenia, 309, 315, 317, 319, 348, 368

of substance use disorders, 155, 158, 160, 161–162, 165, 174

Relaxation therapy, and nicotine dependence, 262

Reminiscence therapy, for Alzheimer's disease and related dementias, 76, 95

Remission, and substance use disorders, 153

Renal effects, of lithium, 512. *See also* Kidneys

Reproductive risk counseling, and bipolar disorder, 542. *See also* Genetic counseling

Research, and future directions

Alzheimer's disease and related dementias and, 123–124

bipolar disorder and, 547–548

eating disorders and, 678–679

major depressive disorder and, 477–478

nicotine dependence and, 284–285

panic disorder and, 608–610

schizophrenia and, 382–383

substance use disorders and, 210–212

Residential treatment facilities

adult psychiatric evaluation and, 10

eating disorders and, **636–637**

substance use disorders and, 147, 172–174

Residual type, of schizophrenia, 311

Respiratory depression, and opioid-related disorders, 205

Respiratory insufficiency, and benzodiazepines, 54

Restraints

adult psychiatric evaluation during use of, 19

Alzheimer's disease and related dementias and, 79, 80, 120–121

delirium and, 47, 61

Restricting subtype, of anorexia nervosa, 646, **647**

Reversible causes, of delirium, **48**

Rewards, and treatment

of nicotine dependence, 261

of substance use disorders, 165

Risk factors

for neuroleptic malignant syndrome, 323

for recurrence of major depressive disorder, **428**

for suicide in schizophrenia patients, 375

for tardive dyskinesia, 324

for violent behavior in schizophrenia patients, 376

Risperidone

Alzheimer's disease and related dementias and, 78, 105, 107

Risperidone *(continued)*
    delirium and, 51
    schizophrenia and, 306, 309, 334–336,
        362–363, 364, 365, 372
    side effects of, 105, 325, 335–336
    tardive dyskinesia and, 324, 325
Role models, and substance use disorders,
    180

SAD (seasonal affective disorder), 444
Safe Return Program, and Alzheimer's
    Association, 89
Safety. *See also* Accidents; Automobiles;
    Suicide and suicidal ideation; Violence
    and violent behavior
    Alzheimer's disease and related
        dementias and, 75–76, 88–89, 116
    delirium and, 46–47
    eating disorders and, 642
    major depressive disorder and, 430, 431
    schizophrenia and, 306
SAMHSA (Substance Abuse and Mental
    Health Services Administration), 212,
    213
SANS (Scale for the Assessment of Negative
    Symptoms), 339
St. John's wort, and major depressive
    disorder, 469
Scale for the Assessment of Negative
    Symptoms (SANS), 339
Schizoaffective disorder, 547
Schizophrenia
    clinical features influencing treatment of,
        310–311, 371–382
    dementia and, 81
    development process for practice
        guideline on, 304
    electroconvulsive therapy for, 344–345,
        367, 370
    epidemiology of, 312–313
    introduction to, 303
    medical conditions and, 381–382
    natural history and course of, 311–312
    nicotine dependence and, 280
    pharmacologic treatments for, 317–344
    psychiatric management and, 306, 309,
        313–317, 361–362, 368–369
    psychosocial interventions for, 306, 309,
        345–349, 368–369
    research directions and, 382–383
    settings for treatment of, 355–359

social and community interventions for,
    349–355
summary of recommendations on,
    305–310
treatment plans for, 359–371
Schools
    eating disorders and, 677–678
    panic disorder and phobias or refusal,
        607
    psychiatric evaluations in, 10
Screening instruments, and delirium, 44. *See
    also* Measurement instruments
Seasonal affective disorder (SAD), 444
Seasonal patterns, of major depressive
    disorder, 455
Secondhand smoke, 250, 278, 281
Sedatives and sedation
    antipsychotics and, 319–320
    delirium and, **48**
    tricyclic antidepressants and, 460
    violent behavior in schizophrenia
        patients and, 376
Seizures. *See also* Epilepsy
    anticonvulsants and, 343
    antipsychotics and, 325, 381–382
    benzodiazepines and, 54
    clozapine and, 332
Selective noradrenaline reuptake inhibitors,
    and major depressive disorder, **424**
Selective serotonin reuptake inhibitors
    (SSRIs)
    alcohol-related disorders and, 185, 192
    Alzheimer's disease and related
        dementias and, 78, 112
    antipsychotics and, 330
    bipolar disorder and, 522
    buspirone and, 110
    eating disorders and, 633, 646, 662–663,
        664, 669
    major depressive disorder and, **424,** 457
    monoamine oxidase inhibitors and, 594
    panic disorder and, 585–587, 601
    side effects of, 111, 461, 586, 601, 669
Selegiline
    Alzheimer's disease and, 77, 97, 101–102,
        116
    schizophrenia and, 372
    side effects of, 102
Self-control training, and alcohol-related
    disorders, 186

Stroke. *See also* Cardiovascular disease
  delirium and, 57
  dementia and, 84, 119
Structured inquiry, and patient interview,
  16, 17
Substance Abuse and Mental Health
  Services Administration (SAMHSA),
  212, 213
Substance dependence, and DSM-IV
  criteria, 152, **249**
Substance use disorders and substance
  abuse. *See also* Alcohol abuse and
  alcoholism; Cocaine use disorders;
  Nicotine dependence; Opioid use
  disorders
  adult psychiatric evaluations and, 10, 12
  assessment of, 145–146, 159
  bipolar disorder and, 538
  clinical factors influencing treatment of,
    175–181
  definition and diagnostic features of,
    153–154
  delirium and, 43, **44**
  dementia and, 85
  development process for practice
    guideline on, 212–213
  DSM-IV criteria for, 152–153
  eating disorders and, 654, 673–674
  epidemiology of, 154–155, 156
  introduction to, 143
  legal and confidentiality issues, 181–182
  major depressive disorder and, 442
  nicotine dependence and, 279–280
  opioid-related disorders and, 208–209
  panic disorder and, 598, 603–604
  pharmacologic treatment of, 146,
    163–164
  psychiatric management of, 146,
    159–163, 169–170
  psychosocial treatments and, 164–169
  as public health problem, 145, 151
  research on, 210–212
  schizophrenia and, 311, 360, 361,
    372–374, 377
  settings for treatment of, 147–148,
    171–175
  summary of recommendations on,
    145–151
  treatment plan formulation and, 146,
    169–170

Succinylcholine, and chemical aversion
  treatment, 164
Sudden death, and antipsychotics, 326–327
Suicide and suicidal ideation. *See also*
  Violence and violent behavior
  alcohol-related disorders and, 191
  Alzheimer's disease and, 88, 110
  bipolar disorder and, 504, 530, 534, 535,
    538
  delirium and, 46–47
  dementia and, 81, 88, 110
  eating disorders and, **636,** 669
  major depressive disorder and, 430, 431,
    440, 441, 442, 445, 452, 455
  opioid-related disorders and, 205
  panic disorder and, 597, 603
  schizophrenia and, 310, 359, 360–361,
    375
  substance use disorders and, 175
  tricyclic antidepressants and, 588
Sundowning, and antipsychotics, 107
Support groups. *See also* Self-help groups
  bipolar disorder and, 529
  eating disorders and, 644, 661, 666–667
  nicotine dependence and, 263
  panic disorder and, 584–585
  schizophrenia and, 348
Supportive-expressive therapy, and
  substance use disorders, 166, 204
Supportive housing, and schizophrenia,
  358–359
Supportive interventions, and delirium, 38,
  49–50, 57
Supportive psychotherapy, for Alzheimer's
  disease and related dementias, 76, 95
Support services, and Alzheimer's disease,
  92–93
Symptom scales, for schizophrenia, 317
Systemic illnesses, and delirium, **42**

Tachycardia, and antipsychotic medications,
  320
Tacrine
  Alzheimer's disease and related dementias
    and, 76–77, 97, 98–100, 116
  delirium and, 55, 58
Tapering
  of benzodiazepines for panic disorder,
    591–592
  of medication for major depressive
    disorder, 439–440

Tardive dyskinesia, and antipsychotics, 78, 106, 324–325

Targeted medication approach, and schizophrenia, 329

Telephone counseling, and nicotine dependence, 262

Temazepam
Alzheimer's disease and related dementias and, 108
delirium and, 60

Temporal course, of delirium and onset of cognitive symptoms, 39, 41

Terminal illnesses, and delirium, 41

Termination, of treatment for opioid-related disorders, 202–203. *See also* Discontinuation

Testosterone, and eating disorders, 676

Tetracyclic antidepressants, and major depressive disorder, **424,** 457

Therapeutic alliance
Alzheimer's disease and related dementias and, 86
bipolar disorder and, 506
delirium and, 48
eating disorders and, 638
major depressive disorder and, 431
nicotine dependence and, 256
panic disorder and, 576
schizophrenia and, 314, 371
substance use disorders and, 160

Therapeutic communities
opioid-related disorders and, 201
substance use disorders and, 173–174

Therapeutic index, of antipsychotics, 326

Thiamine, and alcohol abuse, 149, 190

Thiazide diuretics, and lithium, 511, 512

Thioridazine, and Alzheimer's disease and related dementias, 107

Thiothixene, and Alzheimer's disease and related dementias, 107

Thoughts and thinking, and mental status examination, 14. *See also* Cognition and cognitive impairments

Thyroid hormones
bipolar disorder and, 523, 535, 539
eating disorders and, 651
lithium and, 512
major depressive disorder and supplementation, 466

Timing, of tobacco cessation attempts, 257–258, 273

Tobacco, types of, 283–284. *See also* Nicotine dependence

Tolerance, and substance use disorders, 152, **249**

Torsades de pointes, 52, 53

Toxins and toxicity. *See also* Overdoses; Side effects
anticonvulsants and, 109
antidepressants and, 111–112
antipsychotics and, 105–106
benzodiazepines and, 108
carbamazepine and, 519
cholinesterase inhibitors and, 99
delirium and, **44**
ergoloid mesylates and, 103
lithium and, 341, 513
selegiline and, 102
valproate and, 517
vitamin E supplements and, 100–101

Transdermal nicotine, and nicotine dependence, 247, 248

Transference, and bipolar disorder, 583. *See also* Countertransference

Transitional employment, and schizophrenia, 353–354

Tranylcypromine
Alzheimer's disease and, 113
side effects of, 112

Traumatic brain injuries, and electroconvulsive therapy for delirium, 56

Trazodone
Alzheimer's disease and related dementias and, 78, 79, 109, 112, 113, 115
cocaine-related disorders and, 196
eating disorders and, 668
major depressive disorder and, 458
panic disorder and, 595
side effects of, 112, 462

Treatment. *See* Combined therapy; Length of treatment; Pharmacotherapy; Psychiatric management; Psychosocial treatments; Psychotherapy; Somatic interventions; Treatment plan

Treatment plan, formulation of
adult psychiatric evaluation and, 20
Alzheimer's disease and related dementias and, 115–117
bipolar disorder and, 505, 529–537, 544
delirium and, 57–59

Wernicke's encephalopathy
  alcohol-related disorders and, 193
  delirium and, **48**
White blood cell (WBC) count
  antipsychotics for elderly and, 379
  clozapine and, 332, 333–334
Withdrawal. *See also* Detoxification
  alcohol abuse and, 148, 149, 184,
    189–191
  anxiolytics and panic disorder, 582
  benzodiazepines and, 53, 592
  caffeine and, 259
  cocaine and, 150, 198
  delirium and, 43, **44, 48**
  lithium and, 510
  nicotine dependence and, 247, 249–251,
    252, 257, 265–266, 276, 277, 285

opiates and opioid-related disorders,
  151, 202–203, 206–208
selective serotonin reuptake inhibitors
  and, 586
substance dependence and, 152, 154,
  159, 161, 163, 172
Withdrawal dyskinesia, 324
Women for Sobriety, 188
Work Group on Nicotine Dependence, 263,
  278, 282

Yale-Brown-Cornell Eating Disorder Scale,
  641

Zolpidem, and sleep disturbances in
  Alzheimer's disease patients, 79, 114,
  115
Zung Anxiety Scale, 597